ICD-9-CM
CODING
THEORY AND PRACTICE
with ICD-10

2012

ICD-9-CM
CODING
THEORY AND PRACTICE
with ICD-10

Karla R. Lovaasen, RHIA, CCS, CCS-P
Coding and Consulting Services
Abingdon, Maryland

Jennifer Schwerdtfeger, BS, RHIT, CCS, CPC, CPC-H
Partner, Auditing & Coding Experts, LLC
Crofton, Maryland

ELSEVIER
SAUNDERS

3251 Riverport Lane
St. Louis, Missouri 63043

ICD-9-CM CODING: THEORY AND PRACTICE WITH ICD-10,
2012 EDITION

ISBN: 978-1-4557-0545-0

Notices

Knowledge and best practice in this field are constantly changing. As new research and experience broaden our understanding, changes in research methods, professional practices, or medical treatment may become necessary.

Practitioners and researchers must always rely on their own experience and knowledge in evaluating and using any information, methods, compounds, or experiments described herein. In using such information or methods they should be mindful of their own safety and the safety of others, including parties for whom they have a professional responsibility.

With respect to any drug or pharmaceutical products identified, readers are advised to check the most current information provided (i) on procedures featured or (ii) by the manufacturer of each product to he administered, to verify the recommended dose or formula, the method and duration of administration, and contraindications. It is the responsibility of practitioners, relying on their own experience and knowledge of their patients, to make diagnoses, to determine dosages and the best treatment for each individual patient, and to take all appropriate safety precautions.

To the fullest extent of the law, neither the Publisher nor the authors, contributors, or editors, assume any liability for any injury and/or damage to persons or property as a matter of products liability, negligence or otherwise, or from any use or operation of any methods, products, instructions, or ideas contained in the material herein.

International Standard Book Number: 978-1-4557-0545-0

Publisher: Jeanne R. Olson
Senior Developmental Editor: Jenna Johnson
Publishing Services Manager: Pat Joiner-Myers
Designer: Teresa McBryan

Working together to grow
libraries in developing countries

www.elsevier.com | www.bookaid.org | www.sabre.org

ELSEVIER | BOOK AID International | Sabre Foundation

Last digit is the print number: 9 8 7 6 3 4 3 2 1

Printed in the United States of America

To my husband John, who has more faith in me than I have in myself.
You are the best!

To my children and grandchildren for their ongoing support.

Karla

To the memory of my father, Philip Carter, for his endless
prodding of me to complete this text.

To my husband, children, and grandchildren for sharing me
with the world of publishing.

Jenny

Reviewers

Betty Haar, BS, RHIA
Kirkwood Community College
Cedar Rapids, Iowa

Dorothy M. Hendrix, MEd, RHIT
East Los Angeles College
Monterey Park, California

Karen C. Hoffman, RHIA
Health Information Technology
Southwest Mississippi Community College
Summit, Mississippi

Sandra L. Johnston, MSEd, RHIA, CPC
Clinical Assistant Professor
Health Information Management Program
The University of Kansas Medical Center
Kansas City, Kansas

Mary Juenemann, RHIA, CCS
Health Information Technology Program
Rochester Community and Technical College
Rochester, Minnesota

Jennifer Lamé
Medical Coding and Transcription Instructor
Southwest Wisconsin Technical College
Fennimore, Wisconsin

Celia Lange, RHIT, CCS, CCS-P
Johns Hopkins Bayview Medical Center
Baltimore, Maryland

Sherri Mallett, MEd, RHIA, CCS-P
Adjunct Faculty
Cincinnati State Technical and Community College
Cincinnati, Ohio

Christi Walker
Health Education Instructor
Canadian Valley Technology Center
Yukon, Oklahoma

Joyce S. Waters, MA, RHIA, CCS
Certified ICD10CM/PCS Trainer
Program Chair, Health Information Technology
Athens Technical College
Athens, Georgia

Foreword

It is an honor to have an opportunity to share with you my thoughts and feelings about *ICD-9-CM Coding: Theory and Practice with ICD-10*.

Karla and Jennifer have taken the mystery out of ICD-9-CM and ICD-10-CM/PCS coding by preparing a user-friendly book that meets the needs of not only the student but also the busy instructors. The approach taken by the authors is straightforward, clear, concise, and complete. This book contains the latest in coding assignment and covers a wide variety of coding applications by the use of exercises within the text and the accompanying workbook. The use of color illustrations and photographs further enhances the book and will keep the reader interested.

This is the definitive ICD-9-CM and ICD-10-CM/PCS coding text!

Carol J. Buck
Author/Instructor

Preface

Authoritatively referenced and easy to use for teaching, *ICD-9-CM Coding: Theory and Practice with ICD-10* is the only coding resource designed with instructors and students in mind. This comprehensive guide presents reliable coverage of all three ICD-9-CM volumes in a systematic, straightforward format that guides students through the coding process. With clear examples, challenging review questions, and outstanding instructor support, this innovative resource is not only a valuable coding tool but also a time-saving teaching tool!

ICD-9-CM Coding: Theory and Practice with ICD-10 is intended for those who are learning to code, as well as experienced professionals who wish to have a reference and refresher. Unlike other books in this area, *ICD-9-CM Coding: Theory and Practice with ICD-10* sets out to help students (1) understand why coding is essential and necessary, (2) understand the basics of the health record, and (3) fully understand the rules, guidelines, and functions of ICD-9-CM coding. This book can be used in medical insurance, billing, and coding educational programs; in health information management programs; and as a useful reference for practitioners in the field.

As the implementation date of ICD-10-CM and ICD-10-PCS approaches, this textbook will change accordingly. ICD-10-CM and PCS is still in draft form and therefore still evolving. Because it is still a work in progress, there may be omissions, typos, indexing issues, etc. As of October 1, 2013, many of these issues should be resolved. In the 2012 edition, all exercises and examples are dual coded with ICD-9-CM and ICD-10-CMS/ICD-10-PCS. The ICD-10 2011 draft versions were used to assign codes in this edition. The 2012 edition will also include the ICD-10-CM guidelines in their respective chapters. Chapter 7 provides an introduction to ICD-10-PCS and has been expanded to enhance the teaching and learning of this new procedural coding system. In addition to the above changes, the accompanying workbook has been expanded to include more practice exercises and all answers are now dual coded. These exercises have been added to help the student with applying the guidelines and selecting the principal diagnosis. Several operative reports have also been added to familiarize the student with different types of operative reports and to provide more practice in assigning procedure codes.

ORGANIZATION

The organization of *ICD-9-CM: Theory and Practice with ICD-10* follows the most logical way to learn this material. The early chapters focus on history, the health record as the foundation for coding, and the *Official Guidelines for Coding and Reporting*. A coder must have a basic understanding of this foundational content before moving on to more complicated material. Specifically, Chapter 4 covers the basic steps of ICD-9-CM and ICD-10-CM/PCS coding and the correct process for locating codes in the ICD-9-CM and ICD-10-CM/PCS manual, whereas Chapter 26 is devoted entirely to reimbursement and the role that ICD-9-CM and ICD-10-CM/PCS plays in reimbursement methodologies.

Chapters 8 through 25 cover each chapter of the ICD-9-CM and ICD-10-CM/PCS code book but do not conform to the order of the ICD-9-CM and ICD-10-CM/PCS code book chapters. These chapters are sequenced in this book for the following reasons. The assignment of codes for signs, symptoms, infectious diseases, and V/Z codes may be applied to all chapters in the ICD-9-CM and ICD-10-CM/PCS code book; therefore these are the first coding chapters in this book. Each of these chapters follows a very specific template that will help students learn and instructors teach this complex material, beginning with the corresponding coding guidelines from the *ICD-9-CM Official Guidelines for Coding and Reporting*. This reinforces the importance of the guidelines in accurate code assignment. Following this is a section on anatomy and physiology, with full-color illustrations of the body system discussed in the chapter. This allows for more informed decision making when selecting the correct code and also provides an important review of anatomy and physiology. Key disease conditions are covered and illustrated with examples. References to the *AHA Coding Clinic® for ICD-9-CM* appear throughout each of the coding chapters. *Coding Clinic* is the authority on ICD-9-CM coding, and these references confirm the validity of the content and give students practice using additional information and resources.

Within each coding chapter is a separate list of V/Z codes. V/Z codes are used in all sections of the ICD-9-CM and ICD-10-CM code book, and this list gives students, instructors, and practitioners easy reference to the correct V/Z codes for each section.

Featured in select chapters are common medications and treatment for the related disease conditions. It is important to become familiar with common medications to identify chronic illnesses that may be documented in the health record.

Procedures are another important section of the coding chapters. Common and complex procedures relating to the diagnoses are covered in this section using Volume 3 of the ICD-9-CM code book and ICD-10-PCS.

Finally, each coding chapter has a section on documentation and MS-DRG assignment. This feature brings together all of the steps of ICD-9-CM coding for optimum reimbursement, supported by documentation in the health record.

Chapter 27 completes the picture of facility coding by covering ICD-9-CM coding for outpatient facility services. Most healthcare facilities today treat patients on both an inpatient and an outpatient basis. Coders may be required to code both types of services, and it is important for students to understand the differences.

DISTINCTIVE FEATURES

- Full-color design with illustrations. This helps important content such as anatomy and physiology stand out and come alive and provides visual reinforcement of key concepts.
- References to *AHA Coding Clinic® for ICD-9-CM*. These references verify accuracy and point students to direct citations in *Coding Clinic*, the definitive publication on ICD-9-CM coding.
- Numerous and varied examples and exercises within each chapter. These exercises break the chapter into manageable segments and help students gauge learning while reinforcing important concepts.
- Examples and exercises are coded using ICD-10-CM and ICD-10-PCS, allowing the instructor to introduce the concept of using ICD-10-CM and ICD-10-PCS while still teaching ICD-9-CM.
- Partial answer keys for the textbook and workbook are available on the Evolve website for instant feedback to enhance student learning.

ADDITIONAL RESOURCES

Get the most out of your course with these additional learning and teaching resources.
- Student Workbook. Apply the textbook content and prepare for employment with this study guide! The workbook contains:
  - Application activities that give students hands-on practice applying ICD-9-CM coding to actual health records.
  - Case studies that illustrate common scenarios students will encounter on the job.
- TEACH Instructor Resources. TEACH is the complete curriculum manual, giving instructors everything necessary to enhance an ICD-9-CM course and save time!

- **Lesson plans** tie together related content in the textbook, workbook, and instructor resources and reduce preparation time.
- **Lecture slides and notes** presented in PowerPoint guide instructors through class presentations.
- **Complete answer keys** for every exercise, chapter review, and test bank question enable fast, efficient student assessment.
- **Test banks** help prepare exams instantly with chapter-specific test banks presented in ExamView.

■ Evolve Learning Resources. This companion website contains links to industry updates, reimbursement updates, and important news. The Evolve course management system gives instructors the flexibility of posting course components online.

Acknowledgments

This book was developed to better meet the needs of coding educators, students, and coding professionals.

There are several people who deserve special thanks for their efforts in making this text possible.

Jeanne Olson, Publisher, for stepping in and learning about the world of ICD-9 and ICD-10 coding.

Jenna Johnson, Senior Developmental Editor, for assisting us with the publishing process and the development of the manuscripts.

A special thanks to **Kelly Barnes, RHIT,** for her assistance and support of this textbook and supporting materials. Also, thanks to **Louise Thompson** for her assistance and support of this textbook.

Thanks to all our colleagues who participated in coding discussions and debates about coding issues.

Thanks to **Carol Buck** for her advice and encouragement during this project.

The authors and publisher would like to acknowledge and thank the contributors to the TEACH Instructor Resources and all the textbook reviewers for their constructive comments.

Contents

ICD-9-CM
CODING
THEORY AND PRACTICE
with ICD-10

1

The Rationale for and History of Coding

CHAPTER OUTLINE

Background of Coding
    What Is Coding and What Are Its Applications?
    Nomenclature and Classification
History of Coding
Comparison of ICD-10-CM and ICD-9-CM
Preparation for Transition to ICD-10-CM
Coding Organizations and Credentials
Coding Ethics
Compliance
Confidentiality
Chapter Review Exercise
Chapter Glossary
References

LEARNING OBJECTIVES

1. Describe the application of coding
2. Define nomenclature and classification
3. Identify the historical timeline of coding
4. Explain the difference between ICD-9-CM and ICD-10-CM
5. Delineate coder training needs for transitioning to ICD-10-CM
6. Describe different coding organizations and credentials
7. Recognize the importance of the Standards of Ethical Coding
8. Define compliance as it relates to coding
9. Explain confidentiality as it applies to coding

ABBREVIATIONS/ ACRONYMS

AAPC American Academy of Professional Coders

AHA American Hospital Association

AHIMA American Health Information Management Association

CCA Certified Coding Associate

CCS Certified Coding Specialist

CCS-P Certified Coding Specialist—Physician Based

CEUs continuing education units

CMS Centers for Medicare and Medicaid Services

CPC Certified Professional Coder

CPC-H Certified Professional Coder—Hospital Based

CPT *Current Procedural Terminology*

DRGs diagnosis-related groups

HIPAA Health Insurance Portability and Accountability Act

ICD-9-CM *International Classification of Diseases, 9th Revision, Clinical Modification*

ICD-10-CM *International Classification of Diseases, 10th Revision, Clinical Modification*

ICD-10-PCS *International Classification of Diseases, 10th*

Revision, Procedure Coding System

MS-DRG Medicare Severity diagnosis-related group

NCHS National Center for Health Statistics

OIG Office of the Inspector General

RHIA Registered Health Information Administrator

RHIT Registered Health Information Technician

SNOMED Systematized Nomenclature of Medicine

WHO World Health Organization

BACKGROUND OF CODING

What Is Coding and What Are Its Applications?

As a student in this field, you will often be asked these questions. Why does one study this subject? What type of work does a "coder" do? Basically, medical coding consists of translating **diagnoses** and **procedures** into numbers for the purpose of statistically capturing data. This process is done for us every day in all aspects of daily life. If you buy a banana at the grocery store, the cash register captures that banana as a number, which, in turn, provides data on the number of bananas sold in that store or by that grocery chain; it also yields data of importance to the store on replenishing their inventory, details regarding what time of year the greatest number of bananas are sold, and so forth.

Translation of a disease and/or a procedure into an ICD-9 code is not as simple as it may seem. This process requires a thorough knowledge of anatomy and physiology, disease processes, medical **terminology**, laboratory values, pharmacology, surgical procedures, and last but not least, a myriad of coding rules and guidelines. Diseases and procedures are translated into a coding system known as the *International Classification of Diseases, 9th Revision, Clinical Modification* (ICD-9-CM). This **classification** system has been used worldwide and has been clinically modified for the United States.

Coded data are used for many purposes. Prior to the advent of diagnosis-related groups (DRGs), which are used by Medicare and other payers as the basis for hospital **reimbursement** (payment), coding was used for research and planning. A healthcare provider or facility could use these data to find out how many cases of appendicitis were treated in a year. This information could be used by a healthcare facility in decisions about the possible purchase of more equipment, the addition of an operating room, or the hiring of additional staff, or by the provider to gain additional skills. Since the implementation of DRGs—now known as MS-DRGs—coded data are also used for reimbursement purposes, and they are increasingly used for risk management and quality improvement, as well as in nursing clinical pathways. Coded data were important from the start, but use of these data for reimbursement has elevated the importance of accurate coding to new heights.

Capture of health data through ICD-9 and ICD-10 codes that are used worldwide has proved useful for the study of patterns of disease, disease epidemics, causes of mortality, and treatment modalities. Without the use of a classification system, comparison of data would be impossible.

Nomenclature and Classification

A nomenclature and a classification of diseases are required for development of a coding system. A **nomenclature** is a system of names that are used as preferred terminology, in this case, for diseases and procedures. Often, diseases in different areas of the country or in different countries are identified by dissimilar terminology, which makes the capture of comparative statistical data next to impossible. For example, another name for "amyotrophic lateral sclerosis" is "Lou Gehrig's disease," which is also known as a "motor neuron disease." Nomenclatures of disease were first developed in the United States around 1928. The Systematized Nomenclature of Medicine (SNOMED), published by the College of American Pathologists, is the most up-to-date system in current use.

Classification systems group together similar items for easy storage and retrieval. Within a classification system, items are arranged into groups according to specific criteria. The history of classification systems goes back as far as Hippocrates. During the 17th century, London Bills of Mortality represented the first attempts of scientists to gather statistical data on disease. The ICD-9-CM classification system is a closed system that comprises diseases, injuries, surgeries, and procedures. In a closed classification system a disease, condition, or procedure can be classified in only one place.

HISTORY OF CODING

ICD-9-CM is the coding classification system that is currently in use in the United States. This classification system dates back to Bertillon's Classification of Causes of Death, which was developed in 1893. This system was adopted by the United States in 1898 under the recommendation of the American Public Health Association. System revisions were scheduled to take place every 10 years, and the classification was maintained by the World Health Organization (WHO). Revisions became known as the International Classification of Causes of Death. Over the years, this system has been changed to allow its use not only in mortality reporting but in morbidity reporting as well. Since its inception, this classification has been revised 10 times. The Clinical Modification (CM) was developed in 1977 by the United States to more accurately capture morbidity data for study within the United States, as well as information on operative and diagnostic procedures that were not included in the original publication of ICD. ICD-9-CM, a publication of the U.S. Department of Health and Human Services, consists of three volumes.

Currently, many countries are using ICD-10, which was published in 1993 by the WHO. ICD-10 has also been clinically modified for use in the United States with implementation set for October 1, 2013. ICD-10-CM will replace the 30-year-old ICD-9-CM. The final rule for adoption of ICD-10-CM and ICD-10-PCS was released in January of 2009.

Work on ICD-10 was begun in 1983. The tabular volume was published in 1992, and the instructional volume followed in 1993; the Alphabetic Index was published in 1994. In 1994, the United States began the process of determining whether a clinical modification (CM) would be necessary. A draft version was made available in 2002, updated in July 2007, and updated again in 2009. This version can be found at the National Center for Health Statistics website.

Clinical modifications made to ICD-10 allow a higher level of specificity. Since 1999, ICD-10 has been used in the United States for the reporting of mortality data. A total of 90 countries, including Canada and Australia, are currently using ICD-10.

ICD-9-CM may be updated biannually in April and October. Updates contain additional codes, revised codes, and codes that are deleted. These updates are published in the *Federal Register* (the official daily publication for rules, proposed rules, and notices of U.S. federal agencies and organizations) as a proposed rule and then as a final rule. They are available at the Centers for Medicare and Medicaid Services (CMS) website (www.cms.gov). It is of the utmost importance that code books and coding software (**encoder**) be updated to ensure that coding is accurate and to facilitate accurate reimbursement.

The ICD-9-CM Coordination and Maintenance Committee meets twice a year and is used as a forum for proposals to update ICD-9-CM. This Committee serves in an advisory capacity. Two Federal agencies are responsible for maintenance of ICD-9-CM. The classification of diagnoses is the responsibility of the NCHS (National Center for Health Statistics) and the classification of procedures is the responsibility of CMS (Centers for Medicare and Medicaid Services). The Coordination and Maintenance Committee meetings are open to the public and comments are encouraged. All comments and recommendations are evaluated before a final decision on new codes is issued.

The development and maintenance of the guidelines of ICD-9-CM is the responsibility of the National Center for Health Statistics (NCHS), CMS, the American Hospital Association (AHA), and the American Health Information Management Association (AHIMA), which are also known as the Cooperating Parties. Many publications provide coding advice and information, but only one publication is official. This publication, *AHA Coding Clinic for ICD-9-CM* (referred to as *Coding Clinic*), which is published quarterly by the AHA, provides coding advice and guidelines that have been approved by the Cooperating Parties and must be followed by coders.

Coding Clinic references will be used throughout the text with specific issue information provided, such as 2002:4Q:p126-130. This reference alerts the student of information contained in the fourth quarter 2002 issue and the associated page numbers. The *Coding Clinic* references used throughout this text may be referred to for more detailed information about the subject being referenced. *Coding Clinic* has publications dating back to 1985.

TABLE 1-1 COMPARISON OF ICD-10-CM AND ICD-9-CM*

ICD-9-CM	ICD-10-CM
14,000 codes	69,000 codes
Codes begin with number except for V&E supplementary classification	Codes begin with a letter
	3 to 7 characters
Maximum 5 number code	Codes may end in a number or a letter
All codes end in a number	Both morphology and musculoskeletal codes begin with M
Morphology codes begin with M	
Three tables: Neoplasms, Drugs and Chemicals, Hypertension	Two tables: Neoplasms, Drugs and Chemicals
17 chapters with 2 supplements	21 chapters
1 chapter for Diseases of the Nervous System, Eyes, Ears	3 chapters for Nervous System, Eyes, Ears
No laterality included in codes	Laterality included in codes
Sometimes combine NEC (not elsewhere classified) and NOS (not otherwise specified)	Never combine NEC and NOS
No 7th character extensions	7th character extensions
No placeholder letter X	Placeholder letter X
Excludes notes	Excludes notes 1 and 2

*The index and the tabular of ICD-10-CM are very similar in style to ICD-9-CM.

Unless superseded or clarified by additional *Coding Clinic* references, the original publication of any advice remains in effect. Although reference may be made to advice in an issue from 1994, this may be the most current advice available. A date of 1994 for a given source does not mean that the publication is outdated. As the transition to ICD-10-CM/PCS begins, this textbook will have all examples and exercises coded using ICD-9 and ICD-10.

COMPARISON OF ICD-10-CM AND ICD-9-CM

As noted in Table 1-1, considerable differences can be seen between ICD-10-CM and ICD-9-CM. Most notable is the increase in the number of codes and code categories, the change from numeric to alphanumeric codes with an increase in digits from 5 to 7, and the increase from 17 chapters to 21 chapters.

The best way to appreciate these differences is to view code assignments for the same disease process from both classification systems.

EXAMPLE
| Newborn baby delivered via c-section | V30.01 (ICD-9-CM) |
| Newborn baby delivered via c-section | Z38.01 (ICD-10-CM) |

EXAMPLE
| Displaced spiral closed fracture shaft of left femur, initial encounter 821.01 (ICD-9-CM) |
| Displaced spiral closed fracture shaft of left femur, initial encounter S72.342A (ICD-10-CM) |

PREPARATION FOR TRANSITION TO ICD-10-CM

The steps necessary for transition to ICD-10-CM and ICD-10-PCS involve many different areas within the healthcare system, including Information Systems (IS), Billing, healthcare providers, Utilization Review (UR), Researchers, Compliance, and Accounting, to name a few. Most articles written on the subject recommend a team approach across the facility. Existing coding staff will need to be trained on both ICD-10-CM and ICD-10-PCS.

Reports suggest (see Practice Brief Destination 10: Healthcare Organization Preparation for ICD-10-CM and ICD-10-PCS)[1] that the knowledge base of coders must be broadened so they have detailed knowledge of anatomy and medical terminology, enhanced comprehension of operative reports, and a greater understanding of ICD-10-PCS definitions. It may be necessary to assess the skills of coders before selecting the type of training needed. It has been suggested that training should not take place too early, and probably around 3 months before implementation would be preferable. Aside from more intensive training in anatomy and physiology (A&P) and terminology, the following education on ICD-10-CM is recommended by AHIMA:

- Structure change
- Disease classification
- Definitions
- Guidelines
- ICD-10-PCS

AHIMA is currently offering ICD-10 courses via the Web. *ICD-TEN* is a monthly newsletter to assist in the transition to ICD-10-CM and ICD-10-PCS. The need is great for qualified instructors to teach both of these classification systems to the many users who will need to know them.

AHIMA's Commission on Certification for Health Information and Informatics (CCHIIM) has implemented a new recertification policy specific to ICD-10-CM/PCS. This policy requires that CEU education hours based on ICD-10-CM/PCS content will be required and will be part of the existing CEU requirement. The CEUs required are based on the credential held and are as follows:

RHIT	6 CEUs
RHIA	6 CEUs
CCS-P	12 CEUs
CCS	18 CEUs
CCA	18 CEUs

If a person holds more than one credential, the CEUs necessary are based on the credential requiring the highest number of ICD-10-CM/PCS CEUs. These CEUs should be earned from January 1, 2011 to December 31, 2013. All AHIMA Certified Professionals who completed AHIMA's Academy for ICD-10 prior to January 1, 2011 will be allowed to use those CEU hours to fulfill the ICD-10-CM/PCS CEU requirement.

CODING ORGANIZATIONS AND CREDENTIALS

Coders come from a variety of educational backgrounds. Many coders have attended 4-year college programs in Health Information Administration; others have completed 2-year college programs in Health Information Technology. Some community colleges offer programs geared only to medical coding. Whatever their background, most coders take certification examinations to earn **credentials** (which are certificates that recognize a course of study taken in a specific field and acknowledge that competency is required) and become members of a professional organization. Many employers include a requirement for certification as part of their coding job description.

Coders can work in a variety of settings; most often, they are employed by hospitals, physician offices, outpatient surgical centers, long-term care facilities, and insurance companies. It is predicted that the demand for coding professionals will far exceed the number of coders in the workforce.

The two most well-known professional associations for coders are AHIMA (www.ahima.org) and the American Academy of Professional Coders (AAPC) (www.aapc.com). Both of these organizations offer a variety of coding credentials. AHIMA, which has been in existence for over 75 years, has undergone several name changes along the way to keep up with the ever-changing technological skills, educational requirements, and roles of its members. It boasts a membership of over 60,000. Traditionally, this organization has provided support

TABLE 1-2 CREDENTIALS AND CONTINUING EDUCATION UNIT REQUIREMENTS

Credential	Organization Offering Credential	Education Required	CEUs Required per 2-Year Cycle
CCA	AHIMA	High school diploma or equivalent	20
CCS	AHIMA	High school diploma or equivalent	20
CCS-P	AHIMA	High school diploma or equivalent	20
RHIT	AHIMA	2-Year degree in accredited HIM program	20
RHIA	AHIMA	4-Year degree in accredited HIM program	30
CPC	AAPC	High school diploma or equivalent and 2 years coding experience	36
CPC-H	AAPC	High school diploma or equivalent and 2 years coding experience	36
CPC-P	AAPC	High school diploma or equivalent and 2 years coding experience	36
CPC-A	AAPC	High school diploma or equivalent	36
CPC-H-A	AAPC	High school diploma or equivalent	36
CPC-P-A	AAPC	High school diploma or equivalent	36

for facility coders, but in recent years, it has expanded to include coders who provide services in physician's offices and outpatient settings. AHIMA offers the following credentials:

CCA	Certified Coding Associate
CCS	Certified Coding Specialist
CCS-P	Certified Coding Specialist—Physician Based
RHIT	Registered Health Information Technician
RHIA	Registered Health Information Administrator

AAPC has over 100,000 credentialed members and was started in 1981. It was founded to assist coders in providing services to physicians and offers the following credentials:

CPC	Certified Professional Coder
CPC-H	Certified Professional Coder—Hospital
CPC-P	Certified Professional Coder—Payer
CPC-A	Certified Professional Coder—Apprentice
CPC-H-A	Certified Professional Coder—Hospital Apprentice
CPC-P-A	Certified Professional Coder—Payer Apprentice

To obtain credentials from either organization, a coder must sit for a certification examination and complete college coursework in several areas such as medical terminology and anatomy and physiology. To maintain their credentials, coders must earn continuing education units (CEUs). The number of CEUs required is dependent on the credential(s) of the coder (Table 1-2).

CODING ETHICS

Along with providing credentials, both AHIMA and AAPC have set standards for Coding **Ethics**, which are reprinted in Figures 1-1 and 1-2. (Please see the Evolve companion website for "How to Interpret the Standards of Ethical Coding.") Members of these organizations are expected to abide by these coding standards. A coder who is asked to disregard a guideline to facilitate payment should decline on the basis of these standards, by which coders are bound.

Standards of Ethical Coding

Coding professionals should:

1. Apply accurate, complete, and consistent coding practices for the production of high-quality healthcare data.
2. Report all healthcare data elements (e.g., diagnosis and procedure codes, present on admission indicator, discharge status) required for external reporting purposes (e.g., reimbursement and other administrative uses, population health, quality and patient safety measurement, and research) completely and accurately, in accordance with regulatory and documentation standards and requirements and applicable coding conventions, rules, and guidelines.
3. Assign and report only the codes and data that are clearly and consistently supported by health record documentation in accordance with applicable code set and abstraction conventions, rules, and guidelines.
4. Query provider (physician or other qualified healthcare practitioner) for clarification and additional documentation prior to code assignment when there is conflicting, incomplete, or ambiguous information in the health record regarding a significant reportable condition or procedure or other reportable data element dependent on health record documentation (e.g., present on admission indicator).
5. Refuse to change reported codes or the narratives of codes so that meanings are misrepresented.
6. Refuse to participate in or support coding or documentation practices intended to inappropriately increase payment, qualify for insurance policy coverage, or skew data by means that do not comply with federal and state statutes, regulations, and official rules and guidelines.
7. Facilitate interdisciplinary collaboration in situations supporting proper coding practices.
8. Advance coding knowledge and practice through continuing education.
9. Refuse to participate in or conceal unethical coding or abstraction practices or procedures.
10. Protect the confidentiality of the health record at all times and refuse to access protected health information not required for coding-related activities (examples of coding-related activities include completion of code assignment, other health record data abstraction, coding audits, and educational purposes).
11. Demonstrate behavior that reflects integrity, shows a commitment to ethical and legal coding practices, and fosters trust in professional activities.

Revised and approved by the House of Delegates 09/08

FIGURE 1-1. AHIMA's Standards of Ethical Coding.

AAPC Code of Ethics

Members of the American Academy of Professional Coders (AAPC) shall be dedicated to providing the highest standard of professional coding and billing services to employers, clients, and patients. Professional and personal behavior of AAPC members must be exemplary.

- AAPC members shall maintain the highest standard of personal and professional conduct. Members shall respect the rights of patients, clients, employers, and all other colleagues.

- Members shall use only legal and ethical means in all professional dealings, and shall refuse to cooperate with, or condone by silence, the actions of those who engage in fraudulent, deceptive, or illegal acts.

- Members shall respect and adhere to the laws and regulations of the land, and uphold the mission statement of the AAPC.

- Members shall pursue excellence through continuing education in all areas applicable to their profession.

- Members shall strive to maintain and enhance the dignity, status, competence, and standards of coding for professional services.

- Members shall not exploit professional relationships with patients, employees, clients, or employers for personal gain.

This code of ethical standards for members of the AAPC strives to promote and maintain the highest standard of professional service and conduct among its members. Adherence to these standards assures public confidence in the integrity and service of professional coders who are members of the AAPC.

Failure to adhere to these standards, as determined by AAPC, will result in the loss of credentials and membership with the American Academy of Professional Coders.

FIGURE 1-2. AAPC's Code of Ethical Standards.

COMPLIANCE

Compliance is defined as "acting according to certain accepted standards or, in simple terms, abiding by the rules." In health care, this requires following the rules and guidelines as set forth by the government through Medicare and Medicaid and all professional organizations which a facility or provider may belong to or is participating with, and following the policies and procedures of that organization.

Compliance officers and programs are found in many industries. It wasn't until after the passage of the Health Insurance Portability and Accountability Act of 1996 (HIPAA) that compliance officers became a standard presence in healthcare facilities. HIPAA gave additional funding to the U.S. Department of Health and Human Services, the Office of the Inspector General (OIG), and the U.S. Department of Justice to increase penalties for healthcare fraud and abuse. Ongoing investigations in healthcare institutions across the United States are exploring violations of the False Claim Act and other laws.

As explained in an article by Joette Hanna that appeared in the *Journal of AHIMA*, entitled "Constructing a Coding Compliance Plan,"[2] several steps must be taken if a coding department wishes to ensure that it is in compliance. Coding departments must do the following:

- Abide by AHIMA's Standards of Ethical Coding
- Develop coding policies and procedures
- Develop a working relationship with the billing department
- Develop a coding compliance work plan
- Conduct coding audits
- Develop an action plan based on audit results

Likewise, a practice brief published by AHIMA in 2001, entitled "Developing a Coding Compliance Policy Document,"[3] states that the following bulleted items should be included in a coding compliance plan:

- Policy statement regarding the commitment of the organization to correct assignment and reporting of codes
- The Official Coding Guidelines used by the facility
- The people responsible for code assignment
- What needs to be done when clinical information is not clear enough to assign codes
- If there are payer-specific guidelines, where these may be found
- A procedure for correcting codes that have been assigned incorrectly
- Plan for education on areas of risk as identified by audits
- Identification of essential coding resources that are available and to be used by coding professionals
- Procedure for coding new and/or unusual diagnoses or procedures
- A policy for which procedures will be reported
- Procedure for resolving coding/documentation disputes with physicians
- Procedure for processing claim rejections
- Procedure for handling requests for coding amendments
- Policy that requires coders to have available coding manuals and not just encoder
- Process for review of coding on those records coded with incomplete documentation

CONFIDENTIALITY

Employees in a healthcare setting must be aware of the confidentiality of the information that is all around them. When they take the Hippocratic Oath, physicians swear to maintain patient confidentiality. Likewise, in the Patient Bill of Rights as prepared by the AHA, the patient's right to privacy is stated. The Code of Ethics of the AHIMA also addresses confidentiality when it says, "Members will promote and protect the confidentiality and security of health records and information."

Coders must read a patient's personal medical information before they can code the encounter and/or patient admission. It is important that this information not be shared with anyone, including other employees, unless they have a legitimate need to know to perform their job; patient information should never be discussed in a place where any visitor could overhear.

CHAPTER REVIEW EXERCISE

Write the correct answer(s) in the space(s) provided.

1. What does a coder do?

   _____

2. What coding system is currently used in the United States for inpatient coding?

   _____

3. What does the CM of ICD-9-CM stand for?

   _____

4. List three uses for coded data.

   1. _____
   2. _____
   3. _____

5. What payment system does Medicare use for facility reimbursement?

   _____

6. Describe the difference between a nomenclature and a classification system.

   _____

7. What nomenclature of disease is used in the United States?

   _____

8. Define a closed classification system.

   _____

9. When was the International Classification of Diseases first adopted by the United States?

   _____

10. When and how often is this system (ICD-9-CM) updated?

    _____

11. What four groups constitute the Cooperating Parties?

    1. _____
    2. _____
    3. _____
    4. _____

12. Who publishes official coding advice and guidance?

    _____

13. What organizations award coding credentials?

    _____

14. What is another word that is used in the industry for "following the rules"?

    _____

15. If you were coding a neighbor's record, would it be okay for you to tell your other neighbors the reason the patient was hospitalized?

    _____

16. What does HIPAA stand for?

    _____

17. Most industrialized countries do not use ICD-10.
    A. True
    B. False

18. Coders will require greater technical skill if they are to master ICD-10-CM and ICD-10-PCS.
    A. True
    B. False

CHAPTER GLOSSARY

Classification: grouping together of items as for storage and retrieval.

Compliance: adherence to accepted standards.

Credential: degree, certificate, or award that recognizes a course of study taken in a specific field and that acknowledges the competency required.

Diagnosis: identification of a disease through signs, symptoms, and tests.

Encoder: coding software that is used to assign diagnosis and procedure codes.

Ethics: moral standard.

Federal Register: the official daily publication for rules, proposed rules, and notices of U.S. federal agencies and organizations.

Nomenclature: system of names that are used as the preferred terminology.

Procedure: a diagnostic or therapeutic process performed on a patient.

Reimbursement: payment for healthcare services.

Terminology: words and phrases that apply to a particular field.

REFERENCES

1. American Health Information Management Association. Destination 10: healthcare organization preparation for ICD-10-CM and ICD-10-PCS, *J AHIMA* 75:56A-556D, 2004.
2. Hanna J. Constructing a coding compliance plan, *J AHIMA* 73:48-56, 2002.
3. AHIMA Coding Practice Team. Developing a coding compliance policy document (AHIMA practice brief), *J AHIMA* 72:88A-888C, 2001.

2

The Health Record as the Foundation of Coding

LEARNING OBJECTIVES

1. Explain the purpose of the various forms or reports found in a health record
2. Define "principal diagnosis"
3. Define "principal procedure"
4. Identify reasons for assigning codes for other diagnoses
5. List the basic guidelines for reporting diagnoses/procedures
6. Identify types of documentation acceptable for assigning codes
7. Explain the query process

ABBREVIATIONS/ ACRONYMS

AHQA American Health Quality Association

BPH benign prostatic hypertrophy

CBC complete blood count

CC chief complaint

CMS Centers for Medicare and Medicaid Services

CPT *Current Procedural Terminology*

COPD chronic obstructive pulmonary disease

DOB date of birth

ED Emergency Department

EEG electroencephalogram

EGD esophagogastroduodeno-scopy

EKG electrocardiogram

ER Emergency Room

GERD gastroesophageal reflux disease

H&P history and physical

**ABBREVIATIONS/
ACRONYMS—cont'd**

HPI history of present illness

ICD-9-CM *International Classification of Diseases, 9th Revision, Clinical Modification*

ICD-10-CM *International Classification of Diseases, 10th Revision, Clinical Modification*

ICU intensive care unit

MAR medication administration record

MRA magnetic resonance angiography

MRI magnetic resonance imaging

MS-DRGs Medicare Severity diagnosis-related groups

MVP mitral valve prolapse

NPI National Provider Identifier

OP note operative note

POA present on admission

SOAP Subjective/Objective/Assessment/Plan

TJC The Joint Commission

TPR temperature, pulse, and respiration

UHDDS Uniform Hospital Discharge Data Set

UPIN Unique Physician Identification Number

UTI urinary tract infection

THE HEALTH RECORD

A health record must be maintained for every individual who is assessed or treated. Although Edna Huffman's classic *Health Information Management*[1] book is no longer in print, her definition of the purpose and use of a health record still holds true today. She states, "The main purpose of the medical record is to accurately and adequately document a patient's life and health history, including past and present illnesses and treatments, with emphasis on the events affecting the patient during the current episode of care." Huffman goes on to say, "The medical record must be compiled in a timely manner and contain sufficient data to identify the patient, support the diagnosis or reason for health care encounter, justify the treatment and accurately document the results." According to Abdelhak's *Health Information: Management of a Strategic Resource*,[2] the health record serves five purposes:

1. Describes the patient's health history
2. Serves as a method for clinicians to communicate regarding the plan of care for the patients
3. Serves as a legal document of care and services provided
4. Serves as a source of data
5. Serves as a resource for healthcare practitioner education

The patient's health record in today's environment may be maintained in several formats or **hybrids**. The traditional health record consists of documentation on paper prepared by **healthcare providers** that describes the condition of the patient and the plan and course of treatment. As the world advances through electronic forms of documentation, paper notes become more and more obsolete. Most health records are currently in a state of transition. Some paper documentation and some transcribed or electronically stored documentation may be available. Some facilities have actually achieved a predominantly electronic health record. One of the advantages of storing the record electronically is that many users are able to access the record at the same time. Whether in electronic, paper, or hybrid form, documentation serves as the basis of a health record.

The Centers for Medicare and Medicaid Services (CMS) has provided physicians with *General Principles of Medical Record Documentation*.[3]

■ Medical records should be complete and legible
■ The documentation of each patient encounter should include:
  • Reason for encounter and relevant history
  • Physical examination findings and prior diagnostic test results
  • Assessment, clinical impression, and diagnosis
  • Plan for care
■ Date and legible identity of the observer
■ The rationale for ordering diagnostic and ancillary services (if not documented, should be easily inferred)
■ Past and present diagnoses should be accessible for treating and/or consulting physician
■ Appropriate health risk factors should be identified

- Patient's progress, response to changes in treatment, and revision of diagnosis should be documented
- *Current Procedural Terminology* (CPT) and *International Classification of Diseases, 9th Revision, Clinical Modification* (ICD-9-CM) codes reported on health insurance claim forms should be supported by documentation in the medical record

SECTIONS OF THE HEALTH RECORD

Every facility has its own policies and procedures regarding the organization of the health record. Records will differ slightly depending upon the course of the patient's condition and treatment. If a record were to be organized similarly to a novel that tells a story, the elements discussed in the next sections would be included.

Administrative Data

- Demographic
- Personal data
- Consents

Information contained in this section will facilitate identification of the patient. Some of the UHDDS data elements included are personal identification, date of birth, sex, race, residence, admit date, and discharge date. See Figure 2-1.

Clinical Data

Inpatient records may be organized in a reverse chronological order. The discharge summary may be found at the beginning of the record.
- Emergency room record (when applicable) (see Figure 2-2)
- Admission history and physical (see Figure 2-3)
- Physician orders (see Figures 2-4 and 2-5)
- Progress notes recorded by healthcare providers (see Figure 2-6, *A* and *B*)
- Anesthesia forms (when applicable) (see Figure 2-9)
- Operative report (when applicable) (see Figure 2-10)
- Recovery room notes (when applicable)
- Consultations (when applicable)
- Laboratory test results (when applicable) (see Figure 2-8)
- Radiology report (when applicable) (see Figure 2-11)
- Miscellaneous ancillary reports (when applicable)
- Discharge summary (see Figure 2-12)

Data are collected from the health record as mandated by governmental and nongovernmental agencies. The Joint Commission (TJC) places data requirements and time frames for documentation within the health record. The federal government and state licensing agencies may have similar requirements. Medical staff bylaws often include these documentation requirements. In 1974, the Uniform Hospital Discharge Data Set (UHDDS) mandated that hospitals must report a common core of data. Since that time, the requirements have been revised and will continue to change as necessary. The UHDDS required data elements are listed in Figure 2-1.

Emergency Room Record

The emergency room record is a mini health record. It contains a **chief complaint (CC)**, which is the reason, in the patient's own words, for presentation to the hospital. It contains a history, physical examination, laboratory results, radiology reports (if applicable), plan of care, physician orders, and documentation of any procedures performed. Last but not least, it contains a list of working diagnoses and information on the disposition of the patient. See Figure 2-2 for a sample of an ED (Emergency Department, or also called ER for Emergency Room) record.

Uniform Hospital Discharge Data Set

01. **Personal identification**
02. **Date of birth (month, day, and year)**
03. **Sex**
04. **Race and ethnicity**
05. **Residence (usual residence, full address, and zip code [nine-digit zip code, if available])**
06. **Hospital identification number**
     Three options are given for this institutional number, with the Medicare provider number as the recommended choice. The federal tax identification number of the American Hospital Association number is preferred to creating a new number.
07. **Admission date (month, day, and year)**
08. **Type of admission (scheduled or unscheduled)**
09. **Discharge date (month, day, and year)**
10. **Attending physician identification (NPI)**
11. **Operating physician identification (NPI)**
12. **Principal diagnosis**
     The condition established after study to be chiefly responsible for occasioning the admission of the patient to the hospital for care.
13. **Other diagnoses**
     All conditions that coexist at the time of admission or that develop subsequently that affect the treatment received and/or the length of stay. Diagnoses that relate to an earlier episode and have no bearing on the current hospital stay are excluded.
14. **Qualifier for other diagnoses**
     A qualifier is given for each diagnosis coded under "other diagnoses" to indicate whether the onset of the diagnosis preceded or followed admission to the hospital. The option "uncertain" is permitted.
15. **External cause-of-injury code**
     Hospitals should complete this item whenever there is a diagnosis of an injury, poisoning, or adverse effect.
16. **Birth weight of neonate**
17. **Procedures and dates**
     a. All significant procedures are to be reported. A significant procedure is one that (1) is surgical in nature, (2) carries a procedural risk, (3) carries an anesthetic risk, or (4) requires specialized training.
     b. The date of each significant procedure must be reported.
     c. When multiple procedures are reported, the principal procedure is designated. The principal procedure is one that was performed for definitive treatment rather than one performed for diagnostic or explanatory purposes or was necessary to take care of a complication. If two procedures appear to be principal, then the one most related to the principal diagnosis is selected as the principal procedure.
     d. The UPIN of the person performing the principal procedure must be reported.
18. **Disposition of the patient**
     a. Discharged home (not to home health service)
     b. Discharged to acute care hospital
     c. Discharged to nursing facility
     d. Discharged to home to be under the care of a home health service
     e. Discharged to other health care facility
     f. Left against medical advice
     g. Alive, other; or alive, not stated
     h. Died
19. **Patient's expected source of payment**
     a. Primary source
     b. Other source
20. **Total charges**
     List all charges billed by the hospital for this hospitalization. Professional charges for individual patient care by physicians are excluded.

FIGURE 2-1. Uniform Hospital Discharge Data Set elements.

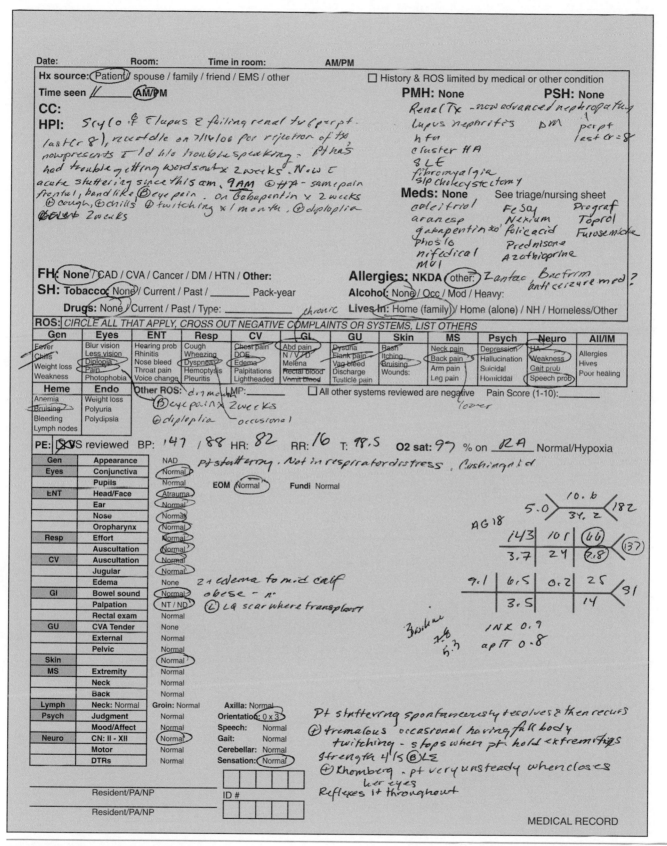

FIGURE 2-2. Emergency Room record.

Continued

MEDICAL DECISION MAKING

PLAN

Head CT
labs

Differential Dx:

1. _Stroke_
2. _uremia_
3. _infection_
4. _drug side effect_

1745
Renal (XH) 39842 codel. will come to eval.

☑ Discussed history, plan or diagnosis with other provider.

Radiology Results: ☐ ED interpretation ☐ Discussed with Radiologist

☐ Prior medical records reviewed.

CT ~ No CT evidence of acute ischemia

☐ Nursing / EMS notes reviewed.

☐ The patient was given: *IM / IV* medications or *IV fluids.*

EKG/Rhythm: NSR / Arrythmia: _____

☐ Patient referred for further care.

ATTENDING PHYSICIAN NOTE: Time seen: _11 0~_ AM / PM

☐ I was present with the resident/midlevel during the patient's history and physical and discussed their management with the resident. I have reviewed the resident's note above and agree with the documented findings and plan of care.

☑ I saw and evaluated the patient. I reviewed the resident/midlevel's note above and agree, in addition to/except that:

Additional findings:

s/p NdT+

↑ most likely delirium

⊖ M/F

→ √ ct

Procedure / Progress Note: Time:_____ AM / PM   **Consult:** _____ Called: _____ AM / PM

No acute neuroissnes per keto
Pt accepted to Medicine For uremia

Provider: _____   __ __ __ __ __ __

Procedures: Central Venous / Intubation / LP / Suture / Chest tube / Nasal Pack / Sedation / Splint / I&D / Other: _____

Diagnosis:

☐ See procedure documentation

1. _Uremia_   4. _____

☐ See additional documentation

2. _____   5. _____

3. _____   6. _____   **Critical Care Time:** _____ minutes

Dispo: Discharge / Admit / Transfer / AMA   **Admission/Transfer Location:** _____
Condition: Stable / Good / Fair / Serious / Expired   **Discharge time:** _____ AM / PM Date: _____

Attendings: _____   __ __ __ __ __ __

MEDICAL RECORD

FIGURE 2-2, cont'd. Emergency Room record.

Admission History and Physical Examination

Admission history and physical documentation normally contains the following elements:
- Chief complaint (CC)
- History of the present illness (HPI)
- Past medical history
- Family medical history
- Social history
- **Review of systems**
- Physical examination
- Impression/Assessment
- Plan

See Figure 2-3 for an example of a history and physical form (H&P).

Physician Orders

This is the area of the record in which the attending **physicians**, as well as physician **consultants**, give directives to the house staff and to nursing and ancillary services. Physician orders are dated, timed, and signed and become part of the record. Verbal orders by physicians are guided by medical staff regulations. See Figure 2-4 for an example of handwritten physician orders and Figure 2-5 for an electronic physician order.

Progress Notes

Progress notes are a record of the course of a patient's hospital care. They are usually written by the attending physician (Figure 2-6, *A*). Academic medical centers may have notes written by medical students, interns, and residents, as well as attending physicians and consultants. Some facilities have integrated progress notes, which allow individuals from several disciplines to write in the same area of the record. An integrated progress note may include notes written by dietitians, physical therapists, respiratory therapists, and nurses.

Progress notes written by the attending physician are recorded on a daily basis; the frequency of such note taking is governed by medical staff regulations. These notes describe how the patient is progressing and put forth the plan of care for the patient. In an electronic patient record, these notes may be dictated and transcribed or typed by physicians themselves. Physicians are usually taught to document progress notes according to the SOAP format. SOAP stands for the following:

    Subjective—The problem in the patient's own words (chief complaint)
    Objective—The physician identifies the history, physical examination, and diagnostic test results
    Assessment—Where the subjective and objective combine for a conclusion
    Plan—Approach the physician is taking to solve the patient's problem
    See Figure 2-6, *B*, for an example of a progress note written in SOAP format.

Nursing Notes

If nursing notes are not integrated, they are often found in their own section of the record on forms that lend themselves to the type of information nurses are required to document. Nursing notes usually consist of an admission note, graphic charts, medication/treatment records, and temperature, pulse, and respiration (TPR) sheets. See Figure 2-7 for an example of an electronic medication administration record (MAR) and Figure 2-8 for an example of laboratory results.

Anesthesia Forms

The anesthesiologist is required to write preanesthesia and postanesthesia notes. The anesthetic agent, amount given, administration technique used, duration of the procedure, amount of blood loss, fluids given, and any complications or additional procedures performed by the anesthesiologist must be documented. See Figure 2-9 for an example of anesthesia documentation.

Text continued on p. 23

ADMISSION NOTE

M.D.:   Pager:

Date: Time:

Chief Complaint:
twitching

History of Present Illness:
This is a 51 year old woman with a history of lupus, lupus nephritis, and cadaveric renal transplant in 2000 who now presents with 2 weeks of worsening twitching. The patient describes starting neurontin for headaches approximately 3 weeks ago. She subsequently noted first subtle twitching of an extremity or her face. The movements have progressed to include difficulty speaking, dysarthria ("I couldn't say what I was thinking") and difficulty walking.

The patient has also noticed worsening fatigue, a change in her skin ("It's ashy") and worsening edema (including LE and peri-orbital).

On Friday the patient called the transplant nurse who recommended she come to the Emergency room. There, she was seen by neuro, who felt most of her symptoms were most likely related to worsening renal failure with gabapentin. They also noted b/l ptosis and findings suggestive of a peripheral neuropathy.

The patient reports no improvement in symptoms since arrival.

ED Course:
As above.

Primary MD:

Emergency Contact:

Code Status:

Review of Systems: ⬭ positive
Constitutional: ~~ABC~~ negative
~~Fevers, Chills, Night Sweats,~~ (Fatigue)
Weight Loss, Weight Gain, Heat Intolerance, Cold Intolerance

Neuro:
(Headache,) ~~Seizures, Syncope, Lightheaded, Vertigo, Dizziness, Tremor, Weakness, Numbness, Tingling~~

HEENT:
~~Vision change,~~ (Diplopia,) Cataracts, Glaucoma, Hearing Loss, Tinnitus, Sinusitis, ~~Sore Throat,~~ Polydipsia, Lymphadenopathy

CV:
~~Chest Pain, Palpitations, Orthopnea,~~ PND Claudication, Exercise Intolerance

Respiratory:
~~SOB,~~ Pleuritic Pain, Wheezing, ~~Cough Sputum,~~ Hemoptysis

GI:
~~Abdominal Pain, Nausea, Vomiting, Diarrhea, Constipation,~~ Jaundice, ~~Melena,~~ BRBPR, Dysphagia, Odynophagia, Reflux, Hematemesis

GU:
~~Dysuria,~~ Frequency, Urgency, Hesitancy, Incontinence, Hematuria, polyuria
LMP _____

Skin/Skeletal:
(Rashes) (Bruising,) Joint Stiffness/Pain, Myalgias

Psych:
~~Depression,~~ Mood Changes, SI, HI, Plan

X All other systems negative

FIGURE 2-3. History and physical.

M.D.:   Pager:

Date: Time:

Past Medical History:
Lupus diagnosed 1991, h/o lupus arthritis and muscle pain
- No prior lupus involvement in brain
- No recent flairs

Social History:

Tobacco: none

Alcohol: none

Illicits: none

Residence: lives with daughter

Occupation: owned her own hair salon, now not working

Family: son and daughter in area

Other:

Allergies:
Zantac –> decreased muscle tone

Medications:
Imuran 150mg po qd
Prednisone 10mg po qd
Prograf 4mg po bid
nexium 40mg po qd
stresstab + zinc
folate 1mg po qd
Fe 300mg po tid
Toprol XL 100mg po qd
Calcitriol 0.5mg po q.o.d.
PhosLo 2 tab po TID
Aranesp 100 q.o.week
Lasix 40mg po bid
Clonidine 0.1mg po bid

Family History:
Mo - Kidney stones
No lupus, no renal failure

T_c afeb	72	140
T_m	HR	BP 80
RR 20	98%	None
Pain 0	SaO$_2$	FiO$_2$
Wt	I/O	Dexi
		Stool

FIGURE 2-3, cont'd. History and physical.

Continued

ADMISSION NOTE

M.D.:   Pager:

Date: Time:

General: Pleasant, NAD. Periodic jerking movements of large muscles, small muscles, and facial muscles	**Affect:** full

HEENT: B/L ptosis, no scleral icterus. MM sl dry. OP clear.

Neck: Neck supple. No LAD.

Chest: CTA B/L	**Skin:** dry
Heart: RR, soft SM at LUSB	**Vasc:**
Abd: Soft, full. BSNA. No ascites	
Ext: Warm, + edema	**Joints:** no effusion or erythema

GU/Rectal: deferred

Neuro: Sensation:

Mental Status: attentive, oriented   Motor: grossly intact. sustained clonus b/l

Cranial Nerves: intact   Coordination:

Reflexes

RDW: 15.4%   MCV: 87.7 FL

Hgb: 10.6 G/DL
WBC: 5030 #/cu mm
HCT: 34.2%
Plat: 182 K/CU MM
11:25 2006/08/18

Na 143 MEQ/L | Cl 101 MEQ/L | BUN 66 MG/DL
K 3.7 MEQ/L | CO2 24 mEq/L | Cr 7.8 MG/DL
Glu 137 MG/DL
11:25 2006/08/18

Ca 9.1 MG/DL | TP 6.5 G/DL | TB 0.2 MG/DL | AST 25 U/L
Mg | Alb 3.5 G/DL | DB | ALT 14 U/L
AlkP 51 U/L
11:25 2006/08/18

L 28.6%   M 5.8%   N 62.6%   E 2.4%   B 0.6%
11:25 2006/08/18

PT 9.4 SECONDS   INR: 0.9*
11:25 2006/08/18

APTT:SECONDS 23.9   APTTr: 0.8 PAT/NORM

EKG:
NSR

Chest XR:
obesity, otherwise clear

FIGURE 2-3, cont'd. History and physical.

ADMISSION NOTE

M.D.:   Pager:

Date: Time:

Radiographic Data:

Impression

51 year old woman with worsening renal failure and muscle twitching.

Plan:

1. Neuro-Muscle twitching is likely due to uremia in the setting of worsened renal function. Suspect contribution of gabapentin, which can cause twitching and is correlated in time. Plan is to start dialysis Monday. Continue prograf (can stop monday per renal).
2. Renal-Continue prograf, nephrovite, phoslo. Renal diet. Renal has seen patient.
3. Rheum-Continue Imuran. No evidence of acute flair, but check ESR & CRP. Continue prednisone.
4. HTN-Continue clonidine, toprol, nifedipine qd.
5. Dispo-See PMD.

DVT Prophylaxis? heparin 5000 units sq bid, stop Sun for dialysis Monday

1. 332.0: Trembling paralysis

2. 586: Renal failure, unspecified

3. 401.9: HTN [Hypertension]

4. 710.0: Lupus nephritis

Date:

FIGURE 2-3, cont'd. History and physical.

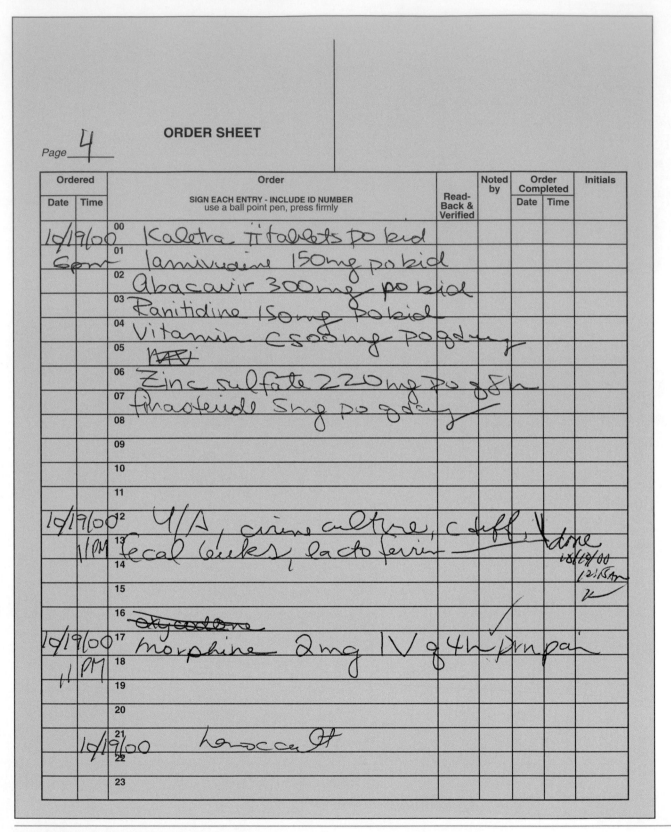

FIGURE 2-4. Handwritten physician orders.

Cumulative Order Summary

Orders: _____

Med Rec No: _____

Location: _____   Birth date: _____   Age: _____

Atn: _____   Sex: _____

ALLERGIES:	Swelling-dexamethasone			
Ord #	**Order name/description**	**Start date**	**Ord status**	**Stop date**
001BXMXJH	**Immunofixation-Electro, Serum LAB**		1 or more final results received	
	Entered DT/TM: _____ _____			
	Auth prescriber: _____			
	Auth prescriber number: _____			
001BXMXJJ	**Immunoglobulins, Serum LAB**		1 or more final results received	
	Entered DT/TM: _____ _____			
	Auth prescriber: _____			
	Auth prescriber number: _____			
001BXNBHF	**Transfuse Red Blood Cells**	_____	Completed _____	

Start date: _____, urgency: when available, transfuse 2 consent obtained units. Transfuse each unit over 2 hours, in dialysis. When the patient is ready and the product is available, call or fax blood bank for delivery.
with dialysis _____

Entered DT/TM: _____

Auth prescriber: _____
Auth prescriber number: _____

FIGURE 2-5. Electronic physician order.

Operative Report

An operative report must be included in the health record for patients who undergo surgical procedures. The operative report should include a preoperative diagnosis, a postoperative diagnosis, dates, names of surgeons, descriptions of findings, procedures performed, and the condition of the patient at completion of the procedure. The operative report should be dictated and should be in the record within 24 hours of completion of surgery. See Figure 2-10 for a sample of a dictated operative report.

Consultations

Consultations are requested by the attending physician who wishes to gain an expert opinion on treatment of a particular aspect of the patient's condition that is outside the expertise of the attending. A preoperative consultation may be requested as part of the determination of the surgical risk of the patient. Information acquired during consults may be integrated within progress notes or recorded on a separate consult form.

Laboratory, Radiology, and Pathology Reports

Laboratory data are often captured electronically and may or may not appear in the paper health record. Laboratory data would include such items as complete blood count (CBC), urinalysis, and metabolic levels. Radiology reports are increasingly captured electronically, and the physician may often find the actual image available electronically. Pathology reports, which are also increasingly found in transcribed reports online, consist of a gross

Text continued on p. 33

PROGRESS NOTES

for addressograph plate

Date	Time	
		∅ c/o
		⊖ flatus / stool in' ostomy
		5-2〉8·7 ∠ 255 INR 1·0
		29·5
		Abdomen c minimal LLQ TTP; ∅ peritoneal signs
		CT reviewed again yesterday c radiologist
		✲✲ Recommend Med-Onc to see pt today!
		— Continue Abx
		— NPO / IVF
		— Start TPN
		— NO Acute surgical indication given
		poor prognosis c exploratory laparotomy
		and high likelihood of short gut
		syndrome if operation performed
		will plan to operate only if pt
		toxic or peritoneal
		Agree c above
		Patient surgically
		Stable

A

FIGURE 2-6. A, Progress notes.

Page 1

Patient information

[can use hospital plate]

Inpatient Progress Note

Evaluation type: ☒ Followup care   ☐ Discharge note

Clinical information

Meds
Lepirudin
Protonix
Odansetron
Dilaudid PCA
Aspart Insulin sliding
                      scale ✓

S| Tearful; c/o pain in abd.

O| VS: 37.1   18 95   108/71   97%

   ⊖ Icterus

   ABD: distended (mod).
        Well appearing Incision
        c/d/i c steristrips

   EXT: ⊖ edema

Assessment & plan:

HD# 10 c Budd Chiari 2° PCV s/p surgical shunt (mesocaval) c bx.

- cont. current management bridging anticoag c Lepirudin
  given h/o HIT. until ~~ok to start~~ coumadin c therapeutic INR
                        chronic

Assistant: _____ _(Signature)_ _____ _(Print)_ MD #: _____ Date: _____
(If involved)   ☐ Fellow   ☐ Resident   ☐ NP   ☐ PA

Attending: _____ _(Signature)_ _____ _(Print)_ MD #: _____ Date/time _____

(7/03)

B

FIGURE 2-6, cont'd. B, SOAP progress note.

Medication Administration Record

Med Rec No: _____
Visit ID No: _____

Location: _____   Age: _____   Sex: _____

Atn DR: _____   Birthday: _____

ALLERGIES: Swelling-dexamethasone

Scheduled

Medications	Doses	Comments
Routine Hydroxychloroquine enteral 200 mg PO bid routine. Administer with food or milk. **Start:** _____ **Stop:** _____	**Ord #: 001BXCBQV** (Continued…) Performed _____ 13:00 _____ (RN) Performed _____ 22:00 _____ (RN)	
Routine Labetalol enteral 400 mg PO bid, routine **Start:** _____ **Stop:** _____	**Ord #: 001BXTZQD** Not performed– _____ 13:00 _____ (RN) Physician request… Canceled	
Routine Levothyroxine enteral 100 mcg PO daily routine **Start:** _____ **Stop:** _____	**Ord #: 001BXBJST** Performed _____ 13:00 _____ (RN)	
Routine Lisinopril enteral 40 mg PO daily routine **Start:** _____ **Stop:** _____	**Ord #: 001BXTKKD** Performed _____ 13:00 _____ (RN)	

FIGURE 2-7. Medication administration record.

Laboratory Results

Component	Low range	High range	Range units	16:00:00
Sodium	135	148	mEq/L	140
Potassium, serum	3.5	5.0	mEq/L	4.3
Chloride	99	111	mEq/L	104
Urea-nitrogen	7	22	mg/dL	11
Glucose	60	99	mg/dL	91*
Creatinine, serum	0.5	1.2	mg/dL	0.5
Calcium	8.4	10.5	mg/dL	9.6
Total protein	6.0	8.2	g/dL	7.4
Albumin	3.5	5.3	g/dL	4.6
Total bilirubin	0.1	1.2	mg/dL	0.3
Alanine amino trans	0	31	U/L	5
Aspartate amino tran	0	31	U/L	16
Alkaline phosphatase	100	320	U/L	92
CO_2	21	31	mEq/L	27
Anion gap	11	20	mEq/L	13
Sun/creat ratio				22
Ast/alt ratio				3.2
Est Gfr (Afr Amer)			mL/min/A	Text*
Est Gfr (non-Afr-Am)			mL/min/A	Text*

FIGURE 2-8. Laboratory results.

Anesthesia Preoperative Assessment

PLEASE WRITE LEGIBLY

PROCEDURE _FEMORAL INTRAMEDULLARY ROD_

DIAGNOSIS _(L) Leg Shortening_

MEDICATIONS _None_

for addressograph plate

PAIN HISTORY ☒ Negative
Intensity (0-10) _____
Location _____
Affect quality of life? ☐ Y ☐ N
Pain meds effective? ☐ Y ☐ N
Alleviating / Aggravating factors

Quality: Sharp / dull / other _____

Onset / duration _____

ALLERGIES (drug/environmental/food) _NKDA_

Anesthesia Issues ☐ Negative
☐ Difficult Airway
  ☐ By exam ☐ By history
  ☐ TMJ problems
☐ Snoring ☐ OSA _mild_
☐ Hoarseness
☐ Nasal obstruction
☐ Stridor/croup
☐ Fam Hx Anesth Problems
☐ Malignant Hyperthermia
☐ Obesity
☐ Post-op nausea/vomiting
☐ Organ transplant _____

Cardiovascular ☒ Negative
☐ Myocard infarct: Date _____
☐ Hypertension
☐ Arrhythmia: type _____
☐ Pacemaker ☐ AICD
☐ Angina: ☐ stable ☐ unstable
☐ CHF: Date ____ EF ___%
☐ Valve disease: _____
  ☐ Mod ☐ Severe
☐ Peripheral vascular disease
☐ Past cardiac surgery _Denies_
☐ Angioplasty
☐ Deep vein thrombus _cyanosis_
☐ Pulmonary embolus _diaphoresis_
☐ Heart murmur
☐ Stress test/cardiac cath _c̄ Activity_
  Detail results below

Pulmonary ☒ Negative
☐ Smoking hx ☐ current ___ppd
☐ Asthma
  ☐ Hospitalized ☐ Steroid use
  ☐ Recent wheezing
☐ COPD/DPD
☐ Cough: active / chronic
☐ Other

Renal ☒ Negative
☐ Renal insufficiency
☐ Dialysis
☐ Other

Hepatic ☒ Negative
☐ Hepatitis
☐ Cirrhosis
☐ Other

Endocrine ☒ Negative
☐ Diabetes
☐ Thyroid
☐ Steroid usage
☐ Other

Infections ☐ Negative
☐ SBE prophylaxis _Immunized to date_
☐ HIV ☐ Sepsis ☐ URI
☐ VRE
☐ MRSA: contact / resp.

Neurologic ☒ Negative
☐ Seizure
☐ Elevated ICP ☐ Shunt
☐ Spinal cord injury
☐ CVA/TIA
☐ Cerebral palsy
☐ Mental retardation
☐ Chronic pain
☐ Neuropathy/paresthesia
☐ Myopathy/muscular dystrophy
☐ Syncope
☐ Hearing loss
☐ Blind: right / left
☐ Other

Gastrointestinal ☒ Negative
☐ GE reflux / hiatal hernia
☐ Bowel obstruction ☐ Ascites
☐ Ulcers
☐ GI bleed
☐ Dysphagia
☐ Other

Hematol/Onc ☒ Negative
☐ Sickle cell disease ☐ Trait
☐ Coagulopathy
☐ Anemia
☐ Past transfusion
☐ Refuses transfusion
☐ Tumor _____
☐ Chemo/Rad therapy

Obstetrics ☐ Negative
☐ Preeclampsia/eclampsia
☐ Placenta previa/abruptio
☐ LMP _7/9/__ ☐ HCG
☐ Other

Drug Use ☒ Negative
☐ ETOH ☐ Daily
  ☐ Never ☐ Occasional
☐ IVDA ☐ Cocaine
☐ Other

Activity Level
☐ Bedridden
☐ Assistance with self-care
☐ <1 flight of stairs
☐ 1–3 flights of stairs
☐ >3 flights of stairs
☒ Able to lie flat one hour

Pediatrics ☐ Negative
☐ Prematurity _FTVD_
☐ Congenital abnl. _in chiari_
☐ Apnea
☐ Passive smoking
☐ Other

Day of Surgery:
NPO since _10 p.m._

DETAILS OF PRESENT ILLNESS AND PAST MEDICAL HISTORY _16 y.o. ♀ for leg length shortening, ∅ PMH._

PREVIOUS SURGERY AND ANESTHESIA ☒ NONE

```
140 | 104 | 11  < 91        4.7 > 124 < 232
4.3 |  27 | 0.5               37.4          hcg ⊖
```

LABS / ECG

BP Range ® 104/60 103/51 P _86_ R _____ T _99.9_ WT _46.4_ (lbs/kg) HT _5' 0"_ (in/cm) Room Air Sat _100%_ Age _16_ M Ⓕ

HISTORY PERFORMED BY: _____ ID Number _____ DATE _____ TIME _____

CHART COPY

page 1 of 2

FIGURE 2-9. Anesthesia record.

Continued

PRE-ANESTHESIA / PRE-OPERATIVE ASSESSMENT
PAGE 2

PLEASE WRITE LEGIBLY

Physical Examination

HEENT _Normocephaly_, _NO oral lesions MP=I_   for addressograph plate

Neck: _supple c FROM midline trachea_

Cardiovascular _RRR S₁S₂ NO murmurs or clicks._

Lungs _Bib CTA_

Pain sites / Pertinent other _A OX3 accompanied by Father NAD._
NPO p̄ 12mn Instructions and directions to CROSS were given to
pt's Father instruction to avoid NSAIDS preop were given as
well to Father

Physical exam performed by: _____ ID Number _____ Date _____ Time _____

ANESTHESIA ATTENDING PRE-ANESTHESIA ASSESSMENT AND CONSENT

Medical record and laboratory data reviewed ☑   Patient examined ☑

Patient is appropriate for the planned anesthesia:
  General ☑   Spinal ☐
  Regional block ☐   Epidural/caudal ☑
  Monitored anesthesia care ☐   Other ☐ _____
  Special monitoring ☐   _____

Planned post-operative care: PACU ☑   ICU ☐   Other ☐

ASA STATUS	1	2	3	4	5	6	E

Airway Assessment:
  Oral excursion: FB   1☐   2☐   3☐
  T-M distance: FB   1☐   2☐
  Dentition: Upper nl☐ dentures☐ caps☐ decayed☐ loose☐
         Lower nl☐ dentures☐ caps☐ decayed☐ loose☐
  Mallampati: I☐   II☐   III☐   IV☐
  Neck Extension: nl☐   7☐   77☐
      Flexion: nl☐   7☐   77☐

16,00g for ® leg shortening   NO All
® leg length discrepancy   NO MOOS
otherwise healthy / ⊖ heart/lungs
ASA I for GOTA/ epidural for p/op analgesia

☐ Informed consent not obtained due to the emergent condition of the patient.

The plan for anesthesia and postoperative pain management, their alternatives, and the risks and benefits of these plans and alternatives have been explained to me and my questions have been answered to my satisfaction. I give my consent.

Signature of Patient / Parent / Guardian, Health Care Agent   Telephone consent witness   Signature of health care provider securing consent

Anesthesiologist Signature _____ **ID Number** _____ **Date** _____ **Time** _____

SURGICAL ATTENDING PRE-OPERATIVE ASSESSMENT--to be completed by surgeon if used as a surgical history and physical

CHIEF COMPLAINT _____

FAMILY HISTORY _____   SOCIAL HISTORY _____

Pre-operative history, physical exam, and pertinent laboratory data reviewed by me with amendments as follows: ☐ NONE

_____
_____
_____

Preoperative diagnosis: _____

Planned procedure: _____

Surgeon Signature _____ ID Number _____ Date _____ Time _____

CHART COPY   page 2 of 2

FIGURE 2-9, cont'd. Anesthesia record.

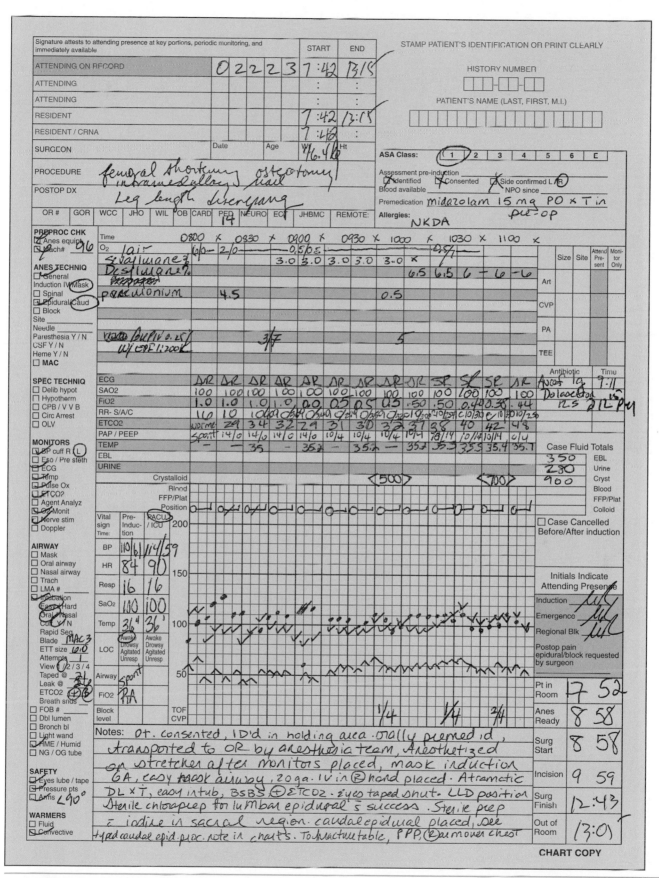

FIGURE 2-9, cont'd. Anesthesia record.

Continued

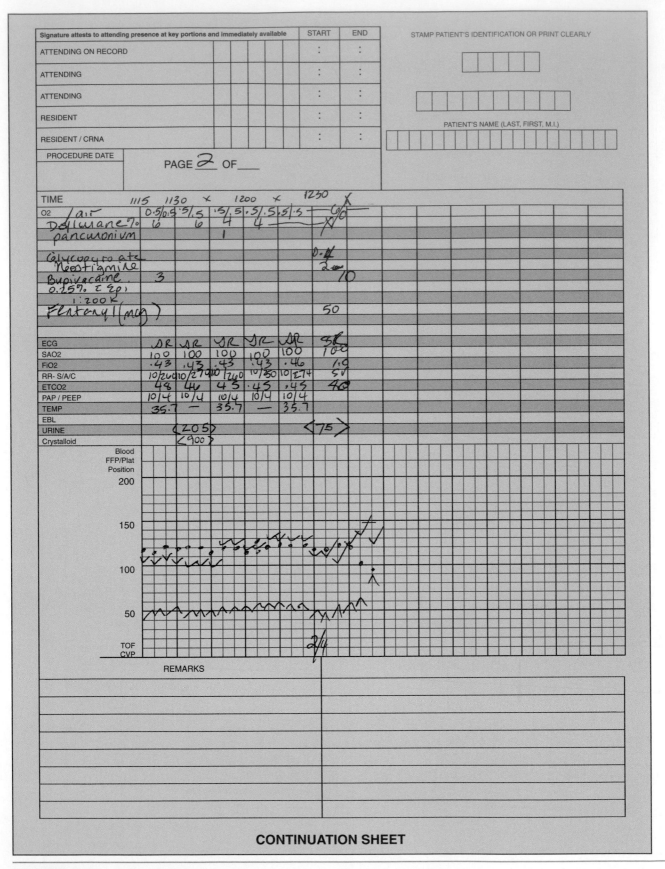

FIGURE 2-9, cont'd. Anesthesia record.

Patient name _____ History # _____

TIME	pH	pCO2	pO2	HCO3	Na	K	Ca	Glu	HGB			

AS A Physical Status Classification
1: A normal, healthy patient
2: A patient with mild systemic disease
3. A patient with severe systemic disease
4: A patient with severe systemic disease that is a threat to life
5. A moribund patient, not expected to survive without the operation
6: A declared dead patient for organ donation
E: An emergency operation

SYMBOLS		POSITION	TABLE FLAT	OTHER POS.
NIBP	X	Supine	○——⌐	Sitting
PULSE	●——●	Prone	○——⌐	Lithotomy
ART BP	╪	Lateral L down	○—⟍	Jackknife
MAP	⤫	Lateral R down	○⟍	

CRITERIA FOR DISCHARGE DIRECTLY TO NURSING UNIT	CRITERIA MET	RETURN TO BASELINE
Level of consciousness–awake, alert appropriately conversant or baseline		
Return to usual pattern of mobility or as appropriate per procedure		
BP within normal range. There is no evidence of severe hyper- or hypotension		
Pulse rate (60–100 adults / 80–150 pediatrics) and rhythm regular or baseline		
Respiratory rate: 12–20 (>3 years); 20–40 (<3 years) and pattern normal		
Oxygen saturation >93% or comparable to baseline		
Ability to swallow secretions or baseline		
Dressings, tubes and drains intact with amount of drainage appropriate for procedure		

DISCHARGE TO: _____ Signature _____ Dr. # _____ Date _____ Time _____

Intraop and Post Anesthesia Notes:

[handwritten notes]

☑ Responsibility for patient management and monitoring after transport and report transferred to: PACU / ICU / Other _____

_____ Date _____ Time _____
Signature _____ Provider No. _____

☐ Transfer of care accepted in ICU:

_____ Date _____ Time _____
Signature _____ Provider No. _____

FIGURE 2-9, cont'd. Anesthesia record.

Operative Report

PATIENT NAME: Sonia Sample
ROOM NUMBER: 222 West
MR NUMBER: 12-34-56

DATE OF PROCEDURE: 04/22/00
PREOPERATIVE DIAGNOSIS: Acute cholecystitis
POSTOPERATIVE DIAGNOSIS: Acute cholecystitis
NAME OF PROCEDURE: 1. Laparoscopic cholecystectomy
2. Intraoperative cystic duct cholangiogram
SURGEON: Claude St. John, M.D.
ASSISTANT: Mark Weiss, D.O.
ANESTHESIOLOGIST: Angela Adams, M.D.
ANESTHESIA: General

DESCRIPTION OF THE OPERATION:

The patient was placed in the supine position under general anesthesia. The oral gastric tube was placed. The Foley catheter was placed. The patient received appropriate antibiotics. The abdomen was prepped with iodine and draped in the usual fashion. Using a midline subumbilical incision, we entered the subcutaneous fat to find the aponeurosis of the rectus abdominis. Two stay sutures were placed 0.5 cm from the midline bilaterally and we left on these sutures, creating an opening in the linea alba.

Under direct vision, the catheter was placed. The Hasson cannula was placed in the abdominal cavity and all was normal except an acute necrotizing and probably gangrenous gallbladder. There were multiple omental adhesions. Three other trocars were placed in the right subcostal plane in the midline, midclavicular line, and midaxillary line using a #10, #5, and #5 mm trocar, respectively. The gallbladder was punctured and emptied of clear white bile indicating a hydrops of the gallbladder. It was grasped at its fundus and at Hartmann's pouch retracted cephalad and to the right, respectively. We found the cystic duct and the cystic artery after circumferential dissection and isolated the cystic duct completely.

When we were sure that this structure was a deep cystic duct, the clip was placed at this most distal aspect to make an opening immediately proximally and we placed a Reddick cholangiocatheter into it via #14 gauge percutaneous catheter. The cholangiogram showed normal arborization of the liver radicals. Normal bifurcation of the common hepatic duct. Normal common hepatic duct. Long large cystic duct. The common bile duct had numerous stones within it. They could not be emptied from the common bile duct. There was good flow into the duodenum.

The impression was choledocholithiasis. This was corroborated by the radiologist. The decision was made to prepare the patient most probably for endoscopic retrograde cholangiopancreatography postoperatively, and no further intervention of the common bile duct was done in this setting.

The cholangiocatheter was removed. An attempt was made to milk the bile out but no stones came out. Three clips were placed on the proximal aspect of the cystic duct and the duct was then cut distally. The artery was isolated and double clipped proximally and single clipped distally and cut in the intervening section. We then peeled the gallbladder off the gallbladder bed with some difficulty because of the intense edema and inflammation. It was then removed from the liver bed completely. Cautery, suctioning and irrigation were used copiously to create a bloodless field. A last check was made and there was no bleeding and no bile leaking. A #15 Jackson-Pratt type drain was placed into Morrison's pouch and brought out through the lateral most port. We then removed, with great difficulty, the gallbladder from the umbilicus. Because of its enormous size and a 3 cm stone within it that was very difficult to macerate, the opening of the umbilicus had to be enlarged.

As this was done, we removed the gallbladder completely and sent it for pathologic section. Two separate figure-of-eight 0 PDS were used to close the abdominal fascia. The Jackson-Pratt drain was then sutured in place with 2.0 nylon. The skin was closed throughout with subcuticular 3-0 PDS after copious irrigation of the subcutaneous plane. Mastisol and Steri-Strips were placed on the wound. The patient remained stable although she did have bigeminy during surgery and was on a Lidocaine drip. She will be going to the intensive care unit but as she left, she was extubated in the recovery room and was fully alert. She is moving all limbs.

I will discuss with the gastroenterologist postoperative endoscopic retrograde cholangiopancreatography.

SPECIMEN: Gallbladder.

Claude St. John, M.D.
CSJ/ld:
D: 04/22/00
T: 04/25/00 9:21 am
CC: Maria Acosta, M.D.

FIGURE 2-10. Operative report.

Radiology Report

EXAM DATE:
HISTORY NUMBER:
AGE: SEX: RACE:
REQUESTER:

EXAM: MHM 1006-MRI, brain w/wo cont w/diff
RESULT:
SYMPTOMS: Acute change in mental status.
MEDICAL/SURGICAL HISTORY: Pancreatic cancer, bacteremia.
SUSPECTED DIAGNOSIS: Mets.

TECHNIQUE: Sagittal T1, axial T2, axial FLAIR, and post-contrast axial and coronal T1 through brain. Magnevist (0.1 mmol/kg) injected intravenously without complication. Diffusion images obtained.

FINDINGS:
Minimal cerebral atrophy with expected ventricular dilatation appropriate for age.

Minimal scattered foci of increased T2 signal are noted in the periventricular and subcortical white matter and brainstem, cerebellar peduncles which are nonspecific but likely reflective of small vessel ischemia. Old lacunar infarcts noted in the posterior limb of the right internal capsule/right thalamus.

No evidence of mass, hemorrhage, midline shift, or abnormal enhancement. Ventricles and sulci are normal in size, shape, and position. No abnormal intra or extra axial fluid collection. Normal flow voids in carotid and basilar arteries. Normal scalp, calvarium, orbits. Trace ethmoid and maxillary sinus disease. Minimal left mastoiditis.

IMPRESSION:
Minimal cerebral atrophy with expected ventricular dilatation appropriate for age.

Chronic ischemic disease.
Old lacunar infarcts.

Minimal left mastoiditis.

FIGURE 2-11. Radiology report.

description of the tissue removed and microscopic evaluation that includes the diagnosis. See Figures 2-8 and 2-11 for examples of these types of reports.

Discharge Summary

The discharge summary (Figure 2-12) is a summary of the patient's stay in the hospital. It should include the following:

- History of the present illness
- Past medical history
- Significant findings
- Pertinent laboratory data
- Procedures performed or treatment rendered
- Final diagnosis
- Discharge instructions; medications and the condition of the patient on discharge

Discharge Summary

PATIENT NAME: Sonia Sample
MR NUMBER: 12-34-56

ADMISSION DATE: 04/19/00
DISCHARGE DATE: 04/27/00
ADMITTING IMPRESSION: Acute abdominal pain, rule out diverticulitis.

HISTORY OF PRESENT ILLNESS:

The patient is a 57-year-old white female who has history of hypertension, valvular heart disease, and cardiomyopathy, who was seen in the emergency room with complaints of acute abdominal pain. On evaluation, she was found to be very tender in the abdomen. She had white blood cell count of 19,000 and was admitted with a diagnosis of rule out diverticulitis.

HOSPITAL COURSE:

CT scan of the abdomen was consistent with cholecystitis and ultrasound of the gallbladder was consistent with cholelithiasis. She was cleared for surgery by cardiologist Dr. Chen and was treated preoperatively with intravenous antibiotics, intravenous fluids, and pain medication. On 4/22/00, the patient underwent laparoscopic cholecystectomy. On 4/26/00, she underwent an endoscopic retrograde cholangiopancreatography. The postoperative course was remarkable for some shortness of breath, otherwise the patient was doing well. She remained very stable, afebrile, and was discharged home.

DISCHARGE DIAGNOSES

1. Cholelithiasis with acute cholecystitis; status post laparoscopic cholecystectomy
2. Mitral valve disorder
3. Hypertensive heart disease with history of angiopathic cardiomyopathy

MEDICATIONS

1. Cozaar
2. Hytrin
3. Lasix
4. Potassium
5. Lanoxin

DIET: The patient is to be on a low-fat diet.

ACTIVITIES: The patient is to be ambulating at home p.r.n.

FOLLOW-UP: Follow-up in two weeks with Dr. St. John and Dr. Glasser.

Medications, diet, activities, and follow-up have all been discussed with the patient and she showed a good understanding

Maria Acosta, M.D.
MA/jw: 11931
D: 05/05/00
T: 05/13/00 1:36 pm

FIGURE 2-12. Discharge summary.

EXERCISE 2-1

Choose the correct answer option or write the correct answer(s) in the space(s) provided.

1. Does every patient encounter have a health record?
   A. Yes
   B. No

2. Is the discharge summary always found in the same place in a health record?
   A. Yes
   B. No

3. List five purposes of a health record.
   1. _____
   2. _____
   3. _____
   4. _____
   5. _____

4. Name an advantage of an electronic patient record.
   _____

5. Name the nonfederal organization that requires reporting of data collected from the health record.
   _____

6. List five elements required by the UHDDS.
   1. _____
   2. _____
   3. _____
   4. _____
   5. _____

7. Where in the record would you find the chief complaint?
   _____

8. If a physician was treating a patient with an antibiotic, where in the record would you look to see that treatment had been discontinued?
   _____

9. Where in the record would you expect to see how the patient was progressing on a daily basis?
   _____

10. Where in the record might you look to find how much blood was lost during surgery?
    _____

UHDDS REPORTING STANDARDS FOR DIAGNOSES AND PROCEDURES

It is the responsibility of a coder to extract from the health record the diagnoses for which a patient is being treated and the procedures that have been performed. The extracting of data from the health record may also be referred to as **abstracting**. To complete this task, a coder must rely on definitions of principal diagnosis, secondary diagnoses, principal procedure, and secondary procedures.

Principal Diagnosis

The **principal diagnosis** is defined as the condition established after study to be chiefly responsible for occasioning the admission of the patient to the hospital for care. This definition is one, if not the most important, concept that a coder must understand and apply. The principal diagnosis, along with the principal procedure, determines the assignment of the Medicare Severity diagnosis-related groups (MS-DRGs), which, in turn, affects reimbursement. Physicians are often not aware of this definition or how it is applied; therefore, the coder must take care to select the correct principal diagnosis after record review.

EXAMPLE

A patient presents to the emergency room with a cough and fever. After the chest x-ray is reviewed, it is determined that the patient has pneumonia.
The principal diagnosis is pneumonia.

EXAMPLE

A patient presents to the emergency room with acute abdominal pain. After the patient is evaluated, he is taken to the OR for an appendectomy. The pathology report reveals an acute appendicitis, which is confirmed by the physician in the discharge summary.
The principal diagnosis is acute appendicitis.

Sometimes, the principal diagnosis is not as easily identifiable as it is in the above two cases. There may be a secondary diagnosis that utilizes more resources during a patient stay but is not the principal diagnosis.

EXAMPLE

A patient is admitted for coronary artery bypass surgery with a diagnosis of coronary artery disease. The surgery is successful, and on the fourth postoperative day, pneumonia develops. The pneumonia is severe, and the patient goes into respiratory failure and must be intubated and treated in the intensive care unit (ICU). The patient remains in the ICU for 10 days because he cannot be weaned from the ventilator. The patient undergoes a tracheostomy procedure and is discharged to a rehab facility.
The principal diagnosis is coronary artery disease, even though most of the treatment was focused on postoperative pneumonia.

Principal Procedure

A **principal procedure** is defined as one that is performed for definitive treatment rather than for diagnostic or exploratory purposes, or a procedure that is necessary to take care of a complication. The principal procedure is sequenced first. If two procedures meet the definition of principal procedure, then the one that is most closely related to the principal diagnosis is the one designated as the principal procedure.

Other Diagnoses

UHDDS requires reporting of other diagnoses that have significance for the specific hospital encounter. Reportable diagnoses are "conditions that coexist at the time of admission, or develop subsequently or affect the treatment received and/or the length of stay. Diagnoses which relate to an earlier episode which have no bearing on the current hospital stay are to be excluded."

This is further clarified in *Coding Clinic* (2000:2Q:p20-21)[4] where "other diagnoses" are defined as additional conditions that affect patient care because they require one or more of the following:

■ Clinical evaluation, or
■ Therapeutic treatment, or
■ Diagnostic procedures, or
■ Extended length of hospital stay, or
■ Increased nursing care and/or monitoring

Second only to an understanding and application of the definition of "principal diagnosis" is the definition of when to code "other diagnoses." Once again, the importance of these secondary diagnoses comes into play in the MS-DRG reimbursement system. Other diagnoses may be identified as complications and/or **comorbidities** under the MS-DRG system, which may affect payment.

Clinical Evaluation

If the condition of a patient is being clinically evaluated, the coder would expect to see some testing and clinical observations, or perhaps a consultation.

EXAMPLE

> During the course of a hospital stay, a patient develops low sodium levels. The physician makes note of this condition and documents that continued laboratory values will be watched. This would constitute clinical evaluation.

Therapeutic Treatment

Medications, physical therapy, and surgery are forms of therapeutic treatment.

EXAMPLE

> The physician documents in the patient's past medical history that the patient has a history of a seizure disorder. The medication list contains the drug Dilantin. The fact that the patient is currently being treated for a seizure disorder with this medication constitutes a reportable secondary diagnosis. Physicians often list conditions in the patient's past medical history for which he or she is currently being treated. The coder should be familiar with medications and the conditions they treat.

Diagnostic Procedures

Often in the course of an inpatient hospital stay, physicians are trying to determine the cause of a sign, symptom, or patient complaint; in these cases, tests are often done to determine the underlying cause. A few examples of types of diagnostic procedures are provided here:

- EKG or ECG (electrocardiogram)
- EEG (electroencephalogram)
- EGD (esophagogastroduodenoscopy)
- Colonoscopy
- Echocardiogram
- MRI (magnetic resonance imaging)
- MRA (magnetic resonance angiography)
- X-rays

EXAMPLE

> A patient presents to the emergency room with pain in the leg after a fall down the stairs. An x-ray is performed that reveals a fracture of the tibia.

Extended Length of Hospital Stay

In some cases, a patient is ready to be discharged from the hospital, but develops a condition that requires more intensive investigation, monitoring, or watchful waiting; this may require an additional night's stay.

Increased Nursing Care and/or Other Monitoring

An example of a situation in which increased nursing care or monitoring might be needed is an electrolyte imbalance that is not significant enough to require treatment, although a physician may order additional laboratory draws for monitoring of this condition. In other cases, a patient may have a decubitus ulcer that requires no physician treatment but does require more intensive nursing care. It is important to remember that if the physician does not document the diagnosis for which care is being rendered, the coder must query the physician before adding the code.

Previous Conditions

Often, in a discharge summary or a history and physical, a physician will list diagnoses and/or procedures from previous admissions that are not applicable to the current hospital stay. These conditions are generally not reported. V codes may be used if this historical condition has an impact on current care or influences treatment.

EXAMPLE

A patient is admitted with acute bronchitis. The patient was admitted two years ago for an appendectomy and has a history of shingles. In the discharge summary, the physician documents acute bronchitis, status post appendectomy, and a history of shingles. In this case, the only diagnosis to be coded is acute bronchitis. V codes may be assigned for any history of or status post conditions.

Reporting of Coexisting Chronic Conditions

Clarification of this guideline is reported in *Coding Clinic* (2000:2Q:p20-21).[4] Often, patients may have multiple chronic conditions when they are admitted to a hospital. *Coding Clinic* says, "Chronic conditions such as, but not limited to, hypertension, congestive heart failure, asthma, emphysema, COPD, Parkinson's disease, and diabetes mellitus are reportable." These chronic conditions may not be specifically treated with medications or procedures; however, they are reported because they may be evaluated and/or monitored.

EXAMPLE

A patient is admitted with benign prostatic hypertrophy (BPH) for a transurethral prostatectomy. The anesthesiologist in the preoperative note documents that the patient has mitral valve prolapse and requires antibiotics prior to undergoing dental procedures. The fact that the patient has mitral valve prolapse and requires antibiotics is a significant factor for the anesthesiologist. This condition is under clinical evaluation by the anesthesiologist and is being treated simultaneously. Therefore, both BPH and mitral valve prolapse (MVP) are reported.

EXAMPLE

A patient is admitted with acute appendicitis. The anesthesiologist and the preoperative consultation indicate that the patient has a history of chronic obstructive pulmonary disease (COPD). The acute appendicitis and the COPD are coded. Refer to *Coding Clinic* (1992:2Q: p16-17)[5]; COPD is a chronic condition that affects patients for the rest of their lives. This, in turn, affects the monitoring and evaluation of this patient.

Integral Versus Nonintegral Conditions

Conditions that are an **integral** part of the disease process are not coded.

EXAMPLE

A patient is admitted to the hospital with a cough. After performing a diagnostic evaluation, the physician determines that the patient has pneumonia. Coughing is a symptom of pneumonia and is not coded.

EXAMPLE

A patient is admitted to the hospital with hypotension, fever, and an elevated white blood count. A blood culture comes back positive, and the physician determines that the patient has sepsis. In this case, only the sepsis and the SIRS are coded; hypotension, fever, and an elevated white blood count are all symptoms of sepsis and are therefore not coded.

Likewise, conditions that are NOT an integral part of the disease process may be coded. Per *Coding Clinic* (1990:2Q:p15)[6]: "Additional conditions that may **not** be associated routinely with a disease process should be coded when present."

EXAMPLE

A patient is admitted to the hospital with a metastatic brain cancer for surgical removal. The patient's history reveals that he has had lung cancer that was surgically removed and now is presenting with seizures, metastatic brain cancer, and headache. Brain cancer is the principal diagnosis, and seizures and history of lung cancer are coded as secondary diagnoses; headache is not reported because it is a symptom of metastatic brain cancer.

Abnormal Findings

Per *Coding Clinic* (2002:2Q:p17-18),[7] "Abnormal findings (laboratory, x-ray, pathologic, and other diagnostic results) are not coded and reported unless the provider indicates their clinical significance. If the findings are outside the normal range and the provider has ordered other tests to evaluate the condition or prescribed treatment, it is appropriate to ask the provider whether the abnormal finding should be added."

EXERCISE 2-2

Write the correct answer(s) in the space(s) provided.

1. What is the most important definition a coder should know?
   _____

2. What determines an MS-DRG?

   _____

3. What is the principal diagnosis in the following scenario?
   A patient is admitted to the hospital with extreme indigestion. A workup ensues, and the patient is found to have GERD (gastroesophageal reflux disease). Three days later, on the day of discharge, the patient is unable to speak. After undergoing MRI, the patient is found to have had a stroke.
   _____

4. A patient is admitted to the hospital with an asthma attack. On his last admission 3 years ago, the diagnosis was community-acquired pneumonia. Is the pneumonia coded, and why or why not?
   _____

5. List five reasons why a secondary diagnosis might be reported.
   1. _____
   2. _____
   3. _____
   4. _____
   5. _____

6. The physician documents seizure disorder in the patient's past medical history. The patient is receiving Tegretol, according to the list of medications. Should the seizure disorder be coded, and why or why not?
   _____

7. A patient has low urine output after undergoing surgery. The attending writes an order for the nursing staff to record urine output. Should the low urine output be coded, and why or why not?
   _____

8. If a patient is not on any drugs for Parkinson's, should this diagnosis be coded?
   _____

9. If a patient has nausea and vomiting that the attending determines to be gastroenteritis, what diagnosis should be coded?
   _____

CODING FROM DOCUMENTATION FOUND IN THE HEALTH RECORD

The usual advice given to a new coder is to begin to code a record by reading the discharge summary. This, in theory, is the summation of what took place during this patient's hospital admission. The discharge summary is similar to a synopsis of a book. By reading this document, the coder should be able to determine the principal diagnosis. However, the caveat is that the documenting physician may not be aware of the definition of a principal diagnosis and may list a diagnosis that does not meet the requirements of this definition.

Following a review of the discharge summary, the coder should move to the ER record (if applicable), which is the beginning of the patient's story. This will reveal the patient's chief complaint. The chief complaint is expressed in the words of the patient and gives the reason why he or she is presenting to the ER. The ER record generally provides to the coder the **admission diagnosis**. The admitting diagnosis may be a symptom, and after examination, a working diagnosis may become apparent. By the time the patient leaves the ER to go to the floor, the emergency room physician will have a working diagnosis or will be aware of a symptom that needs additional workup. If this diagnosis is not clear from the ER record, the admission orders should be reviewed for a diagnosis that is listed as the reason for admission.

If no ER record is available, or after the coder has read the ER record, he or she should move on to the admission history and physical (H&P). Generally, the progress notes are reviewed, followed by the OR reports, laboratory results, radiology reports, consults, and orders. Some documents such as the discharge summary, operative report, or pathology report may not be available at the time of coding. Hospitals may have a policy on whether an inpatient record should be coded without these reports or put on hold until the reports are completed. The following examples show documentation inconsistencies.

EXAMPLE
> The ER form has a listing of common medical conditions. The ER physician will circle any pertinent diagnoses. The physician has circled ESRD (end-stage renal disease) on the ER form. Throughout the body of the health record, no documentation of ESRD is found, nor does any documentation state that the patient is on dialysis or that the patient is awaiting a transplant. The only documentation in the chart is for chronic renal insufficiency (CRI).
> - Differences in coding: with 585.6 (N18.6) or with 585.9 (N18.9)

EXAMPLE
> Throughout a patient's inpatient chart, it is documented that the patient has a history of pneumonia. This is also documented in the past medical history.
> No chest x-ray was performed. Physical exam showed that the lungs were clear. On the discharge summary, pneumonia is documented instead of history of pneumonia.
> - Differences in coding: 486 (J18.9) versus V12.61 (Z87.01)

EXAMPLE
> Throughout a patient's chart, documentation of ESLD (end-stage liver disease) is found, along with the fact that the patient is awaiting a liver transplant. The patient has a history of cirrhosis and hepatitis C.
> One progress note reads:
> Cirrhosis/hep C/ESKD (end-stage kidney disease)
> No documentation in the chart describes any abnormal kidney function. It appears that the physician may have meant to write ESLD instead of ESKD.

It is acceptable to code from any documentation provided by a physician. Physicians (individuals qualified by education and legally authorized to practice medicine) may be referred to as attendings, consulting physicians, interns, and residents. Physicians may include surgeons, anesthesiologists, oncologists, internists, hospitalists, intensivists, family practitioners, and interventionalists. Medical students have not completed their education and are not included in the category of physician. Some medical staff bylaws may accept documentation by other healthcare providers such as nurse practitioners or physician assistants.

Some confusion has arisen as to what exactly may be coded from radiology and pathology reports. *Coding Clinic* (2002:2Q:p18)[8] attempted to clarify this advice. The coder cannot take information from these reports without obtaining confirmation from the attending. *Coding Clinic* stated that "if the attending physician documents breast mass and the pathologist documents carcinoma of the breast, this would be conflicting documentation and the attending must clarify." Additional details (e.g., area of fracture, location of mass) related to confirmed diagnoses may be taken from the x-ray report. The example from *Coding Clinic* (2004:1Q:p20-21)[9] says that if the physician has already documented a femur fracture, the coder may pick up additional details on the site of the fracture from this report.

THE USE OF QUERIES IN THE CODING PROCESS

In 2001, AHIMA published a Practice Brief entitled *Developing a Physician Query Process,*[10] which describes the goal of the query process as "to improve physician documentation and coding professionals' understanding of the unique clinical situation, not to improve reimbursement." A well-established and managed query process ensures data integrity. This Practice Brief was updated in October 2008 with a new Practice Brief entitled *Managing an Effective Query Process.*[11]

Each facility should prepare its own policies and procedures regarding the query process. Some of the best practices for query forms have been recommended by the American Health Quality Association (AHQA). In the October Practice Brief, AHIMA details many items that may be included in a facility policy.

When to Query

A healthcare provider should be queried when documentation is conflicting, incomplete, or ambiguous. The Practice Brief[11] lists six reasons a provider may need to be queried.
1. Clinical indicators of a diagnosis but no documentation of the condition

EXAMPLE In the provider's daily documentation, there is a lab value circled K2.8, and orders are given for potassium supplementation to be added to the IV fluids. It may be necessary in this case to query for a condition.

2. Clinical evidence for a higher degree of specificity or severity

EXAMPLE Physician documents obesity and lists the patient's weight as 345 and height as 5'2". It may be necessary to query for a patient's BMI or degree of obesity.

3. A cause and effect relationship between two conditions or organisms

EXAMPLE Patient has documented ulcer of the toe. There is also documentation of history of diabetes. The physician may be queried as to whether the toe ulcer and the diabetes are related.

4. An underlying cause when admitted with symptoms

EXAMPLE A patient is admitted with chest pain for workup of the underlying cause. The discharge summary lists atypical chest pain as the principal diagnosis. There is evidence in the chart that the patient has and is being treated for GERD. The provider may be queried as to the underlying cause of the chest pain.

5. Only the treatment is documented (without a diagnosis)

EXAMPLE The MAR shows administration of levothyroxine (Synthroid), but no documentation is provided by the provider of a diagnosis. It is noted that a medication is given, but no diagnosis is documented to correspond with the treatment.

6. Present on admission (POA) indicator status is unknown or unclear

EXAMPLE On the third hospital day, the provider documents that the patient's diabetes is uncontrolled. A query is initiated to determine whether the patient's diabetes was uncontrolled at the time of admission.

When Not to Initiate a Query

Do not query a provider's clinical judgment. It is not the coder's responsibility to question a provider's clinical judgment because the documentation in the record does not support the condition.

EXAMPLE Patient presents to the hospital with a cough and fever. The physician documents pneumonia on the discharge summary. The chest x-ray is negative.

Who to Query

The query should be directed to the provider who supplied the documentation in question. This may mean that the query is directed to a consultant, anesthesiologist, or surgeon, among others. Abnormal lab finding queries should be addressed to the attending physician. If there is conflicting documentation between a consultant and an attending physician, the attending physician should be queried for clarification.

Elements of a Query Form

A query should contain the following elements:
- Date of query
- Patient name
- Medical record number
- Account number
- Admission date/date of service
- Specific question needing clarification along with clinical indicators
- Identification of the coder asking the question
- Contact information for the coder initiating the query
- Area for response from provider
- Place for provider signature and date of response
- Instruction for documentation or any correction or addendum in the body of the record

Queries can be forms (Figure 2-13) placed in charts, faxes, and/or electronic communications transmitted via secure e-mail or IT messaging. Facility policy will control where queries are maintained. It is preferable that they become part of the official health record, whether paper or electronic.

It is not advised to use sticky notes, scratch paper, or any note that can be removed and discarded. It is acceptable to use a single query form for multiple queries.

PHYSICIAN QUERY FORM

Patient Name: _____

Patient Number: _____

Admission Date: _____ Discharge Date: _____

Query Date: _____

Dear Dr. _____ :

In order to assign the most appropriate codes that reflect the conditions of your patient, more clarification is required.

From a coding perspective "urosepsis" is a nonspecific term. It may mean that the patient has sepsis localized in the urinary tract, or it may signify that the urinary tract infection has now become generalized sepsis. Please document in the space below or write an addendum to the patient's record the diagnosis that best represents your use of the term "urosepsis."

Physician Response:

_____

_____

_____

_____

_____

_____   _____
Physician signature   Date

Thank you.

Coder Name: _____ Contact #: _____

FIGURE 2-13. Physician query form.

Unacceptable Types of Queries

It is unacceptable to lead a provider to document a particular response. The query should not be directing, prodding, probing, or presumptive. The provider should not be led to make an assumption.

AHIMA in the Practice Brief *Managing an Effective Query Process*[11] has given the following examples of leading queries.

Leading/Unacceptable

EXAMPLE

> Dr. Smith:
> Based on your documentation, this patient has anemia and was transfused 2 units of blood. Also, there was a 10 point dip in hematocrit following surgery. Please document "Acute Blood Loss Anemia," as this patient clearly meets the clinical criteria for this diagnosis.

Acceptable

EXAMPLE

> Dr. Smith:
> In your progress note on 6/20, you documented anemia and ordered transfusion of 2 units of blood. Also, according to the lab work done on xx/xx, the patient had a 10 point drop in hematocrit following surgery. Based on these indications, please document, in the discharge summary, the type of anemia you were treating.

Leading/Unacceptable

EXAMPLE

> Dr. Jones:
> This patient has COPD and is on oxygen every night at home and has been on continuous oxygen since admission. Please document "Chronic Respiratory Failure."

Acceptable

EXAMPLE

> Dr. Jones:
> This patient has COPD and is on oxygen every night at home and has been on continuous oxygen since admission. Based on these indications, please indicate if you were treating one of the following diagnoses:
> - Chronic Respiratory Failure
> - Acute Respiratory Failure
> - Acute on Chronic Respiratory Failure
> - Hypoxia
> - Unable to determine
> - Other _____

In both of the unacceptable examples, the coder was asking for a provider to document a particular diagnosis. No other documentation options were provided other than the one listed. These queries were already assuming a diagnosis, rather than giving the clinical facts and allowing the provider to make a clinical determination. The nonleading way to ask is with open-ended queries or multiple-choice answers with clinically reasonable choices, as well as an "other" option that allows the provider to input something entirely different from the multiple-choice answers given.

It is inappropriate to introduce new information not previously documented in this record. For example, if on a previous admission the provider documents that the patient is HIV positive, but during this stay that diagnosis is not documented, it would be inappropriate to query for "new information" that is not documented during the encounter.

Query forms should steer away from "yes" and "no" answer questions. For POA purposes, when a diagnosis has already been documented, a "yes" or "no" query is unacceptable. Impact on reimbursement should never be indicated on a query form.

Qualifications for Individuals Submitting Queries

In the Practice Brief *Managing an Effective Query Process*,[11] AHIMA suggests that individuals performing queries should be very familiar with the AHIMA Standards of Ethical Coding, as well as have competencies in the following areas:

- Knowledge of healthcare regulations, including reimbursement and documentation requirements
- Clinical knowledge with training in pathophysiology
- Ability to read and analyze all information in a patient's health record
- Established channels of communication with providers and other clinicians
- Demonstrated skills in clinical terminology, coding, and classification systems
- Ability to apply coding conventions, official guidelines, and *Coding Clinic* advice to health record documentation

CHAPTER REVIEW EXERCISE

Write the correct answer(s) in the space(s) provided or choose the correct answer option.

1. When coding a record, where is the best place to begin?

   _____

2. If the discharge summary includes a list of diagnoses, should the coder choose the first in the list as the principal diagnosis?
   A. Yes
   B. No

3. What does TJC stand for?

   _____

4. What does UHDDS stand for?

   _____

5. Which report in the record must be on the record within 24 hours?

   _____

6. What does the term "integral" mean?

   _____

7. Where in the record would a coder find the admitting diagnosis?

   _____

8. Name one reason why a coder would query a physician.

   _____

9. The best place in the record to find the patient's history is in the _____

   _____

10. The beginning of the patient's story is usually the discharge summary.
    A. True
    B. False

11. It is permissible for a coder to use documentation provided by an interventionalist.
    A. True
    B. False

12. Once a physician answers a coding question, it should be thrown in the trash.
    A. True
    B. False

13. Physician queries should have only enough room for a physician to sign and date.
    A. True
    B. False

14. When a coding question is asked, it is very important that the financial impact of the response is included.
    A. True
    B. False

15. It is important that the date and the identity of the physician be included for every note.
    A. True
    B. False

16. Is it important for the record to include documentation that supports a code used in billing?
    A. Yes
    B. No

17. Documentation from a consultant cannot be used to assign codes.
    A. True
    B. False

18. A principal diagnosis is one of the elements that determine an MS-DRG.
    A. True
    B. False

19. An example of a diagnostic procedure is an MRI.
    A. True
    B. False

20. Surgery is a form of therapeutic treatment.
    A. True
    B. False

CHAPTER GLOSSARY

Abstracting: extracting data from the health record.

Admission diagnosis: diagnosis that brings the patient to the hospital. This will often be a symptom.

Chief complaint: the reason, in the patient's own words, for presenting to the hospital.

Comorbidities: preexisting diagnoses or conditions that are present on admission.

Consultant: healthcare provider who is asked to see the patient to provide expert opinion outside the expertise of the requester.

Healthcare provider: person who provides care to a patient.

Hybrid: a combination of formats producing similar results (i.e., paper and electronic records).

Integral: essential part of a disease process.

Physician: licensed medical doctor.

Principal diagnosis: the condition established after study to be chiefly responsible for occasioning the admission of the patient to the hospital for care.

Principal procedure: procedure performed for definitive treatment, rather than for diagnostic or exploratory purposes, or one that was necessary to take care of a complication.

Progress notes: daily recordings by healthcare providers of patient progress.

Review of systems: question-and-answer period that occurs between a patient and a healthcare provider during which any healthcare issues are reviewed.

REFERENCES

1. Huffman E. Health Information Management, 10th ed. Berwyn, IL, Physicians' Record Company, 1994, p 30.
2. Abdelhak M, Grostick S, Hanken MA, Jacobs E (eds). Health Information: Management of a Strategic Resource, 2nd ed. St. Louis, WB Saunders, 2001.
3. Medicare 1995 Documentation Guidelines. General Principles of Medical Record Documentation. Centers for Medicare and Medicaid Services, U.S. Department of Health and Human Services, 1995.
4. American Hospital Association. *Coding Clinic for ICD-9-CM* 2000:2Q:p20-21. Clarification, Reporting of chronic conditions.
5. American Hospital Association. *Coding Clinic for ICD-9-CM* 1992:2Q:p16-17. History of COPD.
6. American Hospital Association. *Coding Clinic for ICD-9-CM* 1990:2Q:p15. Conditions of an integral disease process—guideline.
7. American Hospital Association. *Coding Clinic for ICD-9-CM* 2002:2Q:p17-18. Abnormal findings on radiology reports, inpatient.
8. American Hospital Association. *Coding Clinic for ICD-9-CM* 2002:2Q:p18. Facility-specific coding guidelines.
9. American Hospital Association. *Coding Clinic for ICD-9-CM* 2004:1Q:p20-21. Clarification, Abnormal pathology report.
10. Prophet S. Developing a physician query process (AHIMA practice brief). *J AHIMA* 72:88I-88M, 2001.
11. AHIMA. Managing an effective query process. *J AHIMA* 79:83-88, 2008.

3

ICD-9-CM Format and Conventions

CHAPTER OUTLINE

ICD-9-CM Official Guidelines for Coding and Reporting
ICD-10-CM Official Guidelines for Coding and Reporting
Format of ICD-9-CM and ICD-10-CM Code Books
  Format of Tabular List of Diseases and Injuries
  Format of Alphabetic Index to Diseases and Injuries
Coding Conventions
  Abbreviations
  Punctuation
  Instructional Notes
Appendices
  A. Morphology of Neoplasms
  C. Classification of Drugs by American Hospital Formulary: Service List Number
     and Their ICD-9-CM Equivalents
  D. Classification of Industrial Accidents According to Agency
  E. List of Three-Digit Categories
Chapter Review Exercise
Chapter Glossary

LEARNING OBJECTIVES

1. Identify the format of the ICD-9-CM and ICD-10-CM code book
2. Explain and apply the conventions and guidelines
3. Identify the appendices

ABBREVIATIONS/ ACRONYMS

AHFS *American Hospital Formulary Service*

CPT *Current Procedural Terminology*

DSM-IV *Diagnostic and Statistical Manual of Mental Disorders, Fourth Edition*

ICD-9-CM *International Classification of Diseases, 9th Revision, Clinical Modification*

ICD-10-CM *International Classification of Diseases, 10th Revision, Clinical Modification*

ICD-10-PCS *International Classification of Diseases, 10th Revision, Procedure Coding System*

ICD-O *International Classification of Diseases for Oncology*

MS-DRG Medicare Severity diagnosis-related groups

NEC not elsewhere classifiable

NOS not otherwise specified

WHO World Health Organization

ICD-9-CM

Official
Guidelines for
Coding and
Reporting

Please refer to the companion Evolve website for the most current guidelines.

Section I. Conventions, general coding guidelines, and chapter-specific guidelines

The conventions, general guidelines, and chapter-specific guidelines are applicable to all healthcare settings unless otherwise indicated.

A. Conventions for the ICD-9-CM

The conventions for the ICD-9-CM are the general rules for use of the classification independent of the guidelines. These conventions are incorporated within the index and tabular of the ICD-9-CM as instructional notes. These conventions are as follows:

1. Format

The ICD-9-CM uses an indented format for ease in reference

2. Abbreviations

a. Index abbreviations

NEC   "Not elsewhere classifiable"

This abbreviation in the index represents "other specified"; when a specific code is not available for a condition, the index directs the coder to the "other specified" code in the tabular.

b. Tabular abbreviations

NEC   "Not elsewhere classifiable"

This abbreviation in the tabular represents "other specified". When a specific code is not available for a condition, the tabular includes an NEC entry under a code to identify the code as the "other specified" code.

(See Section I.A.5.a. "Other" codes).

NOS   "Not otherwise specified"

This abbreviation is the equivalent of unspecified.

(See Section I.A.5.b., "Unspecified" codes)

3. Punctuation

[ ] Brackets are used in the tabular list to enclose synonyms, alternative wording or explanatory phrases. Brackets are used in the index to identify manifestation codes. *(See Section I.A.6. "Etiology/manifestations")*

( ) Parentheses are used in both the index and the tabular to enclose supplementary words that may be present or absent in the statement of a disease or procedure without affecting the code number to which it is assigned. The terms within the parentheses are referred to as nonessential modifiers.

: Colons are used in the Tabular list after an incomplete term which needs one or more of the modifiers following the colon to make it assignable to a given category.

4. Includes and Excludes Notes and Inclusion terms

Includes: This note appears immediately under a three-digit code title to further define, or give an example of, the content of the category.

Excludes: An excludes note under a code indicates that the terms excluded from the code are to be coded elsewhere. In some cases the codes for the excluded terms should not be used in conjunction with the code from which it is excluded. An example of this is a congenital condition excluded from an acquired form of the same condition. The congenital and acquired codes should not be used together. In other cases, the excluded terms may be used together with an excluded code. An example of this is when fractures of different bones are coded to different codes. Both codes may be used together if both types of fractures are present.

Inclusion terms: List of terms is included under certain four and five digit codes. These terms are the conditions for which that code number is to be used. The terms may be synonyms of the code title, or, in the case of "other specified" codes, the terms are a list of the various conditions assigned to that code. The inclusion terms are not necessarily exhaustive. Additional terms found only in the index may also be assigned a code.

5. Other and Unspecified codes

a. "Other" codes

Codes titled "other" or "other specified" (usually a code with a 4th digit 8 or a fifth-digit 9 for diagnosis codes) are for use when the information in the medical record provides detail for which a specific code does not exist. Index entries with NEC in the line designate "other" codes in the tabular. These index entries represent specific disease entities for which no specific code exists so the term is included within an "other" code.

b. **"Unspecified" codes**

Codes (usually a code with a 4th digit 9 or a 5th digit 0 for diagnosis codes) titled "unspecified" are used when the information in the medical record is insufficient to assign a more specific code.

6. **Etiology/manifestation convention ("code first," "use additional code," and "in diseases classified elsewhere" notes)**

Certain conditions have both an underlying etiology and multiple body system manifestations due to the underlying etiology. For such conditions, the ICD-9-CM has a coding convention that requires the underlying condition be sequenced first followed by the manifestation. Wherever such a combination exists, there is a "use additional code" note at the etiology code, and a "code first" note at the manifestation code. These instructional notes indicate the proper sequencing order of the codes, etiology followed by manifestation.

In most cases the manifestation codes will have in the code title, "in diseases classified elsewhere." Codes with this title are a component of the etiology/manifestation convention. The code title indicates that it is a manifestation code. "In diseases classified elsewhere" codes are never permitted to be used as first listed or principal diagnosis codes. They must be used in conjunction with an underlying condition code and they must be listed following the underlying condition.

There are manifestation codes that do not have "in diseases classified elsewhere" in the title. For such codes, a "use additional code" note will still be present and the rules for sequencing apply.

In addition to the notes in the Tabular, these conditions also have a specific Index entry structure. In the Index both conditions are listed together with the etiology code first followed by the manifestation codes in brackets. The code in brackets is always to be sequenced second.

The most commonly used etiology/manifestation combinations are the codes for Diabetes mellitus, category 250. For each code under category 250 there is a use additional code note for the manifestation that is specific for that particular diabetic manifestation. Should a patient have more than one manifestation of diabetes, more than one code from category 250 may be used with as many manifestation codes as are needed to fully describe the patient's complete diabetic condition. The category 250 diabetes codes should be sequenced first, followed by the manifestation codes.

"Code first" and "Use additional code" notes are also used as sequencing rules in the classification for certain codes that are not part of an etiology/manifestation combination.

See—Section I.B.9. "Multiple coding for single condition".

7. **"And"**

The word "and" should be interpreted to mean either "and" or "or" when it appears in a title.

8. **"With"**

The word "with" should be interpreted to mean "associated with" or "due to" when it appears in a code title, the Alphabetic Index, or note in an instructional the Tabular List. The word "with" in the alphabetic index is sequenced immediately following the main term, not in alphabetical order.

9. **"See" and "See Also"**

The "see" instruction following a main term in the Index indicates that another term should be referenced. It is necessary to go to the main term referenced with the "see" note to locate the correct code.

A "see also" instruction following a main term in the index instructs that there is another main term that may also be referenced that may provide additional index entries that may be useful. It is not necessary to follow the "see also" note when the original main term provides the necessary code.

ICD-10-CM

Official
Guidelines for
Coding and
Reporting

Please refer to the companion Evolve website for the most current guidelines.
2011
Narrative changes appear in bold text
Items <u>underlined</u> have been moved within the guidelines since the 2010 version
Italics **are used to indicate revisions to heading changes**

The Centers for Medicare and Medicaid Services (CMS) and the National Center for Health Statistics (NCHS), two departments within the U.S. Federal Government's Department of Health and Human Services (DHHS) provide the following guidelines for coding and reporting using the International Classification of Diseases, 10th Revision, Clinical Modification (ICD-10-CM). These guidelines should be used as a companion document to the official version of the ICD-10-CM as published on the NCHS website. The ICD-10-CM is a morbidity classification published by the United States for classifying diagnoses and reason for visits in all health care settings. The ICD-10-CM is based on the ICD-10, the statistical classification of disease published by the World Health Organization (WHO).

These guidelines have been approved by the four organizations that make up the Cooperating Parties for the ICD-10-CM: the American Hospital Association (AHA), the American Health Information Management Association (AHIMA), CMS, and NCHS.

These guidelines are a set of rules that have been developed to accompany and complement the official conventions and instructions provided within the ICD-10-CM itself. The instructions and conventions of the classification take precedence over guidelines. These guidelines are based on the coding and sequencing instructions in **the Tabular List and Alphabetic Index** of ICD-10-CM, but provide additional instruction. Adherence to these guidelines when assigning ICD-10-CM diagnosis codes is required under the Health Insurance Portability and Accountability Act (HIPAA). The diagnosis codes **(Tabular List and Alphabetic Index)** have been adopted under HIPAA for all healthcare settings. A joint effort between the health care provider and the coder is essential to achieve complete and accurate documentation, code assignment, and reporting of diagnoses and procedures. These guidelines have been developed to assist both the healthcare provider and the coder in identifying those diagnoses and procedures that are to be reported. The importance of consistent, complete documentation in the medical record cannot be overemphasized. Without such documentation accurate coding cannot be achieved. The entire record should be reviewed to determine the specific reason for the encounter and the conditions treated.

The term encounter is used for all settings, including hospital admissions. In the context of these guidelines, the term provider is used throughout the guidelines to mean physician or any qualified health care practitioner who is legally accountable for establishing the patient's diagnosis. Only this set of guidelines, approved by the Cooperating Parties, is official.

The guidelines are organized into sections. Section I includes the structure and conventions of the classification and general guidelines that apply to the entire classification, and chapter-specific guidelines that correspond to the chapters as they are arranged in the classification. Section II includes guidelines for selection of principal diagnosis for non-outpatient settings. Section III includes guidelines for reporting additional diagnoses in non-outpatient settings. Section IV is for outpatient coding and reporting. It is necessary to review all sections of the guidelines to fully understand all of the rules and instructions needed to code properly.

Section I. Conventions, general coding guidelines and chapter-specific guidelines
The conventions, general guidelines and chapter-specific guidelines are applicable to all health care settings unless otherwise indicated. The conventions and instructions of the classification take precedence over guidelines.
A. Conventions for the ICD-10-CM
The conventions for the ICD-10-CM are the general rules for use of the classification independent of the guidelines. These conventions are incorporated within the **Alphabetic Index** and **Tabular List** of the ICD-10-CM as instructional notes.
1. The Alphabetic Index and Tabular List
The ICD-10-CM is divided into the **Alphabetic Index**, an alphabetical list of terms and their corresponding code, and the Tabular List, a chronological list of codes divided into chapters based on body system or condition (Figures 3-1 and 3-2). **The Alphabetic Index consists of the following parts: the Index of Diseases and Injury, the Table of Neoplasms and the Table of Drugs and Chemicals.**

See Section I.C2. General guidelines
See Section I.C.19. Adverse effects, poisoning, underdosing and toxic effects

2. Format and Structure:

The ICD-10-CM Tabular List contains categories, subcategories and codes. Characters for categories, subcategories and codes may be either a letter or a number. All categories are 3 characters. A three-character category that has no further subdivision is equivalent to a code. Subcategories are either 4 or 5 characters. Codes may be **3,** 4, 5, 6 or 7 characters. That is, each level of subdivision after a category is a subcategory. The final level of subdivision is a code. Codes that have applicable 7th characters are still referred to as codes, not subcategories. A code that has an applicable 7th character is considered invalid without the 7th character.

The ICD-10-CM uses an indented format for ease in reference

3. Use of codes for reporting purposes

For reporting purposes only codes are permissible, not categories or subcategories, and any applicable 7th character is required.

In the Alphabetic Index of ICD-10-CM a dash (-) is used to indicate that there are further digits that need to be assigned for a valid code. In Figures 3-1 and 3-2, note that C50.91 would be an invalid code. A sixth digit is necessary to identify left, right, or unspecified breast. All codes must be assigned to the final level of subdivision. A valid code is at least three characters, but could be four, five, six, or seven characters.

4. Placeholder character

The ICD-10-CM utilizes a placeholder character "X". The "X" is used as a placeholder at certain codes to allow for future expansion. An example of this is at the poisoning, adverse effect and underdosing codes, categories T36-T50. Where a placeholder exists, the X must be used in order for the code to be considered a valid code (Figure 3-3).

Disease, diseased *(Continued)*
  breast (*see also* Disorder, breast) N64.9
    cystic (chronic) – *see* Mastopathy,
        cystic
    fibrocystic – *see* Mastopathy, cystic
    Paget's (M8540/3)
      female, unspecified side C50.91-
      male, unspecified side C50.92-
      specified NEC N64.8
  Breda's – *see* Yaws
  Bretonneau's (diphtheritic malignant
      angina) A36.0

FIGURE 3-1. Alphabetic Index entry for Paget's disease, female breast.

● C50.9 **Malignant neoplasm of breast of unspecified site**

  ● C50.91 **Malignant neoplasm of breast of unspecified site, female**

      ❑ C50.911 **Malignant neoplasm of unspecified site of right female breast**

      ❑ C50.912 **Malignant neoplasm of unspecified site of left female breast**

      ❑ C50.919 **Malignant neoplasm of unspecified site of unspecified female breast**

FIGURE 3-2. Tabular List entry for Paget's disease, female breast.

5. **7th Characters**

Certain ICD-10-CM categories have applicable 7th characters. The applicable 7th character is required for all codes within the category, or as the notes in the Tabular List instruct. The 7th character must always be the 7th character in the data field. If a code that requires a 7th character is not 6 characters, a placeholder X must be used to fill in the empty characters (see Figure 3-3).

6. **Abbreviations**

    a. *Alphabetic* **Index abbreviations**

        NEC   "Not elsewhere classifiable"

            This abbreviation in the **Alphabetic Index** represents "other specified". When a specific code is not available for a condition, the **Alphabetic Index** directs the coder to the "other specified" code in the **Tabular List**.

        NOS   **"Not otherwise specified"**

            This abbreviation is the equivalent of unspecified.

    b. **Tabular** *List* **abbreviations**

        NEC   "Not elsewhere classifiable"

            This abbreviation in the **Tabular List** represents "other specified". When a specific code is not available for a condition the **Tabular List** includes an NEC entry under a code to identify the code as the "other specified" code.

        NOS   "Not otherwise specified"

            This abbreviation is the equivalent of unspecified.

7. **Punctuation**

    [ ]   Brackets are used in the **Tabular List** to enclose synonyms, alternative wording or explanatory phrases. Brackets are used in the **Alphabetic Index** to identify manifestation codes.

    ( )   Parentheses are used in both the **Alphabetic Index** and **Tabular List** to enclose supplementary words that may be present or absent in the statement of a disease or procedure without affecting the code number to which it is assigned. The terms within the parentheses are referred to as nonessential modifiers.

    :   Colons are used in the Tabular List after an incomplete term which needs one or more of the modifiers following the colon to make it assignable to a given category.

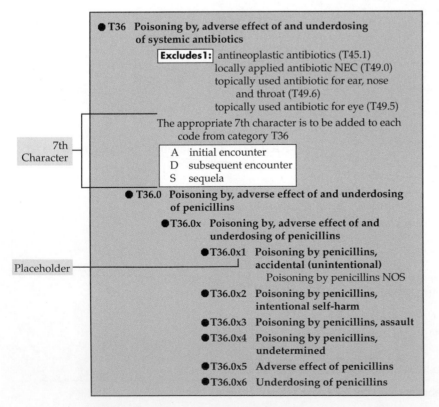

FIGURE 3-3. Placeholder in ICD-10-CM.

8. **Use of "and"**

   When the term "and" is used in a narrative statement it represents and/or.

9. **Other and Unspecified codes**

   a. **"Other" codes**

   Codes titled "other" or "other specified" are for use when the information in the medical record provides detail for which a specific code does not exist. **Alphabetic Index** entries with NEC in the line designate "other" codes in the **Tabular List**. These **Alphabetic Index** entries represent specific disease entities for which no specific code exists so the term is included within an "other" code.

   b. **"Unspecified" codes**

   Codes titled "unspecified" are for use when the information in the medical record is insufficient to assign a more specific code. For those categories for which an unspecified code is not provided, the "other specified" code may represent both other and unspecified.

10. **Includes Notes**

    This note appears immediately under a three **character** code title to further define, or give examples of, the content of the category.

11. **Inclusion terms**

    List of terms is included under some codes. These terms are the conditions for which that code is to be used. The terms may be synonyms of the code title, or, in the case of "other specified" codes, the terms are a list of the various conditions assigned to that code. The inclusion terms are not necessarily exhaustive. Additional terms found only in the **Alphabetic Index** may also be assigned to a code.

12. **Excludes Notes**

    The ICD-10-CM has two types of excludes notes. Each type of note has a different definition for use but they are all similar in that they indicate that codes excluded from each other are independent of each other.

    a. **Excludes1**

    A type 1 Excludes note is a pure excludes note. It means "NOT CODED HERE!" An Excludes1 note indicates that the code excluded should never be used at the same time as the code above the Excludes1 note. An Excludes1 is used when two conditions cannot occur together, such as a congenital form versus an acquired form of the same condition (Figures 3-4 and 3-5).

    b. **Excludes2**

    A type 2 excludes note represents "Not included here". An excludes2 note indicates that the condition excluded is not part of the condition represented by the code, but a patient may have both conditions at the same time. When an Excludes2 note appears under a code, it is acceptable to use both the code and the excluded code together, when appropriate (see Figure 3-5).

●N28 **Other disorders of kidney and ureter, not elsewhere classified**

   N28.0 **Ischemia and infarction of kidney**
       Renal artery embolism
       Renal artery obstruction
       Renal artery occlusion
       Renal artery thrombosis
       Renal infarct

       Excludes1: atherosclerosis of renal artery
                 (extrarenal part) (I70.1)
               congenital stenosis of renal
                 artery (Q27.1)
               Goldblatt's kidney (I70.1)

   N28.1 **Cyst of kidney, acquired**
       Cyst (multiple)(solitary) of kidney, acquired
       Excludes1: cystic kidney disease (congenital)
                 (Q61.-)

FIGURE 3-4. Example of Excludes1 note.

FIGURE 3-5. Example of Excludes1 and Excludes2 notes.

13. **Etiology/manifestation convention ("code first", "use additional code" and "in diseases classified elsewhere" notes)**

    Certain conditions have both an underlying etiology and multiple body system manifestations due to the underlying etiology. For such conditions, the ICD-10-CM has a coding convention that requires the underlying condition be sequenced first followed by the manifestation. Wherever such a combination exists, there is a "use additional code" note at the etiology code, and a "code first" note at the manifestation code. These instructional notes indicate the proper sequencing order of the codes, etiology followed by manifestation.

    In most cases the manifestation codes will have in the code title, "in diseases classified elsewhere." Codes with this title are a component of the etiology/ manifestation convention. The code title indicates that it is a manifestation code. "In diseases classified elsewhere" codes are never permitted to be used as **first-listed** or principal diagnosis codes. They must be used in conjunction with an underlying condition code and they must be listed following the underlying condition. See category F02, Dementia in other diseases classified elsewhere, for an example of this convention.

    There are manifestation codes that do not have "in diseases classified elsewhere" in the title. For such codes a "use additional code" note will still be present and the rules for sequencing apply.

    In addition to the notes in the **Tabular List**, these conditions also have a specific **Alphabetic Index** entry structure. In the **Alphabetic Index** both conditions are listed together with the etiology code first followed by the manifestation codes in brackets. The code in brackets is always to be sequenced second.

    An example of the etiology/manifestation convention is dementia in Parkinson's disease. In the **Alphabetic Index**, code G20 is listed first, followed by code F02.80 or F02.81 in brackets. Code G20 represents the underlying etiology, Parkinson's disease, and must be sequenced first, whereas codes F02.80 and F02.81 represent the manifestation of dementia in diseases classified elsewhere, with or without behavioral disturbance.

    "Code first" and "Use additional code" notes are also used as sequencing rules in the classification for certain codes that are not part of an etiology/manifestation combination.

    See Section I.B.7. Multiple coding for a single condition.

14. **"And"**

    The word "and" should be interpreted to mean either "and" or "or" when it appears in a title.

15. **"With"**

    The word "with" should be interpreted to mean "associated with" or "due to" when it appears in a code title, the Alphabetic Index, or an instructional note in the Tabular List.

    The word "with" in the Alphabetic Index is sequenced immediately following the main term, not in alphabetical order.

16. **"See" and "See Also"**

    The "see" instruction following a main term in the **Alphabetic Index** indicates that another term should be referenced. It is necessary to go to the main term referenced with the "see" note to locate the correct code.

```
Failure, failed (Continued)
   respiration, respiratory J96.9 ◄────────
      acute J96.0
         with chronic J96.2
      center G93.8
      chronic J96.1
         with acute J96.2
      newborn P28.5
      postprocedural J95.82
```

FIGURE 3-6. Alphabetic Index default code for respiratory failure.

A "see also" instruction following a main term in the **Alphabetic Index** instructs that there is another main term that may also be referenced that may provide additional **Alphabetic Index** entries that may be useful. It is not necessary to follow the "see also" note when the original main term provides the necessary code.

17. **"Code also note"**

A "code also" note instructs that two codes may be required to fully describe a condition, but this note does not provide sequencing direction.

18. **Default codes**

A code listed next to a main term in the ICD-10-CM **Alphabetic Index** is referred to as a default code. The default code represents that condition that is most commonly associated with the main term, or is the unspecified code for the condition. If a condition is documented in a medical record (for example, appendicitis) without any additional information, such as acute or chronic, the default code should be assigned (Figure 3-6).

19. **Syndromes**

Follow the Alphabetic Index guidance when coding syndromes. In the absence of **Alphabetic Index** guidance, assign codes for the documented manifestations of the syndrome.

FORMAT OF ICD-9-CM AND ICD-10-CM CODE BOOKS

The ICD-9-CM code book contains three volumes:

- Volume 1 Tabular List of Diseases and Injuries
- Volume 2 Alphabetic Index of Diseases and Injuries
- Volume 3 Tabular List and Alphabetic Index of Procedures

Volume 2 (Alphabetic Index) is usually found at the front of the code book and is followed by Volume 1 (Tabular List) and then Volume 3 (Index and Tabular for Procedures).

Several publishers have a variety of ICD-9-CM code books available. Code books are available for use in physician offices that include only Volumes 1 and 2 because ICD-9-CM procedure codes (Volume 3) are not used by physicians. (Physicians use CPT codes to bill for services and procedures.) Expert versions may contain reimbursement edits, color-coded information, Medicare code edits, and age and sex edits. Some books are updated with replacement pages quarterly and may include references to *Coding Clinic* articles. At the beginning of a code book, information is usually provided that explains the conventions used in that version.

The **ICD-10-CM** codebook is also divided into two parts: an Alphabetic Index and a Tabular List. The Alphabetic Index lists terms and corresponding codes in alphabetic order. The main index is the Index to Diseases and Injuries, and there is an additional index to External Causes of Injury. There are two tables located in the main index: the Neoplasm table and the Table of Drugs and Chemicals. The Tabular List is an alphanumeric listing of codes that are divided into chapters based on body system or conditions.

There is an additional book for procedures, which is entitled **ICD-10-PCS**.

TABLE 3-1 ICD-9-CM TABLE OF CONTENTS FOR TABULAR LIST

Diseases: Tabular List, Volume 1
1. Infectious and Parasitic Diseases (001-139)
2. Neoplasms (140-239)
3. Endocrine, Nutritional and Metabolic Diseases, and Immunity Disorders (240-279)
4. Diseases of the Blood and Blood-Forming Organs (280-289)
5. Mental Disorders (290-319)
6. Diseases of the Nervous System and Sense Organs (320-389)
7. Diseases of the Circulatory System (390-459)
8. Diseases of the Respiratory System (460-519)
9. Diseases of the Digestive System (520-579)
10. Diseases of the Genitourinary System (580-629)
11. Complications of Pregnancy, Childbirth, and the Puerperium (630-679)
12. Diseases of the Skin and Subcutaneous Tissue (680-709)
13. Diseases of the Musculoskeletal System and Connective Tissue (710-739)
14. Congenital Anomalies (740-759)
15. Certain Conditions Originating in the Perinatal Period (760-779)
16. Symptoms, Signs, and Ill-Defined Conditions (780-799)
17. Injury and Poisoning (800-999)

V Codes—Supplementary Classification of Factors Influencing Health Status and Contact With Health Services (V01-V89)

E Codes—Supplementary Classification of External Causes of Injury and Poisoning (E800-E999)

TABLE 3-2 ICD-10-CM TABLE OF CONTENTS FOR TABULAR LIST

ICD-10-CM Tabular List of Diseases and Injuries
1. Certain Infectious and Parasitic Diseases (A00-B99)
2. Neoplasms (C00-D49)
3. Diseases of the Blood and Blood-Forming Organs and Certain Disorders Involving the Immune Mechanism (D50-D89)
4. Endocrine, Nutritional, and Metabolic Diseases (E00-E90)
5. Mental and Behavioral Disorders (F01-F99)
6. Diseases of the Nervous System (G00-G99)
7. Diseases of the Eye and Adnexa (H00-H59)
8. Diseases of the Ear and Mastoid Process (H60-H95)
9. Diseases of the Circulatory System (I00-I99)
10. Diseases of the Respiratory System (J00-J99)
11. Diseases of the Digestive System (K00-K94)
12. Diseases of the Skin and Subcutaneous Tissue (L00-L99)
13. Diseases of the Musculoskeletal System and Connective Tissue (M00-M99)
14. Diseases of the Genitourinary System (N00-N99)
15. Pregnancy, Childbirth, and the Puerperium (O00-O99)
16. Certain Conditions Originating in the Perinatal Period (P00-P96)
17. Congenital Malformations, Deformations, and Chromosomal Abnormalities (Q00-Q99)
18. Symptoms, Signs, and Abnormal Clinical and Laboratory Findings (R00-R99)
19. Injury, Poisoning, and Certain Other Consequences of External Causes (S00-T88)
20. External Causes of Morbidity (V01-Y99)
21. Factors Influencing Health Status and Contact with Health Services (Z00-Z99)

Format of Tabular List of Diseases and Injuries

In ICD-9-CM, Volume 1, the Tabular List of Diseases and Injuries (Table 3-1) consists of 17 chapters. Most of these chapters are classified by body system or **etiology** (cause of disease).

Within each chapter, the codes are divided as follows:
- Sections
- Categories
- Subcategories
- Subclassifications

In ICD-10-CM, the Tabular List of Diseases and Injuries consists of 21 chapters (Table 3-2). Most of the chapters are based on body systems; however, some are based on conditions. Within each chapter, codes are divided as follows:

- Blocks/Sections
- Categories
- Subcategories
- Valid codes

Sections and Blocks

In ICD-9-CM, a **section** consists of a group of three-digit categories that represent diseases or conditions that are similar (Figure 3-7).

Each chapter in ICD-10-CM is divided into section/blocks. A section/block is a group of three-digit categories that represent diseases or conditions that are similar (Table 3-3). A "block" is also known as a "subchapter."

Categories

Categories are represented in ICD-9-CM by single three-digit codes that describe a disease or a similarly related group of conditions (see Figure 3-7). A category may be an assignable code; however, if it is subcategorized, then the three-digit code is not assignable.

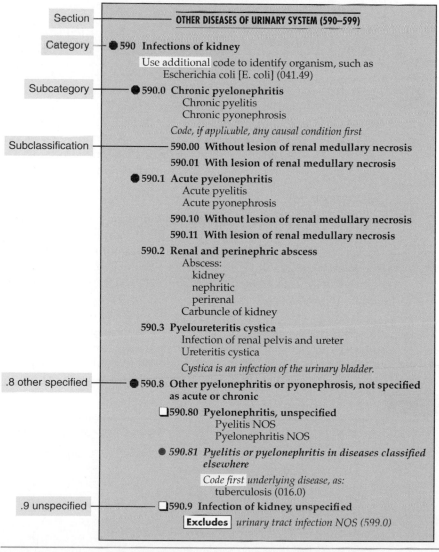

FIGURE 3-7. Divisions within the Tabular List.

TABLE 3-3 SECTIONS/BLOCKS FOR THE NERVOUS SYSTEM CHAPTER OF ICD-10-CM

G00-G09	Inflammatory diseases of the central nervous system
G10-G13	Systemic atrophies primarily affecting the central nervous system
G20-G26	Extrapyramidal and movement disorders
G30-G32	Other degenerative diseases of the nervous system
G35-G37	Demyelinating diseases of the central nervous system
G40-G47	Episodic and paroxysmal disorders
G50-G59	Nerve, nerve root, and plexus disorders
G60-G64	Polyneuropathies and other disorders of the peripheral nervous system
G70-G73	Diseases of myoneural junction and muscle
G80-G83	Cerebral palsy and other paralytic syndromes
G89-G99	Other disorders of the nervous system

● E70.33 Albinism with hematologic abnormality
    E70.330 Chediak-Higashi syndrome
    E70.331 Hermansky-Pudlak syndrome
    E70.338 Other albinism with hematologic abnormality
    ● E70.339 Albinism with hematologic abnormality, unspecified
E70.39 Other specified albinism
    Piebaldism

FIGURE 3-8. Example of sixth-character subclassification in ICD-10-CM.

In ICD-10-CM, the first character of a three-digit category is a letter, and each letter is associated with a particular chapter except for D and H. The letter D can be found in ICD-10-CM Chapters 2 and 3, the letter H can be found in both ICD-10-CM Chapters 7 and 8, and ICD-10-CM Chapter 19 uses two letters, S and T. The second and third characters are numbers. Most three-character categories are divided into four- or five-character subcategories. If a three-character category is not subdivided, it is a valid three-digit code.

Subcategories

Subcategories in ICD-9-CM consist of four-digit codes that provide additional information or specificity. The specificity may provide insight to the etiology of the disease, as well as to the location of the disease or to the manifestation. A **manifestation** is a symptom or condition that is the result of a disease. A fourth digit of .8 usually is used for other specified conditions for that category (see Figure 3-7). A fourth digit of .9 is usually used for unspecified conditions of that category (see Figure 3-7).

In ICD-10-CM, subcategories can be either four or five characters or further subdivided into five or six characters (Figure 3-8). Subcategory characters can be either letters or numbers. Codes may be up to seven characters long. The last level of subdivision becomes the final code. The final character may be a number or a letter.

EXERCISE 3-1

Identify the following as a chapter, section, category, or subcategory.

1. Diseases of Veins and Lymphatics, and Other Disease of Circulatory System (451-459) _____

2. Diseases of the Circulatory System (390-459) _____

3. 452 Portal vein thrombosis _____

4. 453 Other venous embolism and thrombosis _____

5. 453.0 Budd-Chiari syndrome _____

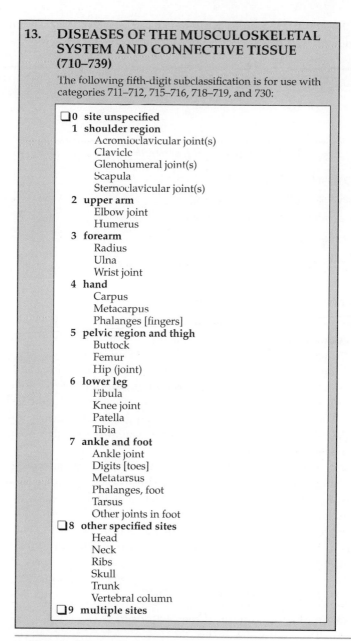

13. DISEASES OF THE MUSCULOSKELETAL SYSTEM AND CONNECTIVE TISSUE (710–739)

The following fifth-digit subclassification is for use with categories 711–712, 715–716, 718–719, and 730:

❏0 **site unspecified**
  1 **shoulder region**
      Acromioclavicular joint(s)
      Clavicle
      Glenohumeral joint(s)
      Scapula
      Sternoclavicular joint(s)
  2 **upper arm**
      Elbow joint
      Humerus
  3 **forearm**
      Radius
      Ulna
      Wrist joint
  4 **hand**
      Carpus
      Metacarpus
      Phalanges [fingers]
  5 **pelvic region and thigh**
      Buttock
      Femur
      Hip (joint)
  6 **lower leg**
      Fibula
      Knee joint
      Patella
      Tibia
  7 **ankle and foot**
      Ankle joint
      Digits [toes]
      Metatarsus
      Phalanges, foot
      Tarsus
      Other joints in foot
❏8 **other specified sites**
      Head
      Neck
      Ribs
      Skull
      Trunk
      Vertebral column
❏9 **multiple sites**

FIGURE 3-9. Fifth-digit subclassifications.

Subclassification

Fifth-digit **subclassifications** provide even greater specificity in ICD-9-CM. Instructions on the use of fifth digits may appear at the beginning of a chapter, a section, or third- and fourth-digit categories (Figure 3-9).

The letter *x* (lowercase) in ICD-10-CM is a dummy placeholder. It is used in the fifth-character position and in certain sixth-character code positions. These dummy placeholders are to be used for future code expansion.

EXAMPLE   T36.0x1A, Poisoning by penicillins, accidental, initial encounter

Some categories in ICD-10-CM have seventh-character extensions, and this seventh character is required for all codes in that category. These seventh-character extensions are widely used in Chapter 19. If a code in these categories is not six characters in length, a dummy placeholder of "x" must be added before the seventh character.

EXAMPLE | Sprain of ribs, subsequent encounter, S23.41xD.

EXERCISE 3-2

Using Figure 3-9, assign the appropriate fifth-digit subclassifications.

1. Pyogenic arthritis left knee   711.0 _____
2. Localized osteoarthritis right wrist   715.3 _____
3. Traumatic arthropathy, right ankle   716.1 _____
4. Pain shoulder joint   719.4 _____
5. Swelling elbow joint   719.0 _____

Supplementary Classifications

There are two sections of supplementary classifications in ICD-9-CM:

■ Supplementary Classification of Factors Influencing Health Status and Contact With Health Services (V01-V89)
■ Supplementary Classification of External Causes of Injury and Poisoning (E800-E999)

Both supplementary classifications contain alphanumeric codes. One of the classifications is found following the Tabular List for Diseases and Injuries and is entitled Supplementary Classification of Factors Influencing Health Status and Contact With Health Services (V01-V89), or V codes. V codes are available to code encounters for circumstances other than disease or injury.

The second supplement is the Supplementary Classification of External Causes of Injury and Poisoning (E800-E999), or E codes. These codes are located after the V codes. The E codes are used as a supplement to ICD-9-CM diagnosis codes to provide data on cause, intent, and place of an injury or poisoning.

There are no supplementary classifications in ICD-10-CM. The two supplementary classifications in ICD-9-CM were moved to the main classification in ICD-10-CM.

Format of Alphabetic Index to Diseases and Injuries

The Alphabetic Index contains three sections in ICD-9-CM:

■ Index to Diseases and Injuries
■ Table of Drugs and Chemicals
■ Alphabetic Index to External Causes of Injury and Poisoning (E codes)

Two tables are located within the Alphabetic Index. These tables are used for further clarification of subterms under the main term entries of Hypertension and Neoplasm. These tables are discussed in their respective chapters.

The Alphabetic Index in ICD-10-CM contains the following:

■ ICD-10-CM Index to Diseases and Injuries
  • Neoplasm Table
  • Table of Drugs and Chemicals
■ ICD-10-CM Index to External Causes

Index to Diseases and Injuries

Three levels of indentation are used in the Alphabetic Index. These include the following:

■ Main terms
■ Subterms
■ Carryover lines

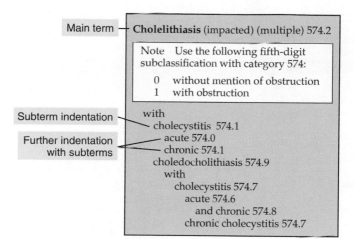

Main term — **Cholelithiasis** (impacted) (multiple) 574.2

> Note   Use the following fifth-digit
> subclassification with category 574:
>
> 0   without mention of obstruction
> 1   with obstruction

Subterm indentation —— with
                            cholecystitis 574.1
Further indentation —— acute 574.0
   with subterms —— chronic 574.1
                        choledocholithiasis 574.9
                            with
                                cholecystitis 574.7
                                    acute 574.6
                                        and chronic 574.8
                                chronic cholecystitis 574.7

FIGURE 3-10. Various levels of indentation in the Index. The bold term is the main term, and the various subterms are listed below.

Deficiency, deficient
   3-beta-hydroxysteroid dehydrogenase
      255.2
   6-phosphogluconic dehydrogenase
      (anemia) 282.2
   11-beta-hydroxylase 255.2
   17-alpha-hydroxylase 255.2
   18-hydroxysteroid dehydrogenase 255.2
   20-alpha-hydroxylase 255.2
   21-hydroxylase 255.2
   AAT (alpha-1 antitrypsin) 273.4
   abdominal muscle syndrome 756.79

FIGURE 3-11. Numerical entries in the Alphabetic Index.

The **main terms** are identified by bold print and are set flush with the left margin of each column (Figure 3-10). Alphabetization rules apply in locating main terms and subterms in the Alphabetic Index. Numerical entries appear first under the main term or subterm (Figure 3-11). Main terms usually are identified by disease conditions and nouns. The main term is not a body part or site.

EXAMPLE   The patient has been admitted with deep vein thrombosis. The main term is "thrombosis." "Deep" is a location and "vein" refers to a body part.

EXAMPLE   The patient is being treated for adhesive bursitis of the shoulder.
    The main term is "bursitis." "Adhesive" describes the type of bursitis and "shoulder" is a body part (Figure 3-12).

EXERCISE 3-3

Underline the main terms to be located in the Alphabetic Index in the following diagnosis statements.

1. Decubitus ulcer of the heel   _____
2. Acute anterior wall myocardial infarction   _____
3. Respiratory anthrax   _____
4. Endometriosis of the ovary   _____
5. Gouty arthritis   _____

```
Bursitis NEC 727.3
   Achilles tendon 726.71
   adhesive 726.90
      shoulder 726.0  ←
   ankle 726.79
   buttock 726.5
   calcaneal 726.79
   collateral ligament
      fibular 726.63
      tibial 726.62
   Duplay's 726.2
```

FIGURE 3-12. Main term and essential modifiers.

```
Fever 780.6
→  with chills 780.6
      in malarial regions (see also Malaria)
         084.6
   abortus NEC 023.9
   aden 061
```

FIGURE 3-13. Connecting term "with" follows the main term.

The subterms are indented to the right under the main term. They are not bolded and begin with a lowercase letter. **Subterms** modify the main term and sometimes are called essential modifiers. These terms provide greater specificity to the disease or injury. It is possible for a subterm to be followed by additional subterm(s). These additional subterms are indented even farther to the right than are subterms (refer to Figure 3-10).

Some subterms are called "**connecting words**". This means that there is a relationship between a main term or a subterm and an associated condition or etiology. Connecting words "with" and "without" are located before any other subterms (Figure 3-13). Additional connecting words include the following:

- Associated with
- Due to
- In
- With
- With mention of

EXERCISE 3-4

Using the Alphabetic Index only, assign codes to the following conditions.

1. Asthma due to detergent _____

2. Cholelithiasis with acute cholecystitis _____

3. Syphilitic Parkinsonism associated with orthostatic hypotension _____

4. Cystocele in pregnancy _____

5. List the subterms for coryza. _____

Carryover lines are used when an entry will not fit on a single line. These are indented to the right even farther than a subterm to avoid confusion (Figure 3-14).

Fenestration, fenestrated - *see also* Imperfect, closure
   aorta-pulmonary 745.0
   aorticopulmonary 745.0
   aortopulmonary 745.0
   cusps, heart valve NEC 746.89
      pulmonary 746.09
   hymen 752.49
   pulmonic cusps 746.09

FIGURE 3-14. Carryover line.

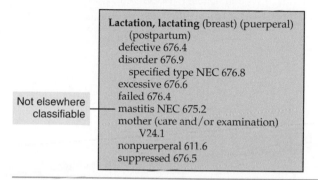

Lactation, lactating (breast) (puerperal)
    (postpartum)
   defective 676.4
   disorder 676.9
     specified type NEC 676.8
   excessive 676.6
   failed 676.4
   mastitis NEC 675.2
   mother (care and/or examination)
     V24.1
   nonpuerperal 611.6
   suppressed 676.5

Not elsewhere classifiable

FIGURE 3-15. The Index entry for lactating mastitis "not elsewhere classifiable" (NEC) is coded to 675.2.

CODING CONVENTIONS

Coding **conventions** are addressed by the Official Guidelines for Coding and Reporting in both ICD-9-CM and ICD-10-CM. It is important for coders to understand these conventions so that accurate assignment of codes can be ensured.

Conventions include the following:

- Abbreviations
- Punctuation/symbols
- Instructional notes
- Linking terms
- Cross-references

Abbreviations

In ICD-9-CM, the two main abbreviations are

- NEC—not elsewhere classifiable
- NOS—not otherwise specified

NEC is used differently in the Alphabetic Index than in the Tabular List. In the Alphabetic Index, NEC represents "other specified." When a specific disease or condition is documented and no specific code is available, the Index will direct the coder with the abbreviation "NEC" to an "other specified" code (Figure 3-15).

The **NEC** abbreviation in the Tabular List means "other specified" or "not elsewhere classifiable" and often is classified to the final digit of 8. The code title may not fully describe the documented disease process or condition (Figure 3-16).

NOS is a Tabular List abbreviation that means "unspecified" (see Figure 3-16). These codes are to be used only when the documentation in the health record does not provide adequate information. The unspecified code often appears as the code following the main term in the Alphabetic Index. The subterms should be reviewed to determine whether a more specific code is available.

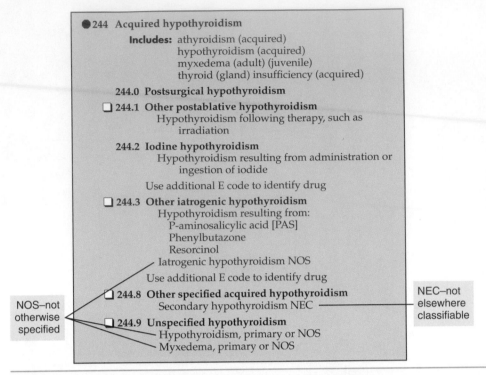

FIGURE 3-16. Examples of NEC and NOS from the Tabular.

There are two types of abbreviations in ICD-10-CM:

■ Index Abbreviation
  • NEC
■ Tabular Abbreviation
  • NEC
  • NOS

Both the Alphabetic Index and Tabular List use the abbreviation NEC, which stands for "not elsewhere classifiable," and what it means is "other specified." When a specific code is unavailable for a condition, the Index will direct the coder to the other specified code. The same applies for the Tabular, which will include an NEC entry for the other specified code.

The abbreviation NOS stands for "not otherwise specified," which means "unspecified".

Punctuation

Brackets

Square brackets [ ] are used in the Tabular List to enclose synonyms, alternative wording, or explanatory phrases (Figure 3-17).

Slanted brackets *[ ]* are used in the Alphabetic Index to identify manifestation codes (Figure 3-18). The code in brackets is always sequenced second.

In ICD-10-CM there is only one type of bracket, used in the index to identify manifestation codes and in the Tabular to enclose synonyms, alternative wording, or explanatory phrases.

Parentheses

Parentheses are used in both the Alphabetic Index and the Tabular List to enclose supplementary words. The presence or absence of these terms does not affect code assignment, so they are called nonessential modifiers. A **nonessential modifier** is a term that is enclosed

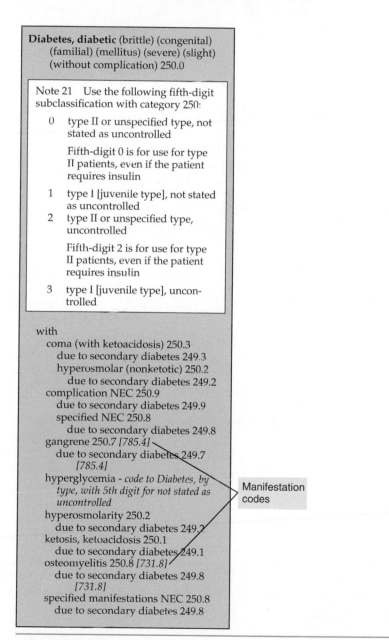

429.2 Cardiovascular disease, unspecified
    Arteriosclerotic cardiovascular disease [ASCVD] —— Abbreviation
    Cardiovascular arteriosclerosis
    Cardiovascular:
        degeneration (with mention of arteriosclerosis)
        disease (with mention of arteriosclerosis)
        sclerosis (with mention of arteriosclerosis)
    Use additional code to identify presence of
      arteriosclerosis
    Excludes *that due to hypertension (402.0–402.9)*

FIGURE 3-17. Square brackets used to enclose abbreviation.

Diabetes, diabetic (brittle) (congenital) (familial) (mellitus) (severe) (slight) (without complication) 250.0

Note 21   Use the following fifth-digit subclassification with category 250:

  0   type II or unspecified type, not stated as uncontrolled

      Fifth-digit 0 is for use for type II patients, even if the patient requires insulin

  1   type I [juvenile type], not stated as uncontrolled
  2   type II or unspecified type, uncontrolled

      Fifth-digit 2 is for use for type II patients, even if the patient requires insulin

  3   type I [juvenile type], uncontrolled

with
  coma (with ketoacidosis) 250.3
    due to secondary diabetes 249.3
    hyperosmolar (nonketotic) 250.2
      due to secondary diabetes 249.2
  complication NEC 250.9
    due to secondary diabetes 249.9
    specified NEC 250.8
      due to secondary diabetes 249.8
  gangrene 250.7 *[785.4]*
    due to secondary diabetes 249.7 *[785.4]*
  hyperglycemia - *code to Diabetes, by type, with 5th digit for not stated as uncontrolled*
  hyperosmolarity 250.2
    due to secondary diabetes 249.2
  ketosis, ketoacidosis 250.1
    due to secondary diabetes 249.1
  osteomyelitis 250.8 *[731.8]*
    due to secondary diabetes 249.8 *[731.8]*
  specified manifestations NEC 250.8
    due to secondary diabetes 249.8

Manifestation codes

FIGURE 3-18. Index entry of diabetic manifestation codes enclosed by slanted brackets.

Nonessential modifiers

Pneumonia (acute) (Alpenstich) (benign)
(bilateral) (brain) (cerebral) (circumscribed) (congestive) (creeping) (delayed resolution) (double) (epidemic)
(fever) (flash) (fulminant) (fungoid)
(granulomatous) (hemorrhagic)
(incipient) (infantile) (infectious)
(infiltration) (insular) (intermittent)
(latent) (lobe) (migratory) (newborn)
(organized) (overwhelming) (primary) (progressive) (pseudolobar)
(purulent) (resolved) (secondary) (senile) (septic) (suppurative) (terminal)
(true) (unresolved) (vesicular) 486
    with influenza, flu, or grippe 487.0
    adenoviral 480.0
    adynamic 514
    alba 090.0
    allergic 518.3
    alveolar - *see* Pneumonia, lobar
    anaerobes 482.81
    anthrax 022.1 [484.5]
    apex, apical - *see* Pneumonia, lobar
    ascaris 127.0 [484.8]

FIGURE 3-19. The use of parentheses in the Index for the diagnosis of pneumonia. Multiple nonessential modifiers are used.

Nonessential modifiers

552.3 Diaphragmatic hernia with obstruction
    Hernia:
        hiatal (esophageal) (sliding) specified as
            incarcerated, irreducible, strangulated, or
            causing obstruction
        paraesophageal specified as incarcerated,
            irreducible, strangulated, or causing
            obstruction
        Thoracic stomach specified as incarcerated,
            irreducible, strangulated, or causing obstruction

FIGURE 3-20. The nonessential modifier in the Tabular for an incarcerated hiatal or diaphragmatic hernia.

in parentheses following a main term or a subterm, whose presence or absence has no effect on code assignment. These are "take it or leave it" terms. Sometimes, the subterm can be found among the nonessential modifiers (Figures 3-19 and 3-20). Parentheses are used in the same manner in both the ICD-9-CM and the ICD-10-CM.

If the diagnostic statement is "double pneumonia," (see Figure 3-19), since "double" is a nonessential modifier, it is assigned the same code as "pneumonia" (486). The word "double" makes absolutely no difference in assignment of the code for "double pneumonia."

Also, if the diagnostic statement (see Figure 3-20) is "sliding hiatal hernia with obstruc-tion," the term "sliding" is a nonessential modifier and would not make any difference in assignment of the code.

EXERCISE 3-5

Using ICD-9-CM, Volume 2, Alphabetic Index, locate the following main terms, and identify whether the bolded subterm is an essential or a nonessential modifier.

1. **Primary** glaucoma _____

2. **Narrow-angle** glaucoma _____

3. **Essential** hypertension _____

4. **Filarial** infestation _____

5. **Thyrotoxic** exophthalmos _____

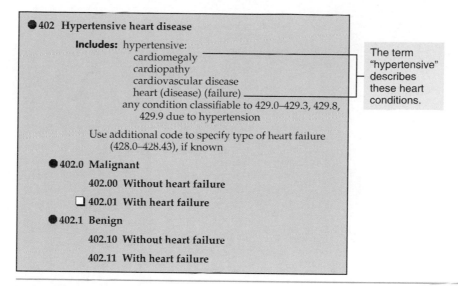

FIGURE 3-21. Colon used within "Includes" note.

FIGURE 3-22. Braces.

Colons

Colons are used in the Tabular List after an incomplete term that needs one or more modifiers following the colon to make it assignable to a given category. Colons also are used in both Inclusion and Exclusion notes to indicate that one of the words from the indented list must be present for the note to apply (Figure 3-21).

In Figure 3-21, the term "hypertensive" is used to describe various heart conditions. The colon helps to save space and means the same as if it was written in this way in both the ICD-9-CM and the ICD-10-CM:

- Hypertensive cardiomegaly
- Hypertensive cardiopathy
- Hypertensive cardiovascular disease
- Hypertensive heart disease or failure

Braces

The purpose of the brace is to save printing space by reducing the repetition of words. A brace is used to enclose a series of terms, each of which is modified by a statement that appears to the right of the brace (Figure 3-22).

Braces are not used in ICD-10-CM.

Instructional Notes

Notes with instructions are found in all three volumes of ICD-9-CM. General notes may be found in the Alphabetic Index and the Tabular List. These notes provide additional information (Figure 3-23). Other types of instructional notes are "Inclusion"; "Exclusion"; "code first"; "use additional code"; and "code, if applicable, any causal condition first."

Fracture (abduction) (adduction)
(avulsion) (compression) (crush)
(dislocation) (oblique) (separation)
(closed) 829.0

Note   For fracture of any of the following sites with fracture of other
bones, *see* Fracture, multiple.

"Closed" includes the following descriptions of fractures, with or without
delayed healing, unless they are specified as open or compound:

comminuted
depressed
elevated
fissured
greenstick
impacted
linear
simple
slipped epiphysis
spiral
unspecified

"Open" includes the following descriptions of fractures, with or without
delayed healing:

compound
infected
missile
puncture
with foreign body

For late effect of fracture, *see* Late, effect, fracture, by site.

FIGURE 3-23. General notes found in the Alphabetic Index.

Inclusion Notes

"Inclusion" notes in the ICD-9-CM are termed "Includes" notes in the ICD-10-CM and are used for the same purpose in both. An Includes note is an instructional note that appears immediately under a three-digit code title or category. The purpose of the Includes note is to give examples or further define the content of the category (Figure 3-24).

Inclusion Terms

According to the guidelines, Inclusion terms are a list of terms that are found under some fourth- and fifth-digit codes (Figure 3-25). These terms may be synonyms or various other conditions that are assigned to the code. Inclusion terms do not necessarily constitute a comprehensive list. Additional terms found only in the Alphabetic Index and not in the Tabular List may be assigned a code without mention in the Inclusion terms. In these instances, the Index should be trusted. Inclusion terms are used in the same manner in both the ICD-9-CM and the ICD-10-CM.

Exclusion Notes

An Excludes note is an instructional note that may appear after any code in the Tabular List. One of the purposes of the Excludes note is to direct the coder to another code.

EXAMPLE

The patient has COPD with asthma. Under category 496, an exclusion note indicates that COPD with asthma is coded to 493.2 (Figure 3-26). After verifying 493.2 in the Tabular List, note that a fifth digit is necessary for a valid code assignment.

In ICD-10-CM, J44- includes asthma with chronic obstructive pulmonary disease, but there is an instructional note to code also the type of asthma, if applicable (J45.-).

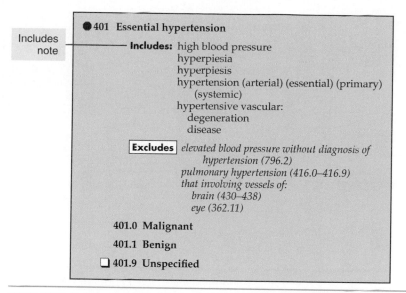

FIGURE 3-24. This "Includes" note is found under category 401, Essential hypertension.

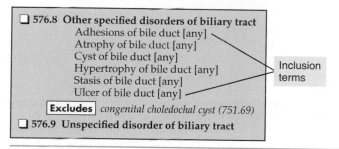

FIGURE 3-25. Inclusion terms.

FIGURE 3-26. Exclusion note.

Another purpose of an Exclusion note is to instruct the coder that the excluded terms should not be used along with the code that is assigned. The example given in the guidelines is that only one code should be assigned for a condition that has different codes for congenital and acquired (Figure 3-27).

Exclusion notes also are used to instruct the coder that an additional code may be required because this code is excluded from a particular code.

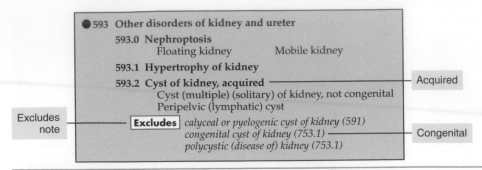

FIGURE 3-27. Example of a congenital cyst of the kidney that is excluded from the acquired form of a kidney cyst.

EXAMPLE

A patient has hypertension and pulmonary hypertension. Under the category 401 code for hypertension is an Exclusion note for pulmonary hypertension. In this case, two codes must be assigned: one for hypertension (401.9 [I10]) and another to identify pulmonary hypertension (416.8 [I27.2]) (Figure 3-28).

ICD-10-CM has two types of "Excludes" notes:

■ Excludes1
An Excludes1 note is used to indicate that two conditions cannot occur together. If a certain condition is excluded, it means it cannot be coded here.

EXAMPLE

Patient presents to the hospital with severe constipation. The doctor diagnoses the patient with congenital megacolon. Code K59.3 excludes congenital megacolon, directing the coder to Q43.1

■ Excludes2
An Excludes2 note is used to indicate that the condition is not represented by the code, "not included here." In the case of the Excludes2 note, it would be acceptable to use two codes as appropriate.

EXAMPLE

Patient presents to the hospital with stomach pain. The doctor diagnoses the patient with diverticulitis of the colon and the appendix. This would require two codes, one for the colon and one for the appendix. See the Excludes note under K57.

EXERCISE 3-6

Using the Tabular List, answer the following questions.

1. Is bronchitis due to fumes and vapors assigned code 490? _____
   If not, what code is assigned? _____

2. Is chronic sinusitis assigned code category 461? _____
   If not, what code is assigned? _____

3. Is gangrenous tonsillitis assigned to code category 463? _____
   If not, what code is assigned? _____

4. Is hypertensive cardiomegaly included in code category 402? _____
   If not, what code is assigned? _____

5. Are tics due to Tourette's syndrome included in code category 333.3? _____
   If not, what code is assigned? _____

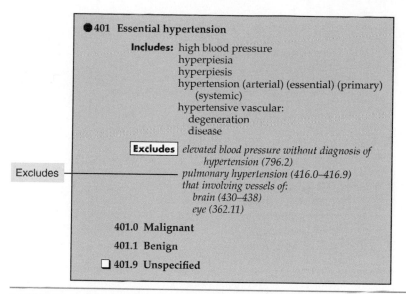

FIGURE 3-28. Exclusion note directing the coder to another code.

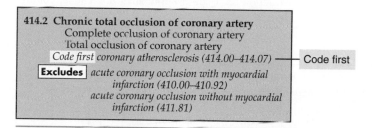

FIGURE 3-29. Instructional note to code first underlying disease.

Etiology and Manifestation Convention

The following instructional notes are designed to instruct the coder regarding proper sequencing of etiology and manifestation codes. The etiology code will include an instructional note to use an additional code to identify a given manifestation. The manifestation code will have an instructional note to code first the etiology code.

An instructional note to *"code first underlying disease"* is used in the Tabular List. The purpose of this is to instruct the coder that there may be a code for the etiology and if so it is to be sequenced first (Figure 3-29).

EXAMPLE   Patient with chronic total occlusion of the coronary artery with coronary atherosclerosis, 414.01, 414.2, codes must be sequenced in this order (I25.10, I25.82).

Code 414.2 includes an instructional note to code the underlying disease first. In this case, the underlying disease is coronary atherosclerosis.

An instructional note to *"code, if applicable, any causal condition first"* is used in the Tabular List. The purpose of this note is to instruct the coder to sequence the causal condition (etiology) first. Different from the instructional note "code first underlying disease," if no causal condition is present or documented, the code may be sequenced first (Figure 3-30).

EXAMPLE   Patient has ulcer of right ankle due to diabetes, type II, 250.80, 707.13, codes must be sequenced in this order (E11.622, L97.319).

● **707.1 Ulcer of lower limbs, except pressure ulcer**
Ulcer, chronic, of lower limb:
  neurogenic of lower limb
  trophic of lower limb

Code if applicable, any causal condition first: ◄
  atherosclerosis of the extremities with ulceration
    (440.23)
  chronic venous hypertension with ulcer (459.31)
  chronic venous hypertension with ulcer and
    inflammation (459.33)
  diabetes mellitus (250.80–250.83)
  postphlebitic syndrome with ulcer (459.11)
  postphlebitic syndrome with ulcer and
    inflammation (459.13)
☐ **707.10 Ulcer of lower limb, unspecified**
707.11 Ulcer of thigh
707.12 Ulcer of calf
707.13 Ulcer of ankle
707.14 Ulcer of heel and midfoot
  Plantar surface of midfoot
707.15 Ulcer of other part of foot
  Toes
707.19 Ulcer of other part of lower limb

FIGURE 3-30. Instruction to "Code if applicable, any causal condition first."

● **599 Other disorders of urethra and urinary tract**
☐ **599.0 Urinary tract infection, site not specified**
| **Excludes** | *Candidiasis of urinary tract (112.2)* |
| | *urinary tract infection of newborn (771.82)* |
| Use additional code to identify organism, such as ◄ |
| Escherichia coli [E. coli] (041.49) |

FIGURE 3-31. Instructional note to use an additional code.

Code 707.1 includes an instructional note to code first any applicable causal condition. In this case, the causal condition is diabetes.

An instructional note to "use additional code" is found in the Tabular List. The purpose of this is to instruct the coder to use an additional code to provide a complete picture of the diagnosis or condition. These codes should be assigned only if they are documented by the provider (Figure 3-31).

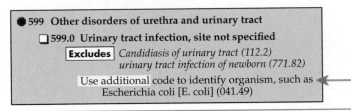

EXAMPLE Patient has a urinary tract infection due to *Escherichia coli*, 599.0, 041.49 must be sequenced in this order (N39.0, B96.2).

The "use additional code" note instructs the coder to assign an additional code for the organism.

In the Alphabetic Index, some manifestation codes are enclosed in slanted brackets. The etiology code is listed first and is sequenced first. The manifestation code is assigned as an additional code. These code conventions are the same for ICD-9-CM and ICD-10-CM. The Index entry for diabetes is a good example of the use of etiology and manifestation codes (Figure 3-32). In ICD-10-CM the etiology and manifestation convention remains consistent with ICD-9-CM.

Diabetes, diabetic *(Continued)*
    Lancereaux's (diabetes mellitus with
        marked emaciation) 250.8 *[261]*
        due to secondary diabetes 249.8
            [261]
    latent (chemical) - *see* Diabetes, second-
        ary
        complicating pregnancy, childbirth,
            or puerperium 648.8
    lipoidosis 250.8 *[272.7]*
        due to secondary diabetes 249.8
            [272.7]
    macular edema 250.5 *[362.07]*
        due to secondary diabetes 249.5
            [362.07]
    microaneurysms, retinal 250.5 *[362.01]*
        due to secondary diabetes 249.5
            [362.01]
    mononeuropathy 250.6 *[355.9]*
        due to secondary diabetes 249.6
            [355.9]
    neonatal, transient 775.1
    nephropathy 250.4 *[583.81]* ────── Diabetic nephropathy
        due to secondary diabetes 249.4   250.4X *[583.81]*
            [581.81]

FIGURE 3-32. Slanted brackets enclosing manifestation code.

EXERCISE 3-7

Using the Tabular List and instructional notes, assign and sequence the following code(s).

1. See category 331 and assign code(s) for a patient who has _____
   Alzheimer's disease with behavioral disturbances.

2. See code 484.3 and assign code(s) for a patient with _____
   pneumonia due to whooping cough.

3. See code 707.1 and assign code(s) for a patient with _____
   atherosclerosis of the left lower extremities with a toe ulcer.

4. See code 600.91 and assign code(s) for a patient with _____
   hyperplasia of the prostate with urinary retention.

5. See code 456.2 and assign code(s) for a patient with _____
   bleeding esophageal varices and cirrhosis of the liver.

Linking Terms

As in the Index, terms such as "and," "with," "due to," and "in" are used to link terms. These terms have special definitions within ICD-9-CM and code assignment.

The term "and" means "and/or" when it appears in a code title in the Tabular List. The code 474.8, Other chronic disease of tonsils and adenoids, could mean any of the following:

■ Chronic disease of tonsils
■ Chronic disease of adenoids
■ Chronic disease of tonsils and adenoids

The term "with" (with "mention of," "associated," and "in") indicates that both elements in the title must be present and documented for this code to be assigned.

EXAMPLE | Viral pneumonia with influenza is assigned codes 487.0 and 480.9 (Figure 3-33). Both the pneumonia and the influenza must be present for code 487.0 to be assigned (J10.08, J12.9).

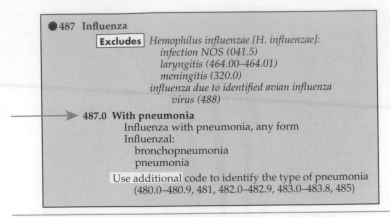

FIGURE 3-33. Influenza with pneumonia.

```
Cataract (Continued)
  complicated NEC 366.30
  congenital 743.30
    capsular or subcapsular 743.31
    cortical 743.32
    nuclear 743.33
    specified type NEC 743.39
    total or subtotal 743.34
    zonular 743.32
  coronary (congenital) 743.39
    acquired 366.12
  cupuliform 366.14
  diabetic 250.5 [366.41]
  drug-induced 366.45
  due to
    chalcosis 360.24 [366.34]
    chronic choroiditis (see also Choroidi-
      tis) 363.20 [366.32]
    degenerative myopia 360.21 [366.34]
    glaucoma (see also Glaucoma) 365.9
      [366.31]
    infection, intraocular NEC 366.32
    inflammatory ocular disorder NEC
      366.32
    iridocyclitis, chronic 364.10 [366.33]
    pigmentary retinal dystrophy 362.74
      [366.34]
    radiation 366.46
```

FIGURE 3-34. "Due to" indicates a relationship between the cataract and subsequent subterms.

The term "due to" indicates a causal relationship between two conditions. It is found in both the Alphabetic Index and the Tabular List. If it is documented that a condition is due to another condition and there is an Alphabetic Index entry for the subterm "due to," the coder must follow the Index (Figure 3-34).

Cross-References

Cross-reference terms are used in the Alphabetic Index to instruct a coder to look elsewhere prior to code assignment. These terms include "*see*," "*see also*," "*see* category," and "*see* condition" (Figure 3-35).

The term "*see*" is a mandatory instruction that advises the coder to go to another main term (Figure 3-36).

The term "*see also*" instructs the coder about the possibility that a better main term may appear elsewhere in the Alphabetic Index. If the specific diagnosis cannot be completely

Hereditary - *see* condition
Heredodegeneration 330.9
    macular 362.70
Heredopathia atactica polyneuritiformis
    356.3

FIGURE 3-35. Under the main term "Hereditary," mandatory instructions are given to "*see*" condition.

Angioblastoma (M9161/1) - *see* Neo-
    plasm, connective tissue, uncertain
    behavior

FIGURE 3-36. Cross-reference to "*see*" another main term.

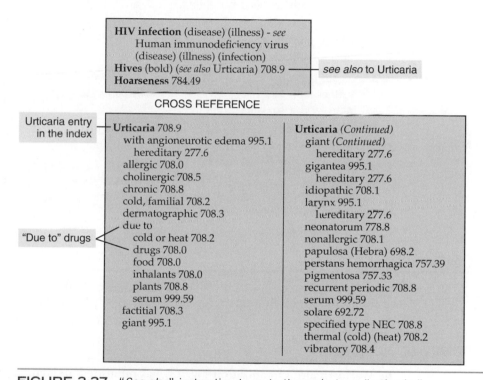

FIGURE 3-37. "*See also*" instruction to go to the main term "urticaria."

identified by the subterms, it may be necessary to follow the "see also" instruction (Figure 3-37).

If a patient has hives because of use of a medication, in the Alphabetic Index, the only code available for the main term "hives" is 708.9. If the "*see also*" instruction is not followed, the wrong code would be assigned. When you go to "urticaria" in the Index, several subterm selections are available, including 708.0 for "urticaria due to a drug" (see Figure 3-37).

A "code also" note instructs the coder that two codes may be required to fully describe a condition. "Code also" notes do not give sequencing instruction.

Default Codes

In the ICD-10-CM Alphabetic Index, if a code is listed next to the main term, it is the default code. A default code may represent a condition that is most commonly associated with the main term or is the unspecified term for that condition. For example, if pneumonia is documented in a medical record, and no additional information or specificity is supplied, such as aspiration or viral, the default code is J18.9.

Syndromes

To code syndromes, the guidance supplied by the Alphabetic Index must be followed. Should there be no guidance in the Index, codes should be assigned for the manifestations of the syndrome that have been documented.

EXERCISE 3-8

Using the Alphabetic Index, answer the following questions.

1. Locate the main term "arthropathy" in the Index. Is there another term for "arthropathy" that may be located in the Index, and if so, what is the term?   _____

2. Locate the main term "climacteric" in the Index. Is there another term for "climacteric" that may be located in the Index, and if so, what is the term?   _____

3. Locate the main term "Endamebiasis" in the Index. Is there another term for "Endamebiasis" that may be located in the Index, and if so, what is the term?   _____

4. Locate the main term "enteric" in the Index. Is there another term for "enteric" that may be located in the Index, and if so, what is the term?   _____

5. Locate the main term "late effect of phlebitis of the intracranial venous sinuses." What cross-reference is given?   _____

APPENDICES

As noted at the beginning of the chapter, book content and format may vary depending on the publisher. The following are the most commonly found appendices.

A. Morphology of Neoplasms

The World Health Organization (WHO) has published an adaptation of the International Classification of Diseases for Oncology (ICD-O). The ICD-O contains codes for the **topography** (location) and morphology of tumors. **Morphology** is the study of neoplasms. Morphology codes consist of five digits; the first four identify the histologic type, and the fifth indicates its behavior (Figure 3-38). Not all facilities use "M codes." These are discussed in greater detail in Chapter 15 of this textbook, Neoplasms.

C. Classification of Drugs by American Hospital Formulary: Service List Number and Their ICD-9-CM Equivalents

Appendix C contains codes from the American Hospital Formulary Services (AHFS) along with corresponding codes from ICD-9-CM (Figure 3-39).

A division of the AFHS regularly publishes a coded listing of drugs. These AHFS codes have as many as five digits. Each code has a number, then a colon, and can include up to four additional digits to provide specificity. An associated ICD-9-CM poisoning code follows the drug. The American Hospital Formulary list can be useful to the coder in assigning appropriate ICD-9-CM poisoning codes.

M805-M808	**Papillary and squamous cell neoplasms**
M8050/0	*Papilloma NOS (except Papilloma of urinary bladder M8120/1)*
M8050/2	*Papillary carcinoma in situ*
M8050/3	*Papillary carcinoma NOS*
M8051/0	*Verrucous papilloma*
M8051/3	*Verrucous carcinoma NOS*
M8052/0	*Squamous cell papilloma*
M8052/3	*Papillary squamous cell carcinoma*
M8053/0	*Inverted papilloma*
M8060/0	*Papillomatosis NOS*
M8070/2	*Squamous cell carcinoma in situ NOS*
M8070/3	*Squamous cell carcinoma NOS*
M8070/6	*Squamous cell carcinoma, metastatic NOS*
M8071/3	*Squamous cell carcinoma, keratinizing type NOS*
M8072/3	*Squamous cell carcinoma, large cell, nonkeratinizing type*
M8073/3	*Squamous cell carcinoma, small cell, nonkeratinizing type*
M8074/3	*Squamous cell carcinoma, spindle cell type*
M8075/3	*Adenoid squamous cell carcinoma*
M8076/2	*Squamous cell carcinoma in situ with questionable stromal invasion*
M8076/3	*Squamous cell carcinoma, microinvasive*
M8080/2	*Queyrat's erythroplasia*
M8081/2	*Bowen's disease*
M8082/3	*Lymphoepithelial carcinoma*

FIGURE 3-38. Example from Appendix A, Morphology of Neoplasms.

24:00	**CARDIOVASCULAR DRUGS**	
24:04	Cardiac Drugs	972.9
	cardiotonic agents	972.1
	rhythm regulators	972.0
24:06	Antilipemic Agents	972.2
	thyroid derivatives	962.7
24:08	Hypotensive Agents	972.6
	adrenergic blocking agents	971.3
	ganglion-blocking agents	972.3
	vasodilators	972.5
24:12	Vasodilating Agents	972.5
	coronary	972.4
	nicotinic acid derivatives	972.2
24:16	Sclerosing Agents	972.7

FIGURE 3-39. Example from Appendix C, Classification of Drugs by American Hospital Formulary Service List Number and Their ICD-9-CM Equivalents.

D. Classification of Industrial Accidents According to Agency

Appendix D contains three-digit codes for use in identifying occupational hazards. These codes can be very useful in assessment of statistical data and analysis of occupational hazards.

The subsection is divided into the following categories:

- Machines
- Means of Transport and Lifting Equipment
- Other Equipment
- Materials, Substances, and Radiations
- Working Environment
- Other Agencies, Not Elsewhere Classified
- Agencies Not Classified for Lack of Sufficient Data

E. List of Three-Digit Categories

Appendix E is a complete listing of all the three-digit code categories used in the ICD-9-CM. All fourth- and fifth-digit codes can be condensed back down to the three-digit categories. This allows for comparability of worldwide data with the use of ICD-9.

CHAPTER REVIEW EXERCISE

Match the term, symbol, or punctuation with the appropriate description.

_____ 1. Appendix that contains a listing of all three-digit code categories

_____ 2. Stands for "not otherwise specified"

_____ 3. Appendix that contains the Morphology of Neoplasm codes

_____ 4. Used in both the Index and the Tabular to enclose supplementary words that may be present or absent in the statement of a disease or procedure, without affecting the code number to which it is assigned

_____ 5. Used in the Tabular List after an incomplete term that needs one or more of the modifiers to make it assignable to a given category

_____ 6. This note appears immediately under a three-digit code title to further define, or give examples of, the content of the category

_____ 7. A note under a code indicates that the terms excluded from the code are to be coded elsewhere

_____ 8. A word that should be interpreted to mean either "and" or "or" when it appears in a title

_____ 9. Appendix that was deleted October 1, 2004

_____ 10. List of terms that is included under particular four- and five-digit codes

_____ 11. Stands for "not elsewhere classifiable"

_____ 12. Term that is used to indicate that no code should be assigned

A. Omit code	**G.** See category	**M.** Use additional code
B. ( )	**H.** Inclusion terms	**N.** Appendix A
C. NOS	**I.** See also	**O.** Appendix B
D. Includes	**J.** Etiology	**P.** Appendix C
E. NEC	**K.** Excludes	**Q.** Appendix D
F. :	**L.** And	**R.** Appendix E

Using ICD-9-CM, Volume 1, Tabular List, locate the first pages of Chapter 8, and answer the following questions about the chapter.

13. The name of the chapter: _____

14. The name of the first section: _____

15. The description of the first category: _____

16. The description of the first subcategory: _____

17. The description of the first subclassification: _____

18. What instructional note applies to the entire chapter? _____

19. What Excludes note applies to the first section? _____

Underline the main terms to be located in the Alphabetic Index in the following diagnostic statements.

20. Profound anemia _____

21. Chronic prostatitis _____

22. Mild protein-calorie malnutrition _____

23. Granuloma lung _____

24. Pain in shoulder _____

Using the Alphabetic Index, locate the following main terms and identify whether the bolded subterm is an essential or a nonessential modifier.

25. **Immature** cataract   _____

26. **Senile** cataract   _____

27. **Contact** dermatitis   _____

28. **Classical** migraine   _____

29. **Congential** strabismus   _____

Using the Alphabetic Index, answer the following questions.

30. Locate the main term "acquired immune deficiency syndrome" in   _____
    the Index. Is there another term for "acquired immune deficiency
    syndrome" that may be located in the Index, and if so, what is
    the term?

31. Locate the main term "malarial" in the Index. Is there another   _____
    term for "malarial" that may be located in the Index, and if so,
    what is the term?

Using the Tabular List, answer the following questions.

32. Is acute exacerbation of chronic myeloid leukemia assigned code   _____
    205.00?

    If not, what code is assigned?   _____

33. Is rupture of the esophagus assigned code 530.4?   _____

    If not, what code is assigned?   _____

Using the Tabular List and instructional notes, assign and sequence the following code(s).

34. See category 331 and assign code(s) for a patient who has Pick's   _____
    disease with behavioral disturbances.

35. See code 484.6 and assign code(s) for a patient with pneumonia   _____
    due to aspergillosis.

36. See code 707.1 and assign code(s) for a patient with   _____
    atherosclerosis of the lower extremities with an ankle ulcer.

CHAPTER GLOSSARY

Carryover line: used when an entry will not fit on a single line.

Category: a single three-digit code that describes a disease or a similarly related group of conditions.

Connecting words: subterms that denote a relationship between a main term or a subterm and an associated condition or etiology.

Conventions: general rules for use in classification that must be followed for accurate coding.

Etiology: cause or origin of a disease or condition.

ICD-10-CM: *International Classification of Diseases, 10th Revision, Clinical Modification.*

ICD-10-PCS: *International Classification of Diseases, 10th Revision, Procedure Coding System.*

Main term: term that identifies disease conditions or injuries, it is identified in bold print and set flush with the left margin of each column in the Alphabetic Index.

Manifestation: symptom of a condition that is the result of a disease.

Morphology: the study of neoplasms.

NEC: abbreviation for "not elsewhere classifiable" that means "other specified."

Nonessential modifier: term that is enclosed in parentheses; its presence or absence does not affect code assignment.

NOS: abbreviation for "not otherwise specified" that means "unspecified."

Section: consists of a group of three-digit categories that represent diseases or conditions that are similar.

See: a mandatory cross-reference that advises the coder to go to another main term.

See also: cross-reference that instructs the coder about the possibility that there may be a better main term elsewhere in the Alphabetic Index.

Subcategory: a fourth-digit code that provides additional information or specificity.

Subclassification: a fifth-digit code that provides even greater specificity.

Subterms: give more specific information about a main term. Subterms identify site, type, or etiology of a disease condition or injury. Also, modifiers that are indented to the right of the main term.

Topography: location.

4

Basic Steps of Coding

LEARNING OBJECTIVES

1. Assign a diagnosis or procedure from the Alphabetic Index using main terms, subterms, and essential modifiers
2. Explain the necessity of referencing the Alphabetic Index and the Tabular List
3. Describe basic steps of coding
4. Explain how to use both the Alphabetic Index and the Tabular List

ABBREVIATIONS/ ACRONYMS

CC	Chief Complaint	**ER**	Emergency Room
DS	Discharge Summary	**OR**	Operating Room

BASIC STEPS OF CODING

1. Review the health record.
2. Identify the diagnoses and procedures to be coded.
3. Identify the principal diagnosis and the principal procedure.
4. Identify main term(s) in the Alphabetic Index.
5. Review any subterms under the main term in the Alphabetic Index.
6. Follow any cross-reference instructions, such as "*see also.*"
7. Verify in the Tabular List the code(s) selected from the Alphabetic Index.
8. Refer to any instructional notation in the Tabular List.
9. Assign codes to the highest level of specificity.
10. Assign codes to the diagnoses and procedures, reporting all applicable codes, and sequence in accordance with the guidelines.

REVIEW OF THE HEALTH RECORD

As described in Chapter 2 of this textbook, the first step in coding the **principal diagnosis** (condition established after study to be chiefly responsible for occasioning admission of the patient to the hospital for care), other reportable diagnoses, and procedures is review of the health record.

The discharge summary (DS), if available, may be the first document to be reviewed for code selection. The coder reads the summary to understand the highlights of this encounter. The **discharge summary** is a synopsis of the events included in a patient's hospital stay. Most pertinent information is contained in the discharge summary. A physician should list the diagnoses and the procedures that were performed during this encounter. The coder should not solely rely on the discharge summary to capture all diagnoses and procedures that occurred during this encounter.

For many reasons, the discharge summary is not the only document from which codes are captured.

- Coders may not have a discharge summary at the time of coding.
- If the patient is in the hospital for a long stay, often the attending physician will focus only on those diagnoses that were treated during the latter part of the stay.
- Physicians list conditions that are not currently under treatment and that appear only in the patient's history.
- Likewise, physicians describe diagnoses as "history of" when, in fact, they represent conditions that are being currently treated.

Most coders start the coding process as they begin their document review. A coder is continually trying to determine the principal diagnosis during the record review. Clues to determination of the principal diagnosis can be found in the ER record or in the admitting orders. Physicians, in their admitting orders, give a reason for admitting the patient. When evaluating an ER record, a coder first looks for the **chief complaint** (CC), which is the reason in the patient's own words for presenting to the hospital.

EXAMPLE

> CC: I have a bad cough, fever, and headache, and my throat is so sore I can't even swallow liquids.

As the coder continues the review of the ER document, the ER physician provides a diagnosis for admission to the hospital. The **admitting diagnosis** is the condition that requires the patient to be hospitalized. This condition may be a sign or a symptom that requires testing and evaluation to determine a diagnosis. This may be a known diagnosis or a probable diagnosis, or it may include a differential diagnosis. In the previous example, the ER physician might document, "Admit patient to the hospital for possible pneumonia, and dehydration." In this case, the pneumonia has not yet been confirmed, but the dehydration is known.

A **differential diagnosis** occurs when a patient presents with a symptom that could represent a variety of diagnoses. During the patient's stay, a variety of studies may be conducted to rule out or confirm the differential diagnoses.

EXAMPLE

> A patient presents with abdominal pain, and the physician suspects that this might represent appendicitis, gastroenteritis, or cholecystitis. Appendicitis, gastroenteritis, and cholecystitis are differential diagnoses.

A coder continues on through the health record, reviewing all progress notes, operative reports, anesthesiology notes, and consults to arrive at all diagnoses and procedures that need to be captured or reported.

The second most important concept that a coder must remember (after the definition of principal diagnosis and principal procedure) is that once a term has been located in the Alphabetic Index, the code must then be verified in the Tabular Index. This is not the case in ICD-10-PCS, in which you do not need to refer to the Index before referring to the tables.

ALPHABETIC INDEX

The **Alphabetic Index** consists of an Alphabetic Index to Diseases and an Alphabetic Index to Procedures. In ICD-10-PCS, the purpose of the Alphabetic Index is to locate the appropriate table.

Locate the Main Term in the Index to Diseases

Once the coder begins to establish diagnoses and procedures, the first task in selecting a code is to locate the **main term**, which is always identified by bold type, in the Alphabetic Index.

EXAMPLE | Using pneumonia as the principal diagnosis, locate this term in the Alphabetic Index. The code for pneumonia is 486 (J18.9) (Figure 4-1).

EXERCISE 4-1

Using Figure 4-1, assign codes to the following diagnoses:

1. Aspiration <u>pneumonia</u>
2. <u>Pneumonia</u> due to *Klebsiella pneumoniae*
3. Mycoplasma <u>pneumonia</u>
4. Varicella <u>pneumonia</u>
5. Viral <u>pneumonia</u>

After the main term, "pneumonia," in the Alphabetic Index, is a long list of **nonessential modifiers** (words in parentheses). Remember that nonessential modifiers have no effect on the main term. They are "take it or leave it" terms. Sometimes, the subterm that a coder is searching for can be found among the nonessential modifiers.

EXAMPLE | Granulomatous pneumonia is coded to 486 (J18.9).
Acute pneumonia, 486 (J18.9).
Fulminant pneumonia, 486 (J18.9). (See Figure 4-1.)

In locating the main term, the coder must remember that main terms are usually identified by disease conditions and nouns. They are not body parts or sites. If a physician documents *Klebsiella pneumoniae* pneumonia, the noun is the main term and the one to be located in the Alphabetic Index. To find *Klebsiella pneumoniae* in the Alphabetic Index, the coder goes to "pneumonia" and looks for the subterm, "*Klebsiella*" (Figure 4-2).

Subterms are modifiers of main terms, and in contrast to nonessential modifiers, they do have an effect on the appropriate code assignment. To determine the main term, the coder must decide what condition the patient has (in this case, pneumonia), which is the main term; subterms are modifiers of the main term, which in this case is *Klebsiella pneumoniae*.

EXAMPLE | If a patient has a diagnosis of hiatal hernia, the main term is "hernia," and the subterm is "hiatal."
The main terms usually are nouns and/or disease conditions. The main terms below are underlined.
Gastric <u>upset</u>
Chronic <u>mastoiditis</u>
<u>Herpes</u> simplex

EXAMPLE | The patient has a diagnosis of appendicitis, and the operative report (OR) describes the procedure as a laparoscopic appendectomy.
Look up "appendectomy" in the Alphabetic Index and the subterm "laparoscopic," 47.01. In ICD-10-PCS, look up "appendectomy," and the Index directs the user to "excision and resection." Under "resection, appendix," the user is referred to table 0DTJ.

Sometimes, a main term may be found under more than one Index entry (Figure 4-3). This is most often true of **eponyms** (a disease, syndrome, or a procedure, named for a person). Adjectives and anatomic sites do appear as main terms, but they instruct the coder to see the condition (Figure 4-4).

Main term →

Nonessential modifier →

Code for pneumonia →

Subterm →

Pneumonia (acute) (Alpenstich) (benign) (bilateral) (brain) (cerebral) (circumscribed) (congestive) (creeping) (delayed resolution) (double) (epidemic) (fever) (flash) (fulminant) (fungoid) (granulomatous) (hemorrhagic) (incipient) (infantile) (infectious) (infiltration) (insular) (intermittent) (latent) (lobe) (migratory) (newborn) (organized) (overwhelming) (primary) (progressive) (pseudolobar) (purulent) (resolved) (secondary) (senile) (septic) (suppurative) (terminal) (true) (unresolved) (vesicular) 486
with influenza, flu, or grippe 487.0
adenoviral 480.0
adynamic 514
alba 090.0
allergic 518.3
alveolar - see Pneumonia, lobar
anaerobes 482.81
anthrax 022.1 [484.5]
apex, apical - see Pneumonia, lobar
ascaris 127.0 [484.8]
aspiration 507.0
    due to
        aspiration of microorganisms
            bacterial 482.9
                specified type NEC 482.89
            specified organism NEC 483.8
                bacterial NEC 482.89
            viral 480.9
                specified type NEC 480.8
        food (regurgitated) 507.0
        gastric secretions 507.0
        milk 507.0
        oils, essences 507.1
        solids, liquids NEC 507.8
        vomitus 507.0
    fetal 770.18
        due to
            blood 770.16
            clear amniotic fluid 770.14
            meconium 770.12
            postnatal stomach contents 770.86
    newborn 770.18
        due to
            blood 770.16
            clear amniotic fluid 770.14
            meconium 770.12
            postnatal stomach contents 770.86
asthenic 514
atypical (disseminated) (focal) (primary) 486
    with influenza 487.0
bacillus 482.9
    specified type NEC 482.89
bacterial 482.9
    specified type NEC 482.89
Bacteroides (fragilis) (oralis) (melaninogenicus) 482.81
basal, basic, basilar - see Pneumonia, lobar
broncho-, bronchial (confluent) (croupous) (diffuse) (disseminated) (hemorrhagic) (involving lobes) (lobar) (terminal) 485
    with influenza 487.0
    allergic 518.3
    aspiration (see also Pneumonia, aspiration) 507.0
    bacterial 482.9
        specified type NEC 482.89
    capillary 466.19
        with bronchospasm or obstruction 466.19
    chronic (see also Fibrosis, lung) 515
    congenital (infective) 770.0
    diplococcal 481
    Eaton's agent 483.0
    Escherichia coli (E. coli) 482.82
    Friedlander's bacillus 482.0
    Haemophilus influenzae 482.2
    hiberno-vernal 083.0 [484.8]
    hypostatic 514
    influenzal 487.0
    inhalation (see also Pneumonia, aspiration) 507.0
        alveolar 507.0
            due to fumes or vapors (chemical) 506.0

Pneumonia (Continued)
    broncho- (Continued)
        Klebsiella 482.0
        lipid 507.1
            endogenous 516.8
        Mycoplasma (pneumoniae) 483.0
        ornithosis 073.0
        pleuropneumonia-like organisms (PPLO) 483.0
        pneumococcal 481
        Proteus 482.83
        Pseudomonas 482.1
        specified organism NEC 483.8
            bacterial NEC 482.89
        staphylococcal 482.40
            aureus 482.41
            specified type NEC 482.49
        streptococcal - see Pneumonia, streptococcal
        typhoid 002.0 [484.8]
        viral, virus (see also Pneumonia, viral) 480.9
    butyrivibrio (fibriosolvens) 482.81
    candida 112.4
    capillary 466.19
        with bronchospasm or obstruction 466.19
    caseous (see also Tuberculosis) 011.6
    catarrhal - see Pneumonia, broncho-
    central - see Pneumonia, lobar
    chlamydia, chlamydial 483.1
        pneumoniae 483.1
        psittaci 073.0
        specified type NEC 483.1
        trachomatis 483.1
    cholesterol 516.8
    chronic (see also Fibrosis, lung) 515
    cirrhotic (chronic) (see also Fibrosis, lung) 515
    clostridium (haemolyticum) (novyi) NEC 482.81
    confluent - see Pneumonia, broncho-
    congenital (infective) 770.0
        aspiration 770.18
    croupous - see Pneumonia, lobar
    cytomegalic inclusion 078.5 [484.1]
    deglutition (see also Pneumonia, aspiration) 507.0
    desquamative interstitial 516.8
    diffuse - see Pneumonia, broncho-
    diplococcal, diplococcus (broncho-) (lobar) 481
    disseminated (focal) - see Pneumonia, broncho-
    due to
        adenovirus 480.0
        anaerobes 482.81
        Bacterium anitratum 482.83
        Chlamydia, chlamydial 483.1
            pneumoniae 483.1
            psittaci 073.0
            specified type NEC 483.1
            trachomatis 483.1
        coccidioidomycosis 114.0
        Diplococcus (pneumoniae) 481
        Eaton's agent 483.0
        Escherichia coli (E. coli) 482.82
        Friedlander's bacillus 482.0
        fumes or vapors (chemical) (inhalation) 506.0
        fungus NEC 117.9 [484.7]
            coccidioidomycosis 114.0
        Haemophilus influenzae (H. influenzae) 482.2
        Herellea 482.83
        influenza 487.0
        Klebsiella pneumoniae 482.0
        Mycoplasma (pneumoniae) 483.0
        parainfluenza virus 480.2
        pleuropneumonia-like organism (PPLO) 483.0
        Pneumococcus 481
        Pneumocystis carinii 136.3
        Pneumocystis jiroveci 136.3
        Proteus 482.83
        Pseudomonas 482.1
        respiratory syncytial virus 480.1
        rickettsia 083.9 [484.8]
        SARS-associated coronavirus 480.3
    specified
        bacteria NEC 482.89
        organism NEC 483.8
        virus NEC 480.8

Pneumonia (Continued)
    due to (Continued)
        Staphylococcus 482.40
            aureus 482.41
            specified type NEC 482.49
        Streptococcus - see also Pneumonia, streptococcal
            pneumoniae 481
        virus (see also Pneumonia, viral) 480.9
            SARS-associated coronavirus 480.3
    Eaton's agent 483.0
    embolic, embolism (see Embolism, pulmonary)
    eosinophilic 518.3
    Escherichia coli (E. coli) 482.82
    eubacterium 482.81
    fibrinous - see Pneumonia, lobar
    fibroid (chronic) (see also Fibrosis, lung) 515
    fibrous (see also Fibrosis, lung) 515
    Friedländer's bacillus 482.0
    fusobacterium (nucleatum) 482.81
    gangrenous 513.0
    giant cell (see also Pneumonia, viral) 480.9
    gram-negative bacteria NEC 482.83
        anaerobic 482.81
    grippal 487.0
    Hemophilus influenzae (bronchial) (lobar) 482.2
    hypostatic (broncho-) (lobar) 514
    in
        actinomycosis 039.1
        anthrax 022.1 [484.5]
        aspergillosis 117.3 [484.6]
        candidiasis 112.4
        coccidioidomycosis 114.0
        cytomegalic inclusion disease 078.5 [484.1]
        histoplasmosis (see also Histoplasmosis) 115.95
        infectious disease NEC 136.9 [484.8]
        measles 055.1
        mycosis, systemic NEC 117.9 [484.7]
        nocardiasis, nocardiosis 039.1
        ornithosis 073.0
        pneumocystosis 136.3
        psittacosis 073.0
        Q fever 083.0 [484.8]
        salmonellosis 003.22
        toxoplasmosis 130.4
        tularemia 021.2
        typhoid (fever) 002.0 [484.8]
        varicella 052.1
        whooping cough (see also Whooping cough) 033.9 [484.3]
    infective, acquired prenatally 770.0
    influenzal (broncho) (lobar) (virus) 487.0
    inhalation (see also Pneumonia, aspiration) 507.0
        fumes or vapors (chemical) 506.0
    interstitial 516.8
        with influenzal 487.0
        acute 136.3
        chronic (see also Fibrosis, lung) 515
        desquamative 516.8
        hypostatic 514
        lipoid 507.1
        lymphoid 516.8
        plasma cell 136.3
        Pseudomonas 482.1
    intrauterine (infective) 770.0
        aspiration 770.18
        blood 770.16
        clear amniotic fluid 770.14
        meconium 770.12
        postnatal stomach contents 770.86
    Klebsiella pneumoniae 482.0
    Legionnaires' 482.84
    lipid, lipoid (exogenous) (interstitial) 507.1
        endogenous 516.8
    lobar (diplococcal) (disseminated) (double) (interstitial) (pneumococcal, any type) 481
        with influenza 487.0
        bacterial 482.9
            specified type NEC 482.89
        chronic (see also Fibrosis, lung) 515
        Escherichia coli (E. coli) 482.82
        Friedländer's bacillus 482.0
        Hemophilus influenzae (H. influenzae) 482.2
        hypostatic 514
        influenzal 487.0

Pneumonia (Continued)
    lobar (Continued)
        Klebsiella 482.0
        ornithosis 073.0
        Proteus 482.83
        Pseudomonas 482.1
        psittacosis 073.0
        specified organism NEC 483.8
            bacterial NEC 482.89
        staphylococcal 482.40
            aureus 482.41
            specified type NEC 482.49
        streptococcal - see Pneumonia, streptococcal
        viral, virus (see also Pneumonia, viral) 480.9
    lobular (confluent) - see Pneumonia, broncho-
    Löffler's 518.3
    massive - see Pneumonia, lobar
    meconium aspiration 770.12
    metastatic NEC 038.8 [484.8]
    Mycoplasma (pneumoniae) 483.0
    necrotic 513.0
    nitrogen dioxide 506.9
    orthostatic 514
    parainfluenza virus 480.2
    parenchymatous (see also Fibrosis, lung) 515
    passive 514
    patchy - see Pneumonia, broncho
    Peptococcus 482.81
    Peptostreptococcus 482.81
    plasma cell 136.3
    pleurolobar - see Pneumonia, lobar
    pleuropneumonia-like organism (PPLO) 483.0
    pneumococcal (broncho) (lobar) 481
    Pneumocystis (carinii) (jiroveci) 136.3
    postinfectional NEC 136.9 [484.8]
    postmeasles 055.1
    postoperative 997.3
    primary atypical 486
    Proprionibacterium 482.81
    Proteus 482.83
    Pseudomonas 482.1
    psittacosis 073.0
    radiation 508.0
    respiratory syncytial virus 480.1
    resulting from a procedure 997.3
    rheumatic 390 [517.1]
    Salmonella 003.22
    SARS-associated coronavirus 480.3
    segmented, segmental - see Pneumonia, broncho-
    Serratia (marcascens) 482.83
    specified
        bacteria NEC 482.89
        organism NEC 483.8
        virus NEC 480.8
    spirochetal 104.8 [484]
    staphylococcal (broncho) (lobar) 482.40
        aureus 482.41
        specified type NEC 482.49
    static, stasis 514
    streptococcal (broncho) (lobar) NEC 482.30
        Group
            A 482.31
            B 482.32
            specified NEC 482.39
        pneumoniae 481
        specified type NEC 482.39
    Streptococcus pneumoniae 481
    traumatic (complication) (early) (secondary) 958.8
    tuberculous (any) (see also Tuberculosis) 011.6
    tularemic 021.2
    TWAR agent 483.1
    varicella 052.1
    Veillonella 482.81
    viral, virus (broncho) (interstitial) (lobar) 480.9
        with influenza, flu, or grippe 487.0
        adenoviral 480.0
        parainfluenza 480.2
        respiratory syncytial 480.1
        SARS-associated coronavirus 480.3
        specified type NEC 480.8
    white (congenital) 090.0

FIGURE 4-1. Alphabetic Index entry for "pneumonia."

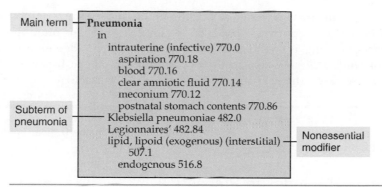

FIGURE 4-2. Example of subterm "Klebsiella," under "pneumonia."

FIGURE 4-3. Example of multiple Alphabetic Index entries for Meckel's diverticulum.

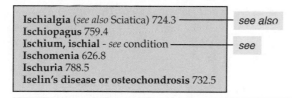

FIGURE 4-4. Example of an anatomic site instructing coder to *see* condition and an instruction to *see also*.

EXAMPLE | Diagnosis of ischial fracture: The Index for "ischial" would direct the coder to go to the condition or, in this case, fracture.
Ischium, ischial—*see* condition

EXAMPLE | Chronic otitis media—look up "chronic" in the Alphabetic Index
Chronic—*see* condition

The term "*see*" is a mandatory direction to look elsewhere in the Alphabetic Index.

Sometimes, the Index will direct the coder to *see also*. This instruction means that if the term cannot be located under the Index entry, the user should go to the *see also* suggested Index entry.

The general rule that main terms identify disease conditions has some exceptions. Some of these exceptions are V/Z codes, which can be found under main terms such as "admission," "examination," and "status." These will be fully covered in Chapter 8 on V/Z codes. Likewise, obstetric conditions can be found under main terms such as "pregnancy," "labor," and "puerperal" and will be covered in Chapter 21 in the section on obstetrics and gynecology. There is also a main term for late effects that can be used to identify residuals of various disease conditions and complications.

Locating a main term may be difficult because of the terminology used by the physician or because an eponym is used. For example, physicians often describe arterial lines used for monitoring as Swan Ganz (pulmonary capillary wedge monitoring). If the user were to look under "Swan Ganz" in the procedural Alphabetic Index, no listing would be found. In these cases, the user should try alternative terminology.

EXAMPLE   Swan Ganz is a pulmonary artery catheter. Try looking under "Catherization, Swan Ganz" in the procedure Alphabetic Index, 89.64. In ICD-10-PCS, "catherization, heart" directs the user to see "measurement" cardiac 4A02.

Locate the Main Term in the Index to Procedures

Just as in diagnoses, once a procedure is determined to have been performed, a coder searches for that procedure in the Alphabetic Index to Procedures. The main terms for procedures are identified by the type of procedure performed and not by the anatomic site. When one is having trouble locating a procedure, it is wise to remember that many procedures can be found under the terms, "excision," "incision," or "removal."

EXAMPLE   <u>Removal</u> of a skin lesion on the back, 86.3 (OHB6XZZ) (Figure 4-5). To locate removal of a skin lesion in ICD-10-CM, locate "excision, skin" in the Alphabetic Index. This entry refers the user to table OHB.

EXAMPLE   Needle <u>biopsy</u> of the liver, 50.11 (OFBO3ZX) (Figure 4-6).

EXERCISE 4-2

Underline all main terms to be located in the Alphabetic Index.

1. Esophageal reflux
2. Tourette's disease
3. Iatrogenic thyroiditis
4. Infantile eczema
5. Coronary artery disease
6. Congestive heart failure
7. Rheumatoid arthritis
8. Atrial fibrillation
9. Sickle cell anemia
10. Coronary artery bypass, one-vessel
11. Inguinal hernia repair
12. Excision herniated disc
13. Balloon angioplasty
14. Open reduction internal fixation
15. Vaginal hysterectomy
16. Calculus of the ureter

TABULAR LIST

Once the code has been selected from the Alphabetic Index, it must then be verified in the **Tabular List**. Sometimes, a code that is selected from the Alphabetic Index does not seem to match what is described in the Tabular List. If this is the case, the user should review the Alphabetic Index and the Tabular List for all exclusion notes and other instructional notes. It may require that the user browse the category in the Tabular List for a more

Excision *(Continued)*
  lesion *(Continued)*
    odontogenic 24.4
    omentum 54.4
    orbit 16.92
    ovary 65.29
      by wedge resection 65.22
        laparoscopic 65.24
      that by laparoscope 65.25
    palate (bony) 27.31
      by wide excision 27.32
      soft 27.49
    pancreas (local) 52.22
      endoscopic 52.21
    parathyroid 06.89
    parotid gland or duct NEC 26.29
    pelvic wall 54.3
    pelvirectal tissue 48.82
    penis 64.2
    pericardium 37.31
    perineum (female) 71.3
      male 86.3
    periprostatic tissue 60.82
    perirectal tissue 48.82
    perirenal tissue 59.91
    peritoneum 54.4
    perivesical tissue 59.91
    pharynx 29.3
      diverticulum 29.32
    pineal gland 07.53
    pinna 18.29
      radical 18.31
    pituitary (gland) - *see?also*Hypophy-
      sectomy, partial 07.63
      by stereotactic radiosurgery
        92.30
        cobalt 60 92.32
        linear accelerator (LINAC)
          92.31
        multi-source 92.32

Excision *(Continued)*
  lesion *(Continued)*
    particle beam 92.33
    particulate 92.33
    radiosurgery NEC 92.39
    single source photon 92.31
    pleura 34.59
    pouch of Douglas 70.32
    preauricular (ear) 18.21
    presacral 54.4
    prostate (transurethral) 60.61
    pulmonary (fibrosis) 32.29
      endoscopic 32.28
    rectovaginal septum 48.82
    rectum 48.35
      polyp (endoscopic) 48.36
    retroperitoneum 54.4
    salivary gland or duct NEC 26.29
      en bloc 26.32
    sclera 12.84
    scrotum 61.3
    sinus (nasal) - *see* Excision, lesion,
      nasal sinus
    Skene's gland 71.3
    skin 86.3 ──────── Excision
      breast 85.21   lesion skin
      nose 21.32
      radical (wide) (involving underly-
        ing or adjacent structure) (with
        flap closure) 86.4
      scrotum 61.3
    skull 01.6
    soft tissue NEC 83.39
      hand 82.29
    spermatic cord 63.3
    sphincter of Oddi 51.62
      endoscopic 51.64
    spinal cord (meninges) 03.4
    spleen (cyst) 41.42
    stomach NEC 43.42

Excision *(Continued)*
  lesion *(Continued)*
    endoscopic 43.41
      polyp 43.41
    polyp (endoscopic) 43.41
    subcutaneous tissue 86.3
      breast 85.21
    subgingival 24.31
    sweat gland 86.3
    tendon 83.39
      hand 82.29
      ocular 15.13
      sheath 83.31
        hand 82.21
    testis 62.2
    thorax 34.4
    thymus 07.81
    thyroid 06.31
      substernal or transsternal route
        06.51
    tongue 25.1
    tonsil 28.92
    trachea 31.5
    tunica vaginalis 61.92
    ureter 56.41
    urethra 58.39
      endoscopic 58.31
    uterine ligament 69.19
    uterosacral ligament 69.19
    uterus 68.29
    vagina 70.33
    vein 38.60
      abdominal 38.67
      head and neck NEC 38.62
      intracranial NEC 38.61
      lower limb 38.69
      thoracic NEC 38.65
      upper limb 38.63
    ventricle (heart) 37.33
    vocal cords 30.09
    vulva 71.3

FIGURE 4-5. Example from entry for "excision, skin lesion" in the Index to Procedures.

representative code. It also may require that the user access *Coding Clinic* for any advice on how to code a specific diagnosis.

EXAMPLE

Documentation in the chart describes the patient as having anorexia. She has been admitted to the psychiatric unit of the hospital.
Look up "Anorexia" in the Alphabetic Index, 783.0 (R63.0).
Go to the Tabular List and review the Excludes notes.
    Because this is a psychiatric admission, reviewing the codes excluded may assist in assigning the correct code.

EXAMPLE

The diagnosis is stated as arteriovenous malformation of the intestine.
Look under "Malformation, colon" in the Alphabetic Index.
This directs the coder to "*see also* Anomaly."
"Anomaly, colon" directs the coder to 751.5 (Q43.9).
    Look up 751.5 in the Tabular, and decide whether this appears to be the correct code.
Look up "arteriovenous malformation" in *Coding Clinic*.
    Coding Clinic (1986:Nov-Dec:p11)[1] directs the coder to use "557.1, Chronic vascular insufficiency of intestine (K55.9)."

Needle biopsy liver

Biopsy (Continued)
joint structure (aspiration) (Continued)
  hand and finger 80.34
  hip 80.35
  knee 80.36
  shoulder 80.31
  specified site NEC 80.39
  spine 80.39
  wrist 80.33
kidney 55.23
  closed 55.23
  open 55.24
  percutaneous (aspiration) (needle) 55.23
labia 71.11
lacrimal
  gland 09.11
  sac 09.12
larynx 31.43
  brush 31.43
  closed (endoscopic) 31.43
  open 31.45
lip 27.23
liver 50.11
  closed 50.11
  laparoscopic 50.19
  open 50.12
  percutaneous (aspiration) (needle) 50.11
lung NEC 33.27
  brush 33.24
  closed (percutaneous) (needle) 33.26
    brush 33.24
    endoscopic 33.27
     brush 33.24
  endoscopic 33.27
    brush 33.24
  open 33.28
  transbronchial 33.27
lymphatic structure (channel) (node) (vessel) 40.11
mediastinum NEC 34.25
  closed 34.25
  open 34.26
  percutaneous (needle) 34.25
meninges (cerebral) NEC 01.11
  closed 01.11
  open 01.12
  percutaneous (needle) 01.11
  spinal 03.32
mesentery 54.23
mouth NEC 27.24

Biopsy (Continued)
muscle 83.21
  extraocular 15.01
  ocular 15.01
nasopharynx 29.12
nerve (cranial) (peripheral) NEC 04.11
  closed 04.11
  open 04.12
  percutaneous (needle) 04.11
  sympathetic 05.11
nose, nasal 21.22
  sinus 22.11
    closed (endoscopic) (needle) 22.11
    open 22.12
ocular muscle or tendon 15.01
omentum
  closed 54.24
  open 54.23
  percutaneous (needle) 54.24
orbit 16.23
  by aspiration 16.22
ovary 65.12
  by aspiration 65.11
  laparoscopic 65.13
palate (bony) 27.21
  soft 27.22
pancreas 52.11
  closed (endoscopic) 52.11
  open 52.12
  percutaneous (aspiration) (needle) 52.11
pancreatic duct 52.14
  closed (endoscopic) 52.14
parathyroid gland 06.13
penis 64.11
perianal tissue 49.22
pericardium 37.24
periprostatic 60.15
perirectal tissue 48.26
perirenal tissue 59.21
peritoneal implant
  closed 54.24
  open 54.23
  percutaneous (needle) 54.24
peritoneum
  closed 54.24
  open 54.23
  percutaneous (needle) 54.24
periurethral tissue 58.24
perivesical tissue 59.21
pharynx, pharyngeal 29.12

Biopsy (Continued)
pineal gland 07.17
pituitary gland 07.15
  transfrontal approach 07.13
  transsphenoidal approach 07.14
pleura, pleural 34.24
prostate NEC 60.11
  closed (transurethral) 60.11
  open 60.12
  percutaneous (needle) 60.11
  transrectal 60.11
rectum 48.24
  brush 48.24
  closed (endoscopic) 48.24
  open 48.25
retroperitoneal tissue 54.24
salivary gland or duct 26.11
  closed (needle) 26.11
  open 26.12
scrotum 61.11
seminal vesicle NEC 60.13
  closed 60.13
  open 60.14
  percutaneous (needle) 60.13
sigmoid colon 45.25
  brush 45.25
  closed (endoscopic) 45.25
  open 45.26
sinus, nasal 22.11
  closed (endoscopic) (needle) 22.11
  open 22.12
skin (punch) 86.11
skull 01.15
soft palate 27.22
soft tissue NEC 83.21
spermatic cord 63.01
sphincter of Oddi 51.14
  closed (endoscopic) 51.14
  open 51.13
spinal cord (meninges) 03.32
spleen 41.32
  closed 41.32
  open 41.33
  percutaneous (aspiration) (needle) 41.32
stomach 44.14
  brush 44.14
  closed (endoscopic) 44.14
  open 44.15
subcutaneous tissue (punch) 86.11
supraglottic mass 29.12
sympathetic nerve 05.11

Biopsy (Continued)
tendon 83.21
  extraocular 15.01
  ocular 15.01
testis NEC 62.11
  closed 62.11
  open 62.12
  percutaneous (needle) 62.11
thymus 07.16
thyroid gland NEC 06.11
  closed 06.11
  open 06.12
  percutaneous (aspiration) (needle) 06.11
    tongue 25.01
  closed (needle) 25.01
  open 25.02
tonsil 28.11
trachea 31.44
  brush 31.44
  closed (endoscopic) 31.44
  open 31.45
tunica vaginalis 61.11
umbilicus 54.22
ureter 56.33
  closed (percutaneous) 56.32
    endoscopic 56.33
  open 56.34
  transurethral 56.33
urethra 58.23
uterus, uterine (endometrial) 68.16
  by
    aspiration curettage 69.59
    dilation and curettage 69.09
  closed (endoscopic) 68.16
  ligaments 68.15
    closed (endoscopic) 68.15
    open 68.14
  open 68.13
uvula 27.22
vagina 70.24
vas deferens 63.01
vein (any site) 38.21
vulva 71.11

FIGURE 4-6. Example from the entry for "needle, biopsy liver" in the Index to Procedures.

The rule of never coding directly from the Alphabetic Index without reviewing the Tabular also applies to never coding from instructional notes within the Tabular without first reviewing the actual Tabular Listing of the code.

EXAMPLE The instructional notes found in category 601 (N41) recommend the use of an additional code to identify the organism Staph (041.1) or Strep (041.0) (B95-B97). If these codes were captured without review of the Tabular, an invalid code would be assigned because both require fifth digits.

CHAPTER REVIEW EXERCISE

Using the Alphabetic Index and the Tabular List, code all the following diagnoses and procedures.

1. Acute subendocardial infarction, initial episode of care _____
2. *Clostridium difficile* enteritis _____
3. Refractory megaloblastic anemia _____
4. Acute suppurative appendicitis with laparoscopic appendectomy _____
5. Stage 3 pressure ulcer of the sacrum treated with excisional debridement _____
6. Abdominal aortic aneurysm _____
7. Small-bowel obstruction treated with left hemicolectomy _____
8. Intractable epilepsy with status epilepticus _____
9. Paroxysmal supraventricular tachycardia _____
10. Streptococcal group A pneumonia _____
11. Deep vein thrombosis of the right femoral vein _____
12. Acute congenital syphilitic laryngotracheitis, 40 years old _____
13. Dysphagia as a late effect of a stroke _____
14. Adhesive bursitis of the right shoulder _____
15. History of cardiovascular disease in the family _____

CHAPTER GLOSSARY

Admitting diagnosis: the condition that requires the patient to be hospitalized.

Alphabetic Index: the index found in the ICD-9-CM book for both disease conditions and procedures.

Chief complaint: the reason, in the patient's own words, for presenting to the hospital.

Differential diagnosis: when a symptom may represent a variety of diagnoses.

Discharge summary: a review of the patient's hospital course. This summary details the reason for admission or tests or procedures performed and how the patient responded.

Eponym: term for a disease, structure, procedure, or syndrome that has been named for a person.

Main term: term that identifies disease conditions or injuries; it is identified in bold print and set flush with the left margin of each column in the Alphabetic Index.

Nonessential modifier: term that is enclosed in parentheses; its presence or absence does not affect code assignment.

Principal diagnosis: condition established after study to be chiefly responsible for occasioning admission of the patient to the hospital for care.

Subterm: gives more specific information about a main term. Subterms identify site, type, or etiology of a disease condition or injury. Also, modifiers that are indented to the right of the main term.

Tabular List: section of the ICD-9-CM book that contains the code listing, along with exclusion or inclusion notes.

REFERENCE

1. American Hospital Association. *Coding Clinic for ICD-9-CM* 1986:Nov-Dec:p11. Arteriovenous (A-V) malformation of colon.

5

General Coding Guidelines for Diagnosis

CHAPTER OUTLINE
ICD-9-CM Official Guidelines for Coding and Reporting
General Coding Guidelines
Late Effects
Present on Admission
ICD-10-CM Official Guidelines for Coding and Reporting
Chapter Review Exercise
Chapter Glossary
Reference

LEARNING OBJECTIVES
1. Apply ICD-9-CM and ICD-10-CM Official Guidelines for Coding and Reporting
2. Sequence ICD-9-CM and ICD-10-CM diagnosis codes as directed by coding guidelines or ICD-9-CM and ICD-10-CM conventions
3. Determine whether signs, symptoms, or manifestations require separate code assignments
4. Assign ICD-9-CM and ICD-10-CM diagnosis codes for late effects

ABBREVIATIONS/ ACRONYMS

AHA American Hospital Association

AHIMA American Health Information Management Association

CABG coronary artery bypass graft

CMS Centers for Medicare and Medicaid Services

DHHS U.S. Department of Health and Human Services

DRA Deficit Reduction Act

GPO Government Printing Office

HAC hospital acquired condition

HIPAA Health Insurance Portability and Accountability Act

ICD-9-CM *International Classification of Diseases, 9th Revision, Clinical Modification*

ICD-10-CM *International Classification of Diseases, 10th Revision, Clinical Modification*

ICD-10-PCS *International Classification of Diseases, 10th Revision, Procedure Coding System*

NCHS National Center for Health Statistics

POA present on admission

ICD-9-CM OFFICIAL GUIDELINES FOR CODING AND REPORTING

The ICD-9-CM Official Guidelines for Coding and Reporting were developed by the cooperating parties to provide further guidance regarding coding and sequencing that is not provided in the ICD-9-CM manual. These guidelines do not cover every situation and have been formatted in a manner that will allow for expansion as new guidelines are developed. The guidelines may be changed each year, and changes may have greater impact in some years than in others.

In this chapter, the coder will review the general guidelines and coding examples as applicable. The convention guidelines with examples were presented in Chapter 3, "ICD-9-CM, Format and Conventions." Chapter-specific guidelines are provided and explained in the respective disease or body system chapter.

Official Guidelines for Coding and Reporting

Please refer to the companion Evolve website for the most current guidelines.

Effective October 1, 2010

Narrative changes appear in bold text

Items underlined have been moved within the guidelines since October 1, 2009

The Centers for Medicare and Medicaid Services (CMS) and the National Center for Health Statistics (NCHS), two departments within the U.S. Federal Government's Department of Health and Human Services (DHHS) provide the following guidelines for coding and reporting using the International Classification of Diseases, 9th Revision, Clinical Modification (ICD-9-CM). These guidelines should be used as a companion document to the official version of the ICD-9-CM as published on CD-ROM by the U.S. Government Printing Office (GPO).

These guidelines have been approved by the four organizations that make up the Cooperating Parties for the ICD-9-CM: the American Hospital Association (AHA), the American Health Information Management Association (AHIMA), CMS, and NCHS. These guidelines are included on the official government version of the ICD-9-CM, and also appear in "*Coding Clinic for ICD-9-CM*" published by the AHA.

These guidelines are a set of rules that have been developed to accompany and complement the official conventions and instructions provided within the ICD-9-CM itself. The instructions and conventions of the classification take precedence over guidelines. These guidelines are based on the coding and sequencing instructions in Volumes I, II and III of ICD-9-CM, but provide additional instruction. Adherence to these guidelines when assigning ICD-9-CM diagnosis and procedure codes is required under the Health Insurance Portability and Accountability Act (HIPAA). The diagnosis codes (Volumes 1-2) have been adopted under HIPAA for all healthcare settings. Volume 3 procedure codes have been adopted for inpatient procedures reported by hospitals. A joint effort between the healthcare provider and the coder is essential to achieve complete and accurate documentation, code assignment, and reporting of diagnoses and procedures. These guidelines have been developed to assist both the healthcare provider and the coder in identifying those diagnoses and procedures that are to be reported. The importance of consistent, complete documentation in the medical record cannot be overemphasized. Without such documentation accurate coding cannot be achieved. The entire record should be reviewed to determine the specific reason for the encounter and the conditions treated.

The term encounter is used for all settings, including hospital admissions. In the context of these guidelines, the term provider is used throughout the guidelines to mean physician or any qualified health care practitioner who is legally accountable for establishing the patient's diagnosis. Only this set of guidelines, approved by the Cooperating Parties, is official.

The guidelines are organized into sections. Section I includes the structure and conventions of the classification and general guidelines that apply to the entire classification, and chapter-specific guidelines that correspond to the chapters as they are arranged in the classification. Section II includes guidelines for selection of principal diagnosis for non-outpatient settings. Section III includes guidelines for reporting additional diagnoses in non-outpatient settings. Section IV is for outpatient coding and reporting.

GENERAL CODING GUIDELINES

General coding guidelines apply to all healthcare settings and to the entire ICD-9-CM and ICD-10-CM classification systems.

Section I. Conventions, general coding guidelines and chapter specific guidelines
  B. General Coding Guidelines
    1. Use of Both Alphabetic Index and Tabular List
      Use both the Alphabetic Index and the Tabular List when locating and assigning a code. Reliance on only the Alphabetic Index or the Tabular List leads to errors in code assignments and less specificity in code selection.

Threatened
    abortion or miscarriage 640.0
        with subsequent abortion (*see also*
            Abortion, spontaneous) 634.9
        affecting fetus 762.1
    labor 644.1
        affecting fetus or newborn 761.8
        premature 644.0
    miscarriage 640.0 ←
        affecting fetus 762.1
    premature
        delivery 644.2
            affecting fetus or newborn 761.8
        labor 644.0
            before 22 completed weeks of
                gestation 640.0

FIGURE 5-1. Alphabetic Index entry for "threatened miscarriage."

EXAMPLE

Patient presents with threatened miscarriage. She is discharged home the next day with viable pregnancy. Threatened miscarriage: Under the main term "threatened" and the subterm "miscarriage" in the Alphabetic Index, code 640.0 is listed. If the coder were to assign this code, it would be an invalid code. Verification in the Tabular List reveals that a fifth digit is required. The correct code assignment for "threatened miscarriage" is 640.03. (See Figures 5-1 and 5-2.)

2. Locate each term in the Alphabetic Index

Locate each term in the Alphabetic Index and verify the code selected in the Tabular List. Read and be guided by instructional notations that appear in both the Alphabetic Index and the Tabular List. (See Figures 5-3 and 5-4.)

Instructional notes can be found in all three volumes. It is important to review the Tabular code category for notes that may apply to the entire category. These notes can be found at the beginning of a chapter, section, code category, or individual code classification. For additional details on various instructional notes, refer to Chapter 3 in this text.

3. Level of Detail in Coding

Diagnosis and procedure codes are to be used at their highest number of digits available.

ICD-9-CM diagnosis codes are composed of codes with either 3, 4, or 5 digits. Codes with three digits are included in ICD-9-CM as the heading of a category of codes that may be further subdivided by the use of fourth and/or fifth digits, which provide greater detail.

A three-digit code is to be used only if it is not further subdivided. Where fourth-digit subcategories and/or fifth-digit subclassifications are provided, they must be assigned. A code is invalid if it has not been coded to the full number of digits required for that code. For example, Acute myocardial infarction, code 410, has fourth digits that describe the location of the infarction (e.g., 410.2, Of inferolateral wall), and fifth digits that identify the episode of care. It would be incorrect to report a code in category 410 without a fourth and fifth digit.

ICD-9-CM Volume 3 procedure codes are composed of codes with either 3 or 4 digits. Codes with two digits are included in ICD-9-CM as the heading of a category of codes that may be further subdivided by the use of third and/or fourth digits, which provide greater detail.

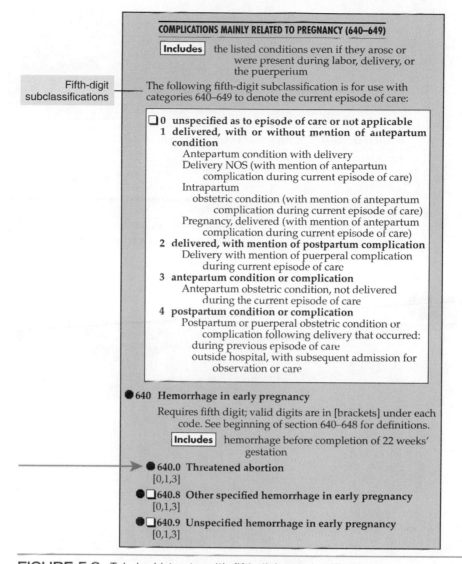

Fifth-digit subclassifications

COMPLICATIONS MAINLY RELATED TO PREGNANCY (640–649)

Includes the listed conditions even if they arose or
were present during labor, delivery, or
the puerperium

The following fifth-digit subclassification is for use with
categories 640–649 to denote the current episode of care:

☐ 0 **unspecified as to episode of care or not applicable**
  1 **delivered, with or without mention of antepartum**
    condition
      Antepartum condition with delivery
      Delivery NOS (with mention of antepartum
        complication during current episode of care)
      Intrapartum
        obstetric condition (with mention of antepartum
          complication during current episode of care)
      Pregnancy, delivered (with mention of antepartum
        complication during current episode of care)
  2 **delivered, with mention of postpartum complication**
      Delivery with mention of puerperal complication
        during current episode of care
  3 **antepartum condition or complication**
      Antepartum obstetric condition, not delivered
        during the current episode of care
  4 **postpartum condition or complication**
      Postpartum or puerperal obstetric condition or
        complication following delivery that occurred:
        during previous episode of care
        outside hospital, with subsequent admission for
          observation or care

● **640 Hemorrhage in early pregnancy**

  Requires fifth digit; valid digits are in [brackets] under each
  code. See beginning of section 640–648 for definitions.

  Includes hemorrhage before completion of 22 weeks'
     gestation

● **640.0 Threatened abortion**
  [0,1,3]

●☐**640.8 Other specified hemorrhage in early pregnancy**
  [0,1,3]

●☐**640.9 Unspecified hemorrhage in early pregnancy**
  [0,1,3]

FIGURE 5-2. Tabular List entry with fifth-digit subclassifications.

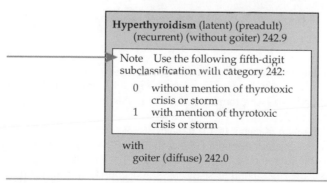

Hyperthyroidism (latent) (preadult)
  (recurrent) (without goiter) 242.9

Note Use the following fifth-digit
subclassification with category 242:

  0 without mention of thyrotoxic
     crisis or storm
  1 with mention of thyrotoxic
     crisis or storm

with
  goiter (diffuse) 242.0

FIGURE 5-3. Instructional note from Alphabetic Index.

> **15. CERTAIN CONDITIONS ORIGINATING IN THE PERINATAL PERIOD (760–779)**
>
> **Includes:** conditions which have their origin in the perinatal period, before birth through the first 28 days after birth, even though death or morbidity occurs later
>
> Use additional code(s) to further specify condition

FIGURE 5-4. Instructional notes from Tabular List.

EXAMPLE

Bronchitis, 490 (three-digit code) (J40).
Chronic bronchitis, 491.9 (four-digit code) (J42).
Emphysematous bronchitis, 491.20 (five-digit code) (J44.9).

EXERCISE 5-1

Using the Alphabetic Index and the Tabular List, assign the appropriate code(s).

1. Status asthmaticus
   Code from Alphabetic Index _____
   Code following verification in Tabular List _____

2. Hairy cell leukemia in remission
   Code from Alphabetic Index _____
   Code following verification in Tabular List _____

3. Closed fracture humerus
   Code from Alphabetic Index _____
   Code following verification in Tabular List _____

4. Epilepsy
   Code from Alphabetic Index _____
   Code following verification in Tabular List _____

5. Right upper quadrant pain
   Code from Alphabetic Index _____
   Code following verification in Tabular List _____

4. **Code or codes from 001.0 through V91.99**
   The appropriate code or codes from 001.0 through **V91.99** must be used to identify diagnoses, symptoms, conditions, problems, complaints, or other reason(s) for the encounter/visit.

5. **Selection of codes 001.0 through 999.9**
   The selection of codes 001.0 through 999.9 will frequently be used to describe the reason for the admission/encounter. These codes are from the section of ICD-9-CM for the classification of diseases and injuries (e.g., infectious and parasitic diseases; neoplasms; symptoms, signs, and ill-defined conditions, etc.).

6. **Signs and symptoms**
   Codes that describe symptoms and signs, as opposed to diagnoses, are acceptable for reporting purposes when a related definitive diagnosis has not been established (confirmed) by the provider. Chapter 16 of ICD-9-CM, Symptoms, Signs, and Ill-defined conditions (codes 780.0-799.9) contain many, but not all codes for symptoms.

EXAMPLE | Pyrexia of unknown origin, 780.60 (R50.9).

7. Conditions that are an integral part of a disease process
Signs and symptoms that are associated routinely with a disease process should not be assigned as additional codes, unless otherwise instructed by the classification.

EXAMPLE | Hematuria due to calculus of kidney, 592.0 (N20.0).
Code 599.70 (R31.9) for "hematuria" would not be assigned because hematuria is integral to a kidney stone. According to *Coding Clinic* (1995:3Q:p8),[1] "hematuria is a usual finding in a patient with renal stones and is considered integral to the condition."

8. Conditions that are not an integral part of a disease process
Additional signs and symptoms that may not be associated routinely with a disease process should be coded when present.

EXAMPLE | Ascites due to cirrhosis of the liver, 571.5, 789.59 (K74.60, R18.8).

Chapter 16 of ICD-9-CM contains most but not all codes used to identify signs and symptoms (780.0 to 799.9).
Signs and symptoms codes are acceptable to code:
- When no definitive diagnosis has been established
- When they are not an integral part of the disease process
- When directed by the classification to assign an additional code

It is not acceptable to code signs or symptoms:
- When a definitive diagnosis has been established
- When they are an integral part of the disease process

EXERCISE 5-2

Identify integral and nonintegral conditions by answering the following questions.

1. List two common symptoms of gallstones. _____
2. List the symptom most commonly associated with costochondritis. _____
3. List two common symptoms of urinary tract infection. _____
4. A patient has osteoarthritis and anemia. The anemia is integral to the osteoarthritis.
   A. True
   B. False
5. A patient has dyspnea caused by congestive heart failure. Dyspnea should be assigned as an additional code.
   A. True
   B. False

> ● **590 Infections of kidney**
>   Use additional code to identify organism, such as
>   Escherichia coli [E. coli] (041.41–041.49)

FIGURE 5-5. Instruction to "Use additional code" if applicable.

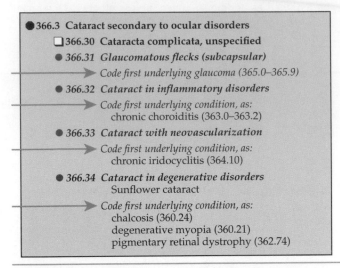

FIGURE 5-6. Examples of "Code first" instructions.

9. Multiple coding for a single condition

In addition to the etiology/manifestation convention that requires two codes to fully describe a single condition that affects multiple body systems, there are other single conditions that also require more than one code. "Use additional code" notes (Figure 5-5) are found in the tabular at codes that are not part of an etiology/manifestation pair where a secondary code is useful to fully describe a condition. The sequencing rule is the same as the etiology/manifestation pair—, "use additional code" indicates that a secondary code should be added.

For example, for infections that are not included in chapter 1, a secondary code from category 041, Bacterial infection in conditions classified elsewhere and of unspecified site, may be required to identify the bacterial organism causing the infection. A "use additional code" note will normally be found at the infectious disease code, indicating a need for the organism code to be added as a secondary code.

EXAMPLE Acute pyelonephritis due to *Escherichia coli (E. coli)*, 590.10, 041.49 (N10, B96.2).

"Code first" notes (Figure 5-6) are also under certain codes that are not specifically manifestation codes but may be due to an underlying cause. When a "code first" note is present and an underlying condition is present the underlying condition should be sequenced first.

"Code, if applicable, any causal condition first", notes indicate that this code may be assigned as a principal diagnosis when the causal condition is unknown or not applicable. If a causal condition is known, then the code for that condition should be sequenced as the principal or first-listed diagnosis.

EXAMPLE Chronic pyelonephritis due to vesicoureteral reflux, 593.70, 590.00 (N11.0).

Pancreatitis 577.0
★ acute (edematous) (hemorrhagic) (re-
        current) 577.0
    annular 577.0
    apoplectic 577.0
    calcereous 577.0
★ chronic (infectious) 577.1
        recurrent 577.1
    cystic 577.2
    fibrous 577.8
    gangrenous 577.0

Acute and chronic are at the same indention level

FIGURE 5-7. Subterms for acute and chronic at the same indention level.

Multiple codes may be needed for late effects, complication codes and obstetric codes to more fully describe a condition. See the specific guidelines for these conditions for further instruction.

10. Acute and Chronic Conditions

If the same condition is described as both acute (subacute) and chronic, and separate subentries exist in the Alphabetic Index at the same indentation level (Figure 5-7), code both and sequence the acute (subacute) code first.

EXAMPLE Acute and chronic pancreatitis, 577.0, 577.1 (K85.9, K86.1).

EXAMPLE Acute and chronic cholecystitis, 575.12 (K81.2).
Separate subterms are included for "acute" and "chronic," but a subterm for "acute and chronic" is also provided.

EXAMPLE Acute and chronic otitis media, 382.9 (H66.90).
Separate subterms are provided for "acute" and "chronic," but they use the same code.

EXERCISE 5-3

Assign and sequence codes to the following conditions.

1. Subacute and chronic appendicitis _____
2. Acute and chronic bronchitis _____
3. Acute and chronic pyelonephritis _____
4. Acute on chronic renal failure _____
5. Acute on chronic respiratory failure _____

11. Combination Code

A combination code is a single code used to classify:
Two diagnoses, or
A diagnosis with an associated secondary process (manifestation)
A diagnosis with an associated complication

Combination codes are identified by referring to subterm entries in the Alphabetic Index and by reading the inclusion and exclusion notes in the Tabular List.

Assign only the combination code when that code fully identifies the diagnostic conditions involved or when the Alphabetic Index so directs. Multiple coding should not be used when the classification provides a combination code that clearly identifies all of the elements documented in the diagnosis. When the combination code lacks necessary specificity in describing the manifestation or complication, an additional code should be used as a secondary code.

EXAMPLE

Pseudomonas pneumonia, 482.1 (J15.1).
    The combination code includes the infection and the organism responsible for the infection (*Pseudomonas*). It would be incorrect to assign separate codes such as 486 (J18.9) for pneumonia and 041.7 (B96.5) to identify the *Pseudomonas* organism.

EXERCISE 5-4

Assign codes to the following conditions.

1. Urinary tract infection due to candidiasis   _____
2. Streptococcal group A pneumonia   _____
3. Food poisoning due to *Salmonella*   _____

12. Late Effects

A late effect is the residual effect (condition produced) after the acute phase of an illness or injury has terminated. There is no time limit on when a late effect code can be used. The residual may be apparent early, such as in cerebrovascular accident cases, or it may occur months or years later, such as that due to a previous injury. Coding of late effects generally requires two codes sequenced in the following order: The condition or nature of the late effect is sequenced first. The late effect code is sequenced second.

EXAMPLE

Paraplegia due to traumatic spinal cord injury (lumbar) suffered in a motor vehicle accident 3 years ago, 344.1 (residual), 907.2 (cause, late effect code), E929.0 (late effect E code) (G82.20, S34.109S, V89.2xxS).

An exception to the above guidelines are those instances where the code for late effect is followed by a manifestation code identified in the Tabular List and title, or the late effect code has been expanded (at the fourth and fifth-digit levels) to include the manifestation(s). The code for the acute phase of an illness or injury that led to the late effect is never used with a code for the late effect.

EXAMPLE

Aphasia due to cerebrovascular accident 4 months ago, 438.11 (I69.320). Includes the residual, aphasia, and describes the cause, cerebrovascular accident.

EXAMPLE

Scoliosis (neuromuscular) due to past history of poliomyelitis, 138, 737.43 (M41.40, B91).
    This is an example of the exception to sequencing the residual first. In the Alphabetic Index, under the main term "scoliosis" and the subterm "due to poliomyelitis," the 138 (cause) is listed first with the scoliosis code 737.43 in brackets. This means that 138 must be sequenced first (Figure 5-8).

13. Impending or Threatened Condition

Code any condition described at the time of discharge as "impending" or "threatened" as follows:
If it did occur, code as confirmed diagnosis.
If it did not occur, reference the Alphabetic Index to determine if the condition has a subentry term for "impending" or "threatened" and also reference main term entries for "Impending" and for "Threatened."
If the subterms are listed, assign the given code.
If the subterms are not listed, code the existing underlying condition(s) and not the condition described as impending or threatened.

Scoliosis (acquired) (postural) 737.30
    congenital 754.2
    due to or associated with
        Charcôt-Marie-Tooth disease 356.1
            [737.43]
        mucopolysaccharidosis 277.5
            [737.43]
        neurofibromatosis 237.71 [737.43]
        osteitis
            deformans 731.0 [737.43]
            fibrosa cystica 252.01 [737.43]
        osteoporosis (see also Osteoporosis)
            733.00 [737.43]
        poliomyelitis 138 [737.43] ★ ◄────────

FIGURE 5-8. Alphabetic Index entry for scoliosis due to poliomyelitis.

Occasionally, conditions will be treated and documented as impending conditions. According to the guidelines, if the diagnosis has been confirmed, it should be coded as an active and current condition. If it is impending or threatened rather than active and current, check the Alphabetic Index to see whether a code is available that describes the impending condition. If no code is available, code the existing underlying condition(s).

EXAMPLE   Impending cerebrovascular accident (CVA), 435.9 (In ICD-10-CM there is no listing under the main term impending—code the underlying condition).

EXAMPLE   Impending fracture of the humerus due to multiple myeloma, 203.00 (C90.00).

14. Reporting Same Diagnosis Code More than Once
Each unique ICD-9-CM diagnosis code may be reported only once for an encounter. This applies to bilateral conditions or two different conditions classified to the same ICD-9-CM diagnosis codes.

EXAMPLE   Primary osteoarthritis both hips, 715.15 (M16.0).

15. Admission/Encounters for Rehabilitation
When the purpose for the admission/encounter is rehabilitation, sequence the appropriate V code from category V57, Care involving use of rehabilitation procedures, as the principal/first-listed diagnosis. The code for the condition for which the service is being performed should be reported an additional diagnosis.
   Only one code from category V57 is required. Code V57.89, Other specified rehabilitation procedures, should be assigned if more than one type of rehabilitation is performed during a single encounter. A procedure code should be reported to identify each type of rehabilitation therapy actually performed.

EXAMPLE   Patient is admitted for rehab following left hip replacement. Patient received physical and occupational therapy. V57.89, V54.81, V43.64, 93.39, 93.83 (Z51.89, Z47.1, Z96.642).

16. Documentation for BMI and Pressure Ulcer Stages

For the Body Mass Index (BMI) and pressure ulcer stage codes, code assignment may be based on medical record documentation from clinicians who are not the patient's provider (i.e., physician or other qualified healthcare practitioner legally accountable for establishing the patient's diagnosis), since this information is typically documented by other clinicians involved in the care of the patient (e.g., a dietitian often documents the BMI and nurses often documents the pressure ulcer stages). However, the associated diagnosis (such as overweight, obesity, or pressure ulcer) must be documented by the patient's provider. If there is conflicting medical record documentation, either from the same clinician or different clinicians, the patient's attending provider should be queried for clarification.

The BMI and pressure ulcer stage codes should only be reported as secondary diagnoses. As with all other secondary diagnosis codes, the BMI and pressure ulcer stage codes should only be assigned when they meet the definition of a reportable additional diagnosis (see Section III, Reporting Additional Diagnoses).

EXAMPLE

The dietitian documents a BMI of 32. The physician documents obesity, 278.00, V85.32 (E66.9, Z68.32).

17. Syndromes

Follow the Alphabetic Index guidance when coding syndromes. In the absence of index guidance, assign codes for the documented manifestations of the syndrome.

EXAMPLE

Patient with Noonan's syndrome with undescended testicles, von Willebrand's, and mild mental retardation, 759.89, 317, 752.51, 286.4 (Q87.1, Q53.20, D68.0, F70).

EXERCISE 5-5

Assign codes to the following conditions.

1. Impending delirium tremens _____
2. Threatened miscarriage _____
3. Impending myocardial infarction _____
4. Impending fracture of femur due to severe osteoporosis _____
5. Impending stroke _____
6. Physician documents sacral pressure ulcer. Nursing documentation indicates stage III. _____
7. Patient is being treated for blackheads and cystic acne. _____
8. Patient has bilateral radial fractures. _____
9. Patient was admitted for physical therapy following a CVA with residual left-sided hemiparesis. _____
10. Physician documents that the patient is overweight. BMI is documented as 29.0. _____

LATE EFFECTS

Late effect codes are not assigned to a separate chapter in the Tabular. A **late effect code** is used when the acute phase of an illness or injury has passed but a residual condition or health problem remains. The residual is coded first, and the appropriate late effects code is assigned to indicate the cause of the residual. In most instances, two codes are assigned —one for the residual that is being treated and the other to indicate the cause. As the guidelines state, no time limit applies, and it is possible that a residual may not be immediately apparent. It is also possible for a patient to have more than one residual condition.

EXAMPLE

> Facial droop as a result of previous stroke (CVA). The CVA late effect codes include the residual and its cause in a combination code, so only one code is necessary, 438.83 (I69.392).

EXAMPLE

> Patient is being treated for arthritis due to previous ankle fracture, 716.17, 905.4, E989 (M12.579, S82.899S).

Sometimes, it may be difficult to determine what is the residual and what is the late effect. The following exercise will help with that differentiation.

EXERCISE 5-6

Write the term(s) that represent the residual and its cause in the following cases on the lines provided, and assign the appropriate codes.

1. Keloid scar left right forearm, resulting from second-degree burns; injury occurred 1 year ago

   Residual: _____   Code: _____

   Cause: _____   Code: _____

2. Traumatic arthritis in the ankle joint due to fracture of the right ankle with a nondisplaced lateral malleolar fracture

   Residual: _____   Code: _____

   Cause: _____   Code: _____

3. Dysphagia due to CVA 3 months ago

   Residual: _____   Code: _____

   Cause: _____   Code: _____

Section II. Selection of Principal Diagnosis

The circumstances of inpatient admission always govern the selection of principal diagnosis. The principal diagnosis is defined in the Uniform Hospital Discharge Data Set (UHDDS) as "that condition established after study to be chiefly responsible for occasioning the admission of the patient to the hospital for care."

The UHDDS definitions are used by hospitals to report inpatient data elements in a standardized manner. These data elements and their definitions can be found in the July 31, 1985, *Federal Register* (Vol. 50, No, 147), pp. 31038-40.

Since that time the application of the UHDDS definitions has been expanded to include all non-outpatient settings (acute care, short term, long term care and psychiatric hospitals; home health agencies; rehab facilities; nursing homes, etc).

In determining principal diagnosis the coding conventions in the ICD-9-CM, Volumes I and II take precedence over these official coding guidelines.
(See Section I.A., Conventions for the ICD-9-CM)

The importance of consistent, complete documentation in the medical record cannot be overemphasized. Without such documentation the application of all coding guidelines is a difficult, if not impossible, task.

A. Codes for symptoms, signs, and ill-defined conditions

Codes for symptoms, signs, and ill-defined conditions from Chapter 16 are not to be used as principal diagnosis when a related definitive diagnosis has been established.

EXAMPLE   Right lower quadrant abdominal pain due to acute appendicitis. The code for the abdominal pain is 789.03 (R10.31) (from Chapter 16), and it is due to acute appendicitis. The only code necessary is 540.9 (K35.80), for acute appendicitis.

B. Two or more interrelated conditions, each potentially meeting the definition for principal diagnosis

When there are two or more interrelated conditions (such as diseases in the same ICD-9-CM chapter or manifestations characteristically associated with a certain disease) potentially meeting the definition of principal diagnosis, either condition may be sequenced first, unless the circumstances of the admission, the therapy provided, the Tabular List, or the Alphabetic Index indicate otherwise.

EXAMPLE   The patient had severe dehydration and hypokalemia that were treated with IV fluids and IV potassium supplements, 276.51, 276.8, or 276.8, 276.51 (E86.0, E87.6, or E87.6, E86.0).

C. Two or more diagnoses that equally meet the definition for principal diagnosis

In the unusual instance when two or more diagnoses equally meet the criteria for principal diagnosis as determined by the circumstances of admission, diagnostic workup and/or therapy provided, and the Alphabetic Index, Tabular List, or another coding guidelines does not provide sequencing direction, any one of the diagnoses may be sequenced first.

EXAMPLE   The patient was admitted with an exacerbation of her chronic obstructive pulmonary disease and decompensation of her congestive heart failure. Either 491.21 (J44.1) or 428.0 (I50.9) could be selected for the principal diagnosis, and the other code would be a secondary diagnosis code.

D. Two or more comparative or contrasting conditions

In those rare instances when two or more contrasting or comparative diagnoses are documented as "either/or" (or similar terminology), they are coded as if the diagnoses were confirmed and the diagnoses are sequenced according to the circumstances of the admission. If no further determination can be made as to which diagnosis should be principal, either diagnosis may be sequenced first.

EXAMPLE   Peptic ulcer disease versus cholecystitis, 533.90, 575.10, or 575.10, 533.90 (K27.9, K81.9, or K81.9, K27.9).

E. A symptom(s) followed by contrasting/comparative diagnoses

When a symptom(s) is followed by contrasting/comparative diagnoses, the symptom code is sequenced first. All the contrasting/comparative diagnoses should be coded as additional diagnoses.

EXAMPLE   Abdominal pain due to peptic ulcer disease versus cholecystitis, 789.00, 533.90, 575.10 (R10.9, K27.9, K81.9).

F. Original treatment plan not carried out

Sequence as the principal diagnosis the condition, which after study occasioned the admission to the hospital, even though treatment may not have been carried out due to unforeseen circumstances.

EXAMPLE

The patient was admitted for cholecystectomy because of cholelithiasis. The patient was noted to be having an exacerbation of congestive heart failure (CHF), so the surgery was canceled and IV Lasix was administered to treat the CHF, 574.20, 428.0, V64.1 (K80.20, I50.9, Z53.09). No procedure code would be assigned because the procedure was canceled before it was started.

G. Complications of surgery and other medical care

When the admission is for treatment of a complication resulting from surgery or other medical care, the complication code is sequenced as the principal diagnosis. If the complication is classified to the 996-999 series and the code lacks the necessary specificity in describing the complication, an additional code for the specific complication should be assigned.

EXAMPLE

The patient was admitted for dehiscence of an abdominal incision, 998.32, E879.9 (T81.31xA, Y83.9).

H. Uncertain Diagnosis

If the diagnosis documented at the time of discharge is qualified as "probable", "suspected", "likely", "questionable", "possible", or "still to be ruled out", or other similar terms indicating uncertainty, code the condition as if it existed or was established. The bases for these guidelines are the diagnostic workup, arrangements for further workup or observation, and initial therapeutic approach that correspond most closely with the established diagnosis.

Note: This guideline is applicable only to inpatient admissions to short-term, acute, long-term care and psychiatric hospitals.

EXAMPLE

Possible adenovirus meningitis, 049.1 (A87.1).

In the chapter-specific guidelines, there are three exceptions to the uncertain diagnosis guideline.

- Code 042 (B20) AIDS should only be assigned for confirmed cases
- Code 488.02 (J09.02) Avian influenza should only be assigned for confirmed cases
- Code 488.12 (J09.12) H1N1 influenza should only be assigned for confirmed cases

I. Admission from Observation Unit

1. Admission Following Medical Observation

When a patient is admitted to an observation unit for a medical condition, which either worsens or does not improve, and is subsequently admitted as an inpatient of the same hospital for this same medical condition, the principal diagnosis would be the medical condition which led to the hospital admission.

EXAMPLE

The patient was admitted for medical observation because of chest pain. After further investigation and testing, it was determined that the patient had a NSTEMI, and the patient was admitted for inpatient care, 410.71 (I21.4).

2. Admission Following Post-Operative Observation

When a patient is admitted to an observation unit to monitor a condition (or complication) that develops following outpatient surgery, and then is subsequently admitted as an inpatient of the same hospital, hospitals should apply the Uniform Hospital Discharge Data Set (UHDDS) definition of principal diagnosis as "that condition established after study to be chiefly responsible for occasioning the admission of the patient to the hospital for care."

J. Admission from Outpatient Surgery

When a patient receives surgery in the hospital's outpatient surgery department and is subsequently admitted for continuing inpatient care at the same hospital, the following guidelines should be followed in selecting the principal diagnosis for the inpatient admission:

- If the reason for the inpatient admission is a complication, assign the complication as the principal diagnosis.

EXAMPLE

The patient was admitted following an outpatient esophagogastroduodenoscopy for gastroesophageal reflux. The patient went into atrial fibrillation in the recovery room and was admitted. 997.1, 427.31, 530.81, E878.8, E849.7, 45.13 (I97.191, I48.0, K21.9, Y83.8, Y92.238, 0DJ08ZZ).

- If no complication, or other condition, is documented as the reason for the inpatient admission, assign the reason for the outpatient surgery as the principal diagnosis.
- If the reason for the inpatient admission is another condition unrelated to the surgery, assign the unrelated condition as the principal diagnosis.

Section III. Reporting Additional Diagnoses

GENERAL RULES FOR OTHER (ADDITIONAL) DIAGNOSES

For reporting purposes the definition for "other diagnoses" is interpreted as additional conditions that affect patient care in terms of requiring:

> clinical evaluation; or
> therapeutic treatment; or
> diagnostic procedures; or
> extended length of hospital stay; or
> increased nursing care and/or monitoring.

The UHDDS item #11-b defines Other Diagnoses as "all conditions that coexist at the time of admission, that develop subsequently, or that affect the treatment received and/or the length of stay. Diagnoses that relate to an earlier episode which have no bearing on the current hospital stay are to be excluded." UHDDS definitions apply to inpatients in acute care, short-term, long term care and psychiatric hospital setting. The UHDDS definitions are used by acute care short-term hospitals to report inpatient data elements in a standardized manner. These data elements and their definitions can be found in the July 31, 1985, Federal Register (Vol. 50, No, 147), pp. 31038-40.

Since that time the application of the UHDDS definitions has been expanded to include all non-outpatient settings (acute care, short term, long term care and psychiatric hospitals; home health agencies; rehab facilities; nursing homes, etc).

The following guidelines are to be applied in designating "other diagnoses" when neither the Alphabetic Index nor the Tabular List in ICD-9-CM provide direction. The listing of the diagnoses in the patient record is the responsibility of the attending provider.

A. Previous conditions

If the provider has included a diagnosis in the final diagnostic statement, such as the discharge summary or the face sheet, it should ordinarily be coded. Some providers include in the diagnostic statement resolved conditions or diagnoses and status-post procedures from previous admission that have no bearing on the current stay. Such conditions are not to be reported and are coded only if required by hospital policy.

However, history codes (V10-V19) may be used as secondary codes if the historical condition or family history has an impact on current care or influences treatment.

EXAMPLE

The patient is being treated for congestive heart failure and has a history of allergy to shellfish. A code is available for history of shellfish allergy, V15.04, but it would not be necessary to assign this code unless facility policy directs the coder to do so. Some physicians list allergies and previous surgeries as diagnoses, 428.0 (I50.9).

EXAMPLE

The patient is being treated for prostate cancer. A significant family history of prostate cancer has been reported, 185, V16.42 (C61, Z80.42).

B. Abnormal findings

Abnormal findings (laboratory, x-ray, pathologic, and other diagnostic results) are not coded and reported unless the provider indicates their clinical significance. If the findings are outside the normal range and the attending provider has ordered other tests to evaluate the condition or prescribed treatment, it is appropriate to ask the provider whether the abnormal finding should be added.

Please note: This differs from the coding practices in the outpatient setting for coding encounters for diagnostic tests that have been interpreted by a provider.

EXAMPLE

Potassium is noted to be low on laboratory testing. Potassium 20 mEq was ordered. Query the physician regarding the significance of the abnormal lab value and subsequent treatment.

C. Uncertain Diagnosis

If the diagnosis documented at the time of discharge is qualified as "probable", "suspected", "likely", "questionable", "possible", or "still to be ruled out" or other similar terms indicating uncertainty, code the condition as if it existed or was established. The bases for these guidelines are the diagnostic workup, arrangements for further workup or observation, and initial therapeutic approach that correspond most closely with the established diagnosis.

Note: This guideline is applicable only to inpatient admissions to short-term, acute, long-term care and psychiatric hospitals.

EXAMPLE

Suspected aspiration pneumonitis, 507.0 (J69.0).

Section IV. Diagnostic Coding and Reporting Guidelines for Outpatient Services

These coding guidelines for outpatient diagnoses have been approved for use by hospitals/providers in coding and reporting hospital-based outpatient services and provider-based office visits.

In the hospital setting, many coders must be familiar with both inpatient and outpatient guidelines. The Diagnostic Coding and Reporting Guidelines for Outpatient Services will be presented in detail in Chapter 27 on coding outpatient encounters.

PRESENT ON ADMISSION

The **Deficit Reduction Act** (DRA) mandates that as of October 1, 2007, all acute-care facilities reimbursed under Medicare Severity diagnosis-related groups (MS-DRGs) must identify and report diagnoses that are present at the time of a patient's admission. This policy change was implemented to save lives and dollars by no longer paying the extra costs of treating preventable errors, injuries, and infections that occur in hospitals. Medicare does not want to pay for conditions they consider preventable, such as pressure ulcers, injuries due to falls, infections caused by genitourinary catheters and central venous lines, or complications such as a sponge left in a patient during surgery.

The **present on admission** (POA) indicator (which follows) is to differentiate between conditions that develop during a particular hospital encounter and conditions that were present at the time of admission. Hospitals will have a 1-year grace period before their payment will be affected by conditions that were not present at the time of admission. Most of these conditions will be identified by a particular ICD-9-CM diagnosis code, and the POA indicator on the UB-04. Coding staff will have to assign POA indicators to the ICD-9-CM codes that are assigned. This requirement places even more importance on accurate and complete documentation within the health record. In some instances it may be necessary to query the physician about whether a condition was present at the time of admission.

The Cooperating Parties have developed POA guidelines that are supplemental to the *ICD-9-CM Official Guidelines for Coding and Reporting* to assist with the application of the POA requirement. The indicators that are reported are the following:

- Y = Yes (present at the time of inpatient admission)
- N = No (not present at the time of inpatient admission)
- U = Unknown (documentation is insufficient to determine whether condition is present on admission)
- W = Clinically undetermined (provider is unable to clinically determine whether condition was present on admission)
- Unreported/Not used (Exempt from POA reporting). Electronic claims will have a "1."

The Centers for Medicare and Medicaid Services (CMS) has identified certain hospital-acquired conditions and will no longer reimburse for the extra costs that are incurred as a result of these conditions. The conditions are identified by the ICD-9-CM/ICD-10-CM codes and a POA indicator of N for no—the condition was not present at the time of admission. This provision is applicable only to hospitals that are reimbursed under the Inpatient Prospective Payment System (IPPS). Some hospitals that would be exempt are:

- Critical Access Hospitals
- Long-Term Care Hospitals
- Maryland Waiver Hospitals
- Cancer Hospitals
- Children's Inpatient Facilities
- Rural Health Clinics
- Federally Qualified Health Centers
- Religious Non-Medical Health Care Institutions
- Inpatient Psychiatric Hospitals
- Inpatient Rehabilitation Facilities
- Veterans Administration/Department of Defense Hospitals

See Table 5-1 for a listing of the **hospital-acquired conditions** (HAC) and their corresponding ICD-9-CM codes.

EXAMPLE

> If a patient was admitted for pneumonia and developed a urinary tract infection due to Foley catheter after admission to the hospital, the codes 996.64, 599.0 (T83.51xA, N39.0), both secondary codes with a POA of N, would be assigned. Both of these codes are CCs for MS-DRG assignment. In this case, neither code would qualify as a CC because it occurred after admission and is considered as reasonably preventable.

EXAMPLE

> If a patient is admitted to the hospital with pneumonia and also had a urinary tract infection due to a Foley catheter, the codes 486, 996.64, 599.0 (J18.9, T83.51xA, N39.0), all with a POA of Y, would be assigned. Both of these secondary codes would qualify as CCs because the condition was present at the time of admission and the hospital would be reimbursed for these conditions.

TABLE 5-1 HACS AND ICD-9-CM CODES

HAC	CC/MCC (ICD-9-CM Codes)
Foreign Object Retained After Surgery	998.4 (CC)
	998.7 (CC)
Air Embolism	999.1 (MCC)
Blood Incompatibility	999.60 (CC)
	999.61 (CC)
	999.62 (CC)
	999.63 (CC)
	999.69 (CC)
Pressure Ulcer Stages III & IV	707.23 (MCC)
	707.24 (MCC)
Falls and Trauma:	Codes within these ranges on the CC/MCC list:
• Fracture	800–829
• Dislocation	830–839
• Intracranial Injury	850–854
• Crushing Injury	925–929
• Burn	940–949
• Other Injuries	991–994
Catheter-Associated Urinary Tract Infection (UTI)	996.64 (CC)
	Also excludes the following from acting as a CC/MCC:
	112.2 (CC)
	590.10 (CC)
	590.11 (MCC)
	590.2 (MCC)
	590.3 (CC)
	590.80 (CC)
	590.81 (CC)
	595.0 (CC)
	597.0 (CC)
	599.0 (CC)
Vascular Catheter-Associated Infection	999.3X (CC)
Manifestations of Poor Glydemic Control:	250.10–250.13 (MCC)
• Diabetic Ketoacidosis	250.20–250.23 (MCC)
• Nonketotic Hyperosmolar Coma	251.0 (CC)
• Hypoglycemic Coma	249.10–249.11 (MCC)
• Secondary Diabetes With Ketoacidosis	249.20–249.21 (MCC)
• Secondary Diabetes with Hyperosmolarity	
Surgical Site Infection, Mediastinitis, Following Coronary Artery Bypass Graft (CABG)	519.2 (MCC)
	And one of the following procedure codes:
	36.10–36.19
Surgical Site Infection Following Certain Orthopedic Procedures:	996.67 (CC)
• Spine	998.59 (CC)
• Neck	And one of the following procedure codes: 81.01–81.08,
• Shoulder	81.23–81.24, 81.31–81.38, 81.83, or 81.85
• Elbow	
Surgical Site Infection Following Bariatric Surgery for Obesity:	*Principal Diagnosis*—278.01
• Laparoscopic Gastric Bypass	998.59 (CC)
• Gastroenterostomy	And one of the following procedure codes: 44.38, 44.39, or
• Laparoscopic Gastric Restrictive Surgery	44.95
Deep Vein Thrombosis and Pulmonary Embolism Following Certain Orthopedic Procedures:	415.11 (MCC)
	415.19 (MCC)
• Total Knee Replacement	453.40–453.42 (MCC)
• Hip Replacement	And one of the following procedure codes: 00.85–00.87,
	81.51–81.52, or 81.54

From http://www.cms.gov/HospitalAcqCond.

Appendix I
Present on Admission Reporting Guidelines

Introduction

These guidelines are to be used as a supplement to the *ICD-9-CM Official Guidelines for Coding and Reporting* to facilitate the assignment of the Present on Admission (POA) indicator for each diagnosis and external cause of injury code reported on claim forms (UB-04 and 837 Institutional).

These guidelines are not intended to replace any guidelines in the main body of the *ICD-9-CM Official Guidelines for Coding and Reporting*. The POA guidelines are not intended to provide guidance on when a condition should be coded, but rather, how to apply the POA indicator to the final set of diagnosis codes that have been assigned in accordance with Sections I, II, and III of the official coding guidelines. Subsequent to the assignment of the ICD-9-CM codes, the POA indicator should then be assigned to those conditions that have been coded.

As stated in the Introduction to the ICD-9-CM Official Guidelines for Coding and Reporting, a joint effort between the healthcare provider and the coder is essential to achieve complete and accurate documentation, code assignment, and reporting of diagnoses and procedures. The importance of consistent, complete documentation in the medical record cannot be overemphasized. Medical record documentation from any provider involved in the care and treatment of the patient may be used to support the determination of whether a condition was present on admission or not. In the context of the official coding guidelines, the term "provider" means a physician or any qualified healthcare practitioner who is legally accountable for establishing the patient's diagnosis.

These guidelines are not a substitute for the provider's clinical judgment as to the determination of whether a condition was/was not present on admission. The provider should be queried regarding issues related to the linking of signs/symptoms, timing of test results, and the timing of findings.

General Reporting Requirements

All claims involving inpatient admissions to general acute care hospitals or other facilities that are subject to a law or regulation mandating collection of present on admission information.

Present on admission is defined as present at the time the order for inpatient admission occurs—conditions that develop during an outpatient encounter, including emergency department, observation, or outpatient surgery, are considered as present on admission.

POA indicator is assigned to principal and secondary diagnoses (as defined in Section II of the Official Guidelines for Coding and Reporting) and the external cause of injury codes.

Issues related to inconsistent, missing, conflicting or unclear documentation must still be resolved by the provider.

If a condition would not be coded and reported based on UHDDS definitions and current official coding guidelines, then the POA indicator would not be reported.

Reporting Options

Y—Yes
N—No
U—Unknown
W—Clinically undetermined
Unreported/Not used (or "1" for Medicare usage)—(Exempt from POA reporting)

Reporting Definitions

Y = present at the time of inpatient admission
N = not present at the time of inpatient admission
U = documentation is insufficient to determine if condition is present on admission
W = provider is unable to clinically determine whether condition was present on admission or not

Timeframe for POA Identification and Documentation

There is no required timeframe as to when a provider (per the definition of "provider" used in these guidelines) must identify or document a condition to be present on admission. In some clinical situations, it may not be possible for a provider to make a definitive diagnosis (or a condition may not be recognized or reported by the patient) for a period of time after admission. In some cases it may be several days before the provider arrives at a definitive diagnosis. This does not mean that the condition was not present on admission. Determination of whether the condition was present on admission or not will be based on the applicable POA guideline as identified in this document, or on the provider's best clinical judgment.

If at the time of code assignment the documentation is unclear as to whether a condition was present on admission or not, it is appropriate to query the provider for clarification.

Assigning the POA Indicator

Condition is on the "Exempt from Reporting" list

Leave the "present on admission" field blank if the condition is on the list of ICD-9-CM codes for which this field is not applicable. This is the only circumstance in which the field may be left blank.

POA Explicitly Documented

Assign Y for any condition the provider explicitly documents as being present on admission.

Assign N for any condition the provider explicitly documents as not present at the time of admission.

Conditions diagnosed prior to inpatient admission

Assign "Y" for conditions that were diagnosed prior to admission (example: hypertension, diabetes mellitus, asthma).

Conditions diagnosed during the admission but clearly present before admission

Assign "Y" for conditions diagnosed during the admission that were clearly present but not diagnosed until after admission occurred.

Diagnoses subsequently confirmed after admission are considered present on admission if at the time of admission they are documented as suspected, possible, rule out, differential diagnosis, or constitute an underlying cause of a symptom that is present at the time of admission.

Condition develops during outpatient encounter prior to inpatient admission

Assign "Y" for any condition that develops during an outpatient encounter prior to a written order for inpatient admission.

Documentation does not indicate whether condition was present on admission

Assign "U" when the medical record documentation is unclear as to whether the condition was present on admission. "U" should not be routinely assigned and used only in very limited circumstances. Coders are encouraged to query the providers when the documentation is unclear.

Documentation states that it cannot be determined whether the condition was or was not present on admission

Assign "W" when the medical record documentation indicates that it cannot be clinically determined whether or not the condition was present on admission.

Chronic condition with acute exacerbation during the admission

If the code is a combination code that identifies both the chronic condition and the acute exacerbation, see POA guidelines pertaining to combination codes.

If the combination code only identifies the chronic condition and not the acute exacerbation (e.g., acute exacerbation of **chronic leukemia**), assign "Y".

Conditions documented as possible, probable, suspected, or rule out at the time of discharge

If the final diagnosis contains a possible, probable, suspected, or rule out diagnosis, and this diagnosis was based on signs, symptoms, or clinical findings suspected at the time of inpatient admission, assign "Y".

If the final diagnosis contains a possible, probable, suspected, or rule out diagnosis, and this diagnosis was based on symptoms or clinical findings that were not present on admission, assign "N".

Conditions documented as impending or threatened at the time of discharge

If the final diagnosis contains an impending or threatened diagnosis, and this diagnosis is based on symptoms or clinical findings that were present on admission, assign "Y".

If the final diagnosis contains an impending or threatened diagnosis, and this diagnosis is based on symptoms or clinical findings that were not present on admission, assign "N".

Acute and chronic conditions

Assign "Y" for acute conditions that are present at time of admission and N for acute conditions that are not present at time of admission.

Assign "Y" for chronic conditions, even though the condition may not be diagnosed until after admission.

If a single code identifies both an acute and chronic condition, see the POA guidelines for combination codes.

Combination codes

Assign "N" if any part of the combination code was not present on admission (e.g., obstructive chronic bronchitis with acute exacerbation and the exacerbation was not present on admission; gastric ulcer that does not start bleeding until after admission; asthma patient develops status asthmaticus after admission).

Assign "Y" if all parts of the combination code were present on admission (e.g., patient with diabetic nephropathy is admitted with uncontrolled diabetes).

If the final diagnosis includes comparative or contrasting diagnoses, and both were present, or suspected, at the time of admission, assign "Y".

For infection codes that include the causal organism, assign "Y" if the infection (or signs of the infection) was present on admission, even though the culture results may not be known until after admission (e.g., patient is admitted with pneumonia and the provider documents pseudomonas as the causal organism a few days later).

Same diagnosis code for two or more conditions

When the same ICD-9-CM diagnosis code applies to two or more conditions during the same encounter (e.g., bilateral condition, or two separate conditions classified to the same ICD-9-CM diagnosis code):

Assign "Y" if all conditions represented by the single ICD-9-CM code were present on admission (e.g., bilateral fracture of the same bone, same site, and both fractures were present on admission).

Assign "N" if any of the conditions represented by the single ICD-9-CM code was not present on admission (e.g., dehydration with hyponatremia is assigned to code 276.1, but only one of these conditions was present on admission).

Obstetrical conditions

Whether or not the patient delivers during the current hospitalization does not affect assignment of the POA indicator. The determining factor for POA assignment is whether the pregnancy complication or obstetrical condition described by the code was present at the time of admission or not.

If the pregnancy complication or obstetrical condition was present on admission (e.g., patient admitted in preterm labor), assign "Y".

If the pregnancy complication or obstetrical condition was not present on admission (e.g., 2nd degree laceration during delivery, postpartum hemorrhage that occurred during current hospitalization, fetal distress develops after admission), assign "N".

If the obstetrical code includes more than one diagnosis and any of the diagnoses identified by the code were not present on admission assign "N".

(e.g., Code 642.7, Pre-eclampsia or eclampsia superimposed on pre-existing hypertension).

If the obstetrical code includes information that is not a diagnosis, do not consider that information in the POA determination.

(e.g., Code 652.1x, Breech or other malpresentation successfully converted to cephalic presentation should be reported as present on admission if the fetus was breech on admission but was converted to cephalic presentation after admission since the conversion to cephalic presentation does not represent a diagnosis, the fact that the conversion occurred after admission has no bearing on the POA determination).

Perinatal conditions

Newborns are not considered to be admitted until after birth. Therefore, any condition present at birth or that developed in utero is considered present at admission and should be assigned "Y". This includes conditions that occur during delivery (e.g., injury during delivery, meconium aspiration, exposure to streptococcus B in the vaginal canal).

Congenital conditions and anomalies*

Assign "Y" for congenital conditions and anomalies. Congenital conditions are always considered present on admission.

External cause of injury codes

Assign "Y" for any E code representing an external cause of injury or poisoning that occurred prior to inpatient admission (e.g., patient fell out of bed at home, patient fell out of bed in emergency room prior to admission)

Assign "N" for any E code representing an external cause of injury or poisoning that occurred during inpatient hospitalization (e.g., patient fell out of hospital bed during hospital stay, patient experienced an adverse reaction to a medication administered after inpatient admission)

---

*In 2010, code categories 740–759 were listed on the Exempt from the Present on Admission requirement. This conflicts with the guideline.

ICD-10-CM

Official Guidelines for Coding and Reporting

Please refer to the companion Evolve website for the most current guidelines.

B. General Coding Guidelines

1. **Locating a code in the ICD-10-CM**

   To select a code in the classification that corresponds to a diagnosis or reason for visit documented in a medical record, first locate the term in the **Alphabetic Index,** and then verify the code in the Tabular List. Read and be guided by instructional notations that appear in both the **Alphabetic Index** and the Tabular List.

   It is essential to use both the **Alphabetic Index** and Tabular List when locating and assigning a code. The **Alphabetic Index** does not always provide the full code. Selection of the full code, including laterality and any applicable 7th character can only be done in the **Tabular List.** A dash (-) at the end of an **Alphabetic Index** entry indicates that additional characters are required. Even if a dash is not included at the **Alphabetic Index** entry, it is necessary to refer to the **Tabular List** to verify that no 7th character is required.

2. **Level of Detail in Coding**

   Diagnosis codes are to be used and reported at their highest number of **characters** available.

   ICD-10-CM diagnosis codes are composed of codes with 3, 4, 5, 6 or 7 **characters.** Codes with three digits are included in ICD-10-CM as the heading of a category of codes that may be further subdivided by the use of fourth and/or fifth **characters and/or sixth characters,** which provide greater detail.

   A three-**character** code is to be used only if it is not further subdivided. A code is invalid if it has not been coded to the full number of characters required for that code, including the 7th character, if applicable.

3. **Code or codes from A00.0 through T88.9, Z00-Z99.8**

   The appropriate code or codes from A00.0 through T88.9, Z00-Z99.8 must be used to identify diagnoses, symptoms, conditions, problems, complaints or other reason(s) for the encounter/visit.

4. **Signs and symptoms**

   Codes that describe symptoms and signs, as opposed to diagnoses, are acceptable for reporting purposes when a related definitive diagnosis has not been established (confirmed) by the provider. Chapter 18 of ICD-10-CM, Symptoms, Signs, and Abnormal Clinical and Laboratory Findings, Not Elsewhere Classified (codes R00.0-R99) contains many, but not all codes for symptoms.

5. **Conditions that are an integral part of a disease process**

   Signs and symptoms that are associated routinely with a disease process should not be assigned as additional codes, unless otherwise instructed by the classification.

6. **Conditions that are not an integral part of a disease process**

   Additional signs and symptoms that may not be associated routinely with a disease process should be coded when present.

7. **Multiple coding for a single condition**

   In addition to the etiology/manifestation convention that requires two codes to fully describe a single condition that affects multiple body systems, there are other single conditions that also require more than one code. "Use additional code" notes are found in the **Tabular List** at codes that are not part of an etiology/manifestation pair where a secondary code is useful to fully describe a condition. The sequencing rule is the same as the etiology/manifestation pair, "use additional code" indicates that a secondary code should be added.

   For example, for bacterial infections that are not included in chapter 1, a secondary code from category B95, Streptococcus, Staphylococcus, and Enterococcus, as the cause of diseases classified elsewhere, or B96, Other bacterial agents as the cause of diseases classified elsewhere, may be required to identify the bacterial organism causing the infection. A "use additional code" note will normally be found at the infectious disease code, indicating a need for the organism code to be added as a secondary code.

   "Code first" notes are also under certain codes that are not specifically manifestation codes but may be due to an underlying cause. When there is a "code first" note and an underlying condition is present, the underlying condition should be sequenced first.

"Code, if applicable, any causal condition first", notes indicate that this code may be assigned as a principal diagnosis when the causal condition is unknown or not applicable. If a causal condition is known, then the code for that condition should be sequenced as the principal or first-listed diagnosis.

Multiple codes may be needed for late effects, complication codes and obstetric codes to more fully describe a condition. See the specific guidelines for these conditions for further instruction.

8. **Acute and Chronic Conditions**

If the same condition is described as both acute (subacute) and chronic, and separate subentries exist in the Alphabetic Index at the same indentation level, code both and sequence the acute (subacute) code first.

9. **Combination Code**

A combination code is a single code used to classify:

Two diagnoses, or

A diagnosis with an associated secondary process (manifestation)

A diagnosis with an associated complication

Combination codes are identified by referring to subterm entries in the Alphabetic Index and by reading the inclusion and exclusion notes in the Tabular List.

Assign only the combination code when that code fully identifies the diagnostic conditions involved or when the Alphabetic Index so directs. Multiple coding should not be used when the classification provides a combination code that clearly identifies all of the elements documented in the diagnosis. When the combination code lacks necessary specificity in describing the manifestation or complication, an additional code should be used as a secondary code.

10. **Late Effects (Sequela)**

A late effect is the residual effect (condition produced) after the acute phase of an illness or injury has terminated. There is no time limit on when a late effect code can be used. The residual may be apparent early, such as in cerebral infarction, or it may occur months or years later, such as that due to a previous injury. Coding of late effects generally requires two codes sequenced in the following order: The condition or nature of the late effect is sequenced first. The late effect code is sequenced second.

An exception to the above guidelines are those instances where the code for late effect is followed by a manifestation code identified in the Tabular List and title, or the late effect code has been expanded (at the fourth, fifth or sixth character levels) to include the manifestation(s). The code for the acute phase of an illness or injury that led to the late effect is never used with a code for the late effect.

See Section I.C.9. Sequelae of cerebrovascular disease

See Section I.C.15. Sequelae of complication of pregnancy, childbirth and the puerperium

See Section I.C.19. Code extensions

11. **Impending or Threatened Condition**

Code any condition described at the time of discharge as "impending" or "threatened" as follows:

If it did occur, code as confirmed diagnosis.

If it did not occur, reference the Alphabetic Index to determine if the condition has a subentry term for "impending" or "threatened" and also reference main term entries for "Impending" and for "Threatened."

If the subterms are listed, assign the given code.

If the subterms are not listed, code the existing underlying condition(s) and not the condition described as impending or threatened.

12. **Reporting Same Diagnosis Code More than Once**

Each unique ICD-10-CM diagnosis code may be reported only once for an encounter. This applies to bilateral conditions when there are no distinct codes identifying laterality or two different conditions classified to the same ICD-10-CM diagnosis code.

13. **Laterality**

For bilateral sites, the final character of the codes in the ICD-10-CM indicates laterality. An unspecified side code is also provided should the side not be identified in the medical record. If no bilateral code is provided and the condition is bilateral, assign separate codes for both the left and right side.

14. **Documentation for BMI and Pressure Ulcer Stages**

For the Body Mass Index (BMI) and pressure ulcer stage codes, code assignment may be based on medical record documentation from clinicians who are not the patient's provider (i.e., physician or other qualified healthcare practitioner legally accountable for establishing the patient's diagnosis), since this information is typically documented by other clinicians involved in the care of the patient (e.g., a dietitian often documents the BMI and nurses often documents the pressure ulcer stages). However, the associated diagnosis (such as overweight, obesity, or pressure ulcer) must be documented by the patient's provider. If there is conflicting medical record documentation, either from the same clinician or different clinicians, the patient's attending provider should be queried for clarification.

The BMI codes should only be reported as secondary diagnoses. As with all other secondary diagnosis codes, the BMI codes should only be assigned when they meet the definition of a reportable additional diagnosis (see Section III, Reporting Additional Diagnoses).

Section II. Selection of Principal Diagnosis

The circumstances of inpatient admission always govern the selection of principal diagnosis. The principal diagnosis is defined in the Uniform Hospital Discharge Data Set (UHDDS) as "that condition established after study to be chiefly responsible for occasioning the admission of the patient to the hospital for care."

The UHDDS definitions are used by hospitals to report inpatient data elements in a standardized manner. These data elements and their definitions can be found in the July 31, 1985, Federal Register (Vol. 50, No, 147), pp. 31038-40.

Since that time the application of the UHDDS definitions has been expanded to include all nonoutpatient settings (acute care, short term, long term care and psychiatric hospitals; home health agencies; rehab facilities; nursing homes, etc).

In determining principal diagnosis the coding conventions in the ICD-10-CM, **the Tabular List and Alphabetic Index** take precedence over these official coding guidelines.
(See Section I.A., Conventions for the ICD-10-CM)

The importance of consistent, complete documentation in the medical record cannot be overemphasized. Without such documentation the application of all coding guidelines is a difficult, if not impossible, task.

A. **Codes for symptoms, signs, and ill-defined conditions**

Codes for symptoms, signs, and ill-defined conditions from Chapter 18 are not to be used as principal diagnosis when a related definitive diagnosis has been established.

B. **Two or more interrelated conditions, each potentially meeting the definition for principal diagnosis.**

When there are two or more interrelated conditions (such as diseases in the same ICD-10-CM chapter or manifestations characteristically associated with a certain disease) potentially meeting the definition of principal diagnosis, either condition may be sequenced first, unless the circumstances of the admission, the therapy provided, the Tabular List, or the Alphabetic Index indicate otherwise.

C. **Two or more diagnoses that equally meet the definition for principal diagnosis**

In the unusual instance when two or more diagnoses equally meet the criteria for principal diagnosis as determined by the circumstances of admission, diagnostic workup and/or therapy provided, and the Alphabetic Index, Tabular List, or another coding guidelines does not provide sequencing direction, any one of the diagnoses may be sequenced first.

D. **Two or more comparative or contrasting conditions**

In those rare instances when two or more contrasting or comparative diagnoses are documented as "either/or" (or similar terminology), they are coded as if the diagnoses were confirmed and the diagnoses are sequenced according to the circumstances of the admission. If no further determination can be made as to which diagnosis should be principal, either diagnosis may be sequenced first.

E. **A symptom(s) followed by contrasting/comparative diagnoses**

When a symptom(s) is followed by contrasting/comparative diagnoses, the symptom code is sequenced first. All the contrasting/comparative diagnoses should be coded as additional diagnoses.

F. Original treatment plan not carried out

Sequence as the principal diagnosis the condition, which after study occasioned the admission to the hospital, even though treatment may not have been carried out due to unforeseen circumstances.

G. Complications of surgery and other medical care

When the admission is for treatment of a complication resulting from surgery or other medical care, the complication code is sequenced as the principal diagnosis. If the complication is classified to the T80-T88 series and the code lacks the necessary specificity in describing the complication, an additional code for the specific complication should be assigned.

H. Uncertain Diagnosis

If the diagnosis documented at the time of discharge is qualified as "probable", "suspected", "likely", "questionable", "possible", or "still to be ruled out", or other similar terms indicating uncertainty, code the condition as if it existed or was established. The bases for these guidelines are the diagnostic workup, arrangements for further workup or observation, and initial therapeutic approach that correspond most closely with the established diagnosis.

   Note: This guideline is applicable only to inpatient admissions to short-term, acute, long-term care and psychiatric hospitals.

I. Admission from Observation Unit

   1. Admission Following Medical Observation

   When a patient is admitted to an observation unit for a medical condition, which either worsens or does not improve, and is subsequently admitted as an inpatient of the same hospital for this same medical condition, the principal diagnosis would be the medical condition which led to the hospital admission.

   2. Admission Following Post-Operative Observation

   When a patient is admitted to an observation unit to monitor a condition (or complication) that develops following outpatient surgery, and then is subsequently admitted as an inpatient of the same hospital, hospitals should apply the Uniform Hospital Discharge Data Set (UHDDS) definition of principal diagnosis as "that condition established after study to be chiefly responsible for occasioning the admission of the patient to the hospital for care."

J. Admission from Outpatient Surgery

When a patient receives surgery in the hospital's outpatient surgery department and is subsequently admitted for continuing inpatient care at the same hospital, the following guidelines should be followed in selecting the principal diagnosis for the inpatient admission:

- If the reason for the inpatient admission is a complication, assign the complication as the principal diagnosis.
- If no complication, or other condition, is documented as the reason for the inpatient admission, assign the reason for the outpatient surgery as the principal diagnosis.
- If the reason for the inpatient admission is another condition unrelated to the surgery, assign the unrelated condition as the principal diagnosis.

Section III. Reporting Additional Diagnoses

GENERAL RULES FOR OTHER (ADDITIONAL) DIAGNOSES

For reporting purposes the definition for "other diagnoses" is interpreted as additional conditions that affect patient care in terms of requiring:

   clinical evaluation; or

   therapeutic treatment; or

   diagnostic procedures; or

   extended length of hospital stay; or

   increased nursing care and/or monitoring.

   The UHDDS item #11-b defines Other Diagnoses as "all conditions that coexist at the time of admission, that develop subsequently, or that affect the treatment received and/or the length of stay. Diagnoses that relate to an earlier episode which have no bearing on the current hospital stay are to be excluded." UHDDS definitions apply to inpatients in acute care, short-term, long term care and psychiatric hospital setting. The UHDDS definitions are used by acute care short-term hospitals to report inpatient data elements in a standardized manner. These data elements and their definitions can be found in the July 31, 1985, Federal Register (Vol. 50, No, 147), pp. 31038-40.

Since that time the application of the UHDDS definitions has been expanded to include all nonoutpatient settings (acute care, short term, long term care and psychiatric hospitals; home health agencies; rehab facilities; nursing homes, etc).

The following guidelines are to be applied in designating "other diagnoses" when neither the Alphabetic Index nor the Tabular List in ICD-10-CM provide direction. The listing of the diagnoses in the patient record is the responsibility of the attending provider.

A. Previous conditions

If the provider has included a diagnosis in the final diagnostic statement, such as the discharge summary or the face sheet, it should ordinarily be coded. Some providers include in the diagnostic statement resolved conditions or diagnoses and status-post procedures from previous admission that have no bearing on the current stay. Such conditions are not to be reported and are coded only if required by hospital policy.

However, history codes (categories Z80-Z87) may be used as secondary codes if the historical condition or family history has an impact on current care or influences treatment.

B. Abnormal findings

Abnormal findings (laboratory, x-ray, pathologic, and other diagnostic results) are not coded and reported unless the provider indicates their clinical significance. If the findings are outside the normal range and the attending provider has ordered other tests to evaluate the condition or prescribed treatment, it is appropriate to ask the provider whether the abnormal finding should be added.

Please note: This differs from the coding practices in the outpatient setting for coding encounters for diagnostic tests that have been interpreted by a provider.

C. Uncertain Diagnosis

If the diagnosis documented at the time of discharge is qualified as "probable", "suspected", "likely", "questionable", "possible", or "still to be ruled out" or other similar terms indicating uncertainty, code the condition as if it existed or was established. The bases for these guidelines are the diagnostic workup, arrangements for further workup or observation, and initial therapeutic approach that correspond most closely with the established diagnosis,

Note: This guideline is applicable only to inpatient admissions to short-term, acute, long-term care and psychiatric hospitals.

CHAPTER REVIEW EXERCISE

Select the correct answer for each of the following:

1. Conditions that are integral to a disease or condition should be coded as additional diagnoses.
   A. True
   B. False

2. When separate codes are used to identify acute and chronic conditions, the chronic code is sequenced first.
   A. True
   B. False

3. Reliance on only the Alphabetic Index or only the Tabular List can lead to errors in code assignments and less specificity in code selection.
   A. True
   B. False

4. A patient has anemia due to chronic renal failure. The anemia is integral to the chronic renal failure.
   A. True
   B. False

5. A patient has right lower quadrant abdominal pain due to acute appendicitis. The abdominal pain should be assigned as an additional code.
   A. True
   B. False

6. In the inpatient setting, it is acceptable to code diagnoses that have not yet been confirmed but that are questionable or suspected at the time of discharge.
   A. True
   B. False

7. If the principal diagnosis was abdominal pain due to acute appendicitis, abdominal pain would be coded as the principal diagnosis.
   A. True
   B. False

Assign codes to the following conditions.

8. Acute exacerbation of asthma

   Code from Alphabetic Index   _____

   Code following verification in Tabular List   _____

9. Non-ST elevation myocardial infarction

   Code from Alphabetic Index   _____

   Code following verification in Tabular List   _____

10. Spastic hemiplegia affecting right dominant side

    Code from Alphabetic Index   _____

    Code following verification in Tabular List   _____

Identify integral and nonintegral conditions by answering the following questions.

11. List two common symptoms of kidney stones.   _____

12. List two common symptoms associated with rheumatoid arthritis.   _____

13. List two common symptoms of acute renal failure.   _____

Assign and sequence codes to the following conditions.

14. Acute and chronic cystitis   _____

15. Acute on chronic oophoritis   _____

16. Acute and chronic prostatitis   _____

17. Viral gastroenteritis   _____

18. Viral meningitis   _____

19. Constrictive pericarditis due to old tuberculosis infection   _____

20. Mild mental retardation due to previous poliomyelitis   _____

CHAPTER GLOSSARY

This chapter is unique in that the glossary definitions are not provided within the chapter. These terms are used within the guidelines without definition. The glossary definitions are provided in this section for quick reference.

Acute: a short and relatively severe course.

Asymptomatic: without any symptoms.

Chronic: persistent over a long period.

Combination code: a single code used to classify two diagnoses; or a diagnosis with an associated secondary process (manifestation); or a diagnosis with an associated complication.

Conventions: general rules for use in classification that must be followed for accurate coding.

Deficit Reduction Act (DRA): mandates all acute-care facilities reimbursed under MS-DRGs to identify and report diagnoses that are present at the time of a patient's admission.

Etiology: cause or origin of a disease or condition.

Late effect code: used when the acute phase of an illness or injury has passed, but a residual condition or health problem remains.

Manifestation: symptom or condition that is the result of a disease.

Present on admission (POA): an indicator to differentiate between conditions that develop during a particular hospital encounter or if a condition was present at the time of admission.

Residual condition or effect: when the acute phase of an illness or injury has passed, but a residual condition or health problem remains.

Sequelae: residual conditions or effects; time when the acute phase of an illness or injury has passed, but residual conditions or health problems remain.

Sign: objective evidence of a disease or of a patient's condition as perceived by the patient's examining physician.

Subacute: somewhat acute; between chronic and acute.

Symptom: subjective evidence of a disease or of a patient's condition as perceived by the patient.

REFERENCE

1. American Hospital Association. *Coding Clinic for ICD-9-CM* 1995:3Q:p8. Hematuria secondary to renal stones.

6

General Coding Guidelines for Procedures in ICD-9-CM

LEARNING OBJECTIVES

1. Identify the format of Volume 3, Tabular List and Alphabetic Index of Procedures
2. Apply the conventions and ICD-9-CM Official Guidelines for Coding and Reporting
3. Define principal procedure
4. Define significant procedures
5. Explain the surgical hierarchy
6. Explain when to code operative approaches and closures
7. Assign codes for canceled or converted to open procedures

8. Compare and contrast endoscopic versus open procedures
9. Discuss the importance of having a hospital policy regarding procedure code assignment
10. Assign procedure codes using ICD-9-CM

ABBREVIATIONS/ ACRONYMS

BMI body mass index

CAS computer assisted surgery

CMS Centers for Medicare and Medicaid Services

COPD chronic obstructive pulmonary disease

CPT *Current Procedural Terminology*

ECMO extracorporeal membrane oxygenation

ER Emergency Room

HCPCS Healthcare Common Procedure Coding System

ICD-9-CM *International Classification of Diseases, 9th Revision, Clinical Modification*

ICD-10-CM *International Classification of Diseases, 10th Revision, Clinical Modification*

ICD-10-PCS *International Classification of Diseases, 10th Revision, Procedure Coding System*

ICU intensive care unit

MCE Medicare Code Editor

MS-DRG Medicare Severity diagnosis-related group

NCHS National Center for Health Statistics

NEC not elsewhere classifiable

NOS not otherwise specified

NPI National Provider Identifier

OB obstetrics

OR Operating Room

UHDDS Uniform Hospital Discharge Data Set

VAD vascular access device

There are only a few references made to procedural coding within the ICD-9-CM Official Guidelines for Coding and Reporting. These will be reviewed briefly in this chapter.

FORMAT OF VOLUME 3, TABULAR LIST AND ALPHABETIC INDEX OF PROCEDURES

The format of Volume 3, Alphabetic Index and Tabular List, follows the same format and conventions that are used in Volume 1, Tabular List of Diseases and Injuries, and Volume 2, Alphabetic Index of Disease and Injuries. These procedural codes are used to code hospital inpatient procedures. ICD-9-CM procedure codes are not used by hospital outpatient departments or by physician practices. Physicians and hospital outpatient services are coded using *Current Procedural Terminology* (CPT) for procedural coding. According to *Coding Clinic* (2008:1Q:p15),[1] "The use of ICD-9-CM procedure codes is restricted to the reporting of inpatient procedures by hospitals." This is in accordance with HIPAA regulations. A hospital may still collect ICD-9-CM procedural data but only for internal or non–claim-related purposes. ICD-10-PCS will only be required for inpatient billing by hospitals. At this time, CMS accepts six procedure codes on a hospital claim. They are considering increasing the number of procedure codes accepted upon conversion to ICD-10-PCS, which will not be used in physicians' offices or other ambulatory settings; those providers will continue to use CPT and the Healthcare Common Procedure Coding System (HCPCS) for billing purposes.

Volume 3 consists of 17 chapters (Table 6-1). Most of these chapters are classified by body system. It should be noted that Chapter 0 contains procedures and interventions that represent new technology.

Alphabetic Index for ICD-9-CM

The location of procedures in the Alphabetic Index can be found under the common name of a procedure (e.g., appendectomy, hysterectomy). However, procedures may be listed under the general type of procedure with terminology such as the following:

TABLE 6-1 **TABLE OF CONTENTS FOR VOLUME 3, PROCEDURES**

Procedures: Volume 3
Index to Procedures
Tabular List of Procedures

- Insertion
- Incision
- Excision
- Clipping
- Repair
- Implantation
- Examination
- Removal

EXERCISE 6-1

Underline the main terms for the following procedures using the Alphabetic Index.

1. Cataract removal
2. Incision and drainage abscess right arm
3. Excisional debridement ulcer ankle
4. Inguinal hernia repair
5. Laparoscopic cholecystectomy

Omit Code

Omit code is an instructional note that is found only in the Alphabetic Index and Tabular List of Volume 3. This instruction denotes that no code is to be assigned. The omit code instruction is generally found under codes that are used for approaches and closures and therefore may be integral to the operative procedure (Figure 6-1). This convention is explained in further detail in this chapter under Operative Approaches and Closures.

Code Also

"Code also" is an instructional note found in Volume 3 that directs the assignment of an additional procedure if it was performed.

EXAMPLE | Aortocoronary bypass, (origin is the aorta with autologous left greater saphenous vein graft, which was harvested via percutaneous endoscopic approach) one coronary vessel with cardiopulmonary bypass, 36.11, 39.61 (Figure 6-2) (021009W, 06BQ4ZZ, 5A1221Z).

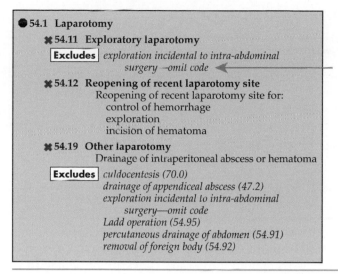

FIGURE 6-1. Instruction to "Omit code" if the laparotomy approach to intra-abdominal surgery is used.

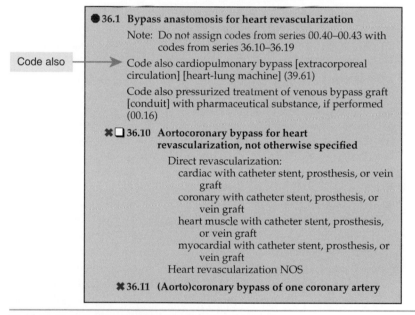

FIGURE 6-2. "Code also" instructional note.

Adjunct Codes

Adjunct codes are assigned as add-on codes to a primary procedure to provide additional information about the primary procedure performed. These codes cannot be used alone and are assigned as a secondary procedure code.

EXAMPLE Percutaneous transluminal coronary angioplasty is performed with drug-eluting stent placement into the LAD for coronary atherosclerosis, 414.01, 00.66, 36.07, 00.45, 00.40 (I25.10, 027034Z).

Codes 00.45 and 00.40 are adjunct vascular system procedure codes. These codes cannot be used alone and are used only to provide more information about the procedure that was performed.

EXERCISE 6-2

Assign and sequence the following procedures using your ICD-9-CM code book.

1. Partial left ventriculectomy with synchronous open mitral valve _____
   repair
2. Total abdominal hysterectomy with bilateral _____
   salpingo-oophorectomy
3. Laparoscopic cholecystectomy _____

UHDDS DEFINITIONS

Uniform Hospital Discharge Data Set (UHDDS) definitions are used by acute care, short-term hospitals to report inpatient data elements in a standardized manner. Definitions that pertain to the assignment of procedure codes are presented in the following sections.

Principal Procedure

A **principal procedure** is one that was performed for definitive treatment rather than for diagnostic or exploratory purposes, or one necessary to take care of a complication. If two procedures appear to meet this definition, then the one most closely related to the principal diagnosis should be selected as the principal procedure.

Significant Procedure

To qualify as a **significant procedure**, one of the following criteria must be met:
- Is surgical in nature
- Carries a procedural risk
- Carries an anesthetic risk
- Requires specialized training

It should be noted that a significant procedure does not have to be performed in an OR. Procedures can be done in the Emergency Room (ER) before admission, at the patient's bedside, in a treatment room, or in an interventional radiology department. These procedures can be easily missed because an operative report describing the procedure may not have been completed. Often, these procedures are documented with a brief, handwritten note on the ER record or in a progress note. Consent for treatment may assist the coder in attempting to verify a procedure, but not all procedures require consent forms. Also, a signed consent form does not confirm that the procedure was actually performed. A complete review of the entire health record is necessary to ensure that all completed procedures have been coded.

Other UHDDS data elements that must be coded include the date of the procedure and the NPI (National Provider Identifier) of the person who performed the procedure. It may be the coder's responsibility to abstract these data elements.

ICD-9-CM

Official Guidelines for Coding and Reporting

Please refer to the companion Evolve site for the most current guidelines.

Under the specific chapter guidelines, there are only a few references to procedure codes. The first is in the OB chapter and references the assignment of the principal diagnosis when a certain procedure was performed. It guides the selection of the principal diagnosis when a vaginal or a cesarean delivery occurs.

Chapter 11: Complications of Pregnancy, Childbirth, and the Puerperium (630-677)
b. Selection of OB Principal or First-listed Diagnosis
   3) Episodes when no delivery occurs
     In episodes when no delivery occurs, the principal diagnosis should correspond to the principal complication of the pregnancy, which necessitated the encounter. Should more than one complication exist, all of which are treated or monitored, any of the complications codes may be sequenced first.

EXAMPLE   Vomiting due to mild hyperemesis gravidarum. Patient is 10 weeks' pregnant, 643.03 (No procedure performed) (O21.0).

---

   4) When a delivery occurs
     When a delivery occurs, the principal diagnosis should correspond to the main circumstances or complication of the delivery. In cases of cesarean delivery, the selection of the principal diagnosis should be the condition established after study that was responsible for the patient's admission. If the patient was admitted with a condition that resulted in the performance of a cesarean procedure, that condition should be selected as the principal diagnosis. If the reason for the admission/encounter was unrelated to the condition resulting in the cesarean delivery, the condition related to the reason for the admission/encounter should be selected as the principal diagnosis, even if a cesarean was preformed.

EXAMPLE   Obstructed labor due to breech position. Lower segment cesarean section was performed with delivery of a single liveborn infant, 660.01, 652.21, V27.0, 74.1 (O64.1xx0, Z37.0, 10D00Z1).

The next reference to procedures involves debridements, which are frequently documented within the physician's progress notes or physical therapy notes.

Chapter 17. Injury and Poisoning (800-999)
d. Coding of Debridement of Wound, Infection, or Burn
   Excisional debridement involves surgical removal or cutting away, as opposed to mechanical (brushing, scrubbing, washing) debridement.
     For coding purposes, excisional debridement is assigned to code 86.22.
     Nonexcisional debridement is assigned to code 86.28.

Excisional debridement, as defined by *Coding Clinic* (1988:4Q:p5),[2] is "the surgical removal or cutting away of devitalized tissue, necrosis, or slough." Excisional debridement may be performed in a variety of settings (Operating Room, Emergency Room, or bedside) and by a variety of healthcare providers (physicians, nurse practitioners, physician assistants, and physical therapists). For a debridement to qualify as excisional, documentation provided by the healthcare provider who performed this service must indicate that the procedure was excisional, per *Coding Clinic* (2008:1Q:p3-4).[3]

According to *Coding Clinic* (1999:1Q:p8-9),[4] when an extensive debridement goes beyond the skin and subcutaneous tissue into the muscle, tendon, and/or bone, it is appropriate to "assign only a code for the deepest layer of debridement when multiple layers of the same site are debrided." If a patient underwent debridement of skin, subcutaneous tissue, muscle, and bone, the bone is the deepest layer, and debridement of the bone, 77.67, is the only procedure code assigned.

Any debridement that does not meet the criteria described for an excisional debridement would be coded as nonexcisional. A **nonexcisional debridement** may be performed by brushing, irrigating, scrubbing, or washing to remove devitalized tissue. Once again, this procedure may be performed in a variety of settings by a variety of healthcare providers.

It is important to remember that if debridement of the skin is performed in preparation for further surgery, the debridement of the skin should not be coded separately. For example, prior to reduction of an open fracture, a debridement may be performed.

EXAMPLE   Excisional debridement of right heel ulcer performed by physical therapist, 707.14, 86.22 (L97.419, 0HBMXZZ).

EXAMPLE   Excisional debridement of gangrenous sacral decubitus ulcer, stage II, by physician, 707.03, 707.22, 785.4, 86.22 (I96, L89.152, 0HB6XZZ).

EXAMPLE   Debridement by scrubbing of the left foot ulcer by physical therapist, 707.15, 86.28 (L97.529, 0HDNXZZ).

The last reference to procedures is in the V code section, Classification of Factors Influencing Health Status and Contact with Health Service. The guideline emphasizes the fact that V codes are not procedure codes.

> **18. Classification of Factors Influencing Health Status and Contact with Health Service (Supplemental VO1-V84)**
> **c. V Codes indicate a reason for an encounter**
> They are not procedure codes. A corresponding procedure code must accompany a V code to describe the procedure performed.

Although V codes can be a reason for an encounter when a procedure is performed, a procedure code is still required in the inpatient setting.

EXAMPLE   A female patient is admitted for elective sterilization. Bilateral endoscopic ligation is performed with a Falope ring, V25.2, 66.29. The V code is the reason for the encounter and the 66.29 identifies the specific procedure that was performed (Z30.2, 0UL74CZ).

PROCEDURE CODES THAT SHOULD BE REPORTED

Any procedures that affect payment or reimbursement must be reported. Other procedures may be reported at a hospital's discretion or in accordance with hospital policy. Encoders (ICD-9-CM coding software) may also have special popup notices that alert the coder about noncovered or limited coverage OR procedures.

Most facilities do not assign codes from the ICD-9-CM procedure Chapter 16, Miscellaneous Diagnostic and Therapeutic Procedures (87-99) for diagnostic tests such as ultrasounds, CT scans, MRIs, etc. Some codes that should be assigned from this chapter include mechanical ventilation, blood transfusions, administration of thrombolytic agents, enteral feedings, and TPN (see Sample policy, Figure 6-3). A facility policy should address which procedure codes should be assigned from this chapter.

After assigning procedure codes, the coder should review the diagnosis codes to ensure the assignment of diagnosis codes that support the performance of a procedure.

Facility Policy

DEPARTMENT:	HEALTH INFORMATION SERVICES
POLICY:	Coding of ICD-9-CM Procedure Codes **POLICY NUMBER:** HIM 03.005
DEVELOPED BY:	Karla Lovaasen, RHIA, CCS, CCS-P
ORIGINATED:	October 2001
REVISED:	10/02 **REVIEWED:** 10/03

SCOPE:	All personnel responsible for performing, supervising or monitoring coding services.
PURPOSE:	To facilitate the coding of ICD-9-CM procedure codes from Volume 3.
POLICY:	To assign procedure codes consistently to optimize reimbursement and capture facility data for quality and statistical monitoring.

PROCEDURE:

Assign ICD-9-CM diagnosis and procedure codes according to UHDDS guidelines and definitions and The Official Guidelines for Coding and Reporting.

ICD-9-CM procedure codes will be assigned to any procedures that are identified as a valid OR procedure or as a non-OR procedure affecting MS-DRG assignment.

Code all procedures that fall within 00.01 and 86.99 EXCEPT insertion of Foley catheter (57.94).

Bilateral procedures will be coded separately. Example: Bilateral knee replacement 81.54, 81.54.

It is not necessary to code minor procedures such as a blood transfusion that is given on multiple days.

Do NOT code procedures that fall within the code range 87.01 to 99.99 EXCEPT:
    Some procedures that fall in this range, but may need to be performed under sedation/anesthesia on certain patients should be coded. Example: A gynecologic exam (89.26) performed under anesthesia due to patient's severe mental retardation.

87.53	Intraoperative cholangiogram
88.40 to 88.58	Arteriography and angiography
88.96	Intraoperative MRI
89.41	Cardiovascular stress test
89.50	Holter monitor
89.62	CVP monitoring
89.64	Swan-Ganz catheterization
92.21 to 92.29	Radiation therapy
92.30 to 92.39	Stereotactic radiosurgery
93.51 to 93.59	Immobilization, pressure and attention to wound
94.24 to 94.27	Psychiatric therapy
94.61 to 94.69	Alcohol/drug detoxification and rehabilitation
95.04	Eye examination under anesthesia
96.01 to 96.09	Nonoperative intubation and irrigation
96.21 to 96.29	Nonoperative dilation and manipulation
96.31 to 96.39	Nonoperative alimentary tract irrigation, cleaning and local instillation
96.49	Prostaglandin instillation
96.51 to 96.52	Irrigation of eye and ear
96.6	Enteral infusion
96.70 to 96.72	Mechanical ventilation
97.01 to 97.05	Nonoperative replacement of gastrointestinal appliances
97.11 to 97.16	Nonoperative replacement of musculoskeletal and integumentary system appliance
97.29	Other nonoperative replacements
98.01 to 98.29	Nonoperative removal of foreign body or calculus
98.51 to 98.59	ESWL
99.00 to 99.09	Transfusion of blood products
99.10 to 99.11	Injections of thrombolytic agent and Rh immune globulin
99.15	TPN
99.20 to 99.29	Injection or infusion of other therapeutic or prophylactic substance (coded primarily in outpatient setting)
99.31 to 99.59	Vaccinations and Inoculations
99.61 to 99.69	Conversions of cardiac rhythm

Any interventional procedures charged by radiology will be assigned a corresponding ICD-9-CM procedure code.

Procedures done at another facility can be coded if they are billed to the patient and/or third party payer by facility.

This policy will be reviewed at least annually to incorporate any procedure code changes that may be effective April and October 1.

FIGURE 6-3. This policy is a sample policy, and any policies should be designed to fit the needs of a facility.

EXAMPLE

> If it was determined that lysis of peritoneal adhesions was sufficient to warrant a procedure code in this male patient, it would make sense that a diagnosis code should be assigned to identify the peritoneal adhesions.
>   Procedure: Lysis of peritoneal adhesions, 54.59 (0DNW0ZZ).
>   Diagnosis: Peritoneal adhesions, 568.0 (K66.0).

The Centers for Medicare and Medicaid Services (CMS) has categorized procedures into different classifications through the Medicare Code Editor (MCE). In some code books, these procedures may be highlighted to facilitate assignment of procedure codes. The **Medicare Code Editor** is software that detects errors in coding on Medicare claims. For example, it would identify a male-only procedure coded on a female patient's record.

During a patient's hospitalization, it may be necessary for a procedure to be performed at an outside facility. This could be for reasons such as the service may not be offered at the admitting hospital or equipment may malfunction. The patient may be transported by ambulance to this outside facility, and after the procedure, returns for continued care at the admitting hospital. In these cases, the admitting hospital may assign procedure codes for services performed at the outside facility. The admitting hospital also would include these charges on the hospital bill, and the admitting hospital would reimburse the outside facility for the procedure.

Valid OR Procedure

A **valid OR procedure** is a procedure that may affect MS-DRG assignment.

EXAMPLE

> Radical vaginal hysterectomy is designated as a valid OR procedure, 68.79 (0UT97ZZ).

Designation of a procedure as a valid OR procedure does not mean that it must be performed in the inpatient setting. Many surgical procedures can be safely performed on an outpatient basis, and many third party payers and/or insurance companies require that certain surgical procedures be performed in an outpatient setting. Repair of direct inguinal hernia is designated as a valid OR procedure, but this procedure is usually performed and billed as an outpatient procedure.

Non-OR Procedure Affecting MS-DRG Assignment

A procedure designated as a "**non-OR procedure affecting MS-DRG assignment**" is a procedure that may affect MS-DRG assignment, even though the procedure is not routinely performed in the OR.

EXAMPLE

> Insertion of a totally implantable vascular access device (VAD), chest (percutaneous approach), 86.07 (0JH63XZ). VADs may be used in patients who require long-term vascular access for chemotherapy, drug administration, or hemodialysis.

In some cases, the procedure code 86.07 will make a difference in MS-DRG assignment; in other cases, it will not.

EXAMPLE

> The patient was admitted with progressive chronic renal failure, stage V. An abdominal VAD was implanted (percutaneously) for future hemodialysis, 585.5, 86.07 (N18.5, 0JH83XZ).

In this case, the codes group to a surgical MS-DRG: MS-DRG 675, Other Kidney & Urinary Tract Procedures without CC/MCC.

> **EXAMPLE** The patient was admitted with primary liver cancer. It was decided to implant (percutaneous) a VAD in the chest for future chemotherapy, 155.0, 86.07 (C22.8, 0JH63XZ).

In this case, the codes group to a medical MS-DRG: MS-DRG 437, Malignancy of Hepatobiliary System or Pancreas without CC/MCC.

Noncovered OR Procedure

Noncovered OR procedure codes are identified by the Medicare Code Editor as procedures for which Medicare does not provide reimbursement.

> **EXAMPLE** Vasectomy (excision of bilateral vas deferens, percutaneous) is identified as a noncovered OR procedure, V25.2, 63.73 (Z30.2, 0VBQ3ZZ).

Sterilization procedures are usually not covered by Medicare. It is possible to assign an MS-DRG, but that does not guarantee payment.

Limited Coverage

Limited coverage procedures are identified by the Medicare Code Editor as procedures covered under limited circumstances.

> **EXAMPLE** Patient with cystic fibrosis had a bilateral lung transplantation (allogenic), 277.02, 33.52 (E84.0, 0BYM0Z0).

For a transplant facility to obtain Medicare coverage for organ transplantation, it must meet preapproved guidelines. Criteria are set forth and updated in *Federal Register* notices.

SURGICAL HIERARCHY

The **MS-DRG grouper** software (computer program that assigns an MS-DRG), using diagnosis and procedure codes, identifies whether a particular patient falls into a medical MS-DRG or a surgical MS-DRG. The MS-DRG grouper is able to determine which procedure is the most resource intensive and assigns the procedure to that particular surgical MS-DRG.

> **EXAMPLE** A patient has an open breast biopsy during the same operative episode as a modified radical mastectomy. The patient also has Crohn's disease. The pathology report confirms that the patient has cancer of the right upper outer quadrant.
> CODE ASSIGNMENTS: 174.4, 555.9, 85.43, 85.12 (C50.411, K50.90, 0HTT0ZZ, 0HBT0ZX)
> (The codes were put into the MS-DRG grouper in this order.)
> MS-DRG: 582, MASTECTOMY FOR MALIGNANCY W CC/MCC

In this case, the patient was admitted and after study was determined to have breast cancer of the right upper outer quadrant. She also has a comorbidity of Crohn's disease. The principal procedure is one that is performed for definitive treatment; in this case, that would be the modified radical mastectomy. The mastectomy is more resource intensive than a breast biopsy. It is appropriate to code the diagnostic breast biopsy as an additional procedure code.

EXAMPLE | CODE ASSIGNMENTS: 174.4, 555.9, 85.12, 85.43 (C50.411, K50.90, 0HTT0ZZ, 0HBT0ZX)
MS-DRG: 582, MASTECTOMY FOR MALIGNANCY W CC/MCC

In this case, all the codes are the same, but the breast biopsy is incorrectly sequenced as the principal procedure instead of the mastectomy. Because of the surgical hierarchy within the grouper, it groups to the mastectomy MS-DRG, so the reimbursement and MS-DRG assignment would be correct. Even if the grouper will automatically arrange the codes to fit the surgical hierarchy, the code should be sequenced as the principal procedure on the basis of the UHDDS definition.

EXAMPLE | CODE ASSIGNMENTS: 555.9, 174.4, 85.43, 85.12 (K50.90, C50.411, 0HTT0ZZ, 0HBT0ZX).
MS-DRG: 983, EXTENSIVE OR PROCEDURE UNRELATED TO PRINCIPAL DIAGNOSIS W/O CC/MCC

In this case, a data entry error was made, and Crohn's disease was incorrectly sequenced as the principal diagnosis, resulting in a 983 MS-DRG assignment. Although MS-DRG 983 may be the correct assignment in some cases, it is not appropriate in this case, and the coder should review the entered codes.

In this case, the principal diagnosis combined with the procedure codes resulted in the MS-DRG assignment. If the data entry error had not been corrected before billing, the facility would have been incorrectly reimbursed.

COMPUTER AND ROBOTIC-ASSISTED SURGERY

Advances in computer technologies have made it possible for computers to be utilized in the performance of diagnostic and therapeutic procedures. **Computer assisted surgery** (CAS) is an adjunct procedure that allows increased visualization and more precise navigation during surgery. CAS may be useful with surgical planning by using preoperative and intraoperative images. The computers identify particular landmarks and then establish spatial relationships between locations on the computer images with the actual corresponding anatomic locations on the patient. Navigation is real-time tracking of instruments during the procedure.

Robotic-assisted surgery is a minimally invasive technique that utilizes robotic arms to manipulate the surgical equipment and tools. A physician sits at a console and controls the joysticks that guide the robot in the performance of the surgical procedure. Unlike CAS, robotic-assisted procedures include the actual performance of the procedure.

EXAMPLE | Patient with prostate cancer had a robotic-assisted radical laparoscopic prostatectomy with pelvic lymphadenectomy (total of three nodes), 185, 60.5, 17.42, 40.3 (C61, 0VT04ZZ, 07BC4ZZ, 8E0W4CZ).

BIOPSIES

Biopsy is a very common diagnostic procedure that is often performed before more definitive treatment is provided. **Biopsy** is defined as "the removal of tissue followed by pathologic examination to establish a precise diagnosis." The entire abnormality is not removed during a biopsy.

If the entire specimen is removed, it is no longer a biopsy but an excision of tissue. The physician may document in the OR report that the lesion was totally removed. Biopsies may be performed in a number of different ways, such as by aspiration, brush, core, endoscopic, excisional, incisional, percutaneous, punch, shave, stereotactic, and washing methods. Different codes may be assigned, depending on the biopsy method used. According to *Coding Clinic* (1984:J-A:p3-4),[5] biopsies that are performed by endoscopy or percutaneous aspiration are coded as "closed" biopsies. An incisional approach for removal of tissue is coded as an "open biopsy." A patient may be undergoing an open abdominal procedure while a percutaneous biopsy of the liver is also performed. Biopsy of the liver would be coded to percutaneous and not to open biopsy, even though the abdominal cavity was open at the time per *Coding Clinic* (1988:4Q:p12).[6]

EXAMPLE | Patient had a diagnostic percutaneous biopsy of the right kidney because of persistent proteinuria, 791.0, 55.23 (R80.1, 0TB03ZX).

EXAMPLE | Patient had a diagnostic open wedge biopsy of the liver and Wilson's disease was confirmed, 275.1, 50.12 (E83.01, 0FB00ZX).

EXAMPLE | The patient was admitted for elective open cholecystectomy for gallstones. An abnormality of the liver (pathology is consistent with patient's chronic hepatitis C) was noted during exploration, and percutaneous biopsy was performed, 574.20, 070.54, 51.22, 50.11 (K80.20, B18.2, 0FT40ZZ, 0FB03ZX).
Cholecystectomy is the principal procedure because it was performed for definitive treatment.

The documentation should be reviewed closely when excisional biopsies are performed. In some instances, the surgeon will document that he/she performed an "excisional biopsy" of a breast mass or lump. Upon reading the OR report and confirming findings through review of the pathology report, the coder may discover that the entire lump or mass was removed. This changes the coding from a biopsy code (85.12) to a lumpectomy code (85.21).

ENDOSCOPIC APPROACHES

Endoscopic examinations and procedures are performed with an instrument that allows examination of any cavity of the body through a rigid or flexible scope. The scope is usually inserted into the body through an orifice or stoma. When a colonoscopy is performed, the anus is the body orifice that allows entry of the scope.

As the scope is inserted and various parts of the body are examined, the coder would not code every body part that is viewed. The coder would code the farthest site that was reached. If a procedure such as a biopsy is performed, only the biopsy code is assigned.

EXAMPLE | A flexible colonoscopy is performed for gastrointestinal bleeding. During the procedure, the physician examines the ascending, transverse, descending, and sigmoid colon, 578.9, 45.23 (K92.2, 0DJD8ZZ).

Only the colonoscopy code is assigned because examination of all these areas is included within that code.

OPERATIVE APPROACHES AND CLOSURES

An important convention in Volume 3 is the "Omit code." Main terms in the Alphabetic Index may be used to identify incisions. If an incision is made only for the purpose of performing further surgery, the instruction "Omit code" is given.

EXAMPLE | Lumbar laminectomy (decompression) (for exploration), 03.09 as operative approach—Omit code.

Other examples of incisions include laparotomy, thoracotomy, arthrotomy, and craniotomy. Often, the surgeon will indicate the approach in the operative procedure statement. Documentation of laparotomy by the physician does not necessarily mean that it should be coded. It is necessary to review the entire operative report to determine the extent of the procedure and to decide what should be coded. Sometimes, a physician will document that an exploratory laparotomy was performed along with an appendectomy for acute appendicitis. It is not necessary to code the exploratory laparotomy. Usually, some component of exploration occurs during a surgical procedure.

EXAMPLE

> Exploratory laparotomy with appendectomy for acute appendicitis, 540.9, 47.09 (K35.80, 0DTJ0ZZ).

The exploratory laparotomy was incidental to the intra-abdominal surgery.

Closure of the operative wound is a routine part of most surgical procedures, so it is not necessary to code this separately. In some instances, a surgical wound is not closed at the time of a surgical operation but is allowed to heal and will be closed at a later date. In this case, a closure would be coded.

EXAMPLE

> A patient is admitted for delayed closure of the laparotomy site, V58.41, 54.62 (Z48.1, 0WQFXZZ).

CLOSED SURGICAL PROCEDURES AND CONVERSION TO OPEN PROCEDURES

As technology has advanced, procedures are increasingly being performed through scopes, which are less invasive than open procedures. This has resulted in quicker recoveries, shorter hospital stays, and fewer complications.

Common closed surgical approaches include laparoscopic, thoracoscopic, and arthroscopic procedures. The **laparoscopic approach** involves use of a laparoscope to examine and perform closed procedures within the abdomen. With a **thoracoscopic approach**, a thoracoscope is used to examine and perform closed procedures within the thorax. The **arthroscopic approach** requires the use of an arthroscope to examine and perform closed procedures within a joint. Closed procedures may be diagnostic and/or therapeutic in nature.

A surgical procedure may start with a closed approach that may need to be converted to an open procedure. V codes describe the conversion from a closed surgical procedure to an open procedure. These codes are found in the Index under the main term, Conversion.

V64.41	Laparoscopic surgical procedure converted to open procedure
V64.42	Thoracoscopic surgical procedure converted to open procedure
V64.43	Arthroscopic surgical procedure converted to open procedure

In the case of conversion from closed to open, assign only the open procedure code. Some reasons for conversion to an open procedure include adhesions, bleeding, technical difficulties due to anatomic body structure and/or inflammatory changes, and injury to an organ.

EXAMPLE

> A patient was admitted for a laparoscopic cholecystectomy for chronic cholecystitis with cholelithiasis. Because of excessive bleeding from the liver bed, the procedure was converted to an open cholecystectomy and the bleeding was controlled, 574.10, 998.11, V64.41, E878.6, E849.7, 51.22 (K80.10, K91.61, Y83.6, Y92.234, 0FT40ZZ, 0FJ44ZZ; ICD-10-PCS guidelines require two procedure codes for a laparoscopic procedure that is converted to an open procedure. There is no diagnosis code to identify the conversion.)

Because the variety of procedures that can be performed via a scope is constantly changing, a code that describes the approach accurately may not be available. In these instances, the open code is used.

EXAMPLE

> A patient is admitted for laparoscopic left nephrectomy as a donor, V59.4, 55.51 (Z52.4, 0TT14ZZ).

Coding Clinic (1992:3Q:p12)[7] states "until specific codes for laparoscopic and thoracoscopic approaches can be created, the codes for open approaches must be applied. Do not assign a separate code for the laparoscopy or thoracoscopy."

It may be the policy of some facilities to assign an additional procedure code for the laparoscopy (54.21) so that data can be collected on the number of laparoscopic procedures performed.

BILATERAL PROCEDURES

A **bilateral procedure** occurs when the same procedure is performed on paired anatomic organs or tissues (i.e., eyes, ears, joints such as shoulder or knee). According to *Coding Clinic* (1988:1Q:p9),[8] "when the same procedures are performed bilaterally and ICD-9-CM provides a single code that identifies the procedure as bilateral, assign that code. When the same procedure is performed bilaterally and ICD-9-CM does not provide a code to identify that procedure as being performed bilaterally, record the procedure code twice. When there is a difference in the procedure performed on one side as opposed to the other side involving different code assignments, report both codes."

The coding of bilateral procedures should be addressed by facility policy. For major procedures such as joint replacements, the coder must assign two codes. As procedures become less invasive, more bilateral procedures may be performed during the same operative episode.

EXAMPLE

> Open repair of bilateral direct and indirect inguinal hernia with synthetic prosthesis, 550.92, 53.16 (K40.20, 0YUA0JZ).

EXAMPLE

> Primary osteoarthritis knees for bilateral total knee synthetic substitute replacement, 715.16, 81.54, 81.54 (M17.0, 0SRC0JZ, 0SRD0JZ).

PLANNED AND CANCELED PROCEDURES

When patients are admitted to the hospital for a scheduled procedure(s), under some circumstances, the procedure(s) may be canceled or not completed. If a patient's procedure is canceled prior to the time that he or she presents to the hospital, no code will be required because no services were provided, no bill was generated, and there is no health record. On some occasions, a patient presents to have a procedure performed, but for whatever reason the procedure has to be canceled. The principal diagnosis in this case is the reason why the patient was going to have the procedure performed. If a complication arose that resulted in the cancellation, a diagnosis code for that condition would be assigned as a secondary diagnosis. Also, V codes describe the reason for the cancellation. They can be located in the Index under the main term, procedure (surgical) not done.

V64.1 (Z53.09)	Surgical or other procedure not carried out because of contraindication (medical reason to delay the procedure)
V64.2 (Z53.20)	Surgical or other procedure not carried out because of patient's decision
V64.3 (Z53.8)	Procedure not carried out for other reasons (staffing, equipment problems, unavailability of OR due to emergency)

EXAMPLE | A patient was admitted for hysterectomy because of uterine fibroids. Shortly after admission, the patient told the nurse that she was having second thoughts and had decided not to go through with the procedure; the patient was discharged, 218.9, V64.2 (D25.9, Z53.29). No procedure code is assigned because the procedure was never started.

EXAMPLE | A patient was admitted for coronary artery bypass grafting because of coronary atherosclerosis of the native arteries. The cardiac surgeon became ill, and the surgery was rescheduled. The patient was discharged, 414.01, V64.3 (I25.10, Z53.8).

EXAMPLE | A patient was admitted for laparoscopic cholecystectomy for cholelithiasis. It was noted that the patient was having an acute exacerbation of his COPD. The patient was treated with steroids and nebulizer treatments and was discharged. The cholecystectomy was rescheduled for next week, 574.20, 491.21, V64.1 (K80.20, J44.1, Z53.09).

Occasionally, a surgical procedure will be started that for whatever reason cannot be completed. The surgical procedure should be coded to the extent that it was performed. These circumstances are different from those surrounding a procedure that is canceled, in that the patient received anesthesia and surgery was begun.

EXAMPLE | A patient was admitted for colon resection because of cancer of the descending colon. A laparotomy incision through subcutaneous tissue and fascia was made, and the patient became unstable with atrial fibrillation. It was decided that the procedure should be terminated and the patient transferred to the ICU for further management. The incision was closed before any definitive surgery could be performed, 153.2, 997.1, 427.31, E878.8, E849.7, 54.0, (C18.6, I97.791, I48.0, Y83.8, Y92.234, 0JJTXZZ).

EXAMPLE | The patient was admitted for colonoscopy, but because of the obstructing lesion, the scope could not be inserted beyond the sigmoid colon. A biopsy specimen of the lesion was taken, and cancer of the sigmoid colon was confirmed, 153.3, 45.25 (sigmoidoscopy with biopsy) (C18.7, 0DBN8ZX).

FACILITY POLICY

Each facility should have its own written policy (see Figure 6-3) regarding the assignment of ICD-9-CM procedure codes. This policy should consider reimbursement, but it should also take into account other uses of a procedure database and how that information can be extracted. It may be necessary to determine what types of procedures are being performed for physician profiles and credentialing. Research is an important aspect of data collection.

As has been stated previously, because not all procedures are performed in the operating room, it may be difficult to locate documentation of all procedures performed. Procedures that are easy to overlook include mechanical ventilation, debridement, lumbar puncture, suturing, ECMO (extracorporeal membrane oxygenation), and procedures performed by interventional radiology.

CHAPTER REVIEW EXERCISE

Complete the following review exercises using ICD-9-CM, Volume 3.

1. If a surgical procedure was canceled because of a medical condition or complication, which V code would be assigned?
   A. V64.1   Surgical or other procedure not carried out because of contraindication
   B. V64.2   Surgical or other procedure not carried out because of patient's decision
   C. V64.3   Procedure not carried out for other reasons
   D. None of the above

2. The principal diagnosis that is assigned when a surgical procedure is canceled is
   A. V64.1   Surgical or other procedure not carried out because of contraindication
   B. V64.2   Surgical or other procedure not carried out because of patient's decision
   C. V64.3   Procedure not carried out for other reasons
   D. None of the above

3. The approach of the surgical procedure should always be coded.
   A. True
   B. False

4. It is not necessary to code closure of a routine surgical incision.
   A. True
   B. False

5. If a procedure has been designated as a valid OR procedure, the procedure should be performed as an inpatient hospital stay.
   A. True
   B. False

6. It is a good idea for facilities to have a policy regarding which procedures are coded and which procedures are not coded.
   A. True
   B. False

7. A biopsy is the removal of tissue and pathologic examination to establish a precise diagnosis.
   A. True
   B. False

8. The surgical hierarchy within an MS-DRG grouper assists with sequencing the most resource-intensive procedure performed.
   A. True
   B. False

9. With the laparoscopic approach, a thoracoscope is used to examine and perform closed procedures within the thorax.
   A. True
   B. False

10. When a procedure is canceled because of a medical contraindication, the principal diagnosis is the medical contraindication and not the reason for which the patient was to undergo the procedure.
    A. True
    B. False

Underline the main terms.

11. Laparoscopic appendectomy
12. Creation of arteriovenous fistula for dialysis
13. Clipping aneurysm of brain
14. Insertion central venous catheter
15. Excision lesion of left eyelid

Assign procedure codes to the following using your ICD-9-CM code book.

16. Low cervical cesarean section with bilateral tubal ligation, Pomeroy technique _____

17. Partial esophagectomy with end-to-end anastomosis _____

18. Excisional debridement (skin right foot) performed by physical therapist _____

19. Robotic-assisted radical abdominal hysterectomy _____

20. Esophagogastroduodenoscopy with biopsy of the esophagus _____

21. Patient was admitted for cardiac ablation for atrial fibrillation. The patient had eaten breakfast so the procedure was canceled and will be rescheduled for a later date. _____

Using the sample facility procedure policy, answer the following questions.

22. Would a code be assigned for TPN? _____

23. Would the code 87.41 be assigned for CT of thorax? _____

24. Absolutely no procedure codes can be assigned unless the procedure is performed at the facility, true or false? _____

25. Would the code 87.53 be assigned for an intraoperative cholangiogram? _____

CHAPTER GLOSSARY

It is important to note that most of these definitions are as defined by ICD-10-PCS.

Adjunct codes: add-on codes to a primary procedure to provide additional information about the primary procedure that was performed.

Arthroscopic approach: an arthroscope is used to examine and perform closed procedures within a joint.

Bilateral procedure: operative procedure performed on paired anatomic organs or tissues during the same operative session.

Biopsy: removal of tissue and pathologic examination to establish a precise diagnosis.

Computer assisted surgery (CAS): adjunctive procedure that allows increased visualization and more precise navigation while remaining minimally invasive.

Endoscopic: examinations and procedures performed with an instrument that examines any cavity of the body through a rigid or flexible scope.

Excisional debridement: surgical removal or cutting away of devitalized tissue, necrosis, or slough.

Laparoscopic approach: uses a laparoscope to examine and perform closed procedures within the abdomen.

Limited coverage: procedures that are identified by the Medicare Code Editor as procedures covered under limited circumstances.

Medicare Code Editor: software that detects errors in coding on Medicare claims.

MS-DRG grouper: software that assigns MS-DRG using diagnosis and procedure codes.

Noncovered OR procedure: procedure code categorized by the Medicare Code Editor as a noncovered operating room procedure for which Medicare does not provide reimbursement.

Nonexcisional debridement: removal of devitalized tissue by brushing, irrigating, scrubbing, or washing.

Non-OR procedure affecting MS-DRG assignment: procedure code recognized by the MS-DRG Grouper as a non–operating room procedure that may affect MS-DRG assignment.

Omit code: an instructional note found in Volume 3 that denotes that no code is to be assigned; it generally is used for coding approaches and closures that are integral to an operative procedure.

Principal procedure: procedure that is performed for definitive treatment, rather than for diagnostic or exploratory purposes, or one performed that was necessary to take care of a complication.

Robotic-assisted surgery: minimally invasive technique that utilizes robotic arms to manipulate the surgical equipment and tools.

Significant procedure: a procedure is considered significant if it is surgical in nature, carries a procedural risk, carries an anesthetic risk, and/or requires specialized training.

Thoracoscopic approach: a thoracoscope is used to examine and perform closed procedures within the thorax.

Valid OR procedure: a procedure that may affect MS-DRG assignment.

REFERENCES

1. American Hospital Association. *Coding Clinic for ICD-9-CM* 2008:1Q:p15. Reporting ICD-9-CM procedure codes for outpatient procedures.
2. American Hospital Association. *Coding Clinic for ICD-9-CM* 1988:4Q:p5. Debridement of wound, excisional vs nonexcisional—Guidelines.
3. American Hospital Association. *Coding Clinic for ICD-9-CM* 2008:1Q:p3-4. Excisional debridement.
4. American Hospital Association. *Coding Clinic for ICD-9-CM* 1999:1Q:p8-9. Extensive wound debridement.
5. American Hospital Association. *Coding Clinic for ICD-9-CM* 1984:J-A:p3-4. Introduction to 1984 revision of UHDDS effective 1/1/86.
6. American Hospital Association. *Coding Clinic for ICD-9-CM* 1988:4Q:p12. Exploratory laparotomy with needle biopsy of liver.
7. American Hospital Association. *Coding Clinic for ICD-9-CM* 1992:3Q:p12. Laparoscopic appendectomy.
8. American Hospital Association. *Coding Clinic for ICD-9-CM* 1988:1Q:p9. Bilateral procedures—Guideline.

7

Introduction to ICD-10-PCS

LEARNING OBJECTIVES

1. Identify the format of ICD-10-PCS, Alphabetic Index and PCS Tables
2. Apply the conventions and ICD-10-PCS Coding Guidelines
3. Discuss the differences between ICD-9-CM, Volume 3, and ICD-10-PCS
4. Explain the use of the General Equivalence Mappings
5. Define the root operations for each section of ICD-10-PCS
6. Define the approaches that are used in ICD-10-PCS
7. Assign procedure codes using ICD-10-PCS

ABBREVIATIONS/ ACRONYMS

CMS Centers for Medicare and Medicaid Services

CPT Current Procedural Terminology

GEMs General Equivalence Mappings

ICD-9-CM International Classification of Diseases, 9th Revision, Clinical Modification

ICD-10-CM International Classification of Diseases, 10th Revision, Clinical Modification

ICD-10-PCS International Classification of Diseases, 10th Revision, Procedure Coding System

NCHS National Center for Health Statistics

NEC not elsewhere classifiable

NOS not otherwise specified

HISTORY OF ICD-10-PCS

In 1992, the Centers for Medicare and Medicaid Services (CMS) funded a project to replace Volume 3 of ICD-9-CM, which was outdated and could not be expanded to classify procedures with more specific detail. 3M Health Information Systems was awarded a contract to develop a new system for procedural coding, ICD-10-PCS (Procedure Coding System). The initial draft was completed in 1998. Since that time, it has been updated to incorporate changes that were made to ICD-9-CM, Volume 3. CMS is responsible for the maintenance of ICD-10-PCS. (Information about ICD-10-PCS is available on the CMS website.)

According to the National Center for Health Statistics (NCHS), the full implementation date for ICD-10-PCS is October 1, 2013.

The ICD-10 Procedure Coding System was developed with four characteristics in mind:
1. Completeness—Each procedure should have its own code.
2. Expandability—New procedure codes should be easily added.
3. Multiaxial—Each code character should have the same meaning across and within body systems.
4. Standardized terminology—ICD-10-PCS will include definitions for terminology used, and multiple meanings will not be associated with the same term.

Other principles followed in the development of ICD-10-PCS include:
- Diagnostic information is not included in the procedure description.
- A "not otherwise specified" (NOS) option is *not* available.
- The "not elsewhere classifiable" (NEC) option is limited.
- All procedures are defined to a high level of specificity.

Differences Between ICD-9-CM and ICD-10-PCS

ICD-9-CM	ICD-10-PCS
Structure is similar to ICD-9 diagnosis codes	Structure is different with the use of tables
Limited number of codes	Expandable with unlimited number of codes
Codes are three to four digits with a decimal	All codes are seven characters, with no decimal after the second digit
Codes are numeric	Codes are alphanumeric
10 different values can be used for each digit, 0 through 9	34 different values can be used for each character, for numbers 0 through 9, and A through Z except for I and O
Combination codes (e.g., tonsillectomy with adenoidectomy)	Separate procedures performed at the same time are coded separately

EXERCISE 7-1

Answer the following questions.

1. ICD-10-PCS is scheduled for full implementation on this date.
   A. October 1, 2012
   B. October 31, 2013
   C. October 1, 2013
   D. October 31, 2012

2. Who is responsible for the maintenance of ICD-10-PCS?
   A. AHIMA
   B. AMA
   C. NCHS
   D. CMS

3. Which of the following is a characteristic of ICD-10-PCS?
   A. Codes are alphanumeric
   B. Similar to ICD-10-CM diagnosis codes
   C. Limited number of codes
   D. Codes are three to four digits

4. The terminology used in ICD-10-PCS is such that multiple meanings can be used for the same term.
   A. True
   B. False

5. ICD-10-PCS is expandable with an unlimited number of codes.
   A. True
   B. False

ICD-9-CM	ICD-10-PCS	Flag
4701	0DTJ4ZZ	10000
4709	0DTJ0ZZ	10000
4709	0DTJ7ZZ	10000
4709	0DTJ8ZZ	10000
4711	0DTJ4ZZ	10000
4719	0DTJ0ZZ	10000
4719	0DTJ7ZZ	10000
4719	0DTJ8ZZ	10000

FIGURE 7-1. GEMs mapping file for ICD-9-CM to ICD-10-PCS.

ICD-10-PCS	ICD-9-CM	Flag
0DTJ0ZZ	4709	10000
0DTJ4ZZ	4701	10000
0DTJ7ZZ	4709	10000
0DTJ8ZZ	4709	10000
0DTK0ZZ	4579	10000
0DTK4ZZ	1739	10000
0DTK7ZZ	4579	10000
0DTK8ZZ	4579	10000

FIGURE 7-2. GEMs mapping file for ICD-10-PCS to ICD-9-CM.

Mapping

Because of the drastic changes in structure and specificity, it is difficult to provide an accurate cross-reference between ICD-9-CM and ICD-10-PCS. As with ICD-10-CM, two sets of procedure code General Equivalence Mappings (GEMs) have been developed. These mappings are a way to find corresponding procedure codes in the two code sets. The GEM files are located on the CMS website, and the two filenames appear below:

1. ICD-9-CM to ICD-10-PCS (forward mapping; Figure 7-1)
2. ICD-10-PCS to ICD-9-CM (backward mapping; Figure 7-2)

EXERCISE 7-2

Using the ICD-9-CM to ICD-10-PCS and ICD-10-PCS to ICD-9-CM GEMs files on the CMS website (Figures 7-1 and 7-2), map the following procedure codes.

1. 45.76 _____
2. 51.23 _____
3. 69.02 _____
4. 0W9B3ZZ _____
5. 0DJ68ZZ _____
6. 0YQ50ZZ _____

ORGANIZATION OF ICD-10-PCS

ICD-10-PCS is divided into 16 sections, the largest being the Medical and Surgical section (value 0). The first character of any procedure code identifies the section that describes the category where the code is located. Sections 1 through 9 are medical- and surgical-related sections. Sections B through D and F through H represent the ancillary sections of ICD-10-PCS. The sections are as follows:

0   Medical and Surgical
1   Obstetrics
2   Placement
3   Administration
4   Measurement and Monitoring
5   Extracorporeal Assistance and Performance
6   Extracorporeal Therapies
7   Osteopathic
8   Other Procedures
9   Chiropractic
B   Imaging
C   Nuclear Medicine
D   Radiation Oncology
F   Physical Rehabilitation and Diagnostic Audiology
G   Mental Health
H   Substance Abuse Treatment

EXERCISE 7-3

Using the ICD-10-PCS, identify the section value for the following.

1.   Radiation oncology   _____
2.   Administration   _____
3.   Other procedure   _____
4.   Obstetrics   _____
5.   Mental health   _____

Alphabetic Index and Tables

The ICD-10-PCS code book comprises the Alphabetic Index and Tables. The ICD-10-PCS Alphabetic Index is not as complete as the Index in ICD-9-CM. Once you have become familiar with the table structure, it may not be necessary to even use the index, which is structured in a way that follows the organization of the tables but may only identify the first three or four characters of the procedure code. The two types of main terms that are listed in the Alphabetic Index are:

- Based on the root operation or general type of procedure
- Common procedure terms

No eponyms or acronyms are used in the Alphabetic Index. The Index is used to assist with the location of the appropriate table that has the information necessary to construct a seven-character procedure code.

EXAMPLE   Alphabetic Index Entry for Appendectomy (Figure 7-3).
    In this example, there are two possible tables, 0DBJ and 0DTJ. The root operation, excision or resection, needs to be determined to find the right table and to assign Characters 4 through 7 for the appropriate code.

All ICD-10-PCS codes are seven characters, with each character representing a particular aspect of the procedure. The meanings of the characters for the Medical and Surgical section are as follows:

Appendectomy
   see Excision, Appendix **0DBJ**
   see Resection, Appendix **0DTJ**
Appendicolysis *see* Release, Appendix **0DNJ**
Appendicotomy *see* Drainage, Appendix **0D9J**

FIGURE 7-3. Alphabetic Index entry for appendectomy.

Section	0 Medical and Surgical
Body System	D Gastrointestinal System
Operation	T Resection: Cutting out or off, without replacement, all of a body part

Body Part	Approach	Device	Qualifier
1 Esophagus, Upper 2 Esophagus, Middle 3 Esophagus, Lower 4 Esophagogastric Junction 5 Esophagus 6 Stomach 7 Stomach, Pylorus 8 Small Intestine 9 Duodenum A Jejunum B Ileum C Ileocecal Valve E Large Intestine F Large Intestine, Right G Large Intestine, Left H Cecum J Appendix K Ascending Colon L Transverse Colon M Descending Colon N Sigmoid Colon P Rectum Q Anus	0 Open 4 Percutaneous Endoscopic 7 Via Natural or Artificial Opening 8 Via Natural or Artificial Opening Endoscopic	Z No Device	Z No Qualifier
R Anal Sphincter S Greater Omentum T Lesser Omentum	0 Open 4 Percutaneous Endoscopic	Z No Device	Z No Qualifier

FIGURE 7-4. Table for resection of gastrointestinal system.

CHARACTER	REPRESENTS
1	Section
2	Body system
3	Root operation
4	Body part
5	Approach
6	Device
7	Qualifier

There are 34 possible values for each character in a code, and a code is assigned from a table based on the documentation of the procedure. The values for characters 1 through 3 are located at the top of each table. Each table has four columns, which contain the applicable values for characters 4 through 7. Each column may have a varying number of rows, and within each row are the applicable values for those characters.

EXAMPLE

Appendectomy (the surgical removal of the appendix).
   The root operation is resection, because all of the appendix is removed without replacement. In the Alphabetic Index, under "Resection," go to Table 0DT (Figure 7-4) and assign Characters 4 through 7. Character 4 is "J," for the appendix. Character 5 is "0," for open, because no other approach was specified. Character 6 is "Z," for no device, and Character 7 is "Z," for no qualifier. Therefore, the ICD-10-PCS code for appendectomy is "0DTJ0ZZ."

CHARACTER 1 SECTION	CHARACTER 2 BODY SYSTEM	CHARACTER 3 OPERATION	CHARACTER 4 BODY PART	CHARACTER 5 APPROACH	CHARACTER 6 DEVICE	CHARACTER 7 QUALIFIER
Medical and Surgical	Gastrointestinal System	Resection	Appendix	Open	No Device	No Qualifier
0	D	T	J	0	Z	Z

EXERCISE 7-4

Answer the following questions about the characters in an ICD-10-PCS code.

1. How many characters are in an ICD-10-PCS code? _____
2. Which character identifies the approach? _____
3. Which character identifies the body part? _____
4. How many characters are given in the Alphabetic Index for a particular code? _____

ICD-10-PCS Coding Guidelines

A draft of the ICD-10-PCS guidelines is available at the Centers for Medicare and Medicaid (CMS) website. The guidelines are divided into three parts:

A. General
B. Medical and Surgical Section
  • Body system guidelines
  • Root operation guidelines
  • Body part guidelines
  • Approach guidelines
  • Device guidelines
C. Other Medical- and Surgical-Related Sections

ICD-10-PCS
Coding Guidelines (2011)

Please refer to the companion Evolve website for the most current guidelines.

These are the draft ICD-10-PCS guidelines. They are grouped into general guidelines and guidelines that apply to a section or sections. Guidelines for the Medical and Surgical section are further grouped by character. The guidelines are numbered sequentially within each category.

A. *Conventions*

A1 ICD-10-PCS codes are composed of seven characters. Each character is an axis of classification that specifies information about the procedure performed. Within a defined code range, a character specifies the same type of information in that axis of classification.
Example: The fifth axis of classification specifies the approach in sections 0 through 4 and 7 through 9 of the system.

A2 One of 34 possible values can be assigned to each axis of classification in the seven-character code: they are the numbers 0 through 9 and the alphabet (except I and O because they are easily confused with the numbers 1 and 0). The number of unique values used in an axis of classification differs as needed.
Example: Where the fifth axis of classification specifies the approach, seven different approach values are currently used to specify the approach.

A3 The valid values for an axis of classification can be added to as needed.
Example: If a significantly distinct type of device is used in a new procedure, a new device value can be added to the system.

A4 As with words in their context, the meaning of any single value is a combination of its axis of classification and any preceding values on which it may be dependent.

Example: The meaning of a body part value in the Medical and Surgical section is always dependent on the body system value. The body part value O in the Central Nervous body system specifies Brain and the body part value O in the Peripheral Nervous body system specifies Cervical Plexus.

A5 As the system is expanded to become increasingly detailed, over time more values will depend on preceding values for their meaning.

Example: In the Lower Joints body system, the device value 3 in the root operation Insertion specifies Infusion Device and the device value 3 in the root operation Fusion specifies Interbody Fusion Device.

A6 The purpose of the alphabetic index is to locate the appropriate table that contains all information necessary to construct a procedure code. The PCS Tables should always be consulted to find the most appropriate valid code.

A7 It is not required to consult the index first before proceeding to the tables to complete the code. A valid code may be chosen directly from the tables.

A8 All seven characters must be specified to be a valid code. If the documentation is incomplete for coding purposes, the physician should be queried for the necessary information.

A9 Within a PCS table, valid codes include all combinations of choices in characters 4 through 7 contained in the same row of the table. In the example below, OJHT3VZ is a valid code, and OJHW3VZ is *not* a valid code.

Section: O Medical and Surgical
Body System: J Subcutaneous Tissue and Fascia
Operation: H Insertion: Putting in a nonbiological appliance that monitors, assists, performs, or prevents a physiological function but does not physically take the place of a body part

Body Part	Approach	Device	Qualifier
S Subcutaneous Tissue and Fascia, Head and Neck V Subcutaneous Tissue and Fascia, Upper Extremity W Subcutaneous Tissue and Fascia, Lower Extremity	O Open 3 Percutaneous	1 Radioactive Element 3 Infusion Device	Z No Qualifier
T Subcutaneous Tissue and Fascia, Trunk	O Open 3 Percutaneous	1 Radioactive Element 3 Infusion Device V Infusion Pump	Z No Qualifier

A10 "And," when used in a code description, means "and/or."

Example: Lower Arm and Wrist Muscle means lower arm and/or wrist muscle.

A11 Many of the terms used to construct PCS codes are defined within the system. It is the coder's responsibility to determine what the documentation in the medical record equates to in the PCS definitions. The physician is not expected to use the terms used in PCS code descriptions, nor is the coder required to query the physician when the correlation between the documentation and the defined PCS terms is clear.

Example: When the physician documents "partial resection" the coder can independently correlate "partial resection" to the root operation Excision without querying the physician for clarification.

B. *Medical and Surgical Section Guidelines (section O)*

  B2. Body System

   General guidelines

   B2.1a The procedure codes in the general anatomical regions body systems should only be used when the procedure is performed on an anatomical region rather than a specific body part (e.g., root operations Control and Detachment, drainage of a body cavity) or on the rare occasion when no information is available to support assignment of a code to a specific body part.

   Example: Control of postoperative hemorrhage is coded to the root operation Control found in the general anatomical regions body systems.

B2.1b Body systems designated as upper or lower contain body parts located above or below the diaphragm respectively.

Example: Vein body parts above the diaphragm are found in the Upper Veins body system; vein body parts below the diaphragm are found in the Lower Veins body system.

B3. Root Operation

General guidelines

B3.1a In order to determine the appropriate root operation, the full definition of the root operation as contained in the PCS Tables must be applied.

B3.1b Components of a procedure specified in the root operation definition and explanation are not coded separately. Procedural steps necessary to reach the operative site and close the operative site are also not coded separately.

Example: Resection of a joint as part of a joint replacement procedure is included in the root operation definition of Replacement and is not coded separately. Laparotomy performed to reach the site of an open liver biopsy is not coded separately.

Multiple procedures

B3.2 During the same operative episode, multiple procedures are coded if:

a. The same root operation is performed on different body parts as defined by distinct values of the body part character.

Example: Diagnostic excision of liver and pancreas are coded separately.

b. The same root operation is repeated at different body sites that are included in the same body part value.

Example: Excision of the sartorius muscle and excision of the gracilis muscle are both included in the upper leg muscle body part value, and multiple procedures are coded.

c. Multiple root operations with distinct objectives are performed on the same body part.

Example: Destruction of sigmoid lesion and bypass of sigmoid colon are coded separately.

d. The intended root operation is attempted using one approach, but is converted to a different approach.

Example: Laparoscopic cholecystectomy converted to an open cholecystectomy is coded as percutaneous endoscopic Inspection and open Resection.

Discontinued procedures

B3.3 If the intended procedure is discontinued, code the procedure to the root operation performed. If a procedure is discontinued before any other root operation is performed, code the root operation Inspection of the body part or anatomical region inspected.

Example: A planned aortic valve replacement procedure is discontinued after the initial thoracotomy and before any incision is made in the heart muscle, when the patient becomes hemodynamically unstable. This procedure is coded as an open Inspection of the mediastinum.

Biopsy followed by more definitive treatment

B3.4 If a diagnostic Excision, Extraction, or Drainage procedure (biopsy) is followed by a more definitive procedure, such as Destruction, Excision or Resection at the same procedure site, both the biopsy and the more definitive treatment are coded.

Example: Biopsy of breast followed by partial mastectomy at the same procedure site, both the biopsy and the partial mastectomy procedure are coded.

Overlapping body layers

B3.5 If the root operations Excision, Repair or Inspection are performed on overlapping layers of the musculoskeletal system, the body part specifying the deepest layer is coded.

Example: Excisional debridement that includes skin and subcutaneous tissue and muscle is coded to the muscle body part.

Bypass procedures

B3.6a Bypass procedures are coded by identifying the body part bypassed "from" and the body part bypassed "to." The fourth character body part specifies the body part bypassed from, and the qualifier specifies the body part bypassed to.

Example: Bypass from stomach to jejunum, stomach is the body part and jejunum is the qualifier.

B3.6b Coronary arteries are classified by number of distinct sites treated, rather than number of coronary arteries or anatomic name of a coronary artery (e.g., left anterior descending). Coronary artery bypass procedures are coded differently than other bypass procedures as described in the previous guideline. Rather than identifying the body part bypassed from, the body part identifies the number of coronary artery sites bypassed to, and the qualifier specifies the vessel bypassed from.

Example: Aortocoronary artery bypass of one site on the left anterior descending coronary artery and one site on the obtuse marginal coronary artery is classified in the body part axis of classification as two coronary artery sites and the qualifier specifies the aorta as the body part bypassed from.

B3.6c If multiple coronary artery sites are bypassed, a separate procedure is coded for each coronary artery site that uses a different device and/or qualifier.

Example: Aortocoronary artery bypass and internal mammary coronary artery bypass are coded separately.

Control vs. more definitive root operations

B3.7 The root operation Control is defined as, "Stopping, or attempting to stop, postprocedural bleeding." If an attempt to stop postprocedural bleeding is initially unsuccessful, and to stop the bleeding requires performing any of the definitive root operations Bypass, Detachment, Excision, Extraction, Reposition, Replacement, or Resection, then that root operation is coded instead of Control.

Example: Resection of spleen to stop postprocedural bleeding is coded to Resection instead of Control.

Excision vs. Resection

B3.8 PCS contains specific body parts for anatomical subdivisions of a body part, such as lobes of the lungs or liver and regions of the intestine. Resection of the specific body part is coded whenever all of the body part is cut out or off, rather than coding Excision of a less specific body part.

Example: Left upper lung lobectomy is coded to Resection of Upper Lung Lobe, Left rather than Excision of Lung, Left.

Excision for graft

B3.9 If an autograft is obtained from a different body part in order to complete the objective of the procedure, a separate procedure is coded.

Example: Coronary bypass with excision of saphenous vein graft, excision of saphenous vein is coded separately.

Fusion procedures of the spine

B3.10a The body part coded for a spinal vertebral joint(s) rendered immobile by a spinal fusion procedure is classified by the level of the spine (e.g. thoracic). There are distinct body part values for a single vertebral joint and for multiple vertebral joints at each spinal level.

Example: Body part values specify Lumbar Vertebral Joint, Lumbar Vertebral Joints, 2 or More and Lumbosacral Vertebral Joint.

B3.10b If multiple vertebral joints are fused, a separate procedure is coded for each vertebral joint that uses a different device and/or qualifier.

Example: Fusion of lumbar vertebral joint, posterior approach, anterior column and fusion of lumbar vertebral joint, posterior approach, posterior column are coded separately.

B3.10c Combinations of devices and materials are often used on a vertebral joint to render the joint immobile. When combinations of devices are used on the same vertebral joint, the device value coded for the procedure is as follows:

- If an interbody fusion device is used to render the joint immobile (alone or containing other material like bone graft), the procedure is coded with the device value Interbody Fusion Device
- If internal fixation is used to render the joint immobile and an interbody fusion device is *not* used, the procedure is coded with the device value Internal Fixation Device

- If bone graft is the *only* device used to render the joint immobile, the procedure is coded with the device value Nonautologous Tissue Substitute or Autologous Tissue Substitute
- If a mixture of autologous and nonautologous bone graft (with or without biological or synthetic extenders or binders) is used to render the joint immobile, code the procedure with the device value Autologous Tissue Substitute.

Examples: Fusion of a vertebral joint using a cage style interbody fusion device containing morsellized bone graft is coded to the device Interbody Fusion Device.

Fusion of a vertebral joint using a bone dowel interbody fusion device made of cadaver bone and packed with a mixture of local morsellized bone and demineralized bone matrix is coded to the device Interbody Fusion Device.

Fusion of a vertebral joint using rigid plates affixed with screws and reinforced with bone cement is coded to the device Internal Fixation Device.

Fusion of a vertebral joint using both autologous bone graft and bone bank bone graft is coded to the device Autologous Tissue Substitute.

Inspection procedures

B3.11a Inspection of a body part(s) performed in order to achieve the objective of a procedure is not coded separately.

Example: Fiberoptic bronchoscopy performed for irrigation of bronchus, only the irrigation procedure is coded.

B3.11b If multiple tubular body parts are inspected, the most distal body part inspected is coded. If multiple non-tubular body parts in a region are inspected, the body part that specifies the entire area inspected is coded.

Examples: Cystoureteroscopy with inspection of bladder and ureters is coded to the ureter body part value.

Exploratory laparotomy with general inspection of abdominal contents is coded to the peritoneal cavity body part value.

B3.11c When both an Inspection procedure and another procedure are performed on the same body part during the same episode, if the Inspection procedure is performed using a different approach than the other procedure, the Inspection procedure is coded separately.

Example: Endoscopic Inspection of the duodenum is coded separately when open Excision of the duodenum is performed during the same procedural episode.

Occlusion vs. Restriction for vessel embolization procedures

B3.12 If the objective of an embolization procedure is to completely close a vessel, the root operation Occlusion is coded. If the objective of an embolization procedure is to narrow the lumen of a vessel, the root operation Restriction is coded.

Examples: Tumor embolization is coded to the root operation Occlusion, because the objective of the procedure is to cut off the blood supply to the vessel.

Embolization of a cerebral aneurysm is coded to the root operation Restriction, because the objective of the procedure is not to close off the vessel entirely, but to narrow the lumen of the vessel at the site of the aneurysm where it is abnormally wide.

Release procedures

B3.13 In the root operation Release, the body part value coded is the body part being freed and not the tissue being manipulated or cut to free the body part.

Example: Lysis of intestinal adhesions is coded to the specific intestine body part value.

Release vs. Division

B3.14 If the sole objective of the procedure is freeing a body part without cutting the body part, the root operation is Release. If the sole objective of the procedure is separating or transecting a body part, the root operation is Division.

Examples: Freeing a nerve root from surrounding scar tissue to relieve pain is coded to the root operation Release. Severing a nerve root to relieve pain is coded to the root operation Division.

Reposition for fracture treatment

B3.15   Reduction of a displaced fracture is coded to the root operation Reposition and the application of a cast or splint in conjunction with the Reposition procedure is not coded separately. Treatment of a nondisplaced fracture is coded to the procedure performed.

Examples: Putting a pin in a nondisplaced fracture is coded to the root operation Insertion.

Casting of a nondisplaced fracture is coded to the root operation Immobilization in the Placement section.

Transplantation vs. Administration

B3.16   Putting in a mature and functioning living body part taken from another individual or animal is coded to the root operation Transplantation. Putting in autologous or nonautologous cells is coded to the Administration section.

Example: Putting in autologous or nonautologous bone marrow, pancreatic islet cells or stem cells is coded to the Administration section.

B4.   Body Part

General guidelines

B4.1a   If a procedure is performed on a portion of a body part that does not have a separate body part value, code the body part value corresponding to the whole body part.

Example: A procedure performed on the alveolar process of the mandible is coded to the mandible body part.

B4.1b   If the prefix "peri" is combined with a body part to identify the site of the procedure, the procedure is coded to the body part named.

Example: A procedure site identified as perirenal is coded to the kidney body part.

Branches of body parts

B4.2   Where a specific branch of a body part does not have its own body part value in PCS, the body part is coded to the closest proximal branch that has a specific body part value.

Example: A procedure performed on the mandibular branch of the trigeminal nerve is coded to the trigeminal nerve body part value

Bilateral body part values

B4.3   Bilateral body part values are available for a limited number of body parts. If the identical procedure is performed on contralateral body parts, and a bilateral body part value exists for that body part, a single procedure is coded using the bilateral body part value. If no bilateral body part value exists, each procedure is coded separately using the appropriate body part value.

Example: The identical procedure performed on both fallopian tubes is coded once using the body part value Fallopian Tube, Bilateral. The identical procedure performed on both knee joints is coded twice using the body part values Knee Joint, Right and Knee Joint, Left.

Coronary arteries

B4.4   The coronary arteries are classified as a single body part that is further specified by number of sites treated and not by name or number of arteries. Separate body part values are used to specify the number of sites treated when the same procedure is performed on multiple sites in the coronary arteries.

Examples: Angioplasty of two distinct sites in the left anterior descending coronary artery with placement of two stents is coded as Dilation of Coronary Arteries, Two Sites, with Intraluminal Device.

Angioplasty of two distinct sites in the left anterior descending coronary artery, one with stent placed and one without, is coded separately as Dilation of Coronary Artery, One Site with Intraluminal Device, and Dilation of Coronary Artery, One Site with no device.

Tendons, ligaments, bursae and fascia near a joint

B4.5   Procedures performed on tendons, ligaments, bursae and fascia supporting a joint are coded to the body part in the respective body system that is the focus of the procedure. Procedures performed on joint structures themselves are coded to the body part in the joint body systems.

Example: Repair of the anterior cruciate ligament of the knee is coded to the knee bursae and ligament body part in the bursae and ligaments body system.

Knee arthroscopy with shaving of articular cartilage is coded to the knee joint body part in the Lower Joints body system.

Skin, subcutaneous tissue and fascia overlying a joint

B4.6 If a procedure is performed on the skin, subcutaneous tissue or fascia overlying a joint, the procedure is coded to the following body part:
- Shoulder is coded to Upper Arm
- Elbow is coded to Lower Arm
- Wrist is coded to Lower Arm
- Hip is coded to Upper Leg
- Knee is coded to Lower Leg
- Ankle is coded to Foot

Fingers and toes

B4.7 If a body system does not contain a separate body part value for fingers, procedures performed on the fingers are coded to the body part value for the hand. If a body system does not contain a separate body part value for toes, procedures performed on the toes are coded to the body part value for the foot.
Example: Excision of finger muscle is coded to one of the hand muscle body part values in the Muscles body system.

B5. Approach

Open approach with percutaneous endoscopic assistance

B5.2 Procedures performed using the open approach with percutaneous endoscopic assistance are coded to the approach Open.
Example: Laparoscopic-assisted sigmoidectomy is coded to the approach Open.

External approach

B5.3a Procedures performed within an orifice on structures that are visible without the aid of any instrumentation are coded to the approach External.
Example: Resection of tonsils is coded to the approach External.

B5.3b Procedures performed indirectly by the application of external force through the intervening body layers are coded to the approach External.
Example: Closed reduction of fracture is coded to the approach External.

Percutaneous procedure via device

B5.4 Procedures performed percutaneously via a device placed for the procedure are coded to the approach Percutaneous.
Example: Fragmentation of kidney stone performed via percutaneous nephrostomy is coded to the approach Percutaneous.

B6. Device

General guidelines

B6.1a A device is coded only if a device remains after the procedure is completed. If no device remains, the device value No Device is coded.

B6.1b Materials such as sutures, ligatures, radiological markers and temporary post-operative wound drains are considered integral to the performance of a procedure and are not coded as devices.

B6.1c Procedures performed on a device only and not on a body part are specified in the root operations Change, Irrigation, Removal and Revision, and are coded to the procedure performed.
Example: Irrigation of percutaneous nephrostomy tube is coded to the root operation Irrigation of indwelling device in the Administration section.

Drainage device

B6.2 A separate procedure to put in a drainage device is coded to the root operation Drainage with the device value Drainage Device.

C. *Obstetric Section Guidelines (section 1)*

Obstetrics Section

Products of conception

C1 Procedures performed on the products of conception are coded to the Obstetrics section. Procedures performed on the pregnant female other than the products of conception are coded to the appropriate root operation in the Medical and Surgical section.
Example: Amniocentesis is coded to the products of conception body part in the Obstetrics section. Repair of obstetric urethral laceration is coded to the urethra body part in the Medical and Surgical section.

Procedures following delivery or abortion

C2 Procedures performed following a delivery or abortion for curettage of the endometrium or evacuation of retained products of conception are all coded in the Obstetrics section, to the root operation Extraction and the body part Products of Conception, Retained. Diagnostic or therapeutic dilation and curettage performed during times other than the postpartum or post-abortion period are all coded in the Medical and Surgical section, to the root operation Extraction and the body part Endometrium.

EXERCISE 7-5

Without the use of reference material, answer the following questions about ICD-10-PCS.

1. It is acceptable to choose a valid code directly from the tables.
   A. True
   B. False

2. Procedures that are performed using an open approach with percutaneous endoscopic assistance are coded to an open approach.
   A. True
   B. False

3. Body systems designated as "upper" contain body parts above the heart.
   A. True
   B. False

4. When a patient is having a hip replacement, a code for the resection of a joint is assigned in addition to the joint replacement code.
   A. True
   B. False

5. Procedures performed on the distal end of the humerus are coded to the Arm body part value.
   A. True
   B. False

6. A closed reduction of a fracture is coded to the manipulation approach.
   A. True
   B. False

7. It is acceptable to choose a valid code directly from the Index.
   A. True
   B. False

8. Body systems designated as "lower" contain body parts below the diaphragm.
   A. True
   B. False

9. If the intended procedure is discontinued, code to the root operation that was intended.
   A. True
   B. False

10. If the identical procedure is performed on contralateral body parts, and a bilateral body part value is available for that body part, a single code with the bilateral body part should be assigned.
    A. True
    B. False

11. When used in a code description, the term "and" means "and/or."
    A. True
    B. False

12. It is acceptable to use a general body part value when the specific body part cannot be determined.
    A. True
    B. False

13. The body site for perirenal is "peritoneum."
    A. True
    B. False

14. A temporary postoperative wound drain is considered a device when assigning a ICD-10-PCS code.
    A. True
    B. False

15. Exploration or inspection of a body part that is integral to the performance of the procedure is not coded separately.
    A. True
    B. False

16. A bone marrow transplant is coded to the root operation transplant.
    A. True
    B. False

17. The root operation to stop postprocedural bleeding is control.
    A. True
    B. False

18. Procedures performed on the skin are coded to the body part values in the body system Skin and breast.
    A. True
    B. False

19. A device is only coded if the device remains after the procedure is completed.
    A. True
    B. False

20. The resection of tonsils is coded to an open approach.
    A. True
    B. False

Medical and Surgical Section

Because the Medical and Surgical section is the largest section, and the section that is used the most, we will use this section to learn more about the structure and standardized definitions that are utilized by ICD-10-PCS. The character value for the Medical and Surgical section is zero (the digit, not the letter *O*). All the codes from the tables in the Medical and Surgical section begin with a zero.

Body Systems

The body systems, or the second character for the Medical and Surgical section, are as follows:

    0 Central nervous system
    1 Peripheral nervous system
    2 Heart and great vessels
    3 Upper arteries
    4 Lower arteries
    5 Upper veins
    6 Lower veins
    7 Lymphatic and hemic system
    8 Eye
    9 Ear, nose, sinus
    B Respiratory system
    C Mouth and throat
    D Gastrointestinal system
    F Hepatobiliary system and pancreas
    G Endocrine system
    H Skin and breast
    J Subcutaneous tissue and fascia

K   Muscles
L   Tendons
M   Bursae and ligaments
N   Head and facial bones
P   Upper bones
Q   Lower bones
R   Upper joints
S   Lower joints
T   Urinary system
U   Female reproductive system
V   Male reproductive system
W   Anatomical regions, general
X   Anatomical regions, upper extremities
Y   Anatomical regions, lower extremities

EXERCISE 7-6

Using reference material if necessary, answer the following questions about ICD-10-PCS.

1. The thoracic nerve is in what body system?   _____

2. The lacrimal gland is in what body system?   _____

3. The cystic duct is in what body system?   _____

Root Operations

The root operation, or the third character, identifies the main objective of the procedure. There is a specific definition for each root operation. Although this is part of the standardization of terminology for ICD-10-PCS, it may not be the terminology used by physicians. According to the guidelines it is the coder's responsibility to determine what the documentation in the medical record equates to in the PCS definitions. Physicians are not expected to use terminology in the same way that has been defined by the PCS. For example, a TURP (transurethral resection of the prostate) includes the word resection. In PCS resection means the cutting out/off without replacing all of a body part. A TURP is not a resection of the whole body part (prostate), so it would be coded to an excision (cutting out/off without replacing some of a body) in PCS. It would be the coder's responsibility to determine this by reading the OR report and being knowledgeable about the surgical procedure. There are 31 root operations for the Medical and Surgical section. The character value for the root operation is in parentheses following the root operation term, and an example of a procedure that fits the root operation is in parentheses following the definition.

Root operations that remove some/all of a body part:

- **Destruction (5):** physical eradication of all or a portion of a body part by the direct use of energy, force, or a destructive agent (ablation of endometriosis)
- **Detachment (6):** cutting off all or a portion of the upper or lower extremities (above-knee amputation)
- **Excision (B):** cutting out or off, without replacement, a portion of a body part (partial nephrectomy)
- **Extraction (D):** pulling or stripping out or off all or a portion of a body part by the use of force (bone marrow biopsy)
- **Resection (T):** cutting out or off, without replacement, all of a body part (total lobectomy of lung)

Root operations that remove solids, fluids, or gases from a body part:

- **Drainage (9):** taking or letting out fluids and/or gases from a body part (paracentesis)
- **Extirpation (C):** taking or cutting out solid matter from a body part (thrombectomy)
- **Fragmentation (F):** breaking solid matter in a body part into pieces (extracorporeal shockwave lithotripsy)

Root operations that involve cutting or separation only:

- **Division (8):** cutting into a body part without draining fluids and/or gases from the body part in order to separate or transect a body part (osteotomy)

- **Release (N):** freeing a body part from an abnormal physical constraint (lysis of adhesions)

Root operations that put in, put back, or move some or all of a body part:

- **Reattachment (M):** putting back in or on all or a portion of a separated body part to its normal location or other suitable location (reattachment of finger)
- **Reposition (S):** moving to its normal location, or other suitable location, all or a portion of a body part (fracture reduction)
- **Transfer (X):** moving, without taking out, all or a portion of a body part to another location to take over the function of all or a portion of a body part (pedicle skin flap)
- **Transplantation (Y):** putting in or on all or a portion of a living body part taken from another individual or animal to physically take the place and/or function of all or a portion of a similar body part (kidney transplant)

Root operations that alter the diameter/route of a tubular body part:

- **Bypass (1):** altering the route of passage of the contents of a tubular body part (CABG)
- **Dilation (7):** expanding an orifice or the lumen of a tubular body part (PTCA)
- **Occlusion (L):** completely closing an orifice or lumen of a tubular body part (tubal ligation)
- **Restriction (V):** partially closing an orifice or lumen of a tubular body part (Nissen fundoplication)

Root operations that always involve a device:

- **Change (2):** taking out or off a device from a body part and putting back an identical or similar device in or on the same body part without cutting or puncturing the skin or a mucous membrane (changing a gastrostomy tube)
- **Insertion (H):** putting in a nonbiological appliance that monitors, assists, performs, or prevents a physiological function but does not physically take the place of a body part (insertion of pacemaker lead)
- **Replacement (R):** putting in or on biological or synthetic material that physically takes the place and/or function of all or a portion of a body part (total knee replacement)
- **Removal (P):** taking out or off a device from a body part (removing a chest tube)
- **Revision (W):** correcting, to the extent possible, a malfunctioning or displaced device (adjustment of knee prosthesis)
- **Supplement (U):** putting in or on biological or synthetic material that physically reinforces and/or augments the function of a portion of a body part (herniorrhaphy with mesh)

Root operations that involve examination only:

- **Inspection (J):** visually and/or manually exploring a body part (diagnostic arthroscopy)
- **Map (K):** locating the route of passage of electrical impulses and/or locating functional areas in a body part (cardiac mapping)

Root operations that include other repair:

- **Control (3):** stopping, or attempting to stop, postprocedural bleeding (control of post-tonsillectomy hemorrhage)
- **Repair (Q):** restoring, to the extent possible, a body part to its normal anatomic structure and function (herniorrhaphy)

The root operation repair is used when the root operation for the procedure performed cannot be classified to a more specific root operation.

Root operations that include other objectives:

- **Alteration (0):** modifying the natural anatomic structure of a body part without affecting the function of the body part (breast augmentation)
- **Creation (4):** making a new structure that does not take over the place of a body part (creation of a vagina in males for sex reassignment)
- **Fusion (G):** joining together portions of an articular body part rendering the articular body part immobile (spinal fusion)

Terms such as "incision" or "anastomosis" are not root operations, as they are always integral to another procedure. The identification and selection of the correct root operation is vital to the selection of the appropriate table.

EXERCISE 7-7

Without using reference material, answer the following questions about ICD-10-PCS.

1. Modifying the natural anatomic structure of a body part without affecting the function of the body part is
   A. alteration
   B. fusion
   C. creation
   D. repair

2. Cutting off all or a portion of the upper or lower extremities is
   A. destruction
   B. fragmentation
   C. detachment
   D. resection

3. Completely closing an orifice or lumen of a tubular body part is
   A. bypass
   B. restriction
   C. dilation
   D. occlusion

4. Freeing a body part from an abnormal physical constraint is
   A. reposition
   B. division
   C. release
   D. transfer

5. Taking or letting out fluids and/or gases from a body part is
   A. extirpation
   B. fragmentation
   C. extraction
   D. drainage

6. Stopping, or attempting to stop, postprocedural bleeding is
   A. inspection
   B. control
   C. mapping
   D. alteration

7. Taking out or off a device from a body part is
   A. replacement
   B. removal
   C. revision
   D. change

8. Moving to its normal location or other suitable location all or a portion of a body part is
   A. reposition
   B. release
   C. transfer
   D. transplantation

9. Cutting out or off, without replacement, a portion of a body part is
   A. resection
   B. excision
   C. destruction
   D. extraction

10. Cutting into a body part without draining fluids and/or gases from the body part in order to separate or transect a body part is
    A. reattachment
    B. release
    C. transfer
    D. division

11. Putting in or on biological or synthetic material that physically reinforces and/or augments the function of a portion of a body part is
    A. restriction
    B. insertion
    C. supplementation
    D. revision

12. Visually and/or manually exploring a body part is
    A. creation
    B. fusion
    C. inspection
    D. mapping

Body Part

The body part, the fourth character, identifies the specific body part on which the procedure was performed. Each body system will have corresponding body parts. Look at the various tables to get an idea about the body parts that are body part values (Figures 7-4 and 7-5).

Approaches

The approach, the fifth character, identifies the operative approach or the method used to reach the operative site. There is a specific definition for each approach. Although this is part of the standardization of terminology for ICD-10-PCS, it may not be the terminology used by physicians. There are seven approaches for the Medical and Surgical section. An example is included in parentheses following the definition. The character value and definition for the approaches are as follows:

0 **Open:** cutting through the skin, mucous membrane, and any other body layers necessary to expose the site of the procedure (abdominal hysterectomy)

3 **Percutaneous:** entry, by puncture or minor incision, of instrumentation through the skin, mucous membrane, and any other body layers necessary to reach the site of the procedure (needle biopsy liver)

Section	0 **Medical and Surgical**			
Body System	B **Respiratory System**			
Operation	5 **Destruction:** Physical eradication of all or a portion of a body part by the direct use of energy, force, or a destructive agent			
Body Part	**Approach**		**Device**	**Qualifier**
1 Trachea 2 Carina 3 Main Bronchus, Right 4 Upper Lobe Bronchus, Right 5 Middle Lobe Bronchus, Right 6 Lower Lobe Bronchus, Right 7 Main Bronchus, Left 8 Upper Lobe Bronchus, Left 9 Lingula Bronchus B Lower Lobe Bronchus, Left C Upper Lung Lobe, Right D Middle Lung Lobe, Right F Lower Lung Lobe, Right G Upper Lung Lobe, Left H Lung Lingula J Lower Lung Lobe, Left K Lung, Right L Lung, Left M Lungs, Bilateral	0 Open 3 Percutaneous 4 Percutaneous Endoscopic 7 Via Natural or Artificial Opening 8 Via Natural or Artificial Opening Endoscopic		**Z** No Device	**Z** No Qualifier
N Pleura, Right P Pleura, Left R Diaphragm, Right S Diaphragm, Left	0 Open 3 Percutaneous 4 Percutaneous Endoscopic		**Z** No Device	**Z** No Qualifier

FIGURE 7-5. Table for destruction of respiratory system.

4 **Percutaneous endoscopic:** entry, by puncture or minor incision, of instrumentation through the skin, mucous membrane, and any other body layers necessary to reach and visualize the site of the procedure (laparoscopic cholecystectomy)

7 **Via natural or artificial opening:** entry of instrumentation through a natural or artificial external opening to reach the site of the procedure (endotracheal intubation)

8 **Via natural or artificial opening endoscopic:** entry of instrumentation through a natural or artificial external opening to reach and visualize the site of the procedure (colonoscopy)

F **Open with percutaneous endoscopic assistance:** cutting through the skin, mucous membrane, and any other body layers necessary to expose the site of the procedure, and entry, by puncture or minor incision, of instrumentation through the skin, mucous membrane, and any other body layers necessary to aid in the performance of the procedure (laparoscopic-assisted vaginal hysterectomy)

X **External:** procedures performed directly on the skin or mucous membrane and procedures performed indirectly by the application of external force through the skin or mucous membrane (tonsillectomy)

The approach is determined by the following three components for procedures performed on an internal body part:

- Access location—specifies the external site through which the site of the procedure is reached, either through skin, mucous membrane, or external orifices
- Method—specifies how the external access location is entered
- Type of instrumentation—specifies the specialized equipment used to perform the procedure

EXERCISE 7-8

Without the use of reference material, answer the following questions about ICD-10-PCS.

1. Entry of instrumentation, by puncture or minor incision, through the skin, mucous membrane, and any other body layers necessary to reach the site of the procedure is
   A. open
   B. percutaneous
   C. percutaneous endoscopic
   D. open with percutaneous endoscopic assistance

2. Cutting through the skin, mucous membrane, and any other body layers necessary to expose the site of the procedure is
   A. open
   B. percutaneous
   C. percutaneous endoscopic
   D. open with percutaneous endoscopic assistance

3. Procedures performed directly on the skin or mucous membrane and procedures performed indirectly by the application of external force through the skin or mucous membrane are
   A. percutaneous
   B. open
   C. via natural or artificial opening
   D. external

Device

The device, the sixth character, identifies a device that remains after the procedure is completed. There are four types of devices:

- Biological or synthetic material that takes the place of all or a portion of a body part
- Biological or synthetic material that assists or prevents a physiological function
- Therapeutic material that is not absorbed by, eliminated by, or incorporated into a body part

Section	0 **Medical and Surgical**		
Body System	0 **Central Nervous System**		
Operation	2 **Change:** Taking out or off a device from a body part and putting back an identical or similar device in or on the same body part without cutting or puncturing the skin or a mucous membrane		

Body Part	Approach	Device	Qualifier
0 Brain **E** Cranial Nerve **U** Spinal Canal	**X** External	**0** Drainage Device **Y** Other Device ⟵	**Z** No Qualifier

FIGURE 7-6. Table for change in central nervous system.

- Mechanical or electronic appliances used to assist, monitor, take the place of, or prevent a physiological function

Specific device values are required with root operations change, insertion, removal, replacement, and revision. Materials that are part of a procedure—such as clips, ligatures, and sutures—are not considered devices. There is a value for other devices (Y; Figure 7-6), which can be used until more specific devices are added to the ICD-10 coding procedural system.

EXERCISE 7-9

Without the use of reference material, answer the following questions about ICD-10-PCS.

1. Sutures are considered a device.
   A. True
   B. False

2. A device is left in place after completion of the procedure.
   A. True
   B. False

3. The root operation insertion always involves a device.
   A. True
   B. False

Qualifier

The qualifier, the seventh character, identifies a unique value for an individual procedure. A qualifier may indicate that a procedure was done for diagnostic purposes (Figure 7-7); in coronary artery bypass procedures, the qualifier identifies the origin of the bypass (Figure 7-8).

Other Medical- and Surgical-Related Procedures

The other medical- and surgical-related procedure sections of ICD-10-PCS include the following:

1 Obstetrics
2 Placement
3 Administration
4 Measurement and monitoring
5 Extracorporeal assistance and performance
6 Extracorporeal therapies
7 Osteopathic
8 Other procedures
9 Chiropractic

Section		0 Medical and Surgical			
Body System		K Muscles			
Operation		B Excision: Cutting out or off, without replacement, a portion of a body part			

Body Part	Approach	Device	Qualifier
0 Head Muscle 1 Facial Muscle 2 Neck Muscle, Right 3 Neck Muscle, Left 4 Tongue, Palate, Pharynx Muscle 5 Shoulder Muscle, Right 6 Shoulder Muscle, Left 7 Upper Arm Muscle, Right 8 Upper Arm Muscle, Left 9 Lower Arm and Wrist Muscle, Right B Lower Arm and Wrist Muscle, Left C Hand Muscle, Right D Hand Muscle, Left F Trunk Muscle, Right G Trunk Muscle, Left H Thorax Muscle, Right J Thorax Muscle, Left K Abdomen Muscle, Right L Abdomen Muscle, Left M Perineum Muscle N Hip Muscle, Right P Hip Muscle, Left Q Upper Leg Muscle, Right R Upper Leg Muscle, Left S Lower Leg Muscle, Right T Lower Leg Muscle, Left V Foot Muscle, Right W Foot Muscle, Left	0 Open 3 Percutaneous 4 Percutaneous Endoscopic	Z No Device	X Diagnostic ← Z No Qualifier

FIGURE 7-7. Table for excision of muscles.

Section		0 Medical and Surgical			
Body System		2 Heart and Great Vessels			
Operation		1 Bypass: Altering the route of passage of the contents of a tubular body part			

Body Part	Approach	Device	Qualifier ←
0 Coronary Artery, One Site 1 Coronary Artery, Two Sites 2 Coronary Artery, Three Sites 3 Coronary Artery, Four or More Sites	0 Open	9 Autologous Venous Tissue A Autologous Arterial Tissue J Synthetic Substitute K Nonautologous Tissue Substitute	3 Coronary Artery 8 Internal Mammary, Right 9 Internal Mammary, Left C Thoracic Artery F Abdominal Artery W Aorta
0 Coronary Artery, One Site 1 Coronary Artery, Two Sites 2 Coronary Artery, Three Sites 3 Coronary Artery, Four or More Sites	0 Open	Z No Device	3 Coronary Artery 8 Internal Mammary, Right 9 Internal Mammary, Left C Thoracic Artery F Abdominal Artery
0 Coronary Artery, One Site 1 Coronary Artery, Two Sites 2 Coronary Artery, Three Sites 3 Coronary Artery, Four or More Sites	3 Percutaneous	4 Drug-eluting Intraluminal Device D Intraluminal Device	4 Coronary Vein
0 Coronary Artery, One Site 1 Coronary Artery, Two Sites 2 Coronary Artery, Three Sites 3 Coronary Artery, Four or More Sites	4 Percutaneous Endoscopic	4 Drug-eluting Intraluminal Device D Intraluminal Device	4 Coronary Vein
0 Coronary Artery, One Site 1 Coronary Artery, Two Sites 2 Coronary Artery, Three Sites 3 Coronary Artery, Four or More Sites	4 Percutaneous Endoscopic	9 Autologous Venous Tissue A Autologous Arterial Tissue J Synthetic Substitute K Nonautologous Tissue Substitute	3 Coronary Artery 8 Internal Mammary, Right 9 Internal Mammary, Left C Thoracic Artery F Abdominal Artery W Aorta
0 Coronary Artery, One Site 1 Coronary Artery, Two Sites 2 Coronary Artery, Three Sites 3 Coronary Artery, Four or More Sites	4 Percutaneous Endoscopic	Z No Device	3 Coronary Artery 8 Internal Mammary, Right 9 Internal Mammary, Left C Thoracic Artery F Abdominal Artery

FIGURE 7-8. Table for bypass of heart and great vessels.

Obstetrics

Obstetrics include only those procedures that are performed on the products of conception. The term "products of conception" refers to all physical components of a pregnancy, including the fetus, amnion, umbilical cord, and placenta, regardless of gestational age. Procedures performed on a pregnant female other than on the products of conception are coded in the Medical and Surgical section. All ICD-10-PCS codes are seven characters, each character representing a particular aspect of the procedure. The meanings of the obstetric procedure characters are as follows:

CHARACTER	REPRESENTS
1	Section
2	Body system
3	Root operation
4	Body part
5	Approach
6	Device
7	Qualifier

Obstetric codes are found in Section 1, so they have a first-character value of 1. The second-character value for body system is Pregnancy. The third character identifies the root operation. The section includes two additional root operations:

- **Abortion (A):** artificially terminating a pregnancy
- **Delivery (E):** assisting the passage of the products of conception from the genital canal

The fourth character classifies the body part. Body part values in this section are:

- Products of conception
- Products of conception, retained
- Products of conception, ectopic

The fifth character identifies the approach; these are defined in the Medical and Surgical section. The sixth character is for the device. The seventh character identifies various qualifiers, such as type of extraction, type of cesarean section, and so on.

EXAMPLE

Manually assisted delivery, 10E0XZZ

CHARACTER 1 SECTION	CHARACTER 2 BODY SYSTEM	CHARACTER 3 OPERATION	CHARACTER 4 BODY PART	CHARACTER 5 APPROACH	CHARACTER 6 DEVICE	CHARACTER 7 QUALIFIER
Obstetrics	Pregnancy	Delivery	Products of Conception	External	No Device	No Qualifier
1	0	E	0	X	7	Z

EXERCISE 7-10

Without the use of reference material, answer the following questions about ICD-10-PCS.

1. Obstetric procedures are any procedure performed on a pregnant woman.
   A. True
   B. False

2. In ICD-10-PCS, "abortion" is defined as "the spontaneous termination of a pregnancy."
   A. True
   B. False

3. Low cervical cesarean section would be identified by the fifth character, the approach.
   A. True
   B. False

Placement

Placement codes include procedures for putting a device in or on a body region for the purpose of protection, immobilization, stretching, compression, or packing. All ICD-10-PCS codes are seven characters, each representing a particular aspect of the procedure. The meanings of the placement procedure characters are as follows:

CHARACTER	REPRESENTS
1	Section
2	Body system
3	Root operation
4	Body region
5	Approach
6	Device
7	Qualifier

Placement codes are found in Section 2, so they have a first-character value of 2. The second-character value, for body system, is either anatomical region or body orifice. The third character identifies the root operation. Section 2 includes five additional root operations:

- **Compression (1):** putting pressure on a body region
- **Dressing (2):** putting material on a body region for protection
- **Immobilization (3):** limiting or preventing motion of a body region
- **Packing (4):** putting material in a body region or orifice
- **Traction (6):** exerting a pulling force on a body region in a distal direction

The fourth-character value classifies body region or natural orifice. The fifth-character value identifies the approach; and because all placement procedures are performed directly on the skin or mucous membranes, or indirectly by applying external force, the approach value is always X, for external. The sixth-character value classifies device. The seventh character is for a qualifier, but it is not used in the Placement section at this time, so the value is always no qualifier(Z).

EXAMPLE

Cast to right lower arm, 2W3CX2Z

CHARACTER 1 SECTION	CHARACTER 2 BODY SYSTEM	CHARACTER 3 OPERATION	CHARACTER 4 BODY REGION	CHARACTER 5 APPROACH	CHARACTER 6 DEVICE	CHARACTER 7 QUALIFIER
Placement	Anatomical Region	Immobilization	Lower Arm, Right	External	Cast	No Qualifier
2	W	3	C	X	2	Z

Administration

Administration codes include procedures for putting in or on a therapeutic, prophylactic, protective, diagnostic, nutritional, or physiological substance. All ICD-10-PCS codes are seven characters, each representing a particular aspect of the procedure. The meanings of the administration procedure characters are as follows:

CHARACTER	REPRESENTS
1	Section
2	Body system
3	Root operation
4	Body system/region
5	Approach
6	Substance
7	Qualifier

Administration codes are found in Section 3, so they have a first-character value of 3. The second character has three values: physiological systems and anatomical regions, circulatory system, or indwelling device. The third-character value identifies the root operation. Section 3 has three root operations:

- **Introduction (0):** putting in or on a therapeutic, diagnostic, nutritional, physiological, or prophylactic substance except blood or blood products
- **Irrigation (1):** putting in or on a cleansing substance
- **Transfusion (2):** putting in blood or blood products

The fourth-character value classifies body system/region. This identifies the site where the substance is administered. The fifth-character value identifies the approach, and each approach is defined in the Medical and Surgical section. Percutaneous is the approach for procedures that are introduced intradermally, subcutaneously, and intramuscularly (e.g., injections). The sixth-character value specifies the substance introduced. The seventh character is for a qualifier that indicates whether the substance used was autologous or nonautologous or to further specify the substance. **Autologous** means originating from the recipient, rather than from a donor, or transferred from the same individual's body, (e.g., a skin graft is taken from one part of the body and transferred to another part of the body on the same individual).

EXAMPLE

Administration of RBCs, nonautologous, via central vein, 30243N1

CHARACTER 1 SECTION	CHARACTER 2 BODY SYSTEM	CHARACTER 3 OPERATION	CHARACTER 4 BODY SYSTEM/ REGION	CHARACTER 5 APPROACH	CHARACTER 6 SUBSTANCE	CHARACTER 7 QUALIFIER
Administration	Circulatory	Transfusion	Central Vein	Percutaneous	Red Blood Cells	Nonautologous
3	0	2	4	3	N	1

EXERCISE 7-11

Without the use of reference material, answer the following questions.

1. Irrigation is a root operation that is found in the Placement section.
   A. True
   B. False

2. Immobilization is limiting or preventing motion of a body region.
   A. True
   B. False

3. In the Administration section, Character 6 identifies the substance being introduced.
   A. True
   B. False

Measurement and Monitoring

Measurement and monitoring codes include procedures for determining the level of a physiological or physical function. All ICD-10-PCS codes are seven characters, each representing a particular aspect of the procedure. The meanings of the measuring and monitoring procedure characters are as follows:

CHARACTER	REPRESENTS
1	Section
2	Body system
3	Root operation
4	Body system
5	Approach
6	Function/Device
7	Qualifier

Measurement and monitoring codes are found in Section 4, so they have a first-character value of 4. The second character has two values, for either physiological systems or physiological devices. The third-character value identifies the root operation. Section 4 has two root operations:

- **Measurement (0):** determining the level of a physiological or physical function at a point in time
- **Monitoring (1):** determining the level of a physiological or physical function repetitively over a period of time

The fourth-character value identifies the body system being measured or monitored. The fifth-character value identifies the approach, and each is defined in the Medical and Surgical section. The sixth-character value specifies the physiological or physical function monitored. The seventh character is for a qualifier used to further specify the body part or a variation of the procedure performed.

EXAMPLE

Holter monitoring, 4A12X45

CHARACTER 1 SECTION	CHARACTER 2 BODY SYSTEM	CHARACTER 3 OPERATION	CHARACTER 4 BODY SYSTEM	CHARACTER 5 APPROACH	CHARACTER 6 FUNCTION/ DEVICE	CHARACTER 7 QUALIFIER
Measurement/ Monitoring 4	Physiological Systems A	Monitoring 1	Cardiac 2	External X	Electrical Activity 4	Ambulatory 5

Extracorporeal Assistance and Performance

Extracorporeal assistance and performance codes are used when equipment outside of the body is used to assist or perform a physiological function. All ICD-10-PCS codes are seven characters, each representing a particular aspect of the procedure. The meanings of the extracorporeal assistance and performance procedure characters are as follows:

CHARACTER	REPRESENTS
1	Section
2	Body system
3	Root operation
4	Body system
5	Duration
6	Function
7	Qualifier

Extracorporeal assistance and performance codes are found in Section 5, so they have a first-character value of 5. The second-character value is for physiological systems. The third-character value identifies the root operation. The section has three root operations:

- **Assistance (0):** taking over a portion of a physiological function by extracorporeal means
- **Performance (1):** completely taking over a physiological function by extracorporeal means
- **Restoration (2):** returning, or attempting to return, a physiological function to its original state by extracorporeal means

The fourth-character value classifies the body system to which the extracorporeal assistance or performance is applied. The fifth-character value identifies the duration of the procedure. The sixth-character value specifies the physiological function assisted or performed during the procedure. The seventh character is a qualifier that specifies the type of equipment used, if any.

EXAMPLE

Mechanical ventilation, continuous for 48 hours, 5A1945Z

CHARACTER 1 SECTION	CHARACTER 2 BODY SYSTEM	CHARACTER 3 OPERATION	CHARACTER 4 BODY SYSTEM	CHARACTER 5 DURATION	CHARACTER 6 FUNCTION	CHARACTER 7 QUALIFIER
Extracorporeal Assistance or Performance	Physiological Systems	Performance	Respiratory	24-96 consecutive hours	Ventilation	No Qualifier
5	A	1	9	4	5	Z

Extracorporeal Therapies

Extracorporeal therapy codes are used when equipment outside of the body is used for a therapeutic purpose that does not involve the assistance or performance of a physiological function. All ICD-10-PCS codes are seven characters, each representing a particular aspect of the procedure. The meanings of the extracorporeal therapies procedure characters are as follows:

CHARACTER	REPRESENTS
1	Section
2	Body system
3	Root operation
4	Body system
5	Duration
6	Qualifier
7	Qualifier

Extracorporeal therapy codes are found in Section 6, so they have a first-character value of 6. The second-character value is for physiological systems. The third-character value identifies the root operation. Section 6 has ten root operations:

- **Atmospheric control (0):** extracorporeal control of atmospheric pressure and composition
- **Decompression (1):** extracorporeal elimination of undissolved gas from body fluids.
- **Electromagnetic therapy (2):** extracorporeal treatment by electromagnetic rays
- **Hyperthermia (3):** extracorporeal raising of body temperature
- **Hypothermia (4):** extracorporeal lowering of body temperature
- **Pheresis (5):** extracorporeal separation of blood products
- **Phototherapy (6):** extracorporeal treatment by light rays
- **Shock wave therapy (9):** extracorporeal treatment by shock waves
- **Ultrasound therapy (7):** extracorporeal treatment by ultrasound
- **Ultraviolet light therapy (8):** extracorporeal treatment by ultraviolet light

The fourth character identifies the body system to which the extracorporeal therapy is performed. The fifth character identifies the duration of the procedure. The sixth-character value is not specified and always has the value no qualifier. The seventh character is a qualifier used for the root operations of pheresis and ultrasound therapy.

EXAMPLE

Plasmapheresis, therapeutic, single encounter, 6A550Z3

CHARACTER 1 SECTION	CHARACTER 2 BODY SYSTEM	CHARACTER 3 OPERATION	CHARACTER 4 BODY SYSTEM	CHARACTER 5 DURATION	CHARACTER 6 QUALIFIER	CHARACTER 7 QUALIFIER
Extracorporeal Therapies	Physiological Systems	Pheresis	Circulatory	Single	No Qualifier	Plasma
6	A	5	5	0	Z	3

Without the use of reference material, answer the following questions about ICD-10-PCS.

1. Hypothermia procedure is a type of extracorporeal therapy.
   A. True
   B. False

2. Measurement is defined as determining the level of physiological or physical function repetitively over a period of time.
   A. True
   B. False

3. Extracorporeal therapy uses equipment outside the body for a therapeutic purpose that does not involve the assistance or performance of a physiological function.
   A. True
   B. False

4. In the extracorporeal assistance and performance section, the definition for "performance" is "completely taking over a physiological function by extracorporeal means."
   A. True
   B. False

5. When a fifth character is used, this specifies the duration of the patient's hospital stay.
   A. True
   B. False

Osteopathic

Osteopathic codes are used for osteopathic procedures. All ICD-10-PCS codes are seven characters, each representing a particular aspect of the procedure. The meanings of the procedure characters for the Osteopathic section are as follows:

CHARACTER	REPRESENTS
1	Section
2	Body system
3	Root operation
4	Body region
5	Approach
6	Method
7	Qualifier

Osteopathic codes are found in Section 7, so they have a first-character value of 7. The second character is for anatomical regions, and the third character identifies the root operation.

Section 7 has only one root operation:

■ **Treatment (0):** manual treatment to eliminate or alleviate somatic dysfunction and related disorders

The fourth character identifies the body region on which the osteopathic treatments are performed. The fifth character identifies the approach, which is always external. The sixth character specifies the method by which the treatment is performed. The seventh character is for a qualifier, but it is not specified in the osteopathic section at this time, so the value is always None(Z).

EXAMPLE

Indirect osteopathic treatment to the lumbar region, 7W03X4Z

CHARACTER 1 SECTION	CHARACTER 2 BODY SYSTEM	CHARACTER 3 OPERATION	CHARACTER 4 BODY REGION	CHARACTER 5 APPROACH	CHARACTER 6 METHOD	CHARACTER 7 QUALIFIER
Osteopathic	Anatomical Regions	Treatment	Lumbar	External	Indirect	No Qualifier
7	W	0	3	X	4	Z

Other Procedures

Other procedure codes are used for a variety of other procedures (e.g., acupuncture, suture removal, and in vitro fertilization). All ICD-10-PCS codes are seven characters, each representing a particular aspect of the procedure. The meanings of the other procedure characters are as follows:

CHARACTER	REPRESENTS
1	Section
2	Body system
3	Root operation
4	Body region
5	Approach
6	Method
7	Qualifier

Other procedure codes are found in Section 8, so they have a first-character value of 8. The second character is for physiological systems and anatomical region, and the third character identifies the root operation.

The section has only one root operation:

- **Other procedures (0):** methodologies that attempt to remediate or cure a disorder or disease

The fourth character specifies the body region on which the procedure is performed. The fifth character identifies the approach, and each is defined in the Medical and Surgical section. The sixth-character value specifies the method by which the procedure is performed. The seventh character is to identify various qualifiers necessary to provide more information about a specific procedure.

EXAMPLE

Suture removal, left calf, 8E0YXY8

CHARACTER 1 SECTION	CHARACTER 2 BODY SYSTEM	CHARACTER 3 OPERATION	CHARACTER 4 BODY REGION	CHARACTER 5 APPROACH	CHARACTER 6 METHOD	CHARACTER 7 QUALIFIER
Other Procedures 8	Anatomical Regions E	Other Procedures 0	Lower Extremity Y	External X	Other Y	Suture Removal 8

Chiropractic

All ICD-10-PCS codes for chiropractic procedures are seven characters, each representing a particular aspect of the procedure. The meanings of the chiropractic procedure characters are as follows:

CHARACTER	REPRESENTS
1	Section
2	Body system
3	Root operation
4	Body region
5	Approach
6	Method
7	Qualifier

Chiropractic codes are found in Section 9, so they have a first-character value of 9. The second character identifies anatomical regions, and the third character identifies the root operation.

Section 9 has only one root operation:

- **Manipulation (B):** manual procedures that involve a directed thrust to move a joint past the physiological range of motion without exceeding the anatomical limit

The fourth character specifies the body region on which the chiropractic manipulation is performed. The fifth character identifies the approach, which is always external. The sixth-character value specifies the method by which the manipulation is performed. The seventh character is for a qualifier, but it is not specified in the chiropractic section at this time, so the value is always None(Z).

EXAMPLE

Chiropractic treatment to cervical spine, short lever specific contact, 9WB1XHZ

CHARACTER 1 SECTION	CHARACTER 2 BODY SYSTEM	CHARACTER 3 OPERATION	CHARACTER 4 BODY REGION	CHARACTER 5 APPROACH	CHARACTER 6 METHOD	CHARACTER 7 QUALIFIER
Chiropractic	Anatomical Regions	Manipulation	Cervical	External	Short lever specific contact	None
9	W	B	1	X	H	Z

EXERCISE 7-13

Without using reference material, answer the following questions about ICD-10-PCS.

1. The approach for chiropractic manipulation is always external.
   A. True
   B. False

2. Acupuncture can be coded in the Other Procedures section of ICD-10-PCS.
   A. True
   B. False

3. Any root operation in the Medical and Surgical section can be used in the Osteopathic section.
   A. True
   B. False

4. The approach for an osteopathic treatment is always external.
   A. True
   B. False

Ancillary Sections

The ancillary sections of ICD-10-PCS include the following:

B   Imaging
C   Nuclear medicine
D   Radiation oncology
F   Physical rehabilitation and diagnostic audiology
G   Mental health
H   Substance abuse treatment

Imaging

Imaging procedures include plain radiography, fluoroscopy, CT, MRI, and ultrasound. All ICD-10-PCS codes are seven characters, each representing a particular aspect of the procedure. The meanings of the imaging procedure characters are as follows:

CHARACTER	REPRESENTS
1	Section
2	Body system
3	Root type
4	Body part
5	Contrast
6	Qualifier
7	Qualifier

Imaging codes are found in Section B, so they have a first-character value of B. Similar to the Medical and Surgical section, the second character value identifies the body system. Instead of root operation, the third character identifies the type of imaging procedure. The root types are as follows:

- Computerized tomography (CT scans) (2)
- Fluoroscopy (1)
- Magnetic resonance imaging (MRI) (3)
- Plain radiography (0)
- Ultrasonography (4)

The fourth character specifies the body part, and the fifth character identifies whether the contrast material used is high or low osmolar when applicable. The sixth and seventh characters identify various qualifiers necessary to provide more information about a specific imaging procedure.

EXAMPLE

CT abdomen and pelvis without contrast, BW21ZZZ

CHARACTER 1 SECTION	CHARACTER 2 BODY SYSTEM	CHARACTER 3 ROOT TYPE	CHARACTER 4 BODY PART	CHARACTER 5 CONTRAST	CHARACTER 6 QUALIFIER	CHARACTER 7 QUALIFIER
Imaging	Anatomical Region	CT	Abdomen and pelvis	None	None	None
B	W	2	1	Z	Z	Z

Nuclear Medicine

Nuclear medicine procedures include nuclear medicine scans and PET scans. Radiation therapy is not included in this section. All ICD-10-PCS codes are seven characters, each representing a particular aspect of the procedure. The meanings of the nuclear medicine procedure characters are as follows:

CHARACTER	REPRESENTS
1	Section
2	Body system
3	Root type
4	Body part
5	Radionuclide
6	Qualifier
7	Qualifier

Nuclear medicine codes are found in Section C, so they have a first-character value of C. Similar to the Medical and Surgical section, the second character here specifies the body system. Instead of root operation, the third character identifies the type of nuclear medicine procedure. The root types are as follows:

- Nonimaging uptake (4)
- Nonimaging probe (5)
- Nonimaging assay (6)
- Planar imaging (1)
- Positron emission tomography (PET scan) (3)
- Systemic therapy (7)
- Tomographic (tomo) imaging (2)

The fourth character specifies body part or body region. The fifth-character value identifies the radionuclide or radiation source. The sixth and seventh characters are for qualifiers, but they are not used in the Nuclear Medicine section at this time, so the value is always None.

EXAMPLE

Whole body PET scan, CW3NYZZ

CHARACTER 1 SECTION	CHARACTER 2 BODY SYSTEM	CHARACTER 3 ROOT TYPE	CHARACTER 4 BODY PART	CHARACTER 5 RADIONUCLIDE	CHARACTER 6 QUALIFIER	CHARACTER 7 QUALIFIER
Nuclear Medicine	Anatomical Region	PET	Whole Body	Other Radionuclide	None	None
C	W	3	N	Y	Z	Z

Radiation Oncology

Radiation oncology includes procedures that introduce radioactive material for the treatment of cancer. All ICD-10-PCS codes used here are seven characters, each representing a particular aspect of the procedure. The meanings of the radiation oncology procedure characters are as follows:

CHARACTER	REPRESENTS
1	Section
2	Body system
3	Root type
4	Body part
5	Modality qualifier
6	Isotope
7	Qualifier

Radiation oncology codes are found in Section D, so they have a first-character value of D. Similar to the Medical and Surgical section, the second character specifies the body system. Instead of root operation, the third character identifies the general modality used (e.g., beam radiation). The fourth-character value specifies the body part that is the focus of the radiation therapy. The fifth-character value, the modality qualifier, specifies the radiation modality used (e.g., photons, electrons). The sixth character specifies the isotopes introduced during the procedure, if applicable. The seventh character is used for other qualifiers.

EXAMPLE

HDR Brachytherapy of prostate using Palladium 103, DV109BZ

CHARACTER 1 SECTION	CHARACTER 2 BODY SYSTEM	CHARACTER 3 MODALITY	CHARACTER 4 BODY PART	CHARACTER 5 MODALITY QUALIFIER	CHARACTER 6 ISOTOPE	CHARACTER 7 QUALIFIER
Radiation Oncology	Male Reproductive	Brachytherapy	Prostate	High Dose Rate	Pd-103	None
D	V	1	0	9	B	Z

EXERCISE 7-14

Without using reference material, answer the following questions about ICD-10-PCS.

1. MRI procedures are located in the Nuclear Medicine section.
   A. True
   B. False

2. Radionuclide is the fifth character in the Nuclear Medicine section.
   A. True
   B. False

3. The first-character value for an imaging procedure is B.
   A. True
   B. False

4. The fourth character specifies the body part that is the focus of the radiation therapy.
   A. True
   B. False

5. Isotope is the seventh-character qualifier in the Radiation Oncology section.
   A. True
   B. False

Physical Rehabilitation and Diagnostic Audiology

Physical rehabilitation procedures include physical therapy, occupational therapy, and speech-language pathology. Diagnostic audiology is also included in this section. All ICD-10-PCS codes are seven characters, each representing a particular aspect of the procedure. The meanings of the physical rehabilitation and diagnostic audiology procedure characters are as follows:

CHARACTER	REPRESENTS
1	Section
2	Section qualifier
3	Root type
4	Body system and region
5	Type qualifier
6	Equipment
7	Qualifier

Physical rehabilitation and diagnostic audiology codes are found in Section F, so they have a first-character value of F. There is a change from body system to section qualifier for the second-character value (e.g., rehabilitation or diagnostic audiology). Instead of root operation, the third character identifies the type of physical rehabilitation and diagnostic audiology procedure. There are four basic root types with 14 different root values. The four basic root types are as follows:

- Assessment
- Caregiver training
- Fittings
- Treatment

The fourth character specifies body part and body region. The fifth character, or type qualifier, further specifies the procedure performed. The sixth character identifies specific equipment used. Character seven is for a qualifier, but it is not used in this section at this time, so the value is always None.

EXAMPLE

Bedside swallow assessment, F00ZHZZ

CHARACTER 1 SECTION	CHARACTER 2 SECTION QUALIFIER	CHARACTER 3 ROOT TYPE	CHARACTER 4 BODY SYSTEM/ REGION	CHARACTER 5 TYPE QUALIFIER	CHARACTER 6 EQUIPMENT	CHARACTER 7 QUALIFIER
Physical Rehab & Diagnostic Audiology	Rehab	Speech Assessment	None	Bedside Swallowing and Oral Function	None	None
F	0	0	Z	H	Z	Z

Mental Health

Mental health procedures are coded in this section. All ICD-10-PCS codes are seven characters, each representing a particular aspect of the procedure. The meanings of the mental health procedure characters are as follows:

CHARACTER	REPRESENTS
1	Section
2	Body system
3	Root type
4	Type qualifier
5	Qualifier
6	Qualifier
7	Qualifier

Mental health codes are found in Section G, so they have a first-character value of G. The second-character value, for body system, has a value of None in this section. And instead of root operation, the third character identifies the type of mental health procedure. The root types are as follows:

■ Psychological tests (1)
■ Crisis intervention (2)
■ Medication management (3)
■ Individual psychotherapy (5)
■ Counseling (6)
■ Family psychotherapy (7)
■ ECT (B)
■ Biofeedback (C)
■ Hypnosis (F)
■ Narcosynthesis (G)
■ Group psychotherapy (H)
■ Light therapy (J)

The fourth-character value is a type qualifier (e.g., educational or vocational counseling). Values for Characters 5, 6, and 7 are for qualifiers but are not used in the Mental Health section at this time, so the value is always None.

EXAMPLE

Family therapy session, GZ72ZZZ

CHARACTER 1 SECTION	CHARACTER 2 BODY SYSTEM	CHARACTER 3 ROOT TYPE	CHARACTER 4 TYPE QUALIFIER	CHARACTER 5 QUALIFIER	CHARACTER 6 QUALIFIER	CHARACTER 7 QUALIFIER
Mental Health	None	Family Psychotherapy	Other Family Psychotherapy	None	None	None
G	Z	7	2	Z	Z	Z

Substance Abuse Treatment Section

Treatments for substance abuse are coded in this section. All ICD-10-PCS codes are seven characters, each representing a particular aspect of the procedure. The meanings of the substance abuse procedure characters are as follows:

CHARACTER	REPRESENTS
1	Section
2	Body system
3	Root type
4	Type qualifier
5	Qualifier
6	Qualifier
7	Qualifier

Substance abuse treatment codes are found in Section H, so they have a first-character value of H. The second-character value for body system has a value of None in this section. And instead of root operation, the third-character value identifies the type of substance abuse procedure. The root types are as follows:

- Detoxification services (2)
- Individual counseling (3)
- Group counseling (4)
- Individual psychotherapy (5)
- Family counseling (6)
- Medication management (8)
- Pharmacotherapy (9)

The fourth-character value is a type qualifier (e.g., cognitive behavioral, 12-step, interpersonal). Values for Characters 5, 6, and 7 are for qualifiers but are not used in the Substance Abuse section at this time, so the value is always None.

EXAMPLE

Medication management for methadone maintenance, HZ81ZZZ

CHARACTER 1 SECTION	CHARACTER 2 BODY SYSTEM	CHARACTER 3 ROOT TYPE	CHARACTER 4 TYPE QUALIFIER	CHARACTER 5 QUALIFIER	CHARACTER 6 QUALIFIER	CHARACTER 7 QUALIFIER
Substance Abuse Treatment	None	Medication Management	Methadone Maintenance	None	None	None
H	Z	8	1	Z	Z	Z

EXERCISE 7-15

Without using reference material, answer the following questions.

1. The seventh character identifies whether the procedure is a physical rehabilitation procedure or a diagnostic audiology procedure.
   A. True
   B. False

2. Equipment is the sixth character in the physical rehabilitation and diagnostic audiology section.
   A. True
   B. False

3. The first-character value for a physical rehabilitation or diagnostic audiology procedure is B.
   A. True
   B. False

4. Hypnosis is a procedure that can be coded in the Mental Health section.
   A. True
   B. False

5. In the Substance Abuse section, Characters 5, 6, and 7 are for qualifiers.
   A. True
   B. False

6. The first-character value for a mental health procedure is G.
   A. True
   B. False

CHAPTER REVIEW EXERCISE

Complete the following review exercises using ICD-10-PCS.

1. CT procedures are located in the Nuclear Medicine section.
   A. True
   B. False

2. Detoxification services can be coded in the Mental Health section.
   A. True
   B. False

3. Obstetric tables include procedures performed on the products of conception only.
   A. True
   B. False

4. In ICD-10-PCS, *abortion* is defined as "spontaneous termination of a pregnancy."
   A. True
   B. False

5. *Irrigation* is defined as "the putting in or on of a cleansing substance."
   A. True
   B. False

6. *Monitoring* is defined as "determining the level of physiological or physical function repetitively over a period of time."
   A. True
   B. False

7. Extracorporeal therapy uses equipment outside the body for a therapeutic purpose that does not involve the assistance or performance of a physiological function.
   A. True
   B. False

8. The approach for an osteopathic treatment is always external.
   A. True
   B. False

9. It is not acceptable to choose a valid code directly from the tables.
   A. True
   B. False

10. The resection of tonsils is coded to an external approach.
    A. True
    B. False

11. The body site for perirenal is kidney.
    A. True
    B. False

12. When a patient is having a knee replacement, a code for the resection of a joint is not assigned but is coded to the joint replacement.
    A. True
    B. False

13. A device is only coded if the device remains after the procedure is completed.
    A. True
    B. False

14. The root operation replacement always involves a device.
    A. True
    B. False

15. The approach for a laparoscopic cholecystectomy is percutaneous endoscopic.
    A. True
    B. False

16. The entry by puncture or minor incision, of instrumentation through the skin, mucous membrane, and any other body layers necessary to reach the operative site is an open approach.
    A. True
    B. False

17. All ICD-10-PCS codes have six characters.
   A. True
   B. False

18. The AMA is responsible for the maintenance of ICD-10-PCS.
   A. True
   B. False

19. Full implementation of the ICD-10-PCS system is scheduled for what date?
   A. October 31, 2013
   B. October 1, 2013
   C. October 1, 2014
   D. October 31, 2014

20. The mapping files that crosswalk ICD-9-CM to ICD-10-PCS are known as
   A. GEMs
   B. ACTs
   C. HIMs
   D. CMS

21. Which of the following is a characteristic of ICD-10-PCS?
   A. Codes have a decimal point.
   B. Codes are similar to ICD-10-CM codes.
   C. There are 34 possible values for a character.
   D. The number of codes is limited.

22. The first character of an ICD-10-PCS code represents
   A. Body part
   B. Approach
   C. Section
   D. Device

Locate the following terms in the Alphabetic Index, and identify the first three to four characters of the ICD-10-PCS code.

23. Brachytherapy, prostate   _____

24. Fragmentation, ureteral stone   _____

25. Kidney transplant   _____

26. Resection, adrenal glands   _____

27. PPN   _____

With the use of the two GEMs files on the CMS website (http://www.cms.gov/ICD10/11b_2011_ICD10PCS.asp#TopOfPage), answer the following.

Map the following procedure codes.

28. 03.51   _____

29. 34.20   _____

30. 38.31   _____

Map the following procedure codes.

31. 0SB00ZZ   _____

32. 0FB00ZX   _____

Assign the appropriate ICD-10-PCS codes to the following procedures in accordance with the coding guidelines.

33. Endometrial ablation via natural opening, endoscopic   _____

34. Above-knee amputation, right mid-shaft femoral region   _____

35. Partial nephrectomy, left   _____

36. Thoracentesis, right pleural cavity, therapeutic   _____

37. ESWL, right ureter   _____

38. Lysis of adhesions, small bowel   _____

39. Bilateral fallopian tubal occlusion, percutaneous   _____

40. Laparoscopic Nissen fundoplication   _____

41. Right inguinal herniorrhaphy with mesh, open   _____

42. Endoscopic dilatation, esophagus   _____

43. Total right hip replacement   _____

44. Open biopsies of liver and pancreas   _____

45. Laparoscopic cholecystectomy converted to open cholecystectomy   _____

46. Fiberoptic bronchoscopy with diagnostic lavage of left main bronchus   _____

47. Closed reduction of right radial fracture   _____

48. Percutaneous aspiration of left perirenal abscess   _____

49. Removal of mole, right upper arm, diagnostic   _____

50. Laparoscopically assisted vaginal hysterectomy   _____

51. Fragmentation of right kidney stone via percutaneous nephrostomy   _____

52. Placement of nasal packing, right nare   _____

53. Packing wound, abdomen wall   _____

54. Nonautologous bone marrow transplant via central venous catheter   _____

55. Mechanical ventilation, less than 24 hours   _____

56. ECMO, circulatory, intermittent–hyperbaric   _____

57. Robotic-assisted laparoscopic abdominal hysterectomy   _____

58. Chiropractic treatment to cervical spine using short lever specific contact   _____

59. Phototherapy with Bili-Lite, single treatment   _____

60. MRI brain   _____

61. Proton radiation therapy for brain metastasis   _____

62. Physical therapy treatment to increase ROM, right shoulder   _____

63. Hypnosis   _____

64. Twelve-step group therapy for alcohol addiction   _____

CHAPTER GLOSSARY

It is important to note that most of these definitions are as defined by ICD-10-PCS.

Abortion: artificially terminating a pregnancy.

Alteration: modifying the natural anatomic structure of a body part without affecting the function of the body part (breast augmentation).

Assistance: taking over a portion of a physiological function by extracorporeal means.

Atmospheric control: extracorporeal control of atmospheric pressure and composition.

Autologous: originating from the recipient, rather than from a donor; tissue transferred from the same individual's body (e.g., a skin graft taken from one part of the body is transferred to another part of the body on the same individual).

Bypass: altering the route of passage of the contents of a tubular body part (CABG).

Change: taking out or off a device from a body part and putting back an identical or similar device in or on the same body part without cutting or puncturing the skin or a mucous membrane (change gastrostomy tube).

Compression: putting pressure on a body region.

Control: stopping, or attempting to stop, postprocedural bleeding (control of post-tonsillectomy hemorrhage).

Creation: making a new structure that does not take the place of a body part (creation of a vagina in males for sex reassignment).

Decompression: extracorporeal elimination of undissolved gas from body fluids.

Delivery: assisting the passage of the products of conception from the genital canal.

Destruction: physical eradication of all or a portion of a body part by the direct use of energy, force, or a destructive agent (ablation of endometriosis).

Detachment: cutting off all or a portion of the upper or lower extremities (above-knee amputation).

Dilation: expanding an orifice or the lumen of a tubular body part (PTCA).

Division: cutting into a body part without draining fluids and/or gases from the body part in order to separate or transect a body part (osteotomy).

Drainage: taking or letting out fluids and/or gases from a body part (paracentesis).

Dressing: putting material on a body region for protection.

Electromagnetic therapy: extracorporeal treatment by electromagnetic rays.

Excision: cutting out or off, without replacement, a portion of a body part (partial nephrectomy).

Extraction: pulling or stripping out or off all or a portion of a body part by the use of force (bone marrow biopsy).

Extirpation: taking or cutting out solid matter from a body part (thrombectomy).

External: procedures performed directly on the skin or mucous membrane and procedures performed indirectly by the application of external force through the skin or mucous membrane (tonsillectomy).

Fragmentation: breaking solid matter in a body part into pieces (extracorporeal shock wave lithotripsy).

Fusion: joining together portions of an articular body part, rendering the articular body part immobile (spinal fusion).

Hyperthermia: extracorporeal raising of body temperature.

Hypothermia: extracorporeal lowering of body temperature.

Immobilization: limiting or preventing motion of a body region.

Insertion: putting in a nonbiological appliance that monitors, assists, performs, or prevents a physiological function but does not physically take the place of a body part (insertion of pacemaker lead).

Inspection: visually and/or manually exploring a body part (diagnostic arthroscopy).

Introduction: putting in or on a therapeutic, diagnostic, nutritional, physiological, or prophylactic substance except blood or blood products.

Irrigation: putting in or on a cleansing substance.

Manipulation: manual procedures that involve a directed thrust to move a joint past the physiological range of motion without exceeding the anatomical limit.

Map: locating the route of passage of electrical impulses and/or locating functional areas in a body part (cardiac mapping).

Measurement: determining the level of a physiological or physical function at a point in time.

Monitoring: determining the level of a physiological or physical function repetitively over a period of time.

Occlusion: completely closing an orifice or lumen of a tubular body part (tubal ligation).

Open: cutting through the skin, mucous membrane, and any other body layers necessary to expose the site of the procedure (abdominal hysterectomy).

Open with percutaneous endoscopic assistance: cutting through the skin, mucous membrane, and any other body layers necessary to expose the site of the procedure, and entry, by puncture or minor incision, of instrumentation through the skin, mucous membrane, and any other body layers necessary to aid in the performance of the procedure (laparoscopic-assisted vaginal hysterectomy).

Other procedures: methodologies that attempt to remediate or cure a disorder or disease.

Packing: putting material in a body region or orifice.

Percutaneous: entry, by puncture or minor incision, of instrumentation through the skin, mucous membrane, and any other body layers necessary to reach the site of the procedure (needle biopsy liver).

Percutaneous endoscopic: entry, by puncture or minor incision, of instrumentation through the skin, mucous membrane, and any other body layers necessary to reach and visualize the site of the procedure (laparoscopic cholecystectomy).

Performance: completely taking over a physiological function by extracorporeal means.

Pheresis: extracorporeal separation of blood products.

Phototherapy: extracorporeal treatment by light rays.

Reattachment: putting back in or on all or a portion of a separated body part to its normal location or other suitable location.

Release: to free a body part from an abnormal physical constraint (lysis of adhesions).

Removal: taking out or off a device from a body part (remove chest tube).

Repair: restoring, to the extent possible, a body part to its normal anatomic structure and function (herniorrhaphy).

Replacement: putting in or on biological or synthetic material that physically takes the place and/or performs the function of all or a portion of a body part (total knee replacement).

Reposition: moving to its normal location, or other suitable location, all or a portion of a body part (fracture reduction).

Resection: cutting out or off, without replacement, all of a body part (total lobectomy of lung).

Restoration: returning, or attempting to return, a physiological function to its original state by extracorporeal means.

Restriction: partially closing an orifice or lumen of a tubular body part (Nissen fundoplication).

Revision: correcting, to the extent possible, a malfunctioning or displaced device (adjustment of knee prosthesis).

Shock wave therapy: extracorporeal treatment by shock waves.

Supplement: putting in or on biological or synthetic material that physically reinforces and/or augments the function of a portion of a body part (herniorrhaphy with mesh).

Traction: exerting a pulling force on a body region in a distal direction.

Transfer: moving, without taking out, all or a portion of a body part to another location to take over the function of all or a portion of a body part (pedicle skin flap).

Transfusion: putting in blood or blood products.

Transplantation: putting in or on all or a portion of a living body part taken from another individual or animal to physically take the place and/or function of all or a portion of a similar body part (kidney transplant).

Treatment: manual treatment to eliminate or alleviate somatic dysfunction and related disorders.

Ultrasound therapy: extracorporeal treatment by ultrasound.

Ultraviolet light therapy: extracorporeal treatment by ultraviolet light.

Via natural or artificial opening: entry of instrumentation through a natural or artificial external opening to reach the site of the procedure (endotracheal intubation).

Via natural or artificial opening endoscopic: entry of instrumentation through a natural or artificial external opening to reach and visualize the site of the procedure (colonoscopy).

8

Symptoms, Signs, and Ill-Defined Conditions, and V Codes

(V Codes and ICD-9-CM Chapter 16, Codes 780-799, and ICD-10-CM Chapters 18 and 21, Codes R00-R99, Z00-Z99)

CHAPTER OUTLINE

ICD-9-CM Official Guidelines for Coding and Reporting
ICD-10-CM Official Guidelines for Coding and Reporting
Guideline Differences Between ICD-9-CM and ICD-10-CM
Major Differences Between ICD-9-CM and ICD-10-CM
Anatomy and Physiology
Disease Conditions
    Symptoms
    Nonspecific Abnormal Findings
    Ill-Defined and Unknown Causes of Morbidity and Mortality
Factors Influencing Health Status and Contact with Health Services (V Codes/Z Codes)
Procedures
Documentation/Reimbursement/MS-DRGs
    Symptoms That Are Integral to a Disease Process
    MS-DRG With and Without MCC/CC
Chapter Review Excrcise
Chapter Glossary
Reference

LEARNING OBJECTIVES

1. Apply and assign the correct ICD-9-CM and ICD-10-CM codes in accordance with Official Guidelines for Coding and Reporting
2. Identify major differences between ICD-9-CM and ICD-10-CM related to the signs and symptoms and V/Z codes
3. Determine when to assign signs and symptoms codes
4. Assign the correct V/Z codes
5. Explain the importance of documentation in relation to MS-DRGs for reimbursement

ABBREVIATIONS/ ACRONYMS

ASCUS atypical squamous cells of undetermined significance

BMI body mass index

COPD chronic obstructive pulmonary disease

CT computerized tomography

CVA cerebrovascular accident

MS-DRG Medicare Severity diagnosis-related group

FUO fever of unknown origin

HGSIL high-grade squamous intraepithelial lesion

HIV human immunodeficiency virus

ICD-9-CM *International Classification of Diseases, 9th Revision, Clinical Modification*

ICD-10-CM *International Classification of Diseases, 10th Revision, Clinical Modification*

ABBREVIATIONS/ ACRONYMS—cont'd

ICD-10-PCS *International Classification of Diseases, 10th Revision, Procedure Coding System*

OR Operating Room
PSA prostate-specific antigen
RW relative weight

SIDS sudden infant death syndrome
UTI urinary tract infection

ICD-9-CM

Official Guidelines for Coding and Reporting

Please refer to the companion Evolve site for the most current guidelines.
16. Chapter 16: Signs, Symptoms and Ill-Defined Conditions (780-799)
Reserved for future guideline expansion

Although there are no guidelines in the Chapter 16 section, there are very specific guidelines in the general coding guideline section that address the coding of signs and symptoms, late effects, and impending conditions. Only guidelines applicable to this chapter are included; therefore, the numbering is not sequential.

B. General Coding Guidelines
6. Signs and symptoms
Codes that describe symptoms and signs, as opposed to diagnoses, are acceptable for reporting purposes when a related definitive diagnosis has not been established (confirmed) by the provider. Chapter 16 of ICD-9-CM, Symptoms, Signs, and Ill-Defined conditions (codes 780.0-799.9) contain many, but not all codes for symptoms.

EXAMPLE Fever of unknown origin, 780.60 (R50.9)

7. Conditions that are an integral part of a disease process
Signs and symptoms that are associated routinely with a disease process should not be assigned as additional codes, unless otherwise instructed by the classification.

EXAMPLE Headache due to classical migraine, 346.00 (G43.109)

8. Conditions that are not an integral part of a disease process
Additional signs and symptoms that may not be associated routinely with a disease process should be coded when present.

EXAMPLE Ascites due to cirrhosis of the liver, 571.5, 789.59 (K74.60, R18.8)

Apply the General Coding Guidelines as found in Chapter 5 and the Procedural Guidelines as found in Chapter 6.

ICD-10-CM	Please refer to the companion Evolve site for the most current guidelines.

ICD-10-CM

Official Guidelines for Coding and Reporting

Please refer to the companion Evolve site for the most current guidelines.

18. **Chapter 18: Symptoms, signs, and abnormal clinical and laboratory findings, not elsewhere classified (R00-R99)**

Chapter 18 includes symptoms, signs, abnormal results of clinical or other investigative procedures, and ill-defined conditions regarding which no diagnosis classifiable elsewhere is recorded. Signs and symptoms that point to a **specific** diagnosis have been assigned to a category in other chapters of the classification.

a. **Use of symptom codes**

Codes that describe symptoms and signs are acceptable for reporting purposes when a related definitive diagnosis has not been established (confirmed) by the provider.

b. **Use of a symptom code with a definitive diagnosis code**

Codes for signs and symptoms may be reported in addition to a related definitive diagnosis when the sign or symptom is not routinely associated with that diagnosis, such as the various signs and symptoms associated with complex syndromes. The definitive diagnosis code should be sequenced before the symptom code.

Signs or symptoms that are associated routinely with a disease process should not be assigned as additional codes, unless otherwise instructed by the classification.

c. **Combination codes that include symptoms**

ICD-10-CM contains a number of combination codes that identify both the definitive diagnosis and common symptoms of that diagnosis. When using one of these combination codes, an additional code should not be assigned for the symptom.

d. **Repeated falls**

Code R29.6, Repeated falls, is for use for encounters when a patient has recently fallen and the reason for the fall is being investigated.

Code Z91.81, History of falling, is for use when a patient has fallen in the past and is at risk for future falls. When appropriate, both codes R29.6 and Z91.81 may be assigned together.

e. *Coma* scale

The coma scale codes (R40.2-) can be used in conjunction with traumatic brain injury codes, **acute cerebrovascular disease** or sequelae of cerebrovascular **disease** codes. These codes are primarily for use by trauma registries, but they may be used in any setting where this information is collected. The coma scale codes should be sequenced after the diagnosis code(s).

These codes, one from each subcategory, are needed to complete the scale. The 7th character indicates when the scale was recorded. The 7th character should match for all three codes.

At a minimum, report the initial score documented on presentation at your facility. This may be a score from the emergency medicine technician (EMT) or in the emergency department. If desired, a facility may choose to capture multiple Glasgow coma scale scores.

f. **Functional quadriplegia**

Functional quadriplegia (code R53.2) is the lack of ability to use one's limbs or to ambulate due to extreme debility. It is not associated with neurologic deficit or injury, and code R53.2 should not be used for cases of neurologic quadriplegia. It should only be assigned if functional quadriplegia is specifically documented in the medical record.

g. **SIRS due to Non-Infectious Process**

The systemic inflammatory response syndrome (SIRS) can develop as a result of certain non-infectious disease processes, such as trauma, malignant neoplasm, or pancreatitis. When SIRS is documented with a noninfectious condition, and no subsequent infection is documented, the code for the underlying condition, such as an injury, should be assigned, followed by code R65.10, Systemic inflammatory response syndrome (SIRS) of non-infectious origin without acute organ dysfunction, or code R65.11, Systemic inflammatory response syndrome (SIRS) of non-infectious origin with acute organ dysfunction. If an associated acute organ dysfunction is documented, the appropriate code(s) for the specific type of organ dysfunction(s) should be assigned in addition to code R65.11. If acute organ dysfunction is documented, but it cannot be determined if the acute organ dysfunction is associated with SIRS or due to another condition (e.g., directly due to the trauma), the provider should be queried.

h. Death NOS

Code R99, Ill-defined and unknown cause of mortality, is only for use in the very limited circumstance when a patient who has already died is brought into an emergency department or other healthcare facility and is pronounced dead upon arrival. It does not represent the discharge disposition of death.

Apply the General Coding Guidelines as found in Chapter 5 and the Procedural Guidelines as found in Chapter 7.

GUIDELINE DIFFERENCES BETWEEN ICD-9-CM AND ICD-10-CM

There are no ICD-9-CM guidelines for Chapter 16. There are a number of guidelines related to Chapter 18 in ICD-10-CM, and the guidelines address when to use symptom codes, as do the general guidelines in ICD-9-CM. There are additional guidelines for the following:

- Repeated falls is coded to a V code in ICD-9-CM, but in ICD-10-CM, it is coded to a symptom code.
- There are ICD-10-CM codes to identify a patient's coma scale.
- A guideline addresses the use of an ICD-10-CM code for functional quadriplegia.
- In ICD-10-CM, SIRS due to noninfectious process is moved from Injury and Poisoning, Chapter 17 in ICD-9-CM, to Chapter 18, Symptoms, Signs, and Abnormal Clinical and Laboratory Findings, Not Elsewhere Classified.
- There is a guideline for the use of code R99, Death NOS, in ICD-10-CM.

The guidelines for V codes and Z codes are fairly similar.

MAJOR DIFFERENCES BETWEEN ICD-9-CM AND ICD-10-CM

A number of Excludes1 notes found in this chapter will be helpful in determining if a symptom code should be assigned. It would be inappropriate to assign R09.2, Respiratory arrest, along with a code I46.-, Cardiac arrest (Figure 8-1).

In ICD-9-CM, the V codes for personal history of malignant neoplasm are only to code a history of primary neoplasm. There are codes to identify a patient's blood type.

ANATOMY AND PHYSIOLOGY

Signs, symptoms, ill-defined conditions, and V codes can affect any of the body systems. The anatomy and physiology of these body systems are outlined in their respective chapters.

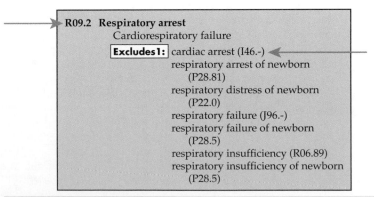

FIGURE 8-1. Excludes1 note in ICD-10-CM.

DISEASE CONDITIONS

Symptoms, Signs, and Ill-Defined Conditions (780-799), Chapter 16 in the ICD-9-CM code book, is divided into the following categories:

CATEGORY	SECTION TITLES
780-789	Symptoms
790-796	Nonspecific Abnormal Findings
797-799	Ill Defined and Unknown Causes of Morbidity and Mortality

Chapter 18 in the ICD-10-CM code book is divided into the following blocks:

CATEGORY	SECTION TITLES
R00-R09	Symptoms and Signs Involving the Circulatory and Respiratory Systems
R10-R19	Symptoms and Signs Involving the Digestive System and Abdomen
R20-R23	Symptoms and Signs Involving the Skin and Subcutaneous Tissue
R25-R29	Symptoms and Signs Involving the Nervous and Musculoskeletal Systems
R30-R39	Symptoms and Signs Involving the Urinary System
R40-R46	Symptoms and Signs Involving Cognition, Perception, Emotional State, and Behavior
R47-R49	Symptoms and Signs Involving Speech and Voice
R50-R69	General Symptoms and Signs
R70-R79	Abnormal Findings on Examination of Blood, without Diagnosis
R80-R82	Abnormal Findings on Examination of Urine, without Diagnosis
R83-R89	Abnormal Findings on Examination of Other Bloody Fluids, Substances, and Tissues, without Diagnosis
R90-R94	Abnormal Findings on Diagnostic Imaging and in Function Studies, without Diagnosis
R97	Abnormal Tumor Markers
R99	Ill-defined and Unknown Cause of Mortality

Chapter 21 in the ICD-10-CM code book is divided into the following blocks:

CATEGORY	SECTION TITLES
Z00-Z13	Persons Encountering Health Services for Examination and Investigation
Z14-Z15	Genetic Carrier and Genetic Susceptibility to Disease
Z16	Infection with Drug-Resistant Microorganisms
Z17	Estrogen Receptor Status
Z20-Z28	Persons with Potential Health Hazards Related to Communicable Disease
Z30-Z39	Persons Encountering Health Services in Circumstances Related to Reproduction
Z40-Z53	Persons Encountering Health Services for Specific Procedures and Health Care
Z55-Z65	Persons with Potential Health Hazards Related to Socioeconomic and Psychosocial Circumstance
Z66	Do Not Resuscitate (DNR) Status
Z67	Blood Type
Z68	Body Mass Index (BMI)
Z69-Z76	Persons Encountering Health Services in Other Circumstances
Z79-Z99	Persons with Potential Health Hazards Related to Family and Personal History and Certain Conditions Influencing Health Status

See Figure 8-2 for details on an instructional note that appears at the very beginning of Chapter 16 of the Tabular List and applies to the entire chapter. This note provides information on the appropriate use of signs and symptoms codes.

In ICD-9-CM the V codes and E codes are found in the supplemental sections of the ICD-9-CM code book, and codes are assigned in the same manner as other codes, that is, by looking up the main term in the Alphabetic Index or E code index and verifying the code in the Tabular. The Tabular List for the V codes is located after the Tabular List for

> ## 16. SYMPTOMS, SIGNS, AND ILL-DEFINED CONDITIONS (780–799)
>
> This section includes symptoms, signs, abnormal results of laboratory or other investigative procedures, and ill-defined conditions regarding which no diagnosis classifiable elsewhere is recorded.
>
> Signs and symptoms that point rather definitely to a given diagnosis are assigned to some category in the preceding part of the classification. In general, categories 780–796 include the more ill-defined conditions and symptoms that point with perhaps equal suspicion to two or more diseases or to two or more systems of the body, and without the necessary study of the case to make a final diagnosis. Practically all categories in this group could be designated as "not otherwise specified," or as "unknown etiology," or as "transient." The Alphabetic Index should be consulted to determine which symptoms and signs are to be allocated here and which to more specific sections of the classification; the residual subcategories numbered .9 are provided for other relevant symptoms which cannot be allocated elsewhere in the classification.
>
> The conditions and signs or symptoms included in categories 780–796 consist of: (a) cases for which no more specific diagnosis can be made even after all facts bearing on the case have been investigated; (b) signs or symptoms existing at the time of initial encounter that proved to be transient and whose causes could not be determined; (c) provisional diagnoses in a patient who failed to return for further investigation or care; (d) cases referred elsewhere for investigation or treatment before the diagnosis was made; (e) cases in which a more precise diagnosis was not available for any other reason; (f) certain symptoms which represent important problems in medical care and which it might be desired to classify in addition to a known cause.

FIGURE 8-2. Instructional note that appears at the beginning of Chapter 16.

Chapter 17, Injury and Poisoning. The Tabular for the E codes follows the V code Tabular List.

A few V code guidelines are explained with the various chapter guidelines; these will be addressed in those chapters. Some of them are repeated in the guidelines for V codes and are reviewed in this chapter. These codes are addressed at the beginning of the book because they apply to all body systems. V codes and signs and symptoms are common throughout this text.

Symptoms

A **symptom** is subjective evidence of a disease or of a patient's condition as perceived by the patient.

EXAMPLE

> The patient presents to the ER complaining of a severe headache. The headache is an example of a symptom because it is a description of the patient's condition as perceived by the patient, 784.0 (R51).

A **sign** is objective evidence of a disease or of a patient's condition as perceived by the patient's examining physician.

EXAMPLE

> The patient has a fever. This can be discerned by noting the patient's elevated temperature, 780.60 (R50.9).

It can be difficult to determine whether a sign or a symptom from Chapter 16 is routinely associated with the disease. It may be necessary to access resource books, such as

Merck's Manual, or the Internet to find the most common symptoms of a disease or condition. As was previously stated in Chapter 5 of this text, signs and symptoms codes are acceptable to code:

■ When no definitive diagnosis has been established
■ When they are not an integral part of the disease process
■ When directed by the classification to assign an additional code

It is not acceptable to code signs or symptoms:

■ When a definitive diagnosis has not been established
■ When they are an integral part of the disease process

EXAMPLE	Fever due to pneumonia, 486 (J18.9).
	Fever is one of the symptoms of pneumonia that is integral to the disease process. Only the pneumonia should be coded.

EXAMPLE	Dehydration due to pneumonia, 486, 276.51 (J18.9, E86.0).
	Although many patients who are admitted to the hospital may be dehydrated, not all patients who have pneumonia become dehydrated.

EXAMPLE	Patient was admitted with right lower quadrant abdominal pain with nausea and vomiting. Patient has a low-grade fever. A diagnosis of acute appendicitis was confirmed upon removal of the patient's appendix in the Operating Room (OR), 540.9, 47.09 (K35.80, 0DTJ0ZZ). The fever, abdominal pain, and nausea/vomiting are all symptoms of appendicitis and are not coded.

EXERCISE 8-1

Assign codes to the following conditions.

1. Alteration in mental status _____
2. Fever of unknown origin (FUO) _____
3. Right upper quadrant abdominal pain due to cholecystitis versus peptic ulcer disease _____
4. Ascites due to cirrhosis of liver _____
5. Oliguria _____
6. Renal colic _____
7. Change in bowel habits _____
8. Substernal chest pain _____
9. Loss of appetite _____
10. Ataxia _____
11. Generalized pain _____
12. Delirium _____

Nonspecific Abnormal Findings

Many times, an abnormality or elevation in a test result will lead to further investigation or repeat performance of certain tests. The patient may be without any signs or symptoms, and no definitive diagnosis may explain the abnormality. Some of the main terms that may be used to assist with location of these codes include "abnormal," "abnormality," "abnormalities," "elevation," and "findings, abnormal, without diagnosis." These abnormal findings must be documented by the physician to be coded. A coder should not code an abnormal finding on the basis of a review of laboratory results or reports of other diagnostic procedures (*Coding Clinic* 1990:2Q:p15-16).[1]

EXAMPLE | Elevated blood pressure. Patient does not have a history of hypertension, 796.2 (R03.0).

EXAMPLE | Abnormal lung x-ray. Patient will be scheduled for a computerized tomography (CT) of the chest, 793.1 (R91).

EXERCISE 8-2

Assign codes to the following conditions.

1. Significant drop in hematocrit   _____
2. Abnormal coagulation profile   _____
3. Proteinuria   _____
4. Abnormal Pap smear with atypical squamous cells of
   undetermined significance (ASCUS)   _____
5. Abnormal mammogram   _____
6. Bacteremia   _____
7. Abnormal lead levels in blood   _____
8. Positive Mantoux test   _____
9. Elevated CA-125   _____
10. Transaminasemia   _____

Ill-Defined and Unknown Causes of Morbidity and Mortality

The title of this section is fitting because the codes included in this section are ill-defined and of unknown causes, ranging from sudden infant death syndrome (SIDS) to decreased libido.

EXAMPLE | Patient is receiving physical therapy for debility, 799.3 (R53.81).

EXERCISE 8-3

Assign codes to the following conditions.

1. Respiratory arrest   _____
2. Sudden infant death syndrome (SIDS)   _____
3. Decreased libido   _____
4. Hypoxia   _____
5. Nervousness   _____

FACTORS INFLUENCING HEALTH STATUS AND CONTACT WITH HEALTH SERVICES (V CODES/Z CODES)

The V codes are located after Chapter 17 in the Tabular List. According to the guidelines, ICD-9-CM provides codes that should be assigned to encounters for circumstances other than a disease or injury. The Supplementary Classification of Factors Influencing Health Status and Contact with Health Services (V01.0-V91.99) is provided to deal with occasions when circumstances other than a disease or injury (codes 001-999) are recorded as a diagnosis or problem. In ICD-10-CM, the Z codes are located in Chapter 21.

18. **Classification of Factors Influencing Health Status and Contact with Health Service (Supplemental V01-V89)**
Note: The chapter specific guidelines provide additional information about the use of V codes for specified encounters.
a. **Introduction**
ICD-9-CM provides codes to deal with encounters for circumstances other than a disease or injury. The Supplementary Classification of Factors Influencing Health Status and Contact with Health Services (V01.0-**V91.99**) is provided to deal with occasions when circumstances other than a disease or injury (codes 001-999) are recorded as a diagnosis or problem.
There are four primary circumstances for the use of V codes:
1) A person who is not currently sick encounters the health services for some specific reason, such as to act as an organ donor, to receive prophylactic care, such as inoculations or health screenings, or to receive counseling on health related issues.

EXAMPLE

The patient was admitted to donate a kidney for a brother's kidney transplant. A right nephrectomy was performed without complication, V59.4, 55.51 (Z52.4, 0TT00ZZ).

2) A person with a resolving disease or injury, or a chronic, long-term condition requiring continuous care, encounters the health care system for specific aftercare of that disease or injury (e.g., dialysis for renal disease; chemotherapy for malignancy; cast change). A diagnosis/symptom code should be used whenever a current, acute, diagnosis is being treated or a sign or symptom is being studied.

EXAMPLE

Patient with hydrocephalus was admitted for removal of ventricular shunt, V53.01, 331.4, 02.43 (Z45.41, G91.9, 00P600Z).

3) Circumstances or problems influence a person's health status but are not in themselves a current illness or injury.

EXAMPLE

A patient was admitted with congestive heart failure and coronary artery disease. The patient has a history of coronary artery bypass graft and a family history of coronary artery disease, 428.0, 414.00, V45.81, V17.3 (I50.9, I25.10, Z95.1, Z82.49).

4) Newborns, to indicate birth status

EXAMPLE

A newborn is delivered by vaginal delivery and receives prophylactic vaccination for hepatitis B before discharge, V30.00, V05.3, 99.55 (Z38.00, Z23, 3E0134Z).

EXAMPLE

Healthy liveborn twins born via cesarean section: Twin A, V30.01 (Z38.31); Twin B V30.01 (Z38.31).

b. V codes use in any healthcare setting
V codes are for use in any healthcare setting. V codes may be used as either a first listed (principal diagnosis code in the inpatient setting) or secondary code, depending on the circumstances of the encounter. Certain V codes may only be used as first listed, others only as secondary codes.
See Section I.C.18.e, V Codes That May Only be Principal/First-Listed Diagnosis.

c. V Codes indicate a reason for an encounter
They are not procedure codes. A corresponding procedure code must accompany a V code to describe the procedure performed.

EXAMPLE A female patient was admitted for elective sterilization and percutaneous endoscopic bilateral tubal occlusion with Falope ring was performed, V25.2, 66.29 (Z30.2, OUL74CZ).

---

d. Categories of V Codes
1) Contact/Exposure
Category V01 indicates contact with or exposure to communicable diseases. These codes are for patients who do not show any sign or symptom of a disease but have been exposed to it by close personal contact with an infected individual or are in an area where a disease is epidemic. These codes may be used as a first listed code to explain an encounter for testing, or, more commonly, as a secondary code to identify a potential risk.

EXAMPLE Exposure to anthrax, V01.81 (Z20.810).

---

2) Inoculations and vaccinations
Categories V03-V06 are for encounters for inoculations and vaccinations. They indicate that a patient is being seen to receive a prophylactic inoculation against a disease. The injection itself must be represented by the appropriate procedure code. A code from V03-V06 may be used as a secondary code if the inoculation is given as a routine part of preventive health care, such as a well-baby visit.

EXAMPLE Vaccination for influenza, V04.81, 99.52 (Z23, 3E0134Z).

---

3) Status
Status codes indicate that a patient is a carrier of a disease, has the sequelae or residual of a past disease or condition, or has another factor influencing a person's health status. This includes such things as the presence of prosthetic or mechanical devices resulting from past treatment. A status code is informative, because the status may affect the course of treatment and its outcome. A status code is distinct from a history code. The history code indicates that the patient no longer has the condition.
A status code should not be used with a diagnosis code from one of the body system chapters, if the diagnosis code includes the information provided by the status code. For example, code V42.1, Heart transplant status, should not be used with code 996.83, Complications of transplanted heart. The status code does not provide additional information. The complication code indicates that the patient is a heart transplant patient.

Assignment of V codes can be problematic because some can be used only as the principal diagnosis, others can be used as both principal and secondary diagnoses, and some can be used only as secondary diagnoses. It can be difficult to locate V codes in the Alphabetic Index. Coders will often say, "I did not know there was a V code for that." It is very important to be familiar with the different types and uses of V codes. Because appropriate main terms are difficult to find in the Alphabetic Index, some common main terms are as follows:

Admission	Donor	Procedure (surgical)
Aftercare	Examination	Prophylactic
Attention to	Fitting of	Replacement
Boarder	Follow-up	Screening
Care (of)	Health, Healthy	Status
Carrier	History	Supervision (of)
Checking	Maintenance	Test
Contraception	Maladjustment	Transplant
Counseling	Observation	Unavailability of medical facilities
Dialysis	Problem	Vaccination

Guidelines for V codes provide a lot of detail and descriptions of the various sections of V codes. It may be necessary to review these guidelines frequently; V codes will also be addressed in most of the following chapters because some V codes are specific to certain body systems.

Screening V codes should be assigned only when the service fits the definition of a screening. A **screening examination** is one that occurs in the absence of any signs or symptoms. It consists of examination of an asymptomatic individual to detect a given disease, typically by means of an inexpensive diagnostic test. There are V codes for prophylactic organ removal. A **prophylactic** measure is the use of medication or treatment to prevent a disease from occurring.

EXAMPLE   Screening mammogram for 45-year-old patient, V76.12 (Z12.31).

EXAMPLE   Screening mammogram in a 45-year-old patient with nipple discharge, 611.79 (N64.52).

In this case, even though it was documented as a screening mammogram, it does not fit the definition because the nipple discharge is a symptom and a reason for the test. It would be inappropriate to assign the screening V code.

Several V codes identify the history of certain conditions. Documentation of a patient's medical and surgical history may be found within the History and Physical or the Admit Note.

Sometimes, documentation in the health record may indicate a history of a particular disease or condition, and the disease or condition is actually a current or active problem. If any question arises as to whether a condition is currently an active problem, a physician query may be necessary.

Relevant family history is often documented. It may be important to code a family history of malignant neoplasm of the breast when a patient has been admitted with breast cancer and is having a mastectomy. In the Index under "History," "Family history" is a subterm, and it may be difficult to locate where the family history subterms start and stop (Figure 8-3).

EXAMPLE   Patient has a past history of chronic obstructive pulmonary disease (COPD). You would not assign a V code to indicate a previous history of a respiratory condition but the code for the active disease. COPD is a chronic condition that cannot be cured, 496 (J44.9).

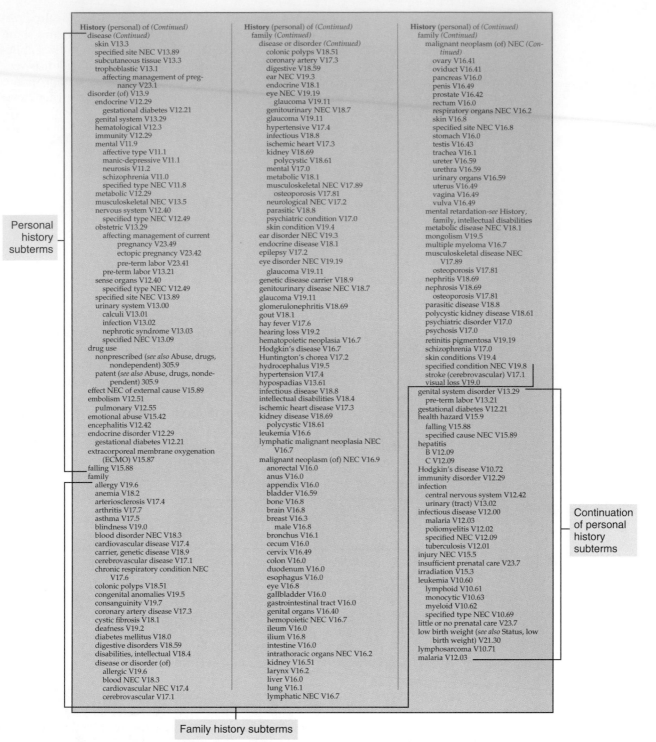

History (personal) of *(Continued)*
  disease *(Continued)*
    skin V13.3
    specified site NEC V13.89
    subcutaneous tissue V13.3
    trophoblastic V13.1
      affecting management of pregnancy V23.1
  disorder (of) V13.9
    endocrine V12.29
      gestational diabetes V12.21
    genital system V13.29
    hematological V12.3
    immunity V12.29
    mental V11.9
      affective type V11.1
      manic-depressive V11.1
      neurosis V11.2
      schizophrenia V11.0
      specified type NEC V11.8
    metabolic V12.29
    musculoskeletal NEC V13.5
    nervous system V12.40
      specified type NEC V12.49
    obstetric V13.29
      affecting management of current
        pregnancy V23.49
        ectopic pregnancy V23.42
        pre-term labor V23.41
      pre-term labor V13.21
    sense organs V12.40
      specified type NEC V12.49
    specified site NEC V13.89
    urinary system V13.00
      calculi V13.01
      infection V13.02
      nephrotic syndrome V13.03
      specified NEC V13.09
  drug use
    nonprescribed (*see also* Abuse, drugs, nondependent) 305.9
    patent (*see also* Abuse, drugs, nondependent) 305.9
  effect NEC of external cause V15.89
  embolism V12.51
    pulmonary V12.55
  emotional abuse V15.42
  encephalitis V12.42
  endocrine disorder V12.29
    gestational diabetes V12.21
  extracorporeal membrane oxygenation (ECMO) V15.87
  falling V15.88
  family
    allergy V19.6
    anemia V18.2
    arteriosclerosis V17.4
    arthritis V17.7
    asthma V17.5
    blindness V19.0
    blood disorder NEC V18.3
    cardiovascular disease V17.4
    carrier, genetic disease V18.9
    cerebrovascular disease V17.1
    chronic respiratory condition NEC V17.6
    colonic polyps V18.51
    congenital anomalies V19.5
    consanguinity V19.7
    coronary artery disease V17.3
    cystic fibrosis V18.1
    deafness V19.2
    diabetes mellitus V18.0
    digestive disorders V18.59
    disabilities, intellectual V18.4
    disease or disorder (of)
      allergic V19.6
      blood NEC V18.3
      cardiovascular NEC V17.4
      cerebrovascular V17.1

Personal history subterms

History (personal) of *(Continued)*
  family *(Continued)*
    disease or disorder *(Continued)*
      colonic polyps V18.51
      coronary artery V17.3
      digestive V18.59
      ear NEC V19.3
      endocrine V18.1
      eye NEC V19.19
        glaucoma V19.11
      genitourinary NEC V18.7
      glaucoma V19.11
      hypertensive V17.4
      infectious V18.8
      ischemic heart V17.3
      kidney V18.69
        polycystic V18.61
      mental V17.0
      metabolic V18.1
      musculoskeletal NEC V17.89
        osteoporosis V17.81
      neurological NEC V17.2
      parasitic V18.8
      psychiatric condition V17.0
      skin condition V19.4
    ear disorder NEC V19.3
    endocrine disease V18.1
    epilepsy V17.2
    eye disorder NEC V19.19
      glaucoma V19.11
    genetic disease carrier V18.9
    genitourinary disease NEC V18.7
    glaucoma V19.11
    glomerulonephritis V18.69
    gout V18.1
    hay fever V17.6
    hearing loss V19.2
    hematopoietic neoplasia V16.7
    Hodgkin's disease V16.7
    Huntington's chorea V17.2
    hydrocephalus V19.5
    hypertension V17.4
    hypospadias V13.61
    infectious disease V18.8
    intellectual disabilities V18.4
    ischemic heart disease V17.3
    kidney disease V18.69
      polycystic V18.61
    leukemia V16.6
    lymphatic malignant neoplasia NEC V16.7
    malignant neoplasm (of) NEC V16.9
      anorectal V16.0
      anus V16.0
      appendix V16.0
      bladder V16.59
      bone V16.8
      brain V16.8
      breast V16.3
        male V16.8
      bronchus V16.1
      cecum V16.0
      cervix V16.49
      colon V16.0
      duodenum V16.0
      esophagus V16.0
      eye V16.8
      gallbladder V16.0
      gastrointestinal tract V16.0
      genital organs V16.40
      hemopoietic NEC V16.7
      ileum V16.0
      ilium V16.8
      intestine V16.0
      intrathoracic organs NEC V16.2
      kidney V16.51
      larynx V16.2
      liver V16.0
      lung V16.1
      lymphatic NEC V16.7

Family history subterms

History (personal) of *(Continued)*
  family *(Continued)*
    malignant neoplasm (of) NEC *(Continued)*
      ovary V16.41
      oviduct V16.41
      pancreas V16.0
      penis V16.49
      prostate V16.42
      rectum V16.0
      respiratory organs NEC V16.2
      skin V16.8
      specified site NEC V16.8
      stomach V16.0
      testis V16.43
      trachea V16.1
      ureter V16.59
      urethra V16.59
      urinary organs V16.59
      uterus V16.49
      vagina V16.49
      vulva V16.49
    mental retardation–*see* History, family, intellectual disabilities
    metabolic disease NEC V18.1
    mongolism V19.5
    multiple myeloma V16.7
    musculoskeletal disease NEC V17.89
      osteoporosis V17.81
    nephritis V18.69
    nephrosis V18.69
      osteoporosis V17.81
    parasitic disease V18.8
    polycystic kidney disease V18.61
    psychiatric disorder V17.0
    psychosis V17.0
    retinitis pigmentosa V19.19
    schizophrenia V17.0
    skin conditions V19.4
    specified condition NEC V19.8
    stroke (cerebrovascular) V17.1
    visual loss V19.0
  genital system disorder V13.29
    pre-term labor V13.21
  gestational diabetes V12.21
  health hazard V15.9
    falling V15.88
    specified cause NEC V15.89
  hepatitis
    B V12.09
    C V12.09
  Hodgkin's disease V10.72
  immunity disorder V12.29
  infection
    central nervous system V12.42
    urinary (tract) V13.02
  infectious disease V12.00
    malaria V12.03
    poliomyelitis V12.02
    specified NEC V12.09
    tuberculosis V12.01
  injury NEC V15.5
  insufficient prenatal care V23.7
  irradiation V15.3
  leukemia V10.60
    lymphoid V10.61
    monocytic V10.63
    myeloid V10.62
    specified type NEC V10.69
  little or no prenatal care V23.7
  low birth weight (*see also* Status, low birth weight) V21.30
  lymphosarcoma V10.71
  malaria V12.03

Continuation of personal history subterms

FIGURE 8-3. Family history subterms.

EXAMPLE   The patient has a history of urinary tract infections (UTIs). In this case, no documentation, such as antibiotic therapy, indicates that the patient currently has a UTI, so a history of UTI V code is appropriate, V13.02 (Z87.440).

EXAMPLE   Patient has a history of thrombocytopenia. The physician documents that the patient still has a low platelet count (thrombocytopenia and low platelets are assigned the same code). A V code is not necessary as the patient continues to be thrombocytopenic, 287.5 (D69.6).

The status V codes/categories are:

V02	Carrier or suspected carrier of infectious diseases
	Carrier status indicates that a person harbors the specific organisms of a disease without manifest symptoms and is capable of transmitting the infection.
V07.5X	**Use** of agents affecting estrogen receptors and estrogen level
	This code indicates when a patient is receiving a drug that affects estrogen receptors and estrogen levels for prevention of cancer.
V08	Asymptomatic HIV infection status
	This code indicates that a patient has tested positive for HIV but has manifested no signs or symptoms of the disease.
V09	Infection with drug-resistant microorganisms
	This category indicates that a patient has an infection that is resistant to drug treatment. Sequence the infection code first.
V21	Constitutional states in development
V22.2	Pregnant state, incidental
	This code is a secondary code only for use when the pregnancy is in no way complicating the reason for visit. Otherwise, a code from the obstetric chapter is required.
V26.5x	Sterilization status
V42	Organ or tissue replaced by transplant
V43	Organ or tissue replaced by other means
V44	Artificial opening status
V45	Other postsurgical states

Assign code V45.87, Transplant organ removal status, to indicate that a transplanted organ has been previously removed. This code should not be assigned for the encounter in which the transplanted organ is removed. The complication necessitating removal of the transplant organ should be assigned for that encounter.
See Section I.C17.f.2. for information on the coding of organ transplant complications.

Assign code V45.88, Status post administration of tPA (rtPA) in a different facility within the last 24 hours prior to admission to the current facility, as a secondary diagnosis when a patient is received by transfer into a facility and documentation indicates they were administered tissue plasminogen activator (tPA) within the last 24 hours prior to admission to the current facility.

This guideline applies even if the patient is still receiving the tPA at the time they are received into the current facility.

The appropriate code for the condition for which the tPA was administered (such as cerebrovascular disease or myocardial infarction) should be assigned first.

Code V45.88 is only applicable to the receiving facility record and not to the transferring facility record.

V46	Other dependence on machines
V49.6	Upper limb amputation status
V49.7	Lower limb amputation status

Note: Categories V42-V46, and subcategories V49.6, V49.7 are for use only if there are no complications or malfunctions of the organ or tissue replaced, the amputation site or the equipment on which the patient is dependent.

V49.81	**Asymptomatic postmenopausal status (age-related) (natural)**
V49.82	Dental sealant status
V49.83	Awaiting organ transplant status
V49.86	**Do not resuscitate status**
	This code may be used when it is documented by the provider that a patient is on do not resuscitate status at any time during the stay.

V49.87   **Physical restraint status**
This code may be used when it is documented by the provider that a patient has been put in restraints during the current encounter. Please note that this code should not be reported when it is documented by the provider that a patient is temporarily restrained during a procedure.

V58.6x   Long-term (current) drug use
Codes from this subcategory indicate a patient's continuous use of a prescribed drug (including such things as aspirin therapy) for the long-term treatment of a condition or for prophylactic use. It is not for use for patients who have addictions to drugs.
This subcategory is not for use of medications for detoxification or maintenance programs to prevent withdrawal symptoms in patients with drug dependence (e.g., methadone maintenance for opiate dependence). Assign the appropriate code for the drug dependence instead.
Assign a code from subcategory V58.6, Long-term (current) drug use, if the patient is receiving a medication for an extended period as a prophylactic measure (such as for the prevention of deep vein thrombosis) or as treatment of a chronic condition (such as arthritis) or a disease requiring a lengthy course of treatment (such as cancer). Do not assign a code from subcategory V58.6 for medication being administered for a brief period of time to treat an acute illness or injury (such as a course of antibiotics to treat acute bronchitis).

V83   Genetic carrier status
Genetic carrier status indicates that a person carries a gene, associated with a particular disease, which may be passed to offspring who may develop that disease. The person does not have the disease and is not at risk of developing the disease.

V84   Genetic susceptibility status
Genetic susceptibility indicates that a person has a gene that increases the risk of that person developing the disease.
Codes from category V84, Genetic susceptibility to disease, should not be used as principal or first-listed codes. If the patient has the condition to which he/she is susceptible, and that condition is the reason for the encounter, the code for the current condition should be sequenced first. If the patient is being seen for follow-up after completed treatment for this condition, and the condition no longer exists, a follow-up code should be sequenced first, followed by the appropriate personal history and genetic susceptibility codes. If the purpose of the encounter is genetic counseling associated with procreative management, a code from subcategory V26.3, Genetic counseling and testing, should be assigned as the first-listed code, followed by a code from category V84. Additional codes should be assigned for any applicable family or personal history.
See Section I.C. 18.d.14 for information on prophylactic organ removal due to a genetic susceptibility.

V85   Body Mass Index (BMI)
V86   Estrogen receptor status
V88   Acquired absence of other organs and tissue
V90   **Retained foreign body**

EXAMPLE   A patient was admitted for myocardial infarction. The patient is status post mitral valve replacement with porcine valve, 410.91, V42.2 (I21.3, Z95.3).

V58.6X is assigned to identify the long-term use of a particular drug or medication. To locate these codes in the Alphabetic Index, the main term is "long-term drug use." These codes should not be used to identify drug abuse or dependence or to identify a medication that is used for a short period during an acute illness or injury. Drugs may be used to prevent a condition as a prophylactic measure or to treat a chronic condition. Sometimes a patient will need to have lab work to monitor the effectiveness of a particular medication or if the medication is causing any adverse effects. Code V58.83 (Z51.81), encounter for therapeutic drug monitoring would be assigned.

EXAMPLE

> Patient has been taking Lipitor for hypercholesterolemia for one year. A hepatic function laboratory test was performed to assess any adverse effects on the patient's liver function. A fasting lipid profile was also done to assess the effectiveness of the Lipitor, V58.83, V58.69, 272.0 (Z51.81, Z79.899, E78.0).

In this example the long-term use of Lipitor is identified with code V58.69, long-term use of other medications, because the patient has been taking it for a year.

EXAMPLE

> Patient was seen in the ER for acute bronchitis. The patient's family physician had seen the patient a couple of days ago and prescribed antibiotics. The patient was instructed to finish the antibiotics and follow-up with family physician, 466.0 (J20.9).

In this example the use of antibiotics is not assigned a V code because it is used only for a short period of time to treat an acute illness.

4) History (of)

There are two types of history V codes, personal and family. Personal history codes explain a patient's past medical condition that no longer exists and is not receiving any treatment, but that has the potential for recurrence, and therefore may require continued monitoring. The exceptions to this general rule are category V14, Personal history of allergy to medicinal agents, and subcategory V15.0, Allergy, other than to medicinal agents. A person who has had an allergic episode to a substance or food in the past should always be considered allergic to the substance.

Family history codes are for use when a patient has a family member(s) who has had a particular disease that causes the patient to be at higher risk of also contracting the disease.

Personal history codes may be used in conjunction with follow-up codes and family history codes may be used in conjunction with screening codes to explain the need for a test or procedure. History codes are also acceptable on any medical record regardless of the reason for visit. A history of an illness, even if no longer present, is important information that may alter the type of treatment ordered.

The history V code categories are:

V10	Personal history of malignant neoplasm
V12	Personal history of certain other diseases
V13	Personal history of other diseases
	Except: V13.4, Personal history of arthritis, and **subcategory** V13.6, **Personal history of congenital (corrected)** malformations. These conditions are life-long so are not true history codes.
V14	Personal history of allergy to medicinal agents
V15	Other personal history presenting hazards to health
	Except: V15.7, Personal history of contraception.
V16	Family history of malignant neoplasm
V17	Family history of certain chronic disabling diseases
V18	Family history of certain other specific diseases
V19	Family history of other conditions
V87	Other specified personal exposures and history presenting hazards to health

EXAMPLE Family history of polycystic kidney disease, V18.61 (Z82.71).

EXAMPLE Personal history of exposure to asbestos, V15.84 (Z77.090).

5) Screening

Screening is the testing for disease or disease precursors in seemingly well individuals so that early detection and treatment can be provided for those who test positive for the disease. Screenings that are recommended for many subgroups in a population include: routine mammograms for women over 40, a fecal occult blood test for everyone over 50, an amniocentesis to rule out a fetal anomaly for pregnant women over 35, because the incidence of breast cancer and colon cancer in these subgroups is higher than in the general population, as is the incidence of Down's syndrome in older mothers.

The testing of a person to rule out or confirm a suspected diagnosis because the patient has some sign or symptom is a diagnostic examination, not a screening. In these cases, the sign or symptom is used to explain the reason for the test.

A screening code may be a first listed code if the reason for the visit is specifically the screening exam. It may also be used as an additional code if the screening is done during an office visit for other health problems. A screening code is not necessary if the screening is inherent to a routine examination, such as a pap smear done during a routine pelvic examination.

Should a condition be discovered during the screening then the code for the condition may be assigned as an additional diagnosis.

The V code indicates that a screening exam is planned. A procedure code is required to confirm that the screening was performed.

The screening V code categories:

| V28 | Antenatal screening |
| V73-V82 | Special screening examinations |

EXAMPLE Screening for prostate cancer, V76.44 (Z12.5).

6) Observation

There are three observation V code categories. They are for use in very limited circumstances when a person is being observed for a suspected condition that is ruled out. The observation codes are not for use if an injury or illness or any signs or symptoms related to the suspected condition are present. In such cases the diagnosis/symptom code is used with the corresponding E code to identify any external cause.

The observation codes are to be used as principal diagnosis only. The only exception to this is when the principal diagnosis is required to be a code from the V30, Live born infant, category. Then the V29 observation code is sequenced after the V30 code. Additional codes may be used in addition to the observation code but only if they are unrelated to the suspected condition being observed.

Codes from subcategory V89.0, Suspected maternal and fetal conditions not found, may either be used as a first listed or as an additional code assignment depending on the case. They are for use in very limited circumstances on a maternal record when an encounter is for a suspected maternal or fetal condition that is ruled out during that encounter (for example, a maternal or fetal condition may be suspected due to an abnormal test result). These codes should not be used when the condition is confirmed. In those cases, the confirmed condition should be coded. In addition, these codes are not for use if an illness or any signs or symptoms related to the suspected condition or problem are present. In such cases the diagnosis/symptom code is used.

Additional codes may be used in addition to the code from subcategory V89.0, but only if they are unrelated to the suspected condition being evaluated.

Codes from subcategory V89.0 may not be used for encounters for antenatal screening of mother. *See Section I.C.18.d., Screening.*

For encounters for suspected fetal condition that are inconclusive following testing and evaluation, assign the appropriate code from category 655, 656, 657 or 658.

The observation V code categories:

V29   Observation and evaluation of newborns for suspected condition not found. For the birth encounter, a code from category V30 should be sequenced before the V29 code.

V71   Observation and evaluation for suspected condition not found

V89   Suspected maternal and fetal conditions not found

EXAMPLE

The driver of a car was admitted for observation after a rollover on the highway, V71.4, E816.0, E849.5 (Z04.1, V48.0xxA, Y92.411).

7) Aftercare

Aftercare visit codes cover situations when the initial treatment of a disease or injury has been performed and the patient requires continued care during the healing or recovery phase, or for the long-term consequences of the disease. The aftercare V code should not be used if treatment is directed at a current, acute disease or injury. The diagnosis code is to be used in these cases. Exceptions to this rule are codes V58.0, Radiotherapy, and codes from subcategory V58.1, Encounter for chemotherapy and immunotherapy for neoplastic conditions. These codes are to be first listed, followed by the diagnosis code when a patient's encounter is solely to receive radiation therapy or chemotherapy for the treatment of a neoplasm. Should a patient receive both chemotherapy and radiation therapy during the same encounter code V58.0 and V58.1 may be used together on a record with either one being sequenced first.

The aftercare codes are generally first listed to explain the specific reason for the encounter. An aftercare code may be used as an additional code when some type of aftercare is provided in addition to the reason for admission and no diagnosis code is applicable. An example of this would be the closure of a colostomy during an encounter for treatment of another condition.

Aftercare codes should be used in conjunction with any other aftercare codes or other diagnosis codes to provide better detail on the specifics of an aftercare encounter visit, unless otherwise directed by the classification. The sequencing of multiple aftercare codes is discretionary.

Certain aftercare V code categories need a secondary diagnosis code to describe the resolving condition or sequelae, for others, the condition is inherent in the code title.

Additional V code aftercare category terms include, fitting and adjustment, and attention to artificial openings.

Status V codes may be used with aftercare V codes to indicate the nature of the aftercare. For example code V45.81, Aortocoronary bypass status, may be used with code V58.73, Aftercare following surgery of the circulatory system, NEC, to indicate the surgery for which the aftercare is being performed. Also, a transplant status code may be used following code V58.44, Aftercare following organ transplant, to identify the organ transplanted. A status code should not be used when the aftercare code indicates the type of status, such as using V55.0, Attention to tracheostomy with V44.0, Tracheostomy status.

See Section I. B.16 Admissions/Encounter for Rehabilitation.

The aftercare V category/codes:

V51.0	Encounter for breast reconstruction following mastectomy
V52	Fitting and adjustment of prosthetic device and implant
V53	Fitting and adjustment of other device
V54	Other orthopedic aftercare
V55	Attention to artificial openings
V56	Encounter for dialysis and dialysis catheter care
V57	Care involving the use of rehabilitation procedures
V58.0	Radiotherapy
V58.11	Encounter for antineoplastic chemotherapy
V58.12	Encounter for antineoplastic immunotherapy
V58.3x	Attention to dressings and sutures
V58.41	Encounter for planned postoperative wound closure
V58.42	Aftercare, surgery, neoplasm
V58.43	Aftercare, surgery, trauma
V58.44	Aftercare involving organ transplant
V58.49	Other specified aftercare following surgery
V58.7x	Aftercare following surgery
V58.81	Fitting and adjustment of vascular catheter
V58.82	Fitting and adjustment of nonvascular catheter
V58.83	Monitoring therapeutic drug
V58.89	Other specified aftercare

EXAMPLE A patient was admitted for takedown of a colostomy placed 3 months ago for diverticular disease. The descending colon was anastomosed to the rectum. Patient still has diverticulosis, V55.3, 562.10, 46.52 (Z43.3, K57.90, 0DQM0ZZ, 0WQFXZ2).

8) Follow-up

The follow-up codes are used to explain continuing surveillance following completed treatment of a disease, condition, or injury. They imply that the condition has been fully treated and no longer exists. They should not be confused with aftercare codes that explain current treatment for a healing condition or its sequelae. Follow-up codes may be used in conjunction with history codes to provide the full picture of the healed condition and its treatment. The follow-up code is sequenced first, followed by the history code.

A follow-up code may be used to explain repeated visits. Should a condition be found to have recurred on the follow-up visit, then the diagnosis code should be used in place of the follow-up code.

The follow-up V code categories:

V24	Postpartum care and evaluation
V67	Follow-up examination

EXAMPLE Routine postpartum follow-up at 6 weeks. No problems or medical issues, V24.2 (Z39.2).

9) Donor

Category V59 is the donor codes. They are used for living individuals who are donating blood or other body tissue. These codes are only for individuals donating for others, not for self donations. They are not for use to identify cadaveric donations.

EXAMPLE Patient is donating a kidney. A left laparoscopic nephrectomy was performed, V59.4, 55.51 (Z52.4, 0TT14ZZ).

10) Counseling

Counseling V codes are used when a patient or family member receives assistance in the aftermath of an illness or injury, or when support is required in coping with family or social problems. They are not necessary for use in conjunction with a diagnosis code when the counseling component of care is considered integral to standard treatment.

The counseling V categories/codes:

V25.0	General counseling and advice for contraceptive management
V26.3	Genetic counseling
V26.4	General counseling and advice for procreative management
V61	Other family circumstances
V65.1	Person consulted on behalf of another person
V65.3	Dietary surveillance and counseling
V65.4	Other counseling, not elsewhere classified

EXAMPLE Dietary counseling for diabetic diet, V65.3, 250.00 (Z71.3, E11.9).

11) Obstetrics and related conditions

See Section I.C.11., the Obstetrics guidelines for further instruction on the use of these codes.

V codes for pregnancy are for use in those circumstances when none of the problems or complications included in the codes from the Obstetrics chapter exist (a routine prenatal visit or postpartum care). Codes V22.0, Supervision of normal first pregnancy, and V22.1, Supervision of other normal pregnancy, are always first listed and are not to be used with any other code from the OB chapter.

The outcome of delivery, category V27, should be included on all maternal delivery records. It is always a secondary code.

V codes for family planning (contraceptive) or procreative management and counseling should be included on an obstetric record either during the pregnancy or the postpartum stage, if applicable.

Obstetrics and related conditions V code categories:

V22	Normal pregnancy
V23	Supervision of high-risk pregnancy
	Except: V23.2, Pregnancy with history of abortion. Code 646.3, **Recurrent pregnancy loss**, from the OB chapter is required to indicate a history of abortion during a pregnancy.
V24	Postpartum care and evaluation
V25	Encounter for contraceptive management
	Except V25.0x
	(See Section I.C.18.d.11, Counseling)
V26	Procreative management
	Except V26.5x, Sterilization status, V26.3 and V26.4
	(See Section I.C.18.d.11., Counseling)
V27	Outcome of delivery
V28	Antenatal screening
	(See Section I.C.18.d.6., Screening)
V91	**Multiple gestation placenta status**

EXAMPLE Vaginal delivery of a single female infant with no complications, 650, V27.0, 73.59 (O80, Z37.0, 10E0XZZ).

12) Newborn, infant and child
See Section I.C.15, the Newborn guidelines for further instruction on the use of these codes.
Newborn V code categories:

V20	Health supervision of infant or child
V29	Observation and evaluation of newborns for suspected condition not found *(See Section I.C.18.d.7, Observation)*
V30-V39	Liveborn infant according to type of birth

EXAMPLE Single liveborn female infant born via vaginal delivery, V30.00 (Z38.00).

13) Routine and administrative examinations
The V codes allow for the description of encounters for routine examinations, such as, a general check-up, or, examinations for administrative purposes, such as, a preemployment physical. The codes are not to be used if the examination is for diagnosis of a suspected condition or for treatment purposes. In such cases the diagnosis code is used. During a routine exam, should a diagnosis or condition be discovered, it should be coded as an additional code. Preexisting and chronic conditions and history codes may also be included as additional codes as long as the examination is for administrative purposes and not focused on any particular condition.

Pre-operative examination V codes are for use only in those situations when a patient is being cleared for surgery and no treatment is given.

The V codes categories/code for routine and administrative examinations:

V20.2	Routine infant or child health check Any injections given should have a corresponding procedure code.
V70	General medical examination
V72	Special investigations and examinations

Codes V72.5 and V72.6 may be used if the reason for the patient encounter is for routine laboratory/radiology testing in the absence of any signs, symptoms, or associated diagnosis. If routine testing is performed during the same encounter as a test to evaluate a sign, symptom, or diagnosis, it is appropriate to assign both the V code and the code describing the reason for the non-routine test.

EXAMPLE Preoperative examination for respiratory clearance for surgery. The patient has emphysema and is scheduled for cholecystectomy for cholelithiasis, V72.82, 492.8, 574.20 (Z01.811, J43.9, K80.20).

14) Miscellaneous V codes
The miscellaneous V codes capture a number of other healthcare encounters that do not fall into one of the other categories. Certain of these codes identify the reason for the encounter, others are for use as additional codes that provide useful information on circumstances that may affect a patient's care and treatment.
Prophylactic Organ Removal
For encounters specifically for prophylactic removal of breasts, ovaries, or another organ due to a genetic susceptibility to cancer or a family history of cancer, the principal or first listed code should be a code from subcategory V50.4, Prophylactic organ removal, followed by the appropriate genetic susceptibility code and the appropriate family history code.

If the patient has a malignancy of one site and is having prophylactic removal at another site to prevent either a new primary malignancy or metastatic disease, a code for the malignancy should also be assigned in addition to a code from subcategory V50.4. A V50.4 code should not be assigned if the patient is having organ removal for treatment of a malignancy, such as the removal of the testes for the treatment of prostate cancer.

Miscellaneous V code categories/codes:

V07	Need for isolation and other prophylactic **or treatment** measures Except V07.5X, **Use** of agents affecting estrogen receptors and estrogen levels
V50	Elective surgery for purposes other than remedying health states
V58.5	Orthodontics
V60	Housing, household, and economic circumstances
V62	Other psychosocial circumstances
V63	Unavailability of other medical facilities for care
V64	Persons encountering health services for specific procedures, not carried out
V66	Convalescence and Palliative Care
V68	Encounters for administrative purposes
V69	Problems related to lifestyle
V85	Body Mass Index

EXAMPLE   A patient was admitted for cosmetic surgery (bilateral silicone breast implants), V50.1, 85.54 (Z41.1, 0HOV0JZ).

15) Nonspecific V codes

Certain V codes are so non-specific, or potentially redundant with other codes in the classification, that there can be little justification for their use in the inpatient setting. Their use in the outpatient setting should be limited to those instances when there is no further documentation to permit more precise coding. Otherwise, any sign or symptom or any other reason for visit that is captured in another code should be used.

Nonspecific V code categories/codes:

V11	Personal history of mental disorder A code from the mental disorders chapter, with an in remission fifth-digit, should be used.
V13.4	Personal history of arthritis
V13.6	Personal history of congenital malformations
V15.7	Personal history of contraception
V23.2	Pregnancy with history of abortion
V40	Mental and behavioral problems
V41	Problems with special senses and other special functions
V47	Other problems with internal organs
V48	Problems with head, neck, and trunk
V49	Problems with limbs and other problems
Exceptions:	
V49.6	Upper limb amputation status
V49.7	Lower limb amputation status
V49.81	**Asymptomatic postmenopausal status (age-related) (natural)**
V49.82	Dental sealant status
V49.83	Awaiting organ transplant status
V49.86	**Do not resuscitate status**
V49.87	**Physical restraints status**
V51.8	Other aftercare involving the use of plastic surgery
V58.2	Blood transfusion, without reported diagnosis
V58.9	Unspecified aftercare
	See Section IV.K. and Section IV.L. of the Outpatient guidelines.

e. V Codes That May Only be Principal/First-Listed Diagnosis

The list of V codes/categories below may only be reported as the principal/first-listed diagnosis, except when there are multiple encounters on the same day and the medical records for the encounters are combined or when there is more than one V code that meets the definition of principal diagnosis (e.g., a patient is admitted to home healthcare for both aftercare and rehabilitation and they equally meet the definition of principal diagnosis). These codes should not be reported if they do not meet the definition of principal or first-listed diagnosis.

See Section II and Section IV.A for information on selection of principal and first-listed diagnosis.

See Section II.C for information on two or more diagnoses that equally meet the definition for principal diagnosis.

V20.X	Health supervision of infant or child
V22.0	Supervision of normal first pregnancy
V22.1	Supervision of other normal pregnancy
V24.X	Postpartum care and examination
V26.81	Encounter for assisted reproductive fertility procedure cycle
V26.82	Encounter for fertility preservation procedure
V30.X	Single liveborn
V31.X	Twin, mate liveborn
V32.X	Twin, mate stillborn
V33.X	Twin, unspecified
V34.X	Other multiple, mates all liveborn
V35.X	Other multiple, mates all stillborn
V36.X	Other multiple, mates live- and stillborn
V37.X	Other multiple, unspecified
V39.X	Unspecified
V46.12	Encounter for respirator dependence during power failure
V46.13	Encounter for weaning from respirator [ventilator]
V51.0	Encounter for breast reconstruction following mastectomy
V56.0	Extracorporeal dialysis
V57.X	Care involving use of rehabilitation procedures
V58.0	Radiotherapy
V58.11	Encounter for antineoplastic chemotherapy
V58.12	Encounter for antineoplastic immunotherapy
V59.X	Donors
V66.0	Convalescence and palliative care following surgery
V66.1	Convalescence and palliative care following radiotherapy
V66.2	Convalescence and palliative care following chemotherapy
V66.3	Convalescence and palliative care following psychotherapy and other treatment for mental disorder
V66.4	Convalescence and palliative care following treatment of fracture
V66.5	Convalescence and palliative care following other treatment
V66.6	Convalescence and palliative care following combined treatment
V66.9	Unspecified convalescence
V68.X	Encounters for administrative purposes
V70.0	Routine general medical examination at a health care facility
V70.1	General psychiatric examination, requested by the authority
V70.2	General psychiatric examination, other and unspecified
V70.3	Other medical examination for administrative purposes
V70.4	Examination for medicolegal reasons
V70.5	Health examination of defined subpopulations
V70.6	Health examination in population surveys
V70.8	Other specified general medical examinations
V70.9	Unspecified general medical examination
V71.X	Observation and evaluation for suspected conditions not found

EXAMPLE Single liveborn infant delivered vaginally, V30.00 (Z38.00)

21. **Chapter 21: Factors influencing health status and contact with health services (Z00-Z99)**
    Note: The chapter specific guidelines provide additional information about the use of Z codes for specified encounters.
    a. **Use of Z codes in any healthcare setting**
       Z codes are for use in any healthcare setting. Z codes may be used as either a **first-listed** (principal diagnosis code in the inpatient setting) or secondary code, depending on the circumstances of the encounter. Certain Z codes may only be used as **first-listed** or principal diagnosis.
    b. **Z Codes indicate a reason for an encounter**
       Z codes are not procedure codes. A corresponding procedure code must accompany a Z code to describe **any** procedure performed.
    c. **Categories of Z Codes**
       1) **Contact/Exposure**
          Category Z20 indicates contact with, and suspected exposure to, communicable diseases. These codes are for patients who do not show any sign or symptom of a disease but are suspected to have been exposed to it by close personal contact with an infected individual or are in an area where a disease is epidemic.
          Category Z77, indicates contact with and suspected exposures hazardous to health.
          Contact/exposure codes may be used as a **first-listed** code to explain an encounter for testing, or, more commonly, as a secondary code to identify a potential risk.
       2) **Inoculations and vaccinations**
          Code Z23 is for encounters for inoculations and vaccinations. It indicates that a patient is being seen to receive a prophylactic inoculation against a disease. Procedure codes are required to identify the actual administration of the injection and the type(s) of immunizations given. Code Z23 may be used as a secondary code if the inoculation is given as a routine part of preventive health care, such as a well-baby visit.
       3) **Status**
          Status codes indicate that a patient is either a carrier of a disease or has the sequelae or residual of a past disease or condition. This includes such things as the presence of prosthetic or mechanical devices resulting from past treatment. A status code is informative, because the status may affect the course of treatment and its outcome. A status code is distinct from a history code. The history code indicates that the patient no longer has the condition.
          A status code should not be used with a diagnosis code from one of the body system chapters, if the diagnosis code includes the information provided by the status code. For example, code Z94.1, Heart transplant status, should not be used with a code from subcategory T86.2, Complications of heart transplant. The status code does not provide additional information. The complication code indicates that the patient is a heart transplant patient.
          For encounters for weaning from a mechanical ventilator, assign **a code from subcategory** J96.1, Chronic respiratory failure, followed by code Z99.11, Dependence on respirator [ventilator] status.

The status Z codes/categories are:

Z14	Genetic carrier

Genetic carrier status indicates that a person carries a gene, associated with a particular disease, which may be passed to offspring who may develop that disease. The person does not have the disease and is not at risk of developing the disease.

Z15	Genetic susceptibility to disease

Genetic susceptibility indicates that a person has a gene that increases the risk of that person developing the disease.

Codes from category Z15 should not be used as principal or first-listed codes. If the patient has the condition to which he/she is susceptible, and that condition is the reason for the encounter, the code for the current condition should be sequenced first. If the patient is being seen for follow-up after completed treatment for this condition, and the condition no longer exists, a follow-up code should be sequenced first, followed by the appropriate personal history and genetic susceptibility codes. If the purpose of the encounter is genetic counseling associated with procreative management, code Z31.5, Encounter for genetic counseling, should be assigned as the first-listed code, followed by a code from category Z15. Additional codes should be assigned for any applicable family or personal history.

Z16	Infection with drug-resistant microorganisms

This code indicates that a patient has an infection that is resistant to drug treatment. Sequence the infection code first.

Z17	Estrogen receptor status
Z18	**Retained foreign body fragments**
Z21	Asymptomatic HIV infection status

This code indicates that a patient has tested positive for HIV but has manifested no signs or symptoms of the disease.

Z22	Carrier of infectious disease

Carrier status indicates that a person harbors the specific organisms of a disease without manifest symptoms and is capable of transmitting the infection.

Z28.3	Underimmunization status
Z33.1	Pregnant state, incidental

This code is a secondary code only for use when the pregnancy is in no way complicating the reason for visit. Otherwise, a code from the obstetric chapter is required.

Z66	Do not resuscitate

This code may be used when it is documented by the provider that a patient is on do not resuscitate status at any time during the stay.

Z67	Blood type
Z68	Body mass index (BMI)
Z74.01	Bed confinement status
Z76.82	Awaiting organ transplant status
Z78	Other specified health status

Code Z78.1, Physical restraint status, may be used when it is documented by the provider that a patient has been put in restraints during the current encounter. Please note that this code should not be reported when it is documented by the provider that a patient is temporarily restrained during a procedure.

Z79	Long-term (current) drug therapy

Codes from this category indicate a patient's continuous use of a prescribed drug (including such things as aspirin therapy) for the long-term treatment of a condition or for prophylactic use. It is not for use for patients who have addictions to drugs. This subcategory is not for use of medications for detoxification or maintenance programs to prevent withdrawal symptoms in patients with drug dependence (e.g., methadone maintenance for opiate dependence). Assign the appropriate code for the drug dependence instead.

Assign a code from Z79 if the patient is receiving a medication for an extended period as a prophylactic measure (such as for the prevention of deep vein thrombosis) or as treatment of a chronic condition (such as arthritis) or a disease requiring a lengthy course of treatment (such as cancer). Do not assign a code from category Z79 for medication being administered for a brief period of time to treat an acute illness or injury (such as a course of antibiotics to treat acute bronchitis).

Z88	Allergy status to drugs, medicaments and biological substances

Except: Z88.9, Allergy status to unspecified drugs, medicaments and biological substances status

Z89	Acquired absence of limb
Z90	Acquired absence of organs, not elsewhere classified
Z91.0-	Allergy status, other than to drugs and biological substances
Z92.82	Status post administration of tPA (rtPA) in a different facility within the last 24 hours prior to admission to a current facility

Assign code Z92.82, Status post administration of tPA (rtPA) in a different facility within the last 24 hours prior to admission to current facility, as a secondary diagnosis when a patient is received by transfer into a facility and documentation indicates they were administered tissue plasminogen activator (tPA) within the last 24 hours prior to admission to the current facility.

This guideline applies even if the patient is still receiving the tPA at the time they are received into the current facility.

The appropriate code for the condition for which the tPA was administered (such as cerebrovascular disease or myocardial infarction) should be assigned first.

Code Z92.82 is only applicable to the receiving facility record and not to the transferring facility record.

Z93	Artificial opening status
Z94	Transplanted organ and tissue status
Z95	Presence of cardiac and vascular implants and grafts
Z96	Presence of other functional implants
Z97	Presence of other devices
Z98	Other postprocedural states

Assign code Z98.85, Transplanted organ removal status, to indicate that a transplanted organ has been previously removed. This code should not be assigned for the encounter in which the transplanted organ is removed. The complication necessitating removal of the transplant organ should be assigned for that encounter.

See section IC19.g.3. for information on the coding of organ transplant complications.

Z99	Dependence on enabling machines and devices, not elsewhere classified

Note: Categories Z89-Z90 and Z93-Z99 are for use only if there are no complications or malfunctions of the organ or tissue replaced, the amputation site or the equipment on which the patient is dependent.

4) History (of)

There are two types of history Z codes, personal and family. Personal history codes explain a patient's past medical condition that no longer exists and is not receiving any treatment, but that has the potential for recurrence, and therefore may require continued monitoring.

Family history codes are for use when a patient has a family member(s) who has had a particular disease that causes the patient to be at higher risk of also contracting the disease.

Personal history codes may be used in conjunction with follow-up codes and family history codes may be used in conjunction with screening codes to explain the need for a test or procedure. History codes are also acceptable on any medical record regardless of the reason for visit. A history of an illness, even if no longer present, is important information that may alter the type of treatment ordered.

The history Z code categories are:

Z80	Family history of primary malignant neoplasm
Z81	Family history of mental and behavioral disorders
Z82	Family history of certain disabilities and chronic diseases (leading to disablement)
Z83	Family history of other specific disorders
Z84	Family history of other conditions
Z85	Personal history of malignant neoplasm
Z86	Personal history of certain other diseases
Z87	Personal history of other diseases and conditions
Z91.4-	Personal history of psychological trauma, not elsewhere classified
Z91.5	Personal history of self-harm
Z91.8-	Other specified personal risk factors, not elsewhere classified
Z92	Personal history of medical treatment
	Except: Z92.0, Personal history of contraception
	Except: Z92.82, Status post administration of tPA (rtPA) in a different facility within the last 24 hours prior to admission to a current facility

5) Screening

Screening is the testing for disease or disease precursors in seemingly well individuals so that early detection and treatment can be provided for those who test positive for the disease (e.g., screening mammogram).

The testing of a person to rule out or confirm a suspected diagnosis because the patient has some sign or symptom is a diagnostic examination, not a screening. In these cases, the sign or symptom is used to explain the reason for the test.

A screening code may be a **first-listed** code if the reason for the visit is specifically the screening exam. It may also be used as an additional code if the screening is done during an office visit for other health problems. A screening code is not necessary if the screening is inherent to a routine examination, such as a pap smear done during a routine pelvic examination.

Should a condition be discovered during the screening then the code for the condition may be assigned as an additional diagnosis.

The Z code indicates that a screening exam is planned. A procedure code is required to confirm that the screening was performed.

The screening Z codes/categories:

Z11	Encounter for screening for infectious and parasitic diseases
Z12	Encounter for screening for malignant neoplasms
Z13	Encounter for screening for other diseases and disorders
	Except: Z13.9, Encounter for screening, unspecified
Z36	Encounter for antenatal screening for mother

6) Observation

There are two observation Z code categories. They are for use in very limited circumstances when a person is being observed for a suspected condition that is ruled out. The observation codes are not for use if an injury or illness or any signs or symptoms related to the suspected condition are present. In such cases the diagnosis/symptom code is used with the corresponding external cause code.

The observation codes are to be used as principal diagnosis only. Additional codes may be used in addition to the observation code but only if they are unrelated to the suspected condition being observed.

Codes from subcategory Z03.7 Encounter for suspected maternal and fetal conditions ruled out, may either be used as a **first-listed** or as an additional code assignment depending on the case. They are for use in very limited circumstances on a maternal record when an encounter is for a suspected maternal or fetal condition that is ruled out during that encounter (for example, a maternal or fetal condition may be suspected due to an abnormal test result). These codes should not be used when the condition is confirmed. In those cases, the confirmed condition should be coded. In addition, these codes are not for use if an illness or any signs or symptoms related to the suspected condition or problem are present. In such cases the diagnosis/symptom code is used.

Additional codes may be used in addition to the code from subcategory Z03.7, but only if they are unrelated to the suspected condition being evaluated.

Codes from subcategory Z03.7 may not be used for encounters for antenatal screening of mother. *See Section I.C.21.c.5, Screening.*

For encounters for suspected fetal condition that are inconclusive following testing and evaluation, assign the appropriate code from category O35, O36, O40 or O41.

The observation Z code categories:

Z03	Encounter for medical observation for suspected diseases and conditions ruled out
Z04	Encounter for examination and observation for other reasons Except: Z04.9, Encounter for examination and observation for unspecified reason

7) Aftercare

Aftercare visit codes cover situations when the initial treatment of a disease has been performed and the patient requires continued care during the healing or recovery phase, or for the long-term consequences of the disease. The aftercare Z code should not be used if treatment is directed at a current, acute disease. The diagnosis code is to be used in these cases. Exceptions to this rule are codes Z51.0, Encounter for antineoplastic radiation therapy, and codes from subcategory Z51.1, Encounter for antineoplastic chemotherapy and immunotherapy. These codes are to be **first-listed**, followed by the diagnosis code when a patient's encounter is solely to receive radiation therapy, chemotherapy, or immunotherapy for the treatment of a neoplasm. If the reason for the encounter is more than one type of antineoplastic therapy, code Z51.0 and a code from subcategory Z51.1 may be assigned together, in which case one of these codes would be reported as a secondary diagnosis.

The aftercare Z codes should also not be used for aftercare for injuries. For aftercare of an injury, assign the acute injury code with the **appropriate** 7th character (**for** subsequent encounter).

The aftercare codes are generally **first-listed** to explain the specific reason for the encounter. An aftercare code may be used as an additional code when some type of aftercare is provided in addition to the reason for admission and no diagnosis code is applicable. An example of this would be the closure of a colostomy during an encounter for treatment of another condition.

Aftercare codes should be used in conjunction with other aftercare codes or diagnosis codes to provide better detail on the specifics of an aftercare encounter visit, unless otherwise directed by the classification. Should a patient receive multiple types of antineoplastic therapy during the same encounter, code Z51.0, Encounter for antineoplastic radiation therapy, and codes from subcategory Z51.1, Encounter for antineoplastic chemotherapy and immunotherapy, may be used together on a record. The sequencing of multiple aftercare codes depends on the circumstances of the encounter.

Certain aftercare Z code categories need a secondary diagnosis code to describe the resolving condition or sequelae. For others, the condition is included in the code title.

Additional Z code aftercare category terms include fitting and adjustment, and attention to artificial openings.

Status Z codes may be used with aftercare Z codes to indicate the nature of the aftercare. For example code Z95.1, Presence of aortocoronary bypass graft, may be used with code Z48.812, Encounter for surgical aftercare following surgery on the circulatory system, to indicate the surgery for which the aftercare is being performed. A status code should not be used when the aftercare code indicates the type of status, such as using Z43.0, Encounter for attention to tracheostomy, with Z93.0, Tracheostomy status.

The aftercare Z category/codes:

Z42	Encounter for plastic and reconstructive surgery following medical procedure or healed injury
Z43	Encounter for attention to artificial openings
Z44	Encounter for fitting and adjustment of external prosthetic device
Z45	Encounter for adjustment and management of implanted device
Z46	Encounter for fitting and adjustment of other devices
Z47	Orthopedic aftercare
Z48	Encounter for other postprocedural aftercare
Z49	Encounter for care involving renal dialysis
Z51	Encounter for other aftercare

8) Follow-up

The follow-up codes are used to explain continuing surveillance following completed treatment of a disease, condition, or injury. They imply that the condition has been fully treated and no longer exists. They should not be confused with aftercare codes, or injury codes with a 7th character **for subsequent encounter**, that explain ongoing care of a healing condition or its sequelae. Follow-up codes may be used in conjunction with history codes to provide the full picture of the healed condition and its treatment. The follow-up code is sequenced first, followed by the history code.

A follow-up code may be used to explain multiple visits. Should a condition be found to have recurred on the follow-up visit, then the **diagnosis** code for the condition should be assigned **in place of the follow-up code**.

The follow-up Z code categories:

Z08	Encounter for follow-up examination after completed treatment for malignant neoplasm
Z09	Encounter for follow-up examination after completed treatment for conditions other than malignant neoplasm
Z39	Encounter for maternal postpartum care and examination

9) Donor

Codes in category Z52, Donors of organs and tissues, are used for living individuals who are donating blood or other body tissue. These codes are only for individuals donating for others, not for self-donations. They are not used to identify cadaveric donations.

10) Counseling

Counseling Z codes are used when a patient or family member receives assistance in the aftermath of an illness or injury, or when support is required in coping with family or social problems. They are not used in conjunction with a diagnosis code when the counseling component of care is considered integral to standard treatment.

The counseling Z codes/categories:

Z30.0-	Encounter for general counseling and advice on contraception
Z31.5	Encounter for genetic counseling
Z31.6-	Encounter for general counseling and advice on procreation
Z32.2	Encounter for childbirth instruction
Z32.3	Encounter for childcare instruction
Z69	Encounter for mental health services for victim and perpetrator of abuse
Z70	Counseling related to sexual attitude, behavior and orientation
Z71	Persons encountering health services for other counseling and medical advice, not elsewhere classified
Z76.81	Expectant mother prebirth pediatrician visit

11) Encounters for Obstetrical and Reproductive Services

See Section I.C.15. Pregnancy, Childbirth, and the Puerperium, for further instruction on the use of these codes.

Z codes for pregnancy are for use in those circumstances when none of the problems or complications included in the codes from the Obstetrics chapter exist (a routine prenatal visit or postpartum care). Codes in category Z34, Encounter for supervision of normal pregnancy, are always **first-listed** and are not to be used with any other code from the OB chapter.

The outcome of delivery, category Z37, should be included on all maternal delivery records. It is always a secondary code. Codes in category Z37 should not be used on the newborn record.

Z codes for family planning (contraceptive) or procreative management and counseling should be included on an obstetric record either during the pregnancy or the postpartum stage, if applicable.

Z codes/categories for obstetrical and reproductive services:

Z30	Encounter for contraceptive management
Z31	Encounter for procreative management
Z32.2	Encounter for childbirth instruction
Z32.3	Encounter for childcare instruction
Z33	Pregnant state
Z34	Encounter for supervision of normal pregnancy
Z36	Encounter for antenatal screening of mother
Z37	Outcome of delivery
Z39	Encounter for maternal postpartum care and examination
Z76.81	Expectant mother prebirth pediatrician visit

12) Newborns and Infants

See Section I.C.16. Newborn (Perinatal) Guidelines, for further instruction on the use of these codes.

Newborn Z codes/categories:

Z76.1	Encounter for health supervision and care of foundling
Z00.1-	Encounter for routine child health examination
Z38	Liveborn infants according to place of birth and type of delivery

13) Routine and administrative examinations

The Z codes allow for the description of encounters for routine examinations, such as, a general check-up, or, examinations for administrative purposes, such as, a pre-employment physical. The codes are not to be used if the examination is for diagnosis of a suspected condition or for treatment purposes. In such cases the diagnosis code is used. During a routine exam, should a diagnosis or condition be discovered, it should be coded as an additional code. Pre-existing and chronic conditions and history codes may also be included as additional codes as long as the examination is for administrative purposes and not focused on any particular condition.

Some of the codes for routine health examinations distinguish between "with" and "without" abnormal findings. Code assignment depends on the information that is known at the time the encounter is being coded. For example, if no abnormal findings were found during the examination, but the encounter is being coded before test results are back, it is acceptable to assign the code for "without abnormal findings." When assigning a code for "with abnormal findings," additional code(s) should be assigned to identify the specific abnormal finding(s).

Pre-operative examination and pre-procedural laboratory examination Z codes are for use only in those situations when a patient is being cleared for a procedure or surgery and no treatment is given.

The Z codes/categories for routine and administrative examinations:

Z00	Encounter for general examination without complaint, suspected or reported diagnosis
Z01	Encounter for other special examination without complaint, suspected or reported diagnosis
Z02	Encounter for administrative examination
	Except: Z02.9, Encounter for administrative examinations, unspecified
Z32.0-	Encounter for pregnancy test

14) Miscellaneous Z codes

The miscellaneous Z codes capture a number of other health care encounters that do not fall into one of the other categories. Certain of these codes identify the reason for the encounter; others are for use as additional codes that provide useful information on circumstances that may affect a patient's care and treatment.

Prophylactic Organ Removal

For encounters specifically for prophylactic removal of an organ (such as prophylactic removal of breasts due to a genetic susceptibility to cancer or a family history of cancer), the principal or **first-listed** code should be a code from category Z40, Encounter for prophylactic surgery, followed by the appropriate codes to identify the associated risk factor (such as genetic susceptibility or family history).

If the patient has a malignancy of one site and is having prophylactic removal at another site to prevent either a new primary malignancy or metastatic disease, a code for the malignancy should also be assigned in addition to a code from subcategory Z40.0, Encounter for prophylactic surgery for risk factors related to malignant neoplasms. A Z40.0 code should not be assigned if the patient is having organ removal for treatment of a malignancy, such as the removal of the testes for the treatment of prostate cancer.

Miscellaneous Z codes/categories:

Z28	Immunization not carried out
	Except: Z28.3, Underimmunization status
Z40	Encounter for prophylactic surgery
Z41	Encounter for procedures for purposes other than remedying health state
	Except: Z41.9, Encounter for procedure for purposes other than remedying health state, unspecified
Z53	Persons encountering health services for specific procedures and treatment, not carried out
Z55	Problems related to education and literacy
Z56	Problems related to employment and unemployment
Z57	Occupational exposure to risk factors
Z58	Problems related to physical environment
Z59	Problems related to housing and economic circumstances
Z60	Problems related to social environment
Z62	Problems related to upbringing
Z63	Other problems related to primary support group, including family circumstances
Z64	Problems related to certain psychosocial circumstances
Z65	Problems related to other psychosocial circumstances
Z72	Problems related to lifestyle
Z73	Problems related to life management difficulty
Z74	Problems related to care provider dependency
	Except: Z74.01, Bed confinement status
Z75	Problems related to medical facilities and other health care
Z76.0	Encounter for issue of repeat prescription
Z76.3	Healthy person accompanying sick person
Z76.4	Other boarder to healthcare facility
Z76.5	Malingerer [conscious simulation]
Z91.1-	Patient's noncompliance with medical treatment and regimen
Z91.89	Other specified personal risk factors, not elsewhere classified

15) Nonspecific Z codes

Certain Z codes are so non-specific, or potentially redundant with other codes in the classification, that there can be little justification for their use in the inpatient setting. Their use in the outpatient setting should be limited to those instances when there is no further documentation to permit more precise coding. Otherwise, any sign or symptom or any other reason for visit that is captured in another code should be used.

Nonspecific Z codes/categories:

Z02.9	Encounter for administrative examinations, unspecified
Z04.9	Encounter for examination and observation for unspecified reason
Z13.9	Encounter for screening, unspecified
Z41.9	Encounter for procedure for purposes other than remedying health state, unspecified
Z52.9	Donor of unspecified organ or tissue
Z86.59	**Personal history of other mental and behavioral disorders**
Z88.9	Allergy status to unspecified drugs, medicaments and biological substances status
Z92.0	Personal history of contraception

16) Z Codes That May Only be Principal/First-Listed Diagnosis

The following Z codes/categories may only be reported as the principal/first-listed diagnosis, except when there are multiple encounters on the same day and the medical records for the encounters are combined:

Z00	Encounter for general examination without complaint, suspected or reported diagnosis
Z01	Encounter for other special examination without complaint, suspected or reported diagnosis
Z02	Encounter for administrative examination
Z03	Encounter for medical observation for suspected diseases and conditions ruled out
Z04	**Encounter for examination and observation for other reasons**
Z33.2	Encounter for elective termination of pregnancy
Z31.81	Encounter for male factor infertility in female patient
Z31.82	Encounter for Rh incompatibility status
Z31.83	Encounter for assisted reproductive fertility procedure cycle
Z31.84	Encounter for fertility preservation procedure
Z34	Encounter for supervision of normal pregnancy
Z39	Encounter for maternal postpartum care and examination
Z38	Liveborn infants according to place of birth and type of delivery
Z42	Encounter for plastic and reconstructive surgery following medical procedure or healed injury
Z51.0	Encounter for antineoplastic radiation therapy
Z51.1-	Encounter for antineoplastic chemotherapy and immunotherapy
Z52	Donors of organs and tissues
	Except: Z52.9, Donor of unspecified organ or tissue
Z76.1	Encounter for health supervision and care of foundling
Z76.2	Encounter for health supervision and care of other healthy infant and child
Z99.12	Encounter for respirator [ventilator] dependence during power failure

EXERCISE 8-4

Assign codes to the following conditions.

1. Patient receives long-term oxygen therapy for emphysema; patient has a history of tobacco abuse   _____

2. Dietary counseling for morbid obesity; body mass index (BMI) is 41   _____

3. Screening for prostate cancer; patient has no signs or symptoms   _____

4. Family history of ischemic heart disease   _____

5. Personal history of malaria   _____

6. History of urinary calculi   _____

7. Personal history of diabetes mellitus, type II; patient currently takes insulin for diabetes   _____

8. Awaiting liver transplant for end-stage liver disease   _____

9. Patient on Coumadin (anticoagulant) because of mechanical heart valve   _____

10. Patient is noncompliant with diet and medications   _____

Using the V code guideline for principal/first-listed diagnosis, select the correct answer.

11. V52.1 Fitting and adjustment of artificial leg
    A. First diagnosis only
    B. First and/or additional diagnosis

12. V51.0 Encounter for breast reconstruction following mastectomy
    A. First diagnosis only
    B. First and/or additional diagnosis

13. V50.2 Routine or ritual circumcision
    A. First diagnosis only
    B. First and/or additional diagnosis

14. V55.3 Attention to colostomy
    A. First diagnosis only
    B. First and/or additional diagnosis

15. V22.0 Supervision of normal first pregnancy
    A. First diagnosis only
    B. First and/or additional diagnosis

PROCEDURES

Procedures can be taken from any of the chapters in Volume 3. When a V/Z code is used as a diagnosis for a given procedure or a reason for the encounter, a procedure code is still necessary to identify that the procedure was performed. It can be confusing when a V/Z code seems to describe a procedure.

EXAMPLE | Patient was admitted for sterilization. A laparoscopic ligation of the fallopian tubes was performed, V25.2, 66.29 (Z30.2, 0UL74ZZ).

EXAMPLE | Patient is donating a kidney. A left laparoscopic nephrectomy was performed, V59.4, 55.51 (Z52.4, 0TT14ZZ).

Assign codes for all diagnoses and procedures.

1. Encounter for dialysis due to end-stage renal disease _____
2. Admission for chemotherapy (via central vein) for ovarian cancer _____
3. Admission for replacement of tracheostomy tube _____
4. Admission following delivery in ambulance _____
5. Encounter for removal of internal fixation device, right femoral shaft _____

DOCUMENTATION/REIMBURSEMENT/MS-DRGs

Often, coding difficulties are due to lack of documentation. Signs and symptoms are often not correlated with a definitive diagnosis in the health record. Sometimes, pathology and other test results are not available at the time of discharge, or when the physician is dictating the discharge summary or reporting the final diagnoses. As a general rule, MS-DRGs that are assigned and have a principal diagnosis from Chapter 16 may have lower reimbursement than an MS-DRG that has a principal diagnosis of a definitive condition or disease.

Frequently missed complications/comorbidities from this chapter include the following:
- Coma
- Shock
- Febrile convulsion
- Gangrene
- Hemoptysis
- Ascites, including malignant ascites
- Cachexia
- V codes for organ replacement/transplant
- Suicidal ideation
- BMI less than 19 or greater than 40 (adult)

Symptoms That Are Integral to a Disease Process

EXAMPLE Patient was admitted with chest pain due to costochondritis, 733.6.

DIAGNOSES	CODES	MS-DRG	RW
Costochondritis	733.6 (M94.0)	206	0.7575
Chest pain due to costochondritis	786.50, 733.6 (R07.9, M94.0)	313	0.5499

In this case, the symptom (chest pain) is due to a specific cause, and the chest pain is an integral part of costochondritis, so to assign a code for the chest pain would be incorrect, and would not be in accordance with the coding guidelines. The hospital would receive less reimbursement.

MS-DRG With and Without MCC/CC

EXAMPLE   Patient was admitted with abdominal pain. The patient has end-stage renal disease on dialysis. No cause was determined for the abdominal pain.

DIAGNOSES	CODES	MS-DRG	RW
Abd pain	789.00 (R10.9)	392	0.7173
Abd pain	789.00	391	1.1550
ESRD	585.6, V45.11 (R10.9, N18.6, Z99.2)		

In this case, the patient has a chronic condition of ESRD so it should be reported as a secondary diagnosis. No cause was determined for the patient's abdominal pain, so assignment of 789.00 (R10.9) symptom code is correct for the principal diagnosis. The hospital receives less reimbursement than it deserves if the 585.6 (N18.6) code for the comorbidity is not assigned.

CHAPTER REVIEW EXERCISE

Assign codes for all diagnoses and procedures.

1. Paresthesia _____
2. Abnormal Pap smear with high-grade squamous intraepithelial lesion (HGSIL) _____
3. History of cardiac arrest _____
4. Anasarca _____
5. Chest pain due to unstable angina _____
6. Adult failure to thrive _____
7. Insulin pump training for Type I diabetic _____
8. Complex febrile seizure _____
9. Cachexia _____
10. History of cleft palate that was corrected with surgical repair _____
11. Debility _____
12. Patient has a gastrostomy tube and receives tube feedings _____
13. Headache due to migraine _____
14. Absence of kidney due to surgical removal _____
15. History of falls _____
16. Fussy baby _____
17. Elevated blood pressure _____
18. Screening mammogram in a high-risk patient with family history of breast cancer _____
19. Anemia with drop in hematocrit _____
20. Elevated prostate-specific antigen (PSA) _____
21. Admission for elective circumcision _____
22. Occult blood in stool _____
23. Screening for bladder cancer in patient with gross hematuria _____
24. Renal colic due to kidney stone _____
25. Abnormal liver function tests _____
26. Changing of gastrostomy tube in patient with dysphagia _____
27. Diarrhea due to gastroenteritis _____
28. Vaccination for influenza _____
29. Patient has type I diabetes mellitus and has an insulin pump _____
30. Prophylactic removal of both ovaries due to strong family history of ovarian cancer and genetic susceptibility. A bilateral salpingo-oophorectomy was performed _____

CHAPTER GLOSSARY

Prophylactic: medication or treatment used to prevent a disease from occurring.

Screening examination: one that occurs in the absence of any signs or symptoms. It involves examination of an asymptomatic individual to detect a given disease, typically by means of an inexpensive diagnostic test.

Sign: objective evidence of a disease or of a patient's condition as perceived by the patient's examining physician.

Symptom: subjective evidence of a disease or of a patient's condition as perceived by the patient.

REFERENCE

1. American Hospital Association. *Coding Clinic for ICD-9-CM* 1990:2Q:p15-16. Abnormal findings—Guidelines.

9

Infectious and Parasitic Diseases

(ICD-9-CM Chapter 1, Codes 001-139, and ICD-10-CM Chapter 1, Codes A00-B99)

LEARNING OBJECTIVES

1. Apply and assign the correct ICD-9-CM and ICD-10-CM codes in accordance with Official Guidelines for Coding and Reporting

2. Identify major differences between ICD-9-CM and ICD-10-CM related to infectious and parasitic diseases

3. Recognize infectious and parasitic diseases

4. Assign the correct V codes and procedure codes related to infectious and parasitic diseases
5. Identify common treatments, medications, laboratory values, and diagnostic tests
6. Explain the importance of documentation as it relates to MS-DRGs for reimbursement

ABBREVIATIONS/ ACRONYMS

AIDS acquired immunodeficiency syndrome

C. DIFF Clostridium difficile

CD4 Cluster of differentiation 4

CDC Centers for Disease Control and Prevention

DMAC disseminated *Mycobacterium avium-intracellulare* complex

EGD esophogastroduodenoscopy

HAART highly active antiretroviral therapy

HIV human immunodeficiency virus

HIVAN HIV-associated nephropathy

HPV Human papilloma virus

HSV herpes simplex virus

ICD-9-CM *International Classification of Diseases, 9th Revision, Clinical Modification*

ICD-10-CM *International Classification of Diseases, 10th Revision, Clinical Modification*

ICD-10-PCS *International Classification of Diseases, 10th Revision, Procedure Coding System*

IVDU intravenous drug use

MAC *Mycobacterium avium-intracellulare* complex

MAI *Mycobacterium avium-intracellulare*

MRSA methicillin-resistant *Staphylococcus aureus*

MSSA methicillin-sensitive *Staphylococcus aureus*

RPR rapid plasma reagin

SARS severe acute respiratory syndrome

SIRS systemic inflammatory response syndrome

STD sexually transmitted disease

TB tuberculosis

UTI urinary tract infection

VDRL Venereal Disease Research Laboratory

VRE vancomycin-resistant enterococcus

ICD-9-CM

Official Guidelines for Coding and Reporting

Please refer to the companion Evolve website for the most current guidelines.

1. Chapter 1: Infectious and Parasitic Diseases (001-139)

    a. Human Immunodeficiency Virus (HIV) Infections

        1) Code only confirmed cases

            Code only confirmed cases of HIV infection/illness. This is an exception of the hospital inpatient guideline Section II, H.

            In this context, "confirmation" does not require documentation of positive serology or culture for HIV; the provider's diagnostic statement that the patient is HIV positive, or has an HIV-related illness is sufficient.

EXAMPLE

Patient with possible human immunodeficiency virus (HIV). Even though in the inpatient setting it is acceptable to code diagnoses that are possible or suspected, in the case of possible HIV, you would not assign 042. You would have to query the physician regarding the patient's exact HIV status. This is one of the only exceptions to coding a diagnosis as if it exists when it is documented as possible or probable.

        2) Selection and sequencing of HIV codes

           (a) Patient admitted for HIV-related condition

                If a patient is admitted for an HIV-related condition, the principal diagnosis should be 042, followed by additional diagnosis codes for all reported HIV-related conditions.

EXAMPLE

The patient was admitted for treatment of Kaposi's sarcoma of the skin. The patient's HIV has been symptomatic for the past year, 042, 176.0 (B20, C46.0).

(b) Patient with HIV disease admitted for unrelated condition

If a patient with HIV disease is admitted for an unrelated condition (such as a traumatic injury), the code for the unrelated condition (e.g., the nature of injury code) should be the principal diagnosis. Other diagnoses would be 042 followed by additional diagnosis codes for all reported HIV-related conditions.

EXAMPLE Initial encounter for traumatic closed-fracture of the left femur in a patient who has acquired immunodeficiency syndrome (AIDS), 821.00, 042, E887 (S72.92xA, B20, W58.xxxA).

(c) Whether the patient is newly diagnosed

Whether the patient is newly diagnosed or has had previous admissions/encounters for HIV conditions is irrelevant to the sequencing decision.

(d) Asymptomatic human immunodeficiency virus

V08 Asymptomatic human immunodeficiency virus [HIV] infection, is to be applied when the patient without any documentation of symptoms is listed as being "HIV positive," "known HIV," "HIV test positive," or similar terminology. Do not use this code if the term "AIDS" is used or if the patient is treated for any HIV-related illness or is described as having any condition(s) resulting from his/her HIV positive status; use 042 in these cases.

EXAMPLE The patient's HIV test last week was positive; the patient is asymptomatic, V08 (Z21).

(e) Patients with inconclusive HIV serology

Patients with inconclusive HIV serology, but no definitive diagnosis or manifestations of the illness, may be assigned code 795.71, Inconclusive serologic test for Human Immunodeficiency Virus [HIV].

(f) Previously diagnosed HIV-related illness

Patients with any known prior diagnosis of an HIV-related illness should be coded to 042. Once a patient had developed an HIV-related illness, the patient should always be assigned code 042 on every subsequent admission/encounter. Patients previously diagnosed with any HIV illness (042) should never be assigned to 795.71 or V08.

EXAMPLE HIV patient with prior history of *Pneumocystis carinii* pneumonia (PCP), 042 (B20). PCP is an opportunistic lung infection that has been identified as an AIDS-defining illness.

(g) HIV Infection in Pregnancy, Childbirth and the Puerperium

During pregnancy, childbirth or the puerperium, a patient admitted (or presenting for a health care encounter) because of an HIV-related illness should receive a principal diagnosis of 647.6X, Other specified infectious and parasitic diseases in the mother classifiable elsewhere, but complicating the pregnancy, childbirth or the puerperium, followed by 042 and the code(s) for the HIV-related illness(es). Codes from Chapter 15 always take sequencing priority.

EXAMPLE The patient is 20 weeks pregnant and is admitted for treatment of esophageal candidiasis due to AIDS, 647.63, 042, 112.84 (098.712, B20, B37.81).

Patients with asymptomatic HIV infection status admitted (or presenting for a health care encounter) during pregnancy, childbirth, or the puerperium should receive codes of 647.6X and V08.

EXAMPLE   A patient at 39 weeks delivered liveborn twins vaginally during her hospital stay. The mother's HIV has remained asymptomatic, 651.01, 647.61, V08, V27.2, 73.59 (O30.003, O98.72, Z21, Z37.2, 10E0XZZ).

(h) Encounters for testing for HIV

If a patient is being seen to determine his/her HIV status, use code V73.89, Screening for other specified viral disease. Use code V69.8, Other problems related to lifestyle, as a secondary code if an asymptomatic patient is in a known high risk group for HIV. Should a patient with signs or symptoms or illness, or a confirmed HIV related diagnosis be tested for HIV, code the signs and symptoms or the diagnosis. An additional counseling code V65.44 may be used if counseling is provided during the encounter for the test.

When a patient returns to be informed of his/her HIV test results use code V65.44, HIV counseling, if the results of the test are negative.

If the results are positive but the patient is asymptomatic use code V08, Asymptomatic HIV infection. If the results are positive and the patient is symptomatic use code 042, HIV infection, with codes for the HIV related symptoms or diagnosis. The HIV counseling code may also be used if counseling is provided for patients with positive test results.

EXAMPLE   Because of high-risk homosexual behavior, the patient is seen in the clinic for HIV screening, V73.89, V69.2 (Z11.4, Z72.52).

EXAMPLE   The patient returns for test results that are negative and is counseled regarding HIV prevention, V65.44 (Z71.7).

EXAMPLE   The patient returns for test results that are positive, and the patient is asymptomatic. She is instructed regarding symptoms to watch for and means of prevention, V08, V65.44 (Z21, Z71.7).

b. Septicemia, Systemic Inflammatory Response Syndrome (SIRS), Sepsis, Severe Sepsis, and Septic Shock

1) SIRS, Septicemia, and Sepsis

(a) The terms *septicemia* and *sepsis* are often used interchangeably by providers, however they are not considered synonymous terms. The following descriptions are provided for reference but do not preclude querying the provider for clarification about terms used in the documentation:

(i) Septicemia generally refers to a systemic disease associated with the presence of pathological microorganisms or toxins in the blood, which can include bacteria, viruses, fungi or other organisms.

(ii) Systemic inflammatory response syndrome (SIRS) generally refers to the systemic response to infection, trauma/burns, or other insult (such as cancer) with symptoms including fever, tachycardia, tachypnea, and leukocytosis.

(iii) Sepsis generally refers to SIRS due to infection.

(iv) Severe sepsis generally refers to sepsis with associated acute organ dysfunction.

(b) The coding of SIRS, Sepsis and severe Sepsis

The coding of SIRS, sepsis and severe sepsis requires a minimum of 2 codes: a code for the underlying cause (such as infection or trauma) and a code from subcategory 995.9 Systemic inflammatory response syndrome (SIRS).

(i) The code for the underlying cause (such as infection or trauma) must be sequenced before the code from subcategory 995.9 Systemic inflammatory response syndrome (SIRS).

(ii) Sepsis and severe sepsis require a code for the systemic infection (038.xx, 112.5, etc.) and either code 995.91, Sepsis, or 995.92, Severe sepsis. If the causal organism is not documented, assign code 038.9, Unspecified septicemia.

(iii) Severe sepsis requires additional code(s) for the associated acute organ dysfunction(s).

(iv) If a patient has sepsis with multiple organ dysfunctions, follow the instructions for coding severe sepsis.

(v) Either the term sepsis or SIRS must be documented to assign a code from subcategory 995.9.

(vi) *See Section I.C.17.g.), Injury and poisoning, for information regarding systemic inflammatory response syndrome (SIRS) due to trauma/burns and other non-infectious processes.*

(c) Due to the complex nature of sepsis and severe sepsis, some cases may require querying the provider prior to assignment of the codes.

2) Sequencing sepsis and severe sepsis

(a) Sepsis and severe sepsis as principal diagnosis

If sepsis or severe sepsis is present on admission, and meets the definition of principal diagnosis, the systemic infection code (e.g., 038.xx, 112.5, etc) should be assigned as the principal diagnosis, followed by code 995.91, Sepsis, or 995.92, Severe sepsis, as required by the sequencing rules in the Tabular List. Codes from subcategory 995.9 can never be assigned as a principal diagnosis. A code should also be assigned for any localized infection, if present.

If the sepsis or severe sepsis is due to a postprocedural infection, see Section I.C.10 for guidelines related to sepsis due to postprocedural infection.

EXAMPLE The patient was admitted and treated for SIRS with sepsis due to streptococcus, group D; the patient has cellulitis of the right leg, 038.0, 995.91, 682.6 (A41.81, L03.115).

(b) Sepsis and severe sepsis as secondary diagnoses

When sepsis or severe sepsis develops during the encounter (it was not present on admission), the systemic infection code and code 995.91 or 995.92 should be assigned as secondary diagnoses.

EXAMPLE The patient was admitted with pneumonia due to *Staphylococcus aureus*. Two days after admission, the patient developed signs of sepsis due to the staph infection, 482.41, 038.11, 995.91 (J15.21, A41.0).

(c) Documentation unclear as to whether sepsis or severe sepsis is present on admission

Sepsis or severe sepsis may be present on admission but the diagnosis may not be confirmed until sometime after admission. If the documentation is not clear whether the sepsis or severe sepsis was present on admission, the provider should be queried.

3) Sepsis/SIRS with Localized Infection

If the reason for admission is both sepsis, severe sepsis, or SIRS and a localized infection, such as pneumonia or cellulitis, a code for the systemic infection (038.xx,

112.5, etc) should be assigned first, then code 995.91 or 995.92, followed by the code for the localized infection. If the patient is admitted with a localized infection, such as pneumonia, and sepsis/SIRS doesn't develop until after admission, see guideline I.C.1.b.2.b).

If the localized infection is postprocedural, *see Section I.C.10 for guidelines related to sepsis due to postprocedural infection.*

EXAMPLE The patient was admitted with pneumonia due to *Staphylococcus aureus* and sepsis due to staph infection, 038.11, 482.41, 995.91 (A41.0, J15.21).

Note: The term urosepsis is a nonspecific term. If that is the only term documented then only code 599.0 should be assigned based on the default for the term in the ICD-9-CM index, in addition to the code for the causal organism if known.

EXAMPLE The patient was treated for UTI due to *E. coli*, 599.0, 041.49, (N39.0, B96.2).

4) **Bacterial Sepsis and Septicemia**
In most cases, it will be a code from category 038, Septicemia, that will be used in conjunction with a code from subcategory 995.9 such as the following:
(a) **Streptococcal sepsis**
If the documentation in the record states streptococcal sepsis, codes 038.0, Streptococcal septicemia, and code 995.91 should be used, in that sequence.
(b) **Streptococcal septicemia**
If the documentation states streptococcal septicemia, only code 038.0 should be assigned, however, the provider should be queried whether the patient has sepsis, an infection with SIRS.
5) **Acute organ dysfunction that is not clearly associated with the sepsis**
If a patient has sepsis and an acute organ dysfunction, but the medical record documentation indicates that the acute organ dysfunction is related to a medical condition other than the sepsis, do not assign code 995.92, Severe sepsis. An acute organ dysfunction must be associated with the sepsis in order to assign the severe sepsis code. If the documentation is not clear as to whether an acute organ dysfunction is related to the sepsis or another medical condition, query the provider.

EXAMPLE The patient was admitted in acute respiratory failure due to *Staphylococcus aureus* pneumonia. The patient also presented with sepsis due to staph infection associated with respiratory failure, 038.11, 482.41, 995.92, 518.81 (A41.0, J15.21, J96.00, R65.20).

6) **Septic shock**
(a) **Sequencing of septic shock**
Septic shock generally refers to circulatory failure associated with severe sepsis, and, therefore, it represents a type of acute organ dysfunction.
For all cases of septic shock, the code for the systemic infection should be sequenced first, followed by codes 995.92 and 785.52. Any additional codes for other acute organ dysfunctions should also be assigned. As noted in the sequencing instructions in the Tabular List, the code for septic shock cannot be assigned as a principal diagnosis.

EXAMPLE The patient was admitted with pneumonia due to *Staphylococcus aureus*. Several days after admission, the patient developed septic shock due to *Staphylococcus* sepsis, 482.41, 038.11, 995.92, 785.52 (J15.21, A41.0, R65.21).

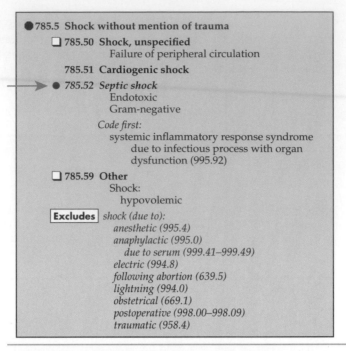

FIGURE 9-1. Tabular entry for septic shock.

(b) Septic Shock without documentation of severe sepsis
Septic shock indicates the presence of severe sepsis.
Code 995.92, Severe sepsis, must be assigned with code 785.52, Septic shock, even if the term severe sepsis is not documented in the record. The "use additional code" note and the "code first" note in the tabular support this guideline. (Figure 9-1)

EXAMPLE The patient was admitted with septic shock and acute renal failure caused by a UTI due to *E. coli*. Discharge summary documents sepsis due to *E. Coli*, 038.42, 995.92, 584.9, 785.52, 599.0 (A41.51, N39.0, R65.21, N17.9).

7) **Sepsis and septic shock complicating abortion and pregnancy**
Sepsis and septic shock complicating abortion, ectopic pregnancy, and molar pregnancy are classified to category codes in Chapter 11 (630-639).
See section I.C.11.

8) **Negative or inconclusive blood cultures**
Negative or inconclusive blood cultures do not preclude a diagnosis of septicemia or sepsis in patients with clinical evidence of the condition, however, the provider should be queried.

9) **Newborn sepsis**
See Section I.C.15.j. for information on the coding of newborn sepsis.

10) **Sepsis due to a Postprocedural Infection**
(a) **Documentation of causal relationship**
As with all postprocedural complications, code assignment is based on the provider's documentation of the relationship between the infection and the procedure.
(b) **Sepsis due to postprocedural infection**
In cases of postprocedural sepsis, the complication code, such as code 998.59, Other postoperative infection, or 674.3x, Other complication of obstetrical surgical wounds should be coded first followed by the appropriate sepsis codes

(systemic infection code and either code 995.91 or 995.92). An additional code(s) for any acute organ dysfunction should also be assigned for cases of severe sepsis.

11) External cause of injury codes with SIRS

Refer to Section I.C.19.a.7 for instruction on the use of external cause of injury codes with codes for SIRS resulting from trauma.

12) Sepsis and Severe Sepsis Associated with Non-infectious Process

In some cases, a non-infectious process, such as trauma, may lead to an infection which can result in sepsis or severe sepsis. If sepsis or severe sepsis is documented as associated with a noninfectious condition, such as a burn or serious injury, and this condition meets the definition for principal diagnosis, the code for the noninfectious condition should be sequenced first, followed by the code for the systemic infection and either code 995.91, Sepsis, or 995.92, Severe sepsis. Additional codes for any associated acute organ dysfunction(s) should also be assigned for cases of severe sepsis. If the sepsis or severe sepsis meets the definition of principal diagnosis, the systemic infection and sepsis codes should be sequenced before the noninfectious condition. When both the associated non-infectious condition and the sepsis or severe sepsis meet the definition of principal diagnosis, either may be assigned as principal diagnosis.

See Section I.C.1.b.2) (a) for guidelines pertaining to sepsis or severe sepsis as the principal diagnosis.

Only one code from subcategory 995.9 should be assigned. Therefore, when a non-infectious condition leads to an infection resulting in sepsis or severe sepsis, assign either code 995.91 or 995.92. Do not additionally assign code 995.93, Systemic inflammatory response syndrome due to non-infectious process without acute organ dysfunction, or 995.94, Systemic inflammatory response syndrome with acute organ dysfunction.

See Section I.C.17.g for information on the coding of SIRS due to trauma/burns or other noninfectious disease processes.

c. Methicillin Resistant Staphylococcus aureus (MRSA) Conditions

1) Selection and sequencing of MRSA codes

(a) Combination codes for MRSA infection

When a patient is diagnosed with an infection that is due to methicillin resistant *Staphylococcus aureus* (MRSA), and that infection has a combination code that includes the causal organism (e.g., septicemia, pneumonia) assign the appropriate code for the condition (e.g., code 038.12, Methicillin resistant Staphylococcus aureus septicemia or code 482.42, Methicillin resistant pneumonia due to Staphylococcus aureus). Do not assign code 041.12, Methicillin resistant Staphylococcus aureus, as an additional code because the code includes the type of infection and the MRSA organism. Do not assign a code from subcategory V09.0, Infection with microorganisms resistant to penicillins, as an additional diagnosis.

See Section C.1.b.1 for instructions on coding and sequencing of septicemia.

EXAMPLE

Patient presents to the hospital with a high fever. Pneumonia is identified on a chest x-ray. Sputum cultures are positive for MRSA. On the discharge summary, the physician documents that patient had pneumonia due to MRSA, 482.42 (J15.21, Z16).

(b) Other codes for MRSA infection

When there is documentation of a current infection (e.g., wound infection, stitch abscess, urinary tract infection) due to MRSA, and that infection does not have a combination code that includes the causal organism, select the appropriate code to identify the condition along with code 041.12, Methicillin resistant Staphylococcus aureus, for the MRSA infection. Do not assign a code from subcategory V09.0, Infection with microorganisms resistant to penicillins.

EXAMPLE | Patient presents to the hospital with an abscess under their left (axilla) arm. It is cultured and grows MRSA. Physician documents that the abscess is due to MRSA, 682.3, 041.12 (L02.412, B95.6, Z16).

(c) Methicillin susceptible Staphylococcus aureus (MSSA) and MRSA colonization

The condition or state of being colonized or carrying MSSA or MRSA is called colonization or carriage, while an individual person is described as being colonized or being a carrier. Colonization means that MSSA or MSRA is present on or in the body without necessarily causing illness. A positive MRSA colonization test might be documented by the provider as "MRSA screen positive" or "MRSA nasal swab positive".

Assign code V02.54, Carrier or suspected carrier, Methicillin resistant Staphylococcus aureus, for patients documented as having MRSA colonization. Assign code V02.53, Carrier or suspected carrier, Methicillin susceptible Staphylococcus aureus, for patient documented as having MSSA colonization. Colonization is not necessarily indicative of a disease process or as the cause of a specific condition the patient may have unless documented as such by the provider.

Code V02.59, Other specified bacterial diseases, should be assigned for other types of staphylococcal colonization (e.g., *S. epidermidis, S. saprophyticus*). Code V02.59 should not be assigned for colonization with any type of *Staphylococcus aureus* (MRSA, MSSA).

EXAMPLE | Due to recent outbreak of MRSA, every patient coming through the Emergency Room has a nasal swab taken to check for carrier status. Patient's swab returns positive for MRSA, V02.54 (Z22.32, Z16).

(d) MRSA colonization and infection

If a patient is documented as having both MRSA colonization and infection during a hospital admission, code V02.54, Carrier or suspected carrier, Methicillin resistant *Staphylococcus aureus*, and a code for the MRSA infection may both be assigned.

EXAMPLE | Patient presents to the hospital with an abscess on the buttock. A culture of the abscess is taken as well as a nasal swab. The culture returns positive for MRSA as well as a positive nasal swab. The physician documents that the abscess is due to MRSA, 682.5, 041.12, V02.54 (L02.31, B95.6, Z16, Z22.32).

Apply the General Coding Guidelines as found in Chapter 5 and the Procedural Guidelines as found in Chapter 6.

ICD-10-CM

Official Guidelines for Coding and Reporting

Please refer to the companion Evolve website for the most current guidelines.

1. Chapter 1: Certain Infectious and Parasitic Diseases (A00-B99)

a. Human Immunodeficiency Virus (HIV) Infections

1) Code only confirmed cases

Code only confirmed cases of HIV infection/illness. This is an exception to the hospital inpatient guideline Section II, H.

In this context, "confirmation" does not require documentation of positive serology or culture for HIV; the provider's diagnostic statement that the patient is HIV positive, or has an HIV-related illness is sufficient.

2) Selection and sequencing of HIV codes

(a) Patient admitted for HIV-related condition

If a patient is admitted for an HIV-related condition, the principal diagnosis should be B20, followed by additional diagnosis codes for all reported HIV-related conditions.

(b) Patient with HIV disease admitted for unrelated condition

If a patient with HIV disease is admitted for an unrelated condition (such as a traumatic injury), the code for the unrelated condition (e.g., the nature of injury code) should be the principal diagnosis. Other diagnoses would be B20 followed by additional diagnosis codes for all reported HIV-related conditions.

(c) Whether the patient is newly diagnosed

Whether the patient is newly diagnosed or has had previous admissions/encounters for HIV conditions is irrelevant to the sequencing decision.

(d) Asymptomatic human immunodeficiency virus

Z21, Asymptomatic human immunodeficiency virus [HIV] infection status, is to be applied when the patient without any documentation of symptoms is listed as being "HIV positive," "known HIV," "HIV test positive," or similar terminology. Do not use this code if the term "AIDS" is used or if the patient is treated for any HIV-related illness or is described as having any condition(s) resulting from his/her HIV positive status; use B20 in these cases.

(e) Patients with inconclusive HIV serology

Patients with inconclusive HIV serology, but no definitive diagnosis or manifestations of the illness, may be assigned code R75, Inconclusive laboratory evidence of human immunodeficiency virus [HIV].

(f) Previously diagnosed HIV-related illness

Patients with any known prior diagnosis of an HIV-related illness should be coded to B20. Once a patient has developed an HIV-related illness, the patient should always be assigned code B20 on every subsequent admission/encounter. Patients previously diagnosed with any HIV illness (B20) should never be assigned to R75 or Z21, Asymptomatic human immunodeficiency virus [HIV] infection status.

(g) HIV Infection in Pregnancy, Childbirth and the Puerperium

During pregnancy, childbirth or the puerperium, a patient admitted (or presenting for a health care encounter) because of an HIV-related illness should receive a principal diagnosis code of O98.7-, Human immunodeficiency [HIV] disease complicating pregnancy, childbirth and the puerperium, followed by B20 and the code(s) for the HIV-related illness(es). Codes from Chapter 15 always take sequencing priority.

Patients with asymptomatic HIV infection status admitted (or presenting for a health care encounter) during pregnancy, childbirth, or the puerperium should receive codes of O98.7- and Z21.

(h) Encounters for testing for HIV

If a patient is being seen to determine his/her HIV status, use code Z11.4, Encounter for screening for human immunodeficiency virus [HIV]. Use additional codes for any associated high risk behavior.

If a patient with signs or symptoms is being seen for HIV testing, code the signs and symptoms. An additional counseling code Z71.7, Human immunodeficiency virus [HIV] counseling, may be used if counseling is provided during the encounter for the test.

When a patient returns to be informed of his/her HIV test results and the test result is negative, use code Z71.7, Human immunodeficiency virus [HIV] counseling.

If the results are positive, see previous guidelines and assign codes as appropriate.

b. Infectious agents as the cause of diseases classified to other chapters

Certain infections are classified in chapters other than Chapter 1 and no organism is identified as part of the infection code. In these instances, it is necessary to use an additional code from Chapter 1 to identify the organism. A code from category B95, Streptococcus, Staphylococcus, and Enterococcus as the cause of diseases classified to other chapters, B96, Other bacterial agents as the cause of diseases classified to other chapters, or B97, Viral agents as the cause of diseases classified to other chapters, is to be used as an additional code to identify the organism. An instructional note will be found at the infection code advising that an additional organism code is required.

c. Infections resistant to antibiotics

Many bacterial infections are resistant to current antibiotics. It is necessary to identify all infections documented as antibiotic resistant. Assign code Z16, Infection with drug resistant microorganisms, following the infection code for these cases.

d. Sepsis, Severe Sepsis, and Septic Shock

1) Coding of Sepsis and Severe Sepsis

(a) Sepsis

For a diagnosis of sepsis, assign the appropriate code for the underlying systemic infection. If the type of infection or causal organism is not further specified, assign code A41.9, Sepsis, unspecified.

A code from subcategory R65.2, Severe sepsis, should not be assigned unless severe sepsis or an associated acute organ dysfunction is documented.

(i) Negative or inconclusive blood cultures and sepsis

Negative or inconclusive blood cultures do not preclude a diagnosis of sepsis in patients with clinical evidence of the condition, however, the provider should be queried.

(ii) Urosepsis

The term urosepsis is a nonspecific term. It is not to be considered synonymous with sepsis. It has no default code in the Alphabetic Index. Should a provider use this term, he/she must be queried for clarification.

(iii) Sepsis with organ dysfunction

If a patient has sepsis and associated acute organ dysfunction or multiple organ dysfunction (MOD), follow the instructions for coding severe sepsis.

(iv) Acute organ dysfunction that is not clearly associated with the sepsis

If a patient has sepsis and an acute organ dysfunction, but the medical record documentation indicates that the acute organ dysfunction is related to a medical condition other than the sepsis, do not assign a code from subcategory R65.2, Severe sepsis. An acute organ dysfunction must be associated with the sepsis in order to assign the severe sepsis code. If the documentation is not clear as to whether an acute organ dysfunction is related to the sepsis or another medical condition, query the provider.

(b) Severe sepsis

The coding of severe sepsis requires a minimum of 2 codes: first a code for the underlying systemic infection, followed by a code from subcategory R65.2, Severe sepsis. If the causal organism is not documented, assign code A41.9, Sepsis, unspecified, for the infection. Additional code(s) for the associated acute organ dysfunction are also required.

Due to the complex nature of severe sepsis, some cases may require querying the provider prior to assignment of the codes.

2) Septic shock

Septic shock is circulatory failure associated with severe sepsis, and therefore, it represents a type of acute organ dysfunction. For all cases of septic shock, the code for the underlying systemic infection should be sequenced first, followed by code R65.21, Severe sepsis with septic shock. Any additional codes for the other acute organ dysfunctions should also be assigned.

Septic shock indicates the presence of severe sepsis. Code R65.21, Severe sepsis with septic shock, must be assigned if septic shock is documented in the medical record, even if the term severe sepsis is not documented.

3) Sequencing of severe sepsis

If severe sepsis is present on admission, and meets the definition of principal diagnosis, the underlying systemic infection should be assigned as principal diagnosis followed by the appropriate code from subcategory R65.2 as required by the sequencing rules in the Tabular List. A code from subcategory R65.2 can never be assigned as a principal diagnosis.

When severe sepsis develops during an encounter (it was not present on admission) the underlying systemic infection and the appropriate code from subcategory R65.2 should be assigned as secondary diagnoses.

Severe sepsis may be present on admission but the diagnosis may not be confirmed until sometime after admission. If the documentation is not clear whether severe sepsis was present on admission, the provider should be queried.

4) Sepsis and severe sepsis with a localized infection

If the reason for admission is both sepsis or severe sepsis and a localized infection, such as pneumonia or cellulitis, a code(s) for the underlying systemic infection should be assigned first and the code for the localized infection should be assigned as a secondary diagnosis. If the patient has severe sepsis, a code from subcategory R65.2 should also be assigned as a secondary diagnosis. If the patient is admitted with a localized infection, such as pneumonia, and sepsis/severe sepsis doesn't develop until after admission, the localized infection should be assigned first, followed by the appropriate sepsis/severe sepsis codes.

5) Sepsis due to a postprocedural infection

Sepsis resulting from a postprocedural infection is a complication of medical care. For such cases, the postprocedural infection code, such as, T80.2, Infections following infusion, transfusion, and therapeutic injection, T81.4, Infection following a procedure, T88.0, Infection following immunization, or O86.0, Infection of obstetric surgical wound, should be coded first, followed by the code for the specific infection. If the patient has severe sepsis the appropriate code from subcategory R65.2 should also be assigned with the additional code(s) for any acute organ dysfunction.

6) Sepsis and severe sepsis associated with a noninfectious process (condition)

In some cases a noninfectious process (condition), such as trauma, may lead to an infection which can result in sepsis or severe sepsis. If sepsis or severe sepsis is documented as associated with a noninfectious condition, such as a burn or serious injury, and this condition meets the definition for principal diagnosis, the code for the noninfectious condition should be sequenced first, followed by the code for the resulting infection. If severe sepsis is present a code from subcategory R65.2 should also be assigned with any associated organ dysfunction(s) codes. It is not necessary to assign a code from subcategory R65.1, Systemic inflammatory response syndrome (SIRS) of non-infectious origin, for these cases.

If the infection meets the definition of principal diagnosis it should be sequenced before the non-infectious condition. When both the associated non-infectious condition and the infection meet the definition of principal diagnosis either may be assigned as principal diagnosis.

Only one code from category R65, Symptoms and signs specifically associated with systemic inflammation and infection, should be assigned. Therefore, when a non-infectious condition leads to an infection resulting in severe sepsis, assign the appropriate code from subcategory R65.2, Severe sepsis. Do not additionally assign a code from subcategory R65.1, Systemic inflammatory response syndrome (SIRS) of non-infectious origin.

See Section I.C.18. SIRS due to non-infectious process

7) Sepsis and septic shock complicating abortion, pregnancy, childbirth, and the puerperium

See Section I.C.15. Sepsis and septic shock complicating abortion, pregnancy, childbirth and the puerperium

8) Newborn sepsis

See Section I.C.16. Newborn sepsis

Apply the General Coding Guidelines as found in Chapter 5 and the Procedural Guidelines as found in Chapter 7.

GUIDELINE DIFFERENCES BETWEEN ICD-9-CM AND ICD-10-CM

- In ICD-10-CM, the term "SIRS" is no longer assigned a separate code when due to an infectious process.
- Septicemia and bacteremia are coded to R78.81 in the chapter on symptoms.
- In ICD-10-CM, urosepsis is not assigned a default code. The use of this term requires a query to the provider.

MAJOR DIFFERENCES BETWEEN ICD-9-CM AND ICD-10-CM

- Streptococcal sore throat in ICD-10-CM has been reclassified to Diseases of the Respiratory System.
- There is an instructional note at the beginning of Chapter 1 in ICD-10-CM to use an additional code (Z16) for any associated drug resistance.
- There is a new block in ICD-10-CM for infections with a predominantly sexual mode of transmission. Many codes from other chapters have been moved to this section.
- In ICD-10-CM, a note under the code for smallpox states the disease has been officially eradicated, but the code is maintained for surveillance purposes.

ANATOMY AND PHYSIOLOGY

This chapter focuses on diseases that are **communicable** (easily spread from one to another) and **parasitic** (organism taking nourishment from another organism) and the organisms that are responsible for the disease conditions. Many times, two codes are required. If a condition is not considered communicable, it will be found in a body system chapter; in this case, an additional code from category 041 or 079 may be assigned to identify causative organisms. To add an additional code identifying the organism, the user should look under the term "infection" in the Alphabetic Index.

EXAMPLE

Acute *Staphylococcus* vaginitis, 616.10, 041.10 (N76.0, B95.8).
To locate the code for *Staphylococcus*, the coder must look under the main term, "Infection," and then under the subterm "*Staphylococcus.*" Sometimes, the organism and the disease condition have a combination code; this is the case for many of the pneumonia codes.
Klebsiella pneumonia, 482.0 (J15.0).

There is no one body system that causes or is affected by infectious disease. These organisms can be found in any or all of the body systems.

DISEASE CONDITIONS

Infectious and Parasitic Diseases (001-139), Chapter 1 in the ICD-9-CM code book, is divided into the following categories:

CATEGORY	SECTION TITLES
001-009	Intestinal Infectious Diseases
010-018	Tuberculosis
020-027	Zoonotic Bacterial Diseases
030-041	Other Bacterial Diseases
042	Human Immunodeficiency Virus (HIV) Infections
045-049	Poliomyelitis and Other Non–Arthropod-Borne Viral Diseases of Central Nervous System
050-058	Viral Diseases Accompanied by Exanthem
060-066	Arthropod-Borne Viral Diseases
070-079	Other Diseases Due to Viruses and Chlamydiae
080-088	Rickettsioses and Other Arthropod-Borne Diseases
090-099	Syphilis and Other Venereal Diseases
100-104	Other Spirochetal Diseases
110-118	Mycoses
120-129	Helminthiases
130-136	Other Infectious and Parasitic Diseases
137-139	Late Effects of Infectious and Parasitic Diseases

Certain Infectious and Parasitic Diseases (A00-B99), Chapter 9 in the ICD-10-CM code book, is divided into the following categories:

CATEGORY	SECTION TITLES
A00-A09	Intestinal Infectious Diseases
A15-A19	Tuberculosis
A20-A28	Certain Zoonotic Bacterial Diseases
A30-A49	Other Bacterial Diseases
A50-A64	Infections with a Predominantly Sexual Mode of Transmission
A65-A69	Other Spirochetal Diseases
A70-A74	Other Diseases Caused by *Chlamydiae*
A75-A79	Rickettsioses
A80-A89	Viral Infections of the Central Nervous System
A90-A99	Arthropod-Borne Viral Fevers and Viral Hemorrhagic Fevers
B00-B09	Viral Infections Characterized by Skin and Mucous Membrane Lesions
B10	Other Human Herpesviruses
B15-B19	Viral Hepatitis
B20-	Human Immunodeficiency Virus (HIV) Disease
B25-B34	Other Viral Diseases
B35-B49	Mycoses
B50-B64	Protozoal Diseases
B65-B83	Helminthiases
B85-B89	Pediculosis, Acariasis, and Other Infestations
B90-B94	Sequelae of Infectious and Parasitic Diseases
B95-B97	Bacterial, Viral, and Other Infectious Agents
B99	Other Infectious Diseases

Intestinal Infectious Diseases

Clostridium difficile

Clostridium difficile, which is also known as *C. diff,* is a leading cause of pseudomembranous colitis. It can be found in the Index under "Enteritis, clostridium, difficile."

C. diff is one of the most common **nosocomial** infections (hospital acquired). In the hospital setting, it may be spread from healthcare worker to patient. Spores associated with this disease can survive up to 70 days. It can also be caused by antibiotic use. This disease is characterized by watery diarrhea and abdominal cramping. The intestinal tract has usually been altered in some way to allow *C. diff* bacteria to flourish.

If a physician suspects *C. diff* (often seen in elderly hospitalized patients), a stool specimen is tested for *C. diff* toxins (cytotoxicity assay). The test results can take between 24 and 48 hours to complete. Treatment depends on the severity of infection. Often, antibiotics are changed or discontinued; however, in severe cases, a patient is treated with metronidazole (Flagyl). Patients with *C. diff* are usually placed on isolation protocol.

EXAMPLE   *Clostridium difficile* colitis, 008.45 (A04.7).

Tuberculosis

Tuberculosis (TB) is an infection caused by *Mycobacterium tuberculosis* (Figure 9-2). These bacteria can attack any part of the body but most often attack the lungs. TB was the leading cause of death in the United States prior to the discovery of medicines to treat the disease. TB was almost eradicated but made a resurgence in the late 1980s.

TB is spread through the air via coughing or sneezing. TB of the lung is the only infectious form of TB. If TB occurs in the bones or kidney, it is not likely to be contagious. TB can be infectious only if it is an active disease. It may be necessary to isolate a patient who is suspected of having this condition, pending confirmation. A form of TB called "latent

FIGURE 9-2. Tuberculosis.

TB" occurs when a person breathes the bacteria but the immune system fights them off, and they remain alive in the body but are inactive. Latent TB can become active TB. Persons with latent TB usually have a positive TB test result.

Active TB usually occurs in the populations whose immune systems are too weak to fight off this disease. This group would include individuals with HIV, individuals with leukemia, substance abusers, young children, and organ transplant recipients.

Coding TB requires the use of a fifth digit. The fifth digits are as follows:

- 0 unspecified
- 1 bacteriological or histological examination not done
- 2 bacteriological or histological examination unknown (at present)
- 3 tubercle bacilli found (in sputum) by microscopy
- 4 tubercle bacilli not found (in sputum) by microscopy, but found by bacterial culture
- 5 tubercle bacilli not found by bacteriological examination, but tuberculosis confirmed histologically
- 6 tubercle bacilli not found by bacteriological or histological examination, but tuberculosis confirmed by other methods [inoculation of animals]

More often than not, a fifth digit of 0, unspecified is assigned because further detail is not documented.

EXAMPLE	Patient admitted for pneumonia due to tuberculosis, which was confirmed by bacterial culture, 011.64 (A15.0).

EXERCISE 9-1

Assign codes to the following conditions.

1. Pyelonephritis caused by tuberculosis   _____

2. Acute miliary tuberculosis   _____

3. Interstitial keratitis caused by tuberculosis; bacterial culture   _____
   performed, results unknown

4. Cavitation of the lung caused by tuberculosis   _____

5. *Salmonella* sepsis   _____

6. Food poisoning caused by *Salmonella* resulting in gastroenteritis   _____

7. Enteritis caused by the rotavirus   _____

8. Norwalk virus   _____

9. Dysentery   _____

10. Giardiasis   _____

Zoonotic Bacterial Diseases

Anthrax

Anthrax is a bacterial infection that is usually found in wild or domestic animals. It is most common in agricultural regions of Central America, Africa, Asia, and the Caribbean. Anthrax occurs in three forms: cutaneous, inhalation, and gastrointestinal. The most serious form is the inhalation type, which causes severe breathing problems that are most often fatal. Since the 9/11 attack on the United States and threats of anthrax attacks, a code was developed for contact or exposure to anthrax.

EXAMPLE   Contact with or exposure to anthrax, V01.81 (Z20.810).

This code can be used for anyone who has been exposed to anthrax or who is closely linked to persons with known exposure. See *Coding Clinic* (2002:4Q:p78).[1]

Other Bacterial Diseases

Mycobacterium Avium *Complex*

Mycobacterium avium complex (MAC) or *Mycobacterium avium-intercellulare* (MAI) is a bacterium that attacks immunocompromised individuals. This bacterium is found in soil and water; an individual who is not immunocompromised does not succumb to the disease. This has been classified as an acquired immunodeficiency syndrome (AIDS)-defining illness. Tests that show high blood levels of the liver enzyme alkaline phosphatase may indicate MAC. Symptoms of this disease include night sweats, weight loss, and diarrhea. Prior to the advent of highly active antiretroviral therapy (**HAART**), which is a group of drugs given to patients with AIDS for prophylaxis, a high incidence of this condition was reported. It generally affects individuals whose T4 cell count is less than 50. A variety of antibiotics are used to treat patients with this disease. Individuals with advanced AIDS often develop disseminated *Mycobacterium avium-intracellulare* complex (DMAC). Per *Coding Clinic* (1997:4Q:p3),[2] the single unique presentation of patients with DMAC is severe anemia.

EXAMPLE   Infection from *Mycobacterium avium*, 031.0 (A31.0).

Meningococcal Infection

Meningococcal infections are caused by the bacterium meningococcus (Figure 9-3). These bacteria may be found in around 10% of the population (in the nose or throat) and cause no ill effects. These people are known as asymptomatic carriers. This bacterium can cause **meningitis**, which is an infection in the fluid of a person's spinal cord and brain. It also can cause septicemia (blood infection), which is known as meningococcal septicemia.

FIGURE 9-3. Bacterial meningitis. The surface of the brain is covered with pus.

EXAMPLE   Meningococcal meningitis, 036.0 (A39.0).

EXAMPLE   Meningococcemia, 036.2 (A39.4).

Septicemia

Septicemia is the presence in the blood of pathologic microorganisms that causes systemic illness. It is also known as blood poisoning. Per *Coding Clinic* (2000:2Q:p5-6),[3] "bacteremia is bacteria in the blood, as confirmed by culture." Bacteremia is a laboratory finding, whereas septicemia is an illness. *Coding Clinic* (2003:4Q:p79-81)[4] gives a detailed explanation of the differences between the terms.

Bacteremia—bacteria in blood 790.7 (R78.81)

Septicemia—systemic disease characterized by the presence of microorganisms or toxins in the blood. These organisms may include bacteria, virus, fungi, and others 038.9 (A41.9)

SIRS—systemic inflammatory response syndrome to infection or trauma. Includes symptoms such as fever, tachycardia, tachypnea, and leukocytosis

Sepsis—SIRS due to infection. Code first 038.X (A41.9) or trauma plus 995.91. Code for causative infection (i.e., pneumonia, cellulitis).

Sepsis with organ failure or severe sepsis—SIRS due to infection with organ failure. Code first 038.XX or causative trauma, 995.92 or 995.94. Then code any organ failure codes.

Septic shock—also known as endotoxic shock and/or Gram-negative shock. It is caused by a failure of the cardiovascular system and therefore meets the definition of severe sepsis.

Code first 038.XX or causative trauma, 995.92 or 995.94, then code 785.2, septic shock, and then code any specified organ failures (A41.9, R65.21).

Urosepsis is an infection of urinary site only. Code 599.0. The Index in ICD-10-CM instructs the user to code to condition.

Sepsis due to urosepsis is an infection of the urinary site that has spread to the blood and has initiated a systemic response, 038.9, 995.91, 599.0 (A41.9, N39.0).

If a physician documents septicemia alone and does not document sepsis, then only a code from 038.XX (A41.9) would be used. It would be appropriate to query the physician for the presence of sepsis.

Sepsis that occurs in the newborn or pregnant patient is governed by coding guidelines found in their respective chapters.

Negative blood cultures do not preclude a diagnosis of sepsis or septicemia in patients who exhibit clinical evidence of these conditions.

EXAMPLE   Patient admitted with pneumonia, fever, and tachycardia. Physician suspects sepsis and orders blood cultures. Two days after admittance, cultures are positive for pneumococcal bacteria and physician confirms pneumococcal sepsis, 038.2, 995.91, 486 (A40.3, J18.9).

EXERCISE 9-2

Assign codes to the following conditions.

1. Respiratory anthrax   _____

2. Cutaneous anthrax   _____

3. *Mycobacterium kansasii*   _____

4. MAI   _____

5. MAC   _____

6. Whooping cough   _____

7. Patient has MAC and is on HAART. What other disease could you query for?   _____

8. Meningococcal infection in the heart muscle   _____

9. Sepsis due to meningococcal bacteria   _____

10. Urosepsis   _____

11. Gonococcal sepsis   _____

12. Severe sepsis with acute respiratory failure   _____

13. Sepsis of the newborn   _____

14. Patient presents with fever, chills, and hypotension. The physician orders blood cultures for suspected sepsis. Results are negative. The discharge summary lists sepsis due to *Escherichia coli*.   _____

15. Patient with SIRS secondary to pneumonia   _____

Bacterial Infection in Conditions Classified Elsewhere and of Unspecified Site

Often, infectious diseases are characterized by a condition and a bacterial organism. When this occurs, it is appropriate to use two codes to fully describe the infection and the causative organism. Practitioners sometimes define organisms as resistant to certain antibiotics. MRSA is methicillin-resistant *Staphylococcus aureus*. If a patient has pneumonia caused by *Staphylococcus aureus* and the organism is resistant to methicillin, it would be coded as 482.41 (J15.21, Z16). Likewise, practitioners may identify organisms that are sensitive to antibiotics, such as MSSA, which is methicillin-sensitive *Staphylococcus aureus*. If a patient has pneumonia caused by *Staphylococcus aureus* that is sensitive to methicillin, it would be coded to 482.41 (J15.21).

EXAMPLE	Urinary tract infection (UTI) caused by *E. coli*, 599.0, 041.49 (N39.0, B96.2).

EXAMPLE	UTI due to strep group D resistant to vancomycin, 599.0, 041.04, V09.80 (N39.0, B95.4, Z16).

Human Immunodeficiency Virus (HIV) Infection

It is important to note that codes within this section are used only when the diagnosis has been confirmed. This is an exception to the hospital inpatient guideline that allows the coding of possible, probable, or suspected diagnoses. This rule is very important because once a person is diagnosed with AIDS, there can be psychological, social, and legal ramifications.

AIDS is an incurable disease of the immune system caused by the **HIV** virus, and it is the final stage of HIV disease. It first appeared in the United States in 1981. In the beginning this virus was seen in the homosexual and intravenous drug user (IVDU) population and later spread to the heterosexual population. The virus is found in and is transmitted by blood, semen, vaginal secretions, and breast milk. Transmission occurs through sexual contact, blood transfusions, needle sharing, or breastfeeding.

People who are infected with the HIV virus may not have any symptoms for up to 10 years. Once the immune system becomes weakened, they become susceptible to opportunistic infections. When HIV infects a person, it most commonly attacks the CD4 cells, which are a type of lymphocyte (white blood cell). Over time, the amount of CD4 cells in a person infected with HIV decreases, which means their immune system is weakened. Normal CD4 counts are between 500 and 1600. When a CD4 count falls below 200 in an HIV-positive individual, it is a sign of AIDS. Often CD4 percentages are used as a basis for determining AIDS. These are percentages of total lymphocytes. When a CD4 percentage falls below 14%, a patient is considered to have AIDS. Once a CD4 count goes below 350 cells/mL, a patient may be at risk to develop herpes, TB, thrush, Kaposi's sarcoma, or non-Hodgkin's lymphoma. When the count goes below 50, a patient may develop *Mycobacterium avium* or cytomegalovirus (CMV).

AIDS may be treated with HAART (highly active antiretroviral therapy). Sometimes drugs are given on a prophylactic basis to prevent opportunistic infections. With the use of today's drugs, a patient's CD4 count can rebound above 200. However, this does not change the fact that he/she has AIDS and should be coded as 042 (B20). For example, it may be documented that a patient's CD4 nadir is 150. **Nadir** means the lowest level a patient's CD4 count has ever been. A patient with a nadir of 150 would be considered to have AIDS.

Once a patient develops AIDS, he or she is always assigned code 042 (B20) from then on. When a patient is admitted for treatment of an HIV-related condition, the principal diagnosis should always be 042 (B20).

EXAMPLE	Patient admitted with Kaposi's sarcoma of subcutaneous tissue. Code first 042, AIDS, then, code 176.1, Kaposi's sarcoma (B20, C46.1).

If a patient is admitted with an AIDS-defining illness (Box 9-1), the principal diagnosis is 042 (B20). Likewise, if a patient is admitted with an HIV-related condition, the principal diagnosis is 042 (B20).

EXAMPLE	A patient presents with severely elevated blood pressure and known hypertension and HIVAN (HIV-associated nephropathy). The patient has end-stage renal disease (ESRD) and is currently on dialysis. The principal diagnosis in this case is 042, 583.9, 403.91, 585.6, V45.11 (B20, N05.9, I12.0, N18.6, Z99.2).

BOX 9-1 LIST OF AIDS-DEFINING CONDITIONS[5]

The Centers for Disease Control and Prevention (CDC) considers a patient to have AIDS if a CD4+ T-cell count is below 200 cells/µl (or a CD4+ T-cell percentage of total lymphocytes is less than 14%) or if the patient has one of the following defining illnesses:

- Conditions included in the 1993 AIDS surveillance case definition
- Candidiasis of bronchi, trachea, or lungs
- Candidiasis, esophageal
- Cervical cancer, invasive
- Coccidioidomycosis, disseminated or extrapulmonary
- Cryptococcosis, extrapulmonary
- Cryptosporidiosis, chronic intestinal (longer than 1 month duration)
- Cytomegalovirus disease (other than liver, spleen, or nodes)
- Cytomegalovirus retinitis (with loss of vision)
- Encephalopathy, HIV-related
- Herpes simplex: chronic ulcer(s) (longer than 1 month duration); or bronchitis, pneumonitis, or esophagitis
- Histoplasmosis, disseminated or extrapulmonary
- Isosporiasis, chronic intestinal (longer than 1 month duration)
- Kaposi's sarcoma
- Lymphoma, Burkitt's (or equivalent term)
- Lymphoma, immunoblastic (or equivalent term)
- Lymphoma, primary, of brain
- *Mycobacterium avium* complex or *Mycobacterium kansasii*, disseminated or extrapulmonary
- *Mycobacterium tuberculosis,* any site (pulmonary or extrapulmonary)
- *Mycobacterium,* other species or unidentified species, disseminated or extrapulmonary
- *Pneumocystis carinii* pneumonia
- Pneumonia, recurrent
- Progressive multifocal leukoencephalopathy
- *Salmonella* septicemia, recurrent
- Toxoplasmosis of brain
- Wasting syndrome due to HIV

When a patient is admitted with a condition unrelated to AIDS, then the code for the unrelated condition is the principal diagnosis.

EXAMPLE A patient with a history of AIDS is admitted in alcohol withdrawal, 291.81, 303.90, 042 (F10.239, B20).

Sometimes, patients test HIV positive but have no symptoms. V08 (Z21) is the code that should be used for these patients. Tests may have inconclusive results; then, the code 795.71 (R75), nonspecific serologic evidence of HIV, should be assigned. This code can be found in the Alphabetic Index under Finding, abnormal, serological, HIV, inconclusive.

EXAMPLE Patient is being treated for thrush and is HIV positive. 112.0, V08 (B37.0, Z21).

AIDS and Pregnancy

If a woman has AIDS and is pregnant, code 647.6X (O98.7-) should be used, along with 042 (B20). Codes from Chapter 15 in the code book always take precedence.

Encounters for Testing for HIV

- Encounter for determining HIV status, V73.89 (Z11.4), Screening for other specified viral disease
- Encounter for counseling for an HIV-negative patient, V65.44 (Z71.7)
- Encounter for an HIV-positive patient who is asymptomatic, V08 (Z21); counseling code may also be used
- Encounter for HIV-positive patient who is symptomatic, 042 (B20); counseling code may also be used

Poliomyelitis and Other Non–Arthropod-Borne Viral Diseases of the Central Nervous System

Poliomyelitis (polio) is a viral disease that affects the nerves and is caused by the poliovirus. It is also known as infantile paralysis. This disease has been nearly eradicated in the United States as the result of mandatory vaccination.

If people are unvaccinated, this disease may be contracted through direct contact with infected persons. The virus usually enters the body through the mouth or nose. Symptoms can resemble the flu, and a person may or may not become paralyzed. Treatment consists of alleviating the symptoms and letting the virus run its course. Essentially three types of polio infection may occur: subclinical infection, nonparalytic, and paralytic. If the spinal cord or the brain is not affected (which is the case 90% of the time), then complete recovery can occur.

EXAMPLE

A patient presents to the hospital with headache, muscle weakness, fever, and muscle spasms of the neck. After a battery of testing, it is determined that the patient has type I acute poliomyelitis, 045.91 (A80.9).

Viral meningitis, also known as aseptic meningitis, is an infection of the fluid in the spinal cord and the fluid around the brain. Viral meningitis is far less serious than bacterial meningitis and is rarely fatal.

No treatment is available for viral meningitis other than relieving the symptoms, which usually consist of headache, stiff neck, and photophobia. Many different viruses may cause meningitis, but most cases are caused by the enteroviruses, and these viruses may be associated with other diseases. Meningitis also may be transmitted via mosquito bites.

EXAMPLE

A patient presents to the hospital with severe headache and stiff neck. A lumbar puncture is performed, and it is determined that the patient has meningitis due to Echo virus, 047.1, 03.31 (A87.0, 009U3ZX).

EXERCISE 9-3

Assign codes to the following conditions.

1. Patient with HIV and CD4 nadir of 100. _____
2. Patient has HIV and a history of invasive cervical cancer. _____
3. Patient is admitted with *Pneumocystis* pneumonia (PCP) and has a history of AIDS. _____
4. Patient is admitted with dehydration and has AIDS. _____
5. Patient is tested for AIDS in the physician's office, and the results are inconclusive. _____
6. Patient is pregnant and is positive for AIDS. _____
7. Patient is admitted with bacteremia and is an AIDS patient. _____
8. Patient is admitted with tuberculosis and has AIDS. _____

9. Patient is admitted with *E coli* sepsis and a CD4 count of 32, with known HIV. _____

10. Patient is admitted with difficulty swallowing; after an esophagogastroduodenoscopy (EGD) was performed, it was discovered that the patient had candidal esophagitis and a history of being HIV positive. _____

Viral Diseases Accompanied by Exanthem

Herpes Zoster

Herpes zoster, or shingles, is a disease that is caused by the same virus that causes chickenpox. Once a person has contracted chickenpox, the virus remains dormant in the body in certain nerves. Shingles usually occurs in people over 50 years of age but sometimes is reported in younger people. It is caused by conditions that weaken the body's immune system such as cancer, aging, and stress.

Shingles starts as a rash that turns into fluid-filled blisters that may become very painful. Sometimes, a case of shingles results in long-term pain known as "postherpetic neuralgia."

EXAMPLE   Shingles with blepharitis, 053.20, 373.00 (B02.39).

EXAMPLE   Trigeminal neuralgia as a result of shingles, 053.12 (B02.22).

Herpes Simplex I and II

Herpes simplex virus is another name for a cold sore or fever blister, also known as HSV type I. The disease manifests as small fluid-filled blisters. It usually occurs on the face but occasionally is noted in the genital area. People usually acquire HSV I during infancy or childhood from people who kiss them or share towels or eating utensils. In type II or genital herpes, sores appear on the vagina, penis, or buttocks (Figure 9-4). Type II is transmitted via sexual intercourse. Antiviral medications are being used to suppress recurrences of herpes.

EXAMPLE   Fever blister, 054.9 (B00.1).

EXAMPLE   Septicemia due to herpes simplex, 054.5 (B00.7).

EXAMPLE   Otitis externa caused by herpes simplex, 054.73 (B00.1).

Arthropod-Borne Viral Diseases

West Nile

West Nile virus is a disease that is spread to individuals by a mosquito bite. People with healthy immune systems may be infected with this disease and have only mild symptoms such as fever or headache. People with weakened immune systems and the elderly may experience complications.

EXAMPLE   West Nile virus, 066.40 (A92.30).

EXAMPLE   West Nile encephalitis, 066.41 (A92.31).

FIGURE 9-4. Genital herpes in the female patient **(A)** and the male patient **(B)**.

Other Diseases Due to Viruses and *Chlamydiae*

Hepatitis

Hepatitis is inflammation of the liver and can be caused by, among other things, several different viruses, namely, A, B, C, D, and E. All of theses strains of hepatitis cause acute viral hepatitis. Only B, C, and D viruses cause chronic hepatitis. In chronic hepatitis, the infection may last a lifetime. Symptoms of hepatitis include fatigue, jaundice, nausea and vomiting, headache, diarrhea, and fever.

Hepatitis A is most commonly spread via food or water that has been contaminated by feces from an infected person. International travelers are at risk for this disease. A vaccine is available. If contracted, this disease usually resolves on its own.

Hepatitis B is spread through contact with infected blood, via sex with an infected person, or during childbirth. A hepatitis B vaccine is available. In the past, this disease may have been acquired during a blood transfusion, but in 1992, testing was instituted to control infection transmitted through the blood supply. Acute hepatitis B usually resolves on its own, but chronic cases require drug treatment. Hepatitis B may cause cirrhosis of the liver, liver failure, and liver cancer. About 10% of those infected with the B virus may become carriers. A carrier will have the B virus in his or her blood for 6 months or longer after the original infection subsides.

Hepatitis C is spread through infected blood, sexual contact, and childbirth. No vaccine is available for this disease; the only way to prevent it is through avoidance of risky behaviors such as needle sharing. Patients with chronic hepatitis C are treated with medications.

Hepatitis D is spread through infected blood. To acquire hepatitis D, a patient must already have a hepatitis B infection. Those with chronic hepatitis D are treated with medications. This form was formerly known as hepatitis delta.

Hepatitis E is spread through food or water that has been contaminated by feces from an infected person; it is unusual in the United Sates. No vaccine is available, and an outbreak usually resolves on its own.

The 070 category for viral hepatitis can be used with the following fifth digits:
- 0 Acute and unspecified, without mention of hepatitis delta
- 1 Acute or unspecified, with hepatitis delta
- 2 Chronic, without mention of hepatitis delta
- 3 Chronic, with hepatitis delta

EXAMPLE

> Patient admitted is jaundiced and has chronic hepatitis B, 070.32 (B18.1).

EXAMPLE

> Patient has elevated liver function tests and was diagnosed with alcoholic hepatitis. Patient drinks alcohol on a daily basis, 571.1, 303.91 (K70.10, F10.20).

Codes are also available for carriers of viral hepatitis B, C, or D. These people have no symptoms, but the condition is identified by laboratory testing.

EXAMPLE

> Hepatitis B carrier, V02.61 (Z22.51).

Rickettsioses and Other Arthropod-Borne Diseases

Lyme disease, also known as borreliosis, is an inflammatory disease caused by bacteria carried by ticks. Ticks acquire this bacterium through biting deer that are infected. It was first reported in the Northeast United States but now has spread throughout the Midwest, as well as the Pacific Coast. The symptoms of this disease resemble the flu and include headache, fever, and muscle aches. Sometimes, a bull's-eye rash appears at the site of the tick bite.

A blood test can be performed to look for antibodies to the bacteria that cause Lyme disease. Treatment for Lyme disease consists of antibiotics and anti-inflammatory medicines. If this disease is left untreated, complications such as Lyme arthritis, heart problems, or neurologic disorders can occur.

EXAMPLE

> A patient presents with severe joint pain. Blood work reveals Lyme disease. The physician documents that the patient has Lyme arthritis, 088.81, 711.80 (A69.23).

EXERCISE 9-4

Assign codes to the following conditions.

1. Shingles _____
2. Stomatitis due to herpes simplex _____
3. Genital herpes _____
4. Mumps _____
5. Hepatitis B _____
6. Acute hepatitis B with hepatitis delta _____
7. Patient is a carrier of hepatitis C _____

FIGURE 9-5. Chancre of primary syphilis.

Syphilis and Other Venereal Diseases

Syphilis

Syphilis is a sexually transmitted disease (STD) that is caused by bacteria. Syphilis is passed through direct contact with syphilis sores. Sores occur in the vagina, penis, anus, or rectum. They can also occur on the lips and in the mouth. Pregnant women can pass syphilis onto their babies. Syphilis occurs in three stages: primary, secondary, and late.

Primary syphilis is revealed by sores called "**chancres**" (Figure 9-5). These sores can last for 3 to 6 weeks. Treatment with a single injection of penicillin can cure the patient at this stage of the disease.

Secondary syphilis, which usually presents as a rash on the palms of the hands and feet, may be accompanied by fever, sore throat, headache, and fatigue. Lesions also may appear in the mouth, vagina, or penis. Sometimes, warty patches called "**condylomata** lata" may appear on the genitalia. These secondary signs eventually disappear even without treatment, but the infection then progresses to late stages.

Late syphilis is the hidden stage of the disease. No signs or symptoms are noted until it begins to damage internal organs, which may occur years later.

A blood test is performed to test for syphilis. This test is called VDRL (Venereal Disease Research Laboratory), or RPR (rapid plasma reagin).

EXAMPLE | Late neurosyphilis with ataxia, 094.0 (A52.11).

EXAMPLE | Two-year-old presents with syphilitic pemphigus, 090.0 (A50.06).

EXAMPLE | Genital chancre, 091.0 (A51.0).

Gonorrhea

Gonorrhea is caused by a bacterium and is transmitted by sexual contact. Women may have no symptoms, but men usually report burning while urinating and discharge from the penis. Gonorrhea is treated with an antibiotic. If gonorrhea is not treated, complications usually occur.

EXAMPLE | Female patient presents with acute gonococcal cervicitis, 098.15 (A54.03).

EXAMPLE | Male patient presents with chronic prostatitis due to gonorrhea, 098.32 (A54.22).

Mycoses

Candidiasis

Candidiasis is caused by *Candida* fungi. These fungi often live harmlessly within the body until a patient's immune system becomes weak or until he or she is taking medications that reduce the native bacteria that control this fungus. Usual spots in which *Candida* infections are found include the following:

Mouth—thrush is found as white plaques on lips, cheeks, or tongue. It can be seen in babies, people with cancer, and diabetics.

Esophagus—often found in patients with AIDS and those on chemotherapy

Cutaneous—found in warm, moist areas that receive little ventilation, such as diaper areas, buttocks, and skin folds of the abdomen or breasts

Vaginal yeast infections are often caused by birth control pills, pregnancy, or frequent douching. Candidal infections are treated according to the area infected. Patients with thrush are generally treated with nystatin swish and swallow, whereas those with candidal esophagitis are treated with fluconazole. Patients with vaginal yeast infection are treated with antifungals such as Monistat, nystatin, or Vagistat.

EXAMPLE Patient is being treated for candidal intertrigo under breast, 112.3 (B37.2).

Late Effects of Infectious and Parasitic Diseases

Some infections result in **sequelae** or late effects of an acute disease that may be due to an inactive condition. Hemoptysis can be a late effect of tuberculosis caused by residual cavitation of the lung. When late effects are coded, two codes are required. Residual conditions/sequelae are coded first, and the cause of the late effect is coded next. If sequelae are unknown or unspecified, the late effect code may be used alone.

EXAMPLE Patient with hemiplegia following acute poliomyelitis, 342.90; hemiplegia, 138 (G81.90, B91).

EXERCISE 9-5

Assign codes to the following conditions.

1. Patient has a chancre on the penis _____
2. Patient presents with condyloma latum _____
3. Latent syphilis with unknown date of infection _____
4. Dementia due to syphilis _____
5. Early congenital syphilis _____
6. Exposure to gonorrhea _____
7. Suspected carrier of gonorrhea _____
8. Yeast infection of the vagina _____
9. Late effect of tuberculosis _____
10. Myalgia as a late effect of Lyme disease _____

FACTORS INFLUENCING HEALTH STATUS AND CONTACT WITH HEALTH SERVICES (V CODES/Z CODES)

In the past, V/Z codes were primarily considered for use in the outpatient setting. This has changed with the addition of more V/Z codes each year. As was discussed in Chapter 8, it may be difficult to locate V/Z codes in the Index. Coders often say, "I did not know there was a V/Z code for that." Refer to Chapter 8 for a listing of common main terms to locate V/Z codes.

A review of the Tabular reveals that some V/Z codes pertain to infectious and parasitic diseases:

V01.0	Contact or exposure to cholera
V01.1	Contact or exposure to tuberculosis
V01.2	Contact or exposure to poliomyelitis
V01.3	Contact or exposure to smallpox
V01.4	Contact or exposure to rubella
V01.5	Contact or exposure to rabies
V01.6	Contact or exposure to venereal diseases
V01.71	Contact or exposure to varicella
V01.79	Contact or exposure to other viral diseases
V01.81	Contact or exposure to anthrax
V01.82	Exposure to severe acute respiratory syndrome (SARS)-associated coronavirus
V01.83	Contact or exposure to *Escherichia coli*
V01.84	Contact or exposure to *meningococcus*
V01.89	Contact or exposure to other communicable diseases
V02.0	Carrier or suspected carrier of cholera
V02.1	Carrier or suspected carrier of typhoid
V02.2	Carrier or suspected carrier of amebiasis
V02.3	Carrier or suspected carrier of other gastrointestinal pathogens
V02.4	Carrier or suspected carrier of diphtheria
V02.51	Carrier or suspected carrier of group B streptococcus
V02.52	Carrier or suspected carrier of other streptococcus
V02.59	Carrier or suspected carrier of other specified bacterial disease
V02.60	Carrier or suspected carrier of viral hepatitis, unspecified
V02.61	Carrier or suspected carrier of hepatitis B
V02.62	Carrier or suspected carrier of hepatitis C
V02.69	Carrier or suspected carrier of other viral hepatitis
V02.7	Carrier or suspected carrier of gonorrhea
V02.8	Carrier or suspected carrier of other venereal diseases
V02.9	Carrier or suspected carrier of another specified infectious organism
V03.81	*Haemophilus influenzae,* type B (Hib)
V03.82	*Streptococcus pneumoniae* (pneumococcus)
V03.89	Other specified vaccination
V04.0	Need for prophylactic vaccination and inoculation against poliomyelitis
V04.1	Need for prophylactic vaccination and inoculation against Smallpox
V04.2	Need for prophylactic vaccination and inoculation against Measles alone
V04.3	Need for prophylactic vaccination and inoculation against Rubella alone
V04.4	Need for prophylactic vaccination and inoculation against Yellow fever
V04.5	Need for prophylactic vaccination and inoculation against Rabies
V04.6	Need for prophylactic vaccination and inoculation against Mumps alone
V04.7	Need for prophylactic vaccination and inoculation against Common cold
V04.81	Need for prophylactic vaccination and inoculation against Influenza
V04.82	Need for prophylactic vaccination and inoculation against Respiratory syncytial virus (RSV)
V04.89	Need for prophylactic vaccination and inoculation against other viral disease
V05.0	Need for prophylactic vaccination and inoculation against arthropod-borne viral encephalitis
V05.1	Need for prophylactic vaccination and inoculation against other arthropod-borne viral diseases

V05.2	Need for prophylactic vaccination and inoculation against Leishmaniasis
V05.3	Need for prophylactic vaccination and inoculation against viral hepatitis
V05.4	Need for prophylactic vaccination and inoculation against Varicella
V05.8	Need for prophylactic vaccination and inoculation against other specified disease
V05.9	Need for prophylactic vaccination and inoculation against unspecified single disease
V06.0	Need for prophylactic vaccination and inoculation against cholera with typhoid-paratyphoid (cholera TAB)
V06.1	Need for prophylactic vaccination and inoculation against diphtheria-tetanus-pertussis, combined (DTP [DtaP])
V06.2	Need for prophylactic vaccination and inoculation against Diphtheria-tetanus-pertussis with typhoid-paratyphoid (DTP-TAB)
V06.3	Need for prophylactic vaccination and inoculation against Diphtheria-tetanus-pertussis with poliomyelitis (DTP + polio)
V06.4	Need for prophylactic vaccination and inoculation against Measles-mumps-rubella (MMR)
V06.5	Need for prophylactic vaccination and inoculation against Tetanus-diphtheria (Td) (DT)
V06.6	Need for prophylactic vaccination and inoculation against *Streptococcus pneumoniae* (pneumococcus) and influenza
V06.8	Need for prophylactic vaccination and inoculation against other combinations
V06.9	Need for prophylactic vaccination and inoculation against unspecified combined vaccine
V07.0	Need for isolation
V07.1	Need for desensitization to allergens
V07.2	Need for prophylactic immunotherapy
V07.31	Need for prophylactic fluoride administration
V07.39	Need for other prophylactic chemotherapy
V07.4	Need for hormone replacement therapy (post menopausal)
V07.8	Need for other specified prophylactic measure
V07.9	Need for unspecified prophylactic measure
V09.0	Infection with microorganisms resistant to penicillins
V09.1	Infection with microorganisms resistant to cephalosporins and other beta-lactam antibiotics
V09.2	Infection with microorganisms resistant to macrolides
V09.3	Infection with microorganisms resistant to tetracyclines
V09.4	Infection with microorganisms resistant to aminoglycosides
V09.50	Infection with microorganisms resistant to quinolones and fluoroquinolones without mention of resistance to multiple quinolones and fluoroquinolones
V09.51	Infection with microorganisms resistant to quinolones and fluoroquinolones with resistance to multiple quinolones and fluoroquinolones
V09.6	Infection with microorganisms resistant to sulfonamides
V09.70	Infection with microorganisms resistant to other specified antimycobacterial agents without mention of resistance to multiple antimycobacterial agents
V09.71	Infection with microorganisms resistant to other specified antimycobacterial agents with resistance to multiple antimycobacterial agents
V09.80	Infection with microorganisms resistant to other specified drugs without mention of multiple drug resistance
V09.81	Infection with microorganisms resistant to other specified drugs without resistance to multiple drugs
V09.90	Infection with drug-resistant microorganism without mention of multiple drug resistance
V09.91	Infection with drug-resistant microorganism with multiple drug resistance

V12.00	Personal history of unspecified infectious and parasitic disease
V12.01	Personal history of tuberculosis
V12.02	Personal history of poliomyelitis
V12.03	Personal history of malaria
V64.00	Vaccination not carried out, unspecified reason
V64.01	Vaccination not carried out because of acute illness
V64.02	Vaccination not carried out because of chronic illness or condition
V64.03	Vaccination not carried out because of immune compromised state
V64.04	Vaccination not carried out because of allergy to vaccine or component
V64.05	Vaccination not carried out because of caregiver refusal
V64.06	Vaccination not carried out because of patient refusal
V64.07	Vaccination not carried out for religious reasons
V64.08	Vaccination not carried out because patient had disease being vaccinated against
V64.09	Vaccination not carried out for other reason
V65.45	Counseling on other sexually transmitted diseases
V71.2	Observation for suspected tuberculosis
V71.82	Observation and evaluation for suspected exposure to anthrax
V73.0	Special screening examination for poliomyelitis
V73.1	Special screening examination for smallpox
V73.2	Special screening examination for measles
V73.3	Special screening examination for rubella
V73.4	Special screening examination for yellow fever
V73.5	Special screening examination for other arthropod-borne viral diseases
V73.6	Special screening examination for trachoma
V73.81	Special screening examination, Human papilloma virus (HPV)
V73.88	Special screening examination for other specified chlamydial diseases
V73.89	Special screening examination for unspecified viral disease
V74.0	Special screening examination for cholera
V74.1	Special screening examination for pulmonary tuberculosis
V74.2	Special screening examination for leprosy (Hansen's disease)
V74.3	Special screening examination for diphtheria
V74.4	Special screening examination for bacterial conjunctivitis
V74.5	Special screening examination for venereal disease
V74.6	Special screening examination for yaws
V74.8	Special screening examination for other specified bacterial and spirochetal diseases
V74.9	Special screening examination for unspecified bacterial and spirochetal disease
V75.0	Special screening examination for rickettsial diseases
V75.1	Special screening examination for malaria
V75.2	Special screening examination for leishmaniasis
V75.3	Special screening examination for Trypanosomiasis
V75.4	Special screening examination for Mycotic infections
V75.5	Special screening examination for Schistosomiasis
V75.6	Special screening examination for Filariasis
V75.7	Special screening examination for Intestinal helminthiasis
V75.8	Special screening examination for Other specified parasitic infections
V75.9	Special screening examination for unspecified infectious disease

EXAMPLE Student presents to health clinic after exposure to meningococcus, V01.84 (Z20.811).

EXAMPLE	Admitted for observation for TB, V71.2 (Z03.89).

EXERCISE 9-6

Assign codes to the following condition.

1. History of malaria   _____

2. Exposure to chickenpox at daycare   _____

3. Patient returning from China; was exposed to SARS   _____

4. Patient needs vaccination for cholera   _____

5. Influenza vaccination not administered because patient is hospitalized with pneumonia   _____

COMMON TREATMENTS

See Table 9-1 for drugs commonly used to treat infectious diseases.

PROCEDURES

There are multiple therapeutic and diagnostic procedures that can be performed for infectious and parasitic diseases. There is no specific procedure chapter for infectious and parasitic diseases.

DOCUMENTATION/REIMBURSEMENT/MS-DRGs

Often, coding difficulties are due to lack of documentation. Sometimes pathology and other test results are not available at the time of discharge or when the physician is dictating the discharge summary or is reporting the final diagnoses.

Frequently missed complications and comorbidities from the Infectious and Parasitic Diseases chapter include the following:

* Sepsis
* Food poisoning
* Intestinal infections
* Herpes
* Post-herpetic conditions
* Viral hepatitis
* Lyme disease
* Candidiasis
* Tuberculosis
* Histoplasmosis

Causative Organism

When coding meningitis, the record should be reviewed for the causative organism.

EXAMPLE	DIAGNOSES	CODE	MS-DRG	RW
	Viral meningitis	047.9 (A87.9)	076	0.9050
	Salmonella meningitis	003.21 (A02.21)	096	1.9247

TABLE 9-1 DRUGS FOR INFECTIOUS DISEASES[6]

Drug Category	Drug Action	Examples	Side Effects	Comments
Antibiotics	Destroy or inhibit the growth of bacterial strains or microorganisms but have not been found to be effective for viral infections	Penicillin V Potassium (Pen-V-K) Tetracycline (Sumycin) Amoxicillin (Amoxil) Cephalosporins (Keflex, Ceclor) Ciprofloxacin (Cipro) Metronidazole (Flagyl) Azithromycin (Zithromax)	Common side effects of any are nausea, GI upset, urticaria	Caution must be used when administering penicillin IM regarding observation after infection for potential of anaphylaxis Cipro: acute infections and prophylactic postanthrax exposure
Antifungals	Inhibit and kill fungal growth	Griseofulvin (Grisactin) Ketoconazole (Nizoral) Clotrimazole (Lotrimin) Fluconazole (Diflucan)	Nausea, vomiting, abdominal pain, itching, urticaria	Some are available in oral form for systemic treatment, others are available in topical form
Antivirals	Inhibit viral growth	Acyclovir (Zovirax) Zidovudine (Retrovir) Amantadine (Symmetrel)	GI disturbances, headache, malaise, insomnia, dizziness	Should be taken at first sign of onset of viral attack for best relief of symptoms
Antiretrovirals	Treat infection by retroviruses	NRTIs (Retrovir, AZT, Epivir, Abacavir) NNRTIs (Sustiva, Viramunde) Protease inhibitors (Kaletra, Norvir)	Often have severe side effects; side effects are many and varied and can include anemia, GI problems, wasting, acidosis, bone problems	Given in combination
Antiprotozoals	Inhibit protozoal infections	Chloroquine HCl (Aralen HCl)	Headache, pruritus, GI disturbances, tinnitus	Also known as antimalarials
Antipyretics	Reduce fever	Acetaminophen (Tylenol) Acetylsalicylic acid (aspirin) Ibuprofen (Motrin)	Toxic doses of acetaminophen may cause irreversible and fatal liver damage	Caution must be exercised when administering Tylenol drops and syrup to infants and children; check dosage for either before administering
Antitubercular	Suppress mycobacterium causing tuberculosis	Isoniazid (INH) Ethambutol (Myambutol)	GI disturbances, hepatic disturbances	Usually given in combination

AIDS and AIDS Manifestations

Coding AIDS, HIV, and any manifestations correctly is very important to MS-DRG assignment.

EXAMPLE

DIAGNOSES	CODE	MS-DRG	RW
AIDS	042 (B20)	977	1.0486
AIDS with candidal esophagitis	042, 112.84 (B20, B37.81)	976	0.8975
AIDS with candidal esophagitis and acute respiratory failure	042, 112.84, 518.81 (B20, B37.81, J96.00)	974	2.5849

For reimbursement purposes, the coder must be aware of possible sepsis on admission. This condition may be suspected at the time of admission, and blood cultures may be taken. Results of the blood cultures may not become positive until several days into the patient's hospital stay. This does not mean that the condition was not present on admission.

CHAPTER REVIEW EXERCISE

Where applicable, assign codes for diagnoses and procedures.

1. Gastroenteritis due to *Salmonella* _____
2. Food poisoning _____
3. UTI due to candidiasis _____
4. Diarrhea due to *Clostridium difficile* _____
5. Rotavirus _____
6. Infectious colitis _____
7. Primary TB; patient in isolation _____
8. TB of the hip bone _____
9. Tuberculosis lichenoides _____
10. Bubonic plague _____
11. Gastrointestinal anthrax _____
12. Whooping cough with pneumonia _____
13. DMAC _____
14. Meningococcal endocarditis _____
15. MSSA sepsis _____
16. *Haemophilus influenzae* septicemia _____
17. Acute prostatitis due to *E. coli* _____
18. HIV positive _____
19. AIDS with Burkitt's lymphoma _____
20. Postherpetic syndrome _____

CHAPTER GLOSSARY

AIDS: acquired immunodeficiency syndrome, an incurable disease of the immune system caused by a virus.

Anthrax: a bacterial infection usually found in wild or domestic animals.

Bacteremia: bacteria in blood, which is a laboratory finding.

Candidiasis: a fungal infection and is also known as a yeast infection.

Chancre: an ulcer that forms during the first stage of syphilis.

Clostridium difficile: microorganisms that are a leading cause of pseudomembranous colitis; also known as *C. diff.*

Communicable: easily spread from one person to another.

Condyloma: wart-type growth found usually in the genital or anal area.

Gonorrhea: disease caused by a bacterium and transmitted by sexual contact.

HAART: highly active antiretroviral therapy, a group of drugs given to AIDS patients for prophylaxis.

Hepatitis: an inflammation of the liver.

Herpes simplex: a virus also known as a *cold sore* or *fever blister.*

Herpes zoster: a disease caused by the same virus that causes chickenpox.

HIV: human immunodeficiency virus, the virus that affects the immune system and can progress to AIDS.

Lyme disease: an inflammatory disease caused by bacteria carried by ticks.

Meningitis: an infection in the fluid of a person's spinal cord and brain.

Mycobacterium avium-intercellulare: a mycobacteria found in soil and water.

Nadir: the lowest level.

Nosocomial: hospital-acquired infection.

Parasitic: organism that lives on or takes nourishment from another organism.

Poliomyelitis: a viral disease that affects the nerves.

Sepsis: SIRS due to infection.

Septic shock: a condition caused by infection and sepsis. It can cause multiple organ failure and death.

Septicemia: the presence in the blood of pathologic microorganisms that cause systemic illness.

Sequelae: late or residual effect of an acute disease.

SIRS: systemic inflammatory response syndrome, which can be caused by infection or trauma.

Syphilis: a sexually transmitted disease (STD) that is caused by bacteria.

Tuberculosis (TB): an infection caused by *Mycobacterium tuberculosis*.

Urosepsis: infection of urinary site

Viral meningitis: a viral infection of the fluid in the spinal cord and around the brain.

West Nile: a viral disease that is spread to individuals by a mosquito bite.

REFERENCES

1. American Hospital Association. *Coding Clinic for ICD-9-CM* 2002:4Q:p78. Contact/exposure.
2. American Hospital Association. *Coding Clinic for ICD-9-CM* 1997:4Q:p3. Disseminated *Mycobacterium avium-intracellulare* complex.
3. American Hospital Association. *Coding Clinic for ICD-9-CM* 2000:2Q:p5-6. Bacteremia vs septicemia.
4. American Hospital Association. *Coding Clinic for ICD-9-CM* 2003:4Q:p79-81. Septicemia, SIRS, sepsis, severe sepsis, and septic shock.
5. Castro KG, Ward JW, Slutsker L, Buehler JW, Jaffe HW, Berkelman RL (National Center for Infectious Diseases Division of HIV/AIDS).

1993 revised classification system for HIV infection and expanded surveillance: Case definition for AIDS among adolescents and adults. *Morb Mortal Wkly Rep*, 41(RR-17), December 18, 1992. Bethesda, Md, Centers for Disease Control and Prevention. Available at: http://www.cdc.gov/mmwr/preview/mmwrhtml/00018871.htm. Accessed April 4, 2008.
6. Modified from Frazier ME, Drzymkowki JW. *Essentials of Human Diseases and Conditions*, 3rd ed. St. Louis, Saunders, 2004, Appendix II, pp 766-767.

Neoplasms

(ICD-9-CM Chapter 2, Codes 140-239, and ICD-10-CM Chapter 2, Codes C00-D49)

LEARNING OBJECTIVES

1. Apply and assign the correct ICD-9-CM and ICD-10-CM codes in accordance with Official Guidelines for Coding and Reporting
2. Identify major differences between ICD-9-CM and ICD-10-CM related to neoplasms

3. Identify pertinent anatomy and physiology for neoplasm
4. Assign the correct M codes
5. Identify neoplastic diseases
6. Assign the correct V/Z codes and procedure codes related to neoplasms
7. Identify common treatments, medications, laboratory values, and diagnostic tests
8. Explain the importance of documentation in relation to MS-DRGs for reimbursement

ABBREVIATIONS/ ACRONYMS

AIDS acquired immunodeficiency syndrome

ALL acute lymphocytic leukemia

BMR biological response modifier

BMT bone marrow transplant

CC chief complaint

CDC Centers for Disease Control and Prevention

CLL chronic lymphocytic leukemia

CML chronic myelogenous leukemia

CNS central nervous system

DCIS ductal carcinoma in situ

FNA fine needle aspiration

HCC hepatocellular carcinoma

ICD-9-CM *International Classification of Diseases, 9th revision, Clinical Modification*

ICD-10-CM *International Classification of Diseases, 10th Revision, Clinical Modification*

ICD-10-PCS *International Classification of Diseases, 10th*

Revision, Procedure Coding System

MS-DRG Medicare severity diagnosis-related group

NHL non-Hodgkin's lymphoma

NSCLC non–small cell lung cancer

RCC renal cell carcinoma

SCLC small cell lung cancer

UHDDS Uniform Hospital Discharge Data Set

ICD-9-CM

Official Guidelines for Coding and Reporting

Please refer to the companion Evolve website for the most current guidelines.

2. Chapter 2: Neoplasms (140-239)

<u>General guidelines</u>

Chapter 2 of the ICD-9-CM contains the codes for most benign and all malignant neoplasms. Certain benign neoplasms, such as prostatic adenomas, may be found in the specific body system chapters. To properly code a neoplasm it is necessary to determine from the record if the neoplasm is benign, in-situ, malignant, or of uncertain histologic behavior. If malignant, any secondary (metastatic) sites should also be determined.

The neoplasm table in the Alphabetic Index should be referenced first. However, if the histological term is documented, that term should be referenced first, rather than going immediately to the Neoplasm Table, in order to determine which column in the Neoplasm Table is appropriate. For example, if the documentation indicates "adenoma," refer to the term in the Alphabetic Index to review the entries under this term and the instructional note to "see also neoplasm, by site, benign." The table provides the proper code based on the type of neoplasm and the site. It is important to select the proper column in the table that corresponds to the type of neoplasm. The tabular should then be referenced to verify that the correct code has been selected from the table and that a more specific site code does not exist. *See Section I. C. 18.d.4. for information regarding V codes for genetic susceptibility to cancer.*

a. Treatment directed at the malignancy

If the treatment is directed at the malignancy, designate the malignancy as the principal diagnosis.

The only exception to this guideline is if a patient admission/encounter is solely for the administration of chemotherapy, immunotherapy or radiation therapy, assign the appropriate V58.x code as the first-listed or principal diagnosis, and the diagnosis or problem for which the service is being performed as a secondary diagnosis.

EXAMPLE

The patient had a prostatectomy and a bilateral pelvic lymphadenectomy for prostate acinar adenocarcinoma. Treatment is directed to the primary cancer of the prostate, 185, 60.5, 40.3 (C61, 0VT00ZZ, 07BC0ZZ).

b. Treatment of secondary site

When a patient is admitted because of a primary neoplasm with metastasis and treatment is directed toward the secondary site only, the secondary neoplasm is designated as the principal diagnosis even though the primary malignancy is still present.

EXAMPLE

Three months ago, the patient was given a diagnosis of small cell lung carcinoma with metastasis to the liver. The patient's primary neoplasm is lung carcinoma; the secondary neoplasm is located in the liver. The patient underwent wedge resection for liver metastasis, 197.7, 162.9, 50.22 (C78.7 C34.90, 0FB00ZZ).

c. Coding and sequencing of complications

Coding and sequencing of complications associated with the malignancies or with the therapy thereof are subject to the following guidelines:

1) Anemia associated with malignancy

When admission/encounter is for management of an anemia associated with the malignancy, and the treatment is only for anemia, the appropriate anemia code (such as code 285.22, Anemia in neoplastic disease) is designated as the principal diagnosis and is followed by the appropriate code(s) for the malignancy.

Code 285.22 may also be used as a secondary code if the patient suffers from anemia and is being treated for the malignancy.

Code 285.22, Anemia in neoplastic disease, and code 285.3, Antineoplastic chemotherapy induced anemia, may both be assigned if anemia in neoplastic disease and anemia due to antineoplastic chemotherapy are both documented.

EXAMPLE

Anemia due to metastatic bone cancer. The patient has a history of primary breast cancer, which was treated with mastectomy 4 years ago. The patient was admitted for transfusion of packed red blood cells (percutaneous peripheral vein), 285.22, 198.5, V10.3, V45.71, 99.04 (C79.51, D63.0, Z85.3, Z90.10, 30233N1. ICD-10-CM instructs to code neoplasm first when anemia is due to neoplasm).

2) Anemia associated with chemotherapy, immunotherapy and radiation therapy

When the admission/encounter is for management of an anemia associated with chemotherapy, immunotherapy or radiotherapy and the only treatment is for the anemia, the anemia is sequenced first followed by code E933.1. The appropriate neoplasm code should be assigned as an additional code.

EXAMPLE

Aplastic anemia due to radiation. The patient is being treated for cancer of the brain. The patient was transfused with 2 units of packed red blood cells (percutaneous peripheral vein), 284.89, 191.9, V15.3, E879.2, 99.04 (D61.2, C71.9, Y84.2, 30233N1).

3) Management of dehydration due to the malignancy

When the admission/encounter is for management of dehydration due to the malignancy or the therapy, or a combination of both, and only the dehydration is being treated (intravenous rehydration), the dehydration is sequenced first, followed by the code(s) for the malignancy.

EXAMPLE

The patient underwent chemotherapy treatment a few days ago, and since that time has become severely dehydrated. The patient is receiving chemo for treatment of cancer of the colon, 276.51, 153.9 (E86.0, C18.9).

4) Treatment of a complication resulting from a surgical procedure
When the admission/encounter is for treatment of a complication resulting from a surgical procedure, designate the complication as the principal or first-listed diagnosis if treatment is directed at resolving the complication.

EXAMPLE | Hernia of colostomy with repair of parastomal hernia. The colostomy was performed 1 year ago during colon cancer resection. The patient is no longer receiving treatment, and the cancer was completely resected, 569.69, V10.05, 46.42 (K94.09, Z85.038, 0WQFXZ2).

d. Primary malignancy previously excised
When a primary malignancy has been previously excised or eradicated from its site and there is no further treatment directed to that site and there is no evidence of any existing primary malignancy, a code from category V10, Personal history of malignant neoplasm, should be used to indicate the former site of the malignancy. Any mention of extension, invasion, or metastasis to another site is coded as a secondary malignant neoplasm to that site. The secondary site may be the principal or first-listed with the V10 code used as a secondary code.

EXAMPLE | The patient had a melanoma removed from his back 4 years ago. The patient is currently being treated for metastatic melanoma of the lung, 197.0, V10.82 (C78.00, Z85.820).

e. Admissions/Encounters involving chemotherapy, immunotherapy and radiation therapy
   1) Episode of care involves surgical removal of neoplasm.
   When an episode of care involves the surgical removal of a neoplasm, primary or secondary site, followed by adjunct chemotherapy or radiation treatment during the same episode of care, the neoplasm code should be assigned as principal or first-listed diagnosis, using codes in the 140-198 series or where appropriate in the 200-203 series.

EXAMPLE | The patient had a modified radical mastectomy for malignant neoplasm of the right (upper outer quadrant) breast with adjunct chemotherapy (percutaneous central vein), 174.4, 85.43, 99.25 (C50.411, 0HTT0ZZ, 3E04305).

   2) Patient admission/encounter solely for administration of chemotherapy, immunotherapy and radiation therapy
   If a patient admission/encounter is solely for the administration of chemotherapy, immunotherapy or radiation therapy assign code V58.0, Encounter for radiation therapy, or V58.11, Encounter for antineoplastic chemotherapy, or V58.12, Encounter for antineoplastic immunotherapy as the first-listed or principal diagnosis. If a patient receives more than one of these therapies during the same admission more than one of these codes may be assigned, in any sequence.

EXAMPLE | The patient was admitted for chemotherapy (percutaneous central vein) treatment of acute lymphocytic leukemia (ALL), V58.11, 204.00, 99.25 (Z51.11, C91.00, 3E04305).

3) Patient admitted for radiotherapy/chemotherapy and immunotherapy and develops complications

When a patient is admitted for the purpose of radiotherapy, immunotherapy or chemotherapy and develops complications such as uncontrolled nausea and vomiting or dehydration, the principal or first-listed diagnosis is V58.0, Encounter for radiotherapy, or V58.11, Encounter for antineoplastic chemotherapy, or V58.12, Encounter for antineoplastic immunotherapy followed by any codes for the complications.

EXAMPLE The patient was admitted for chemotherapy (percutaneous peripheral artery) for lymphoma. Because of nausea and severe vomiting due to the chemotherapy, the patient was also treated for dehydration with IV fluids, V58.11, 202.80, 276.51, 787.01, 99.25 (Z51.11, C85.90, E86.0, T45.1x5A, R11.2, 3E05305).

f. Admission/encounter to determine extent of malignancy

When the reason for admission/encounter is to determine the extent of the malignancy, or for a procedure such as paracentesis or thoracentesis, the primary malignancy or appropriate metastatic site is designated as the principal or first-listed diagnosis, even though chemotherapy or radiotherapy is administered.

EXAMPLE Patient has known carcinoma of the left kidney and left pleural effusion. Patient is admitted to determine if the renal cancer has spread and a thoracentesis is done, which confirms metastasis to the pleura, 197.2, 511.81, 189.0, 34.91 (C78.2, J91.0, C64.1, 0W9B3ZX).

g. Symptoms, signs, and ill-defined conditions listed in Chapter 16 associated with neoplasms

Symptoms, signs, and ill-defined conditions listed in Chapter 16 characteristic of, or associated with, an existing primary or secondary site malignancy cannot be used to replace the malignancy as principal or first-listed diagnosis, regardless of the number of admissions or encounters for treatment and care of the neoplasm.
See section I.C.18.d.14, Encounter for prophylactic organ removal.

EXAMPLE The patient was admitted with a first-time seizure due to brain cancer. The code 780.39 for seizure can be found in Chapter 16, so the brain cancer code would be sequenced as the principal diagnosis, 191.9, 780.39 (C71.9, R56.9). Not all patients with brain cancer develop seizures, so it is appropriate to code the seizure code as a secondary diagnosis.

h. Admission/encounter for pain control/management

See Section I.C.6.a.5 for information on coding admission/encounter for pain control/ management.

i. Malignant neoplasm associated with transplanted organ

A malignant neoplasm of a transplanted organ should be coded as a transplant complication. Assign first the appropriate code from subcategory 996.8, Complications of transplanted organ, followed by code 199.2, Malignant neoplasm associated with transplanted organ. Use an additional code for the specific malignancy.

EXAMPLE Patient was diagnosed with hepatocellular carcinoma. Patient had a liver transplant 2 years ago, 996.82, 199.2, 155.0, E878.0 (T86.49, C80.2, C22.0, Y83.0).

6. **Chapter 6: Diseases of Nervous System and Sense Organs (320-389)**
   a. **Pain—Category 338**
      5) **Neoplasm Related Pain**
         Code 338.3 is assigned to pain documented as being related, associated or due to cancer, primary or secondary malignancy, or tumor. This code is assigned regardless of whether the pain is acute or chronic.

         This code may be assigned as the principal or first-listed code when the stated reason for the admission/encounter is documented as pain control/pain management. The underlying neoplasm should be reported as an additional diagnosis.

         When the reason for the admission/encounter is management of the neoplasm and the pain associated with the neoplasm is also documented, code 338.3 may be assigned as an additional diagnosis.

         See Section I.C.2 for instructions on the sequencing of neoplasms for all other stated reasons for the admission/encounter (except for pain control/pain management).

EXAMPLE | Patient is admitted for pain control due to metastatic bone cancer. Patient has a past history of primary breast cancer, 338.3, 198.5, V10.3 (G89.3, C79.51, Z85.3).

Apply the General Coding Guidelines as found in Chapter 5 and the Procedural Guidelines as found in Chapter 6.

ICD-10-CM

Official Guidelines for Coding and Reporting

Please refer to the companion Evolve website for the most current guidelines.

2. **Chapter 2: Neoplasms (C00-D49)**

   General guidelines

   Chapter 2 of the ICD-10-CM contains the codes for most benign and all malignant neoplasms. Certain benign neoplasms, such as prostatic adenomas, may be found in the specific body system chapters. To properly code a neoplasm it is necessary to determine from the record if the neoplasm is benign, in-situ, malignant, or of uncertain histologic behavior. If malignant, any secondary (metastatic) sites should also be determined.

   The neoplasm table in the Alphabetic Index should be referenced first. However, if the histological term is documented, that term should be referenced first, rather than going immediately to the Neoplasm Table, in order to determine which column in the Neoplasm Table is appropriate. For example, if the documentation indicates "adenoma," refer to the term in the Alphabetic Index to review the entries under this term and the instructional note to "see also neoplasm, by site, benign." The table provides the proper code based on the type of neoplasm and the site. It is important to select the proper column in the table that corresponds to the type of neoplasm. The **Tabular List** should then be referenced to verify that the correct code has been selected from the table and that a more specific site code does not exist.

   See Section I.C.21. Factors influencing health status and contact with health services, Status, for information regarding Z15.0, codes for genetic susceptibility to cancer.

   a. **Treatment directed at the malignancy**

      If the treatment is directed at the malignancy, designate the malignancy as the principal diagnosis.

      The only exception to this guideline is if a patient admission/encounter is solely for the administration of chemotherapy, immunotherapy or radiation therapy, assign the appropriate Z51.– code as the first-listed or principal diagnosis, and the diagnosis or problem for which the service is being performed as a secondary diagnosis.

   b. **Treatment of secondary site**

      When a patient is admitted because of a primary neoplasm with metastasis and treatment is directed toward the secondary site only, the secondary neoplasm is designated as the principal diagnosis even though the primary malignancy is still present.

   c. **Coding and sequencing of complications**

      Coding and sequencing of complications associated with the malignancies or with the therapy thereof are subject to the following guidelines:

1) **Anemia associated with malignancy**

When admission/encounter is for management of an anemia associated with the malignancy, and the treatment is only for anemia, the appropriate code for the malignancy is sequenced as the principal or first-listed diagnosis followed by code D63.0, Anemia in neoplastic disease).

2) **Anemia associated with chemotherapy, immunotherapy and radiation therapy**

When the admission/encounter is for management of an anemia associated with an adverse effect of chemotherapy, immunotherapy or radiotherapy and the only treatment is for the anemia, the appropriate adverse effect code should be sequenced first, followed by the appropriate codes for the anemia and neoplasm.

When the admission/encounter is for management of an anemia associated with an adverse effect of radiotherapy, the anemia code should be sequenced first, followed by the appropriate neoplasm code and code Y84.2, Radiological procedure and radiotherapy as the cause of abnormal reaction of the patient, or of later complication, without mention of misadventure at the time of the procedure.

3) **Management of dehydration due to the malignancy**

When the admission/encounter is for management of dehydration due to the malignancy and only the dehydration is being treated (intravenous rehydration), the dehydration is sequenced first, followed by the code(s) for the malignancy.

4) **Treatment of a complication resulting from a surgical procedure**

When the admission/encounter is for treatment of a complication resulting from a surgical procedure, designate the complication as the principal or first-listed diagnosis if treatment is directed at resolving the complication.

d. **Primary malignancy previously excised**

When a primary malignancy has been previously excised or eradicated from its site and there is no further treatment directed to that site and there is no evidence of any existing primary malignancy, a code from category Z85, Personal history of malignant neoplasm, should be used to indicate the former site of the malignancy. Any mention of extension, invasion, or metastasis to another site is coded as a secondary malignant neoplasm to that site. The secondary site may be the principal or first-listed with the Z85 code used as a secondary code.

e. **Admissions/Encounters involving chemotherapy, immunotherapy and radiation therapy**

1) **Episode of care involves surgical removal of neoplasm**

When an episode of care involves the surgical removal of a neoplasm, primary or secondary site, followed by adjunct chemotherapy or radiation treatment during the same episode of care, the **code for the neoplasm should be assigned as principal or first-listed diagnosis.**

2) **Patient admission/encounter solely for administration of chemotherapy, immunotherapy and radiation therapy**

If a patient admission/encounter is solely for the administration of chemotherapy, immunotherapy or radiation therapy assign code Z51.0, Encounter for antineoplastic radiation therapy, or Z51.11, Encounter for antineoplastic chemotherapy, or Z51.12, Encounter for antineoplastic immunotherapy as the first-listed or principal diagnosis. If a patient receives more than one of these therapies during the same admission more than one of these codes may be assigned, in any sequence.

The malignancy for which the therapy is being administered should be assigned as a secondary diagnosis.

3) **Patient admitted for radiation therapy, chemotherapy or immunotherapy and develops complications**

When a patient is admitted for the purpose of radiotherapy, immunotherapy or chemotherapy and develops complications such as uncontrolled nausea and vomiting or dehydration, the principal or first-listed diagnosis is Z51.0, Encounter for antineoplastic radiation therapy, or Z51.11, Encounter for antineoplastic chemotherapy, or Z51.12, Encounter for antineoplastic immunotherapy followed by any codes for the complications.

f. **Admission/encounter to determine extent of malignancy**

When the reason for admission/encounter is to determine the extent of the malignancy, or for a procedure such as paracentesis or thoracentesis, the primary malignancy or appropriate metastatic site is designated as the principal or first-listed diagnosis, even though chemotherapy or radiotherapy is administered.

g. **Symptoms, signs, and abnormal findings listed in Chapter 18 associated with neoplasms**

Symptoms, signs, and ill-defined conditions listed in Chapter 18 characteristic of, or associated with, an existing primary or secondary site malignancy cannot be used to replace the malignancy as principal or first-listed diagnosis, regardless of the number of admissions or encounters for treatment and care of the neoplasm.

See section I.C.21. Factors influencing health status and contact with health services, Encounter for prophylactic organ removal.

h. **Admission/encounter for pain control/management**

See Section I.C.6. for information on coding admission/encounter for pain control/ management.

i. **Malignancy in two or more noncontiguous sites**

A patient may have more than one malignant tumor in the same organ. These tumors may represent different primaries or metastatic disease, depending on the site. Should the documentation be unclear, the provider should be queried as to the status of each tumor so that the correct codes can be assigned.

j. **Disseminated malignant neoplasm, unspecified**

Code C80.0, Disseminated malignant neoplasm, unspecified, is for use only in those cases where the patient has advanced metastatic disease and no known primary or secondary sites are specified. It should not be used in place of assigning codes for the primary site and all known secondary sites.

k. **Malignant neoplasm without specification of site**

Code C80.1, Malignant **(primary)** neoplasm, unspecified, equates to Cancer, unspecified. This code should only be used when no determination can be made as to the primary site of a malignancy. This code should rarely be used in the inpatient setting.

l. **Sequencing of neoplasm codes**

1) **Encounter for treatment of primary malignancy**

If the reason for the encounter is for treatment of a primary malignancy, assign the malignancy as the principal/**first-listed** diagnosis. The primary site is to be sequenced first, followed by any metastatic sites.

2) **Encounter for treatment of secondary malignancy**

When an encounter is for a primary malignancy with metastasis and treatment is directed toward the metastatic (secondary) site(s) only, the metastatic site(s) is designated as the principal/first listed diagnosis. The primary malignancy is coded as an additional code.

3) **Malignant neoplasm in a pregnant patient**

When a pregnant woman has a malignant neoplasm, a code from subcategory **O9A.1-**, Malignant neoplasm complicating pregnancy, childbirth, and the puerperium, should be **sequenced** first, followed by the appropriate code from Chapter 2 to indicate the type of neoplasm.

4) **Encounter for complication associated with a neoplasm**

When an encounter is for management of a complication associated with a neoplasm, such as dehydration, and the treatment is only for the complication, the complication is coded first, followed by the appropriate code(s) for the neoplasm.

The exception to this guideline is anemia. When the admission/encounter is for management of an anemia associated with the malignancy, and the treatment is only for anemia, the appropriate code for the malignancy is sequenced as the principal or first-listed diagnosis followed by code D63.0, Anemia in neoplastic disease.

5) **Complication from surgical procedure for treatment of a neoplasm**

When an encounter is for treatment of a complication resulting from a surgical procedure performed for the treatment of the neoplasm, designate the complication as the principal/**first-listed** diagnosis. See guideline regarding the coding of a current malignancy versus personal history to determine if the code for the neoplasm should also be assigned.

6) **Pathologic fracture due to a neoplasm**

When an encounter is for a pathological fracture due to a neoplasm, if the focus of treatment is the fracture, a code from subcategory M84.5, Pathological fracture in neoplastic disease, should be sequenced first, followed by the code for the neoplasm.

If the focus of treatment is the neoplasm with an associated pathological fracture, the neoplasm code should be sequenced first, followed by a code from M84.5 for the pathological fracture.

m. Current malignancy versus personal history of malignancy

When a primary malignancy has been excised but further treatment, such as an additional surgery for the malignancy, radiation therapy or chemotherapy is directed to that site, the primary malignancy code should be used until treatment is completed.

When a primary malignancy has been previously excised or eradicated from its site, there is no further treatment (of the malignancy) directed to that site, and there is no evidence of any existing primary malignancy, a code from category Z85, Personal history of malignant neoplasm, should be used to indicate the former site of the malignancy.

See Section I.C.21. Factors influencing health status and contact with health services, History (of)

n. Leukemia, *Multiple Myeloma, and Malignant Plasma Cell Neoplasms* in remission versus personal history

The categories for leukemia, and category C90, Multiple myeloma **and malignant plasma cell neoplasms**, have codes for in remission. There are also codes Z85.6, Personal history of leukemia, and Z85.79, Personal history of other malignant neoplasms of lymphoid, hematopoietic and related tissues. If the documentation is unclear, as to whether the patient is in remission, the provider should be queried.

See Section I.C.21. Factors influencing health status and contact with health services, History (of)

o. Aftercare following surgery for neoplasm

See Section I.C.21. Factors influencing health status and contact with health services, Aftercare

p. Follow-up care for completed treatment of a malignancy

See Section I.C.21. Factors influencing health status and contact with health services, Follow-up

q. Prophylactic organ removal for prevention of malignancy

See Section I.C. 21, Factors influencing health status and contact with health services, Prophylactic organ removal

r. Malignant neoplasm associated with transplanted organ

A malignant neoplasm of a transplanted organ should be coded as a transplant complication. Assign first the appropriate code from category T86.-, Complications of transplanted **organs and tissue**, followed by code C80.2, Malignant neoplasm associated with transplanted organ. Use an additional code for the specific malignancy.

Apply the General Coding Guidelines as found in Chapter 5 and the Procedural Guidelines as found in Chapter 7.

GUIDELINE DIFFERENCES BETWEEN ICD-9-CM AND ICD-10-CM

There are additional ICD-10-CM guidelines that address the following:

■ Malignancy in two or more noncontiguous sites
■ Unspecified disseminated malignant neoplasm
■ Malignant neoplasm without specification of site
■ Current malignancy versus personal history of malignancy
■ Leukemia in remission versus personal history of leukemia
■ Sequencing of neoplasm codes when the encounter is for treatment of:
   • Primary malignancy
   • Secondary malignancy
   • Malignant neoplasm in a pregnant patient
   • Complication associated with a neoplasm
   • Complication from surgical procedure for treatment of a neoplasm
   • Pathologic fracture due to a neoplasm

MAJOR DIFFERENCES BETWEEN ICD-9-CM AND ICD-10-CM

- In ICD-10-CM, when an encounter is for the management of anemia associated with malignancy, the malignancy is sequenced as the principal or first-listed diagnosis because of an instructional note, and there is a guideline that addresses this situation.
- There is a change in terminology for neoplasm codes that could be identified with regard to remission status. The terminology in ICD-9-CM is "without mention of remission," but in ICD-10-CM, "not in remission" is used.

ANATOMY AND PHYSIOLOGY

Neoplasms can affect any of the body systems. The anatomy and physiology of these body systems are outlined in their respective chapters. It is important to understand some of the terminology that is specific to neoplasms and their behavior. According to the National Cancer Institute, the most common cancers in the United States include the following:

- Bladder
- Breast
- Colon and rectal
- Endometrial
- Kidney (renal cell)
- Leukemia
- Lung
- Melanoma
- Non-Hodgkin's lymphoma
- Pancreatic
- Prostate
- Skin (nonmelanoma)
- Thyroid

A **neoplasm** is an abnormal tissue that grows by cellular proliferation more rapidly than normal tissue. Neoplasms show partial or complete lack of structural organization and functional coordination with normal tissue, and they usually form a distinct mass of tissue that may be benign (benign tumor) or malignant (cancer) (Figure 10-1). Both benign and malignant neoplasms are classified according to the type of tissue in which they are found. **Benign** neoplasms are tumors that are not malignant. **Malignancy** is a neoplasm that has the ability to invade adjacent structures and spread to distant sites. **Fibromas** are benign neoplasms of fibrous connective tissue, and **melanomas** are malignant changes of melanin cells. Malignant tumors originating from epithelial tissue (e.g., skin, bronchi, stomach) are called **carcinomas** (Table 10-1). Malignancies of epithelial glandular tissue such as those

FIGURE 10-1. Differences between benign and malignant neoplasms.

TABLE 10-1 CARCINOMA AND THE EPITHELIAL TISSUES FROM WHICH THEY DERIVE[1]

Types of Epithelial Tissue	Malignant Tumor (Carcinoma)
Gastrointestinal Tract	
Colon	Adenocarcinoma of the colon
Esophagus	Esophageal carcinoma
Liver	Hepatocellular carcinoma (hepatoma)
Stomach	Gastric adenocarcinoma
Glandular Tissue	
Adrenal glands	Carcinoma of the adrenals
Breast	Carcinoma of the breast
Pancreas	Carcinoma of the pancreas (pancreatic adenocarcinoma)
Prostate	Carcinoma of the prostate
Thyroid	Carcinoma of the thyroid
Kidney and Bladder	
	Renal cell carcinoma (hypernephroma)
	Transitional cell carcinoma of the bladder
Lung	
	Adenocarcinoma (bronchioloalveolar)
	Large cell carcinoma
	Small (oat) cell carcinoma
	Squamous cell (epidermoid)
Reproductive Organs	
	Adenocarcinoma of the uterus
	Carcinoma of the penis
	Choriocarcinoma of the uterus or testes
	Cystadenocarcinoma (mucinous or serous) of the ovaries
	Seminoma and embryonal cell carcinoma (testes)
	Squamous cell (epidermoid) carcinoma of the vagina or cervix
Skin	
Basal cell layer	Basal cell carcinoma
Melanocyte	Malignant melanoma
Squamous cell layer	Squamous cell carcinoma

found in the breast, prostate, and colon are known as **adenocarcinomas**. Malignant growths of connective tissue (e.g., muscle, cartilage, bone) are called **sarcomas** (Table 10-2). **Lymphomas** form in lymphatic tissue, and **leukemias** are malignancies that arise from white blood cells. A **myeloma** originates within the bone marrow.

The **primary site** is the location at which the neoplasm begins, or originates. It is important for the treating physician to identify the site of origin so that the best treatment course and prognosis can be determined. **Metastasis** is the spread of cancer from one part of the body to another, as is seen when neoplasms occur in parts of the body separate from the site of the primary tumor. Metastasis occurs through dissemination of tumor cells by the lymphatics or blood vessels, or by direct extension through serous cavities or other spaces.

Grading involves pathologic examination of tumor cells. The degree of abnormality of cells determines the grade of cancer (Table 10-3). When the level of cell abnormality is greater, the cancer is of higher grade. Cells that are **well-differentiated** closely resemble mature, specialized cells. Tumor cells that are **undifferentiated** are highly abnormal (i.e., immature and primitive).

Cancerous tissue is classified according to degree of malignancy, from grade 1—barely malignant—to grade 4—highly malignant. In practice, it is not always possible for the pathologist to determine the degree of malignancy, and sometimes it may be difficult even to determine whether a particular tumor tissue is benign or malignant.

TABLE 10-2 SARCOMAS AND THE CONNECTIVE TISSUES FROM WHICH THEY DERIVE[2]

Types of Connective Tissue	Malignant Tumor
Bone	
	Osteosarcoma (osteogenic sarcoma)
	Ewing's sarcoma
Muscle	
Smooth (visceral) muscle	Leiomyosarcoma
Striated (skeletal) muscle	Rhabdomyosarcoma
Cartilage	
	Chondrosarcoma
Fat	
	Liposarcoma
Fibrous Tissue	
	Fibrosarcoma
Blood Vessel Tissue	
	Angiosarcoma
Blood-Forming Tissue	
All leukocytes	Leukemias
Lymphocytes	Hodgkin's disease
Plasma cells	Non-Hodgkin's lymphoma
	Burkitt's lymphoma
	Multiple myeloma
Nerve Tissue	
Embryonic nerve tissue	Neuroblastoma
Glial tissue	Astrocytoma (tumors of glial cells, called "astrocytes")
	Glioblastoma multiforme

TABLE 10-3 GRADES OF NEOPLASMS

Grade 1	Cells slightly abnormal and well-differentiated
Grade 2	Cells more abnormal and moderately differentiated
Grade 3	Cells very abnormal and poorly differentiated
Grade 4	Cells immature and undifferentiated

Staging, a means of categorizing a particular cancer, helps the clinician to determine a particular patient's treatment plan and the need for further therapy. Each type of cancer is staged according to specific characteristics:

- In situ cancers have been diagnosed at the earliest possible stage.
- Stage I or "local" cancers have been diagnosed early and have not spread.
- Stage II has spread into surrounding tissues but not beyond the location of origin.
- Stage III or "regional" cancer has spread to nearby lymph nodes.
- Stage IV or "distant" cancers have spread to other parts of the body and are the most difficult to treat.

See Table 10-4 for an example of how the TNM (tumor-node-metastasis) staging system would be used to classify a lung cancer.

Neoplasm Table

The coding of most neoplasms requires an extra step, which involves use of the Neoplasm Table (Figure 10-2). The main term for the type of neoplasm is located in the Alphabetic Index. All subterms must be reviewed to facilitate assignment of proper codes, including M

TABLE 10-4 INTERNATIONAL TNM STAGING SYSTEMS FOR LUNG CANCER[3]

Stage	TNM Description	5-Year Survival, %
I	T1-T2, N0, M0	60-80
II	T1-T2, N1, M0	25-50
IIIA	T3, N0-N1, M0	25-40
IIIB	T1-T3, N2, M0	10-30
IV	Any T4 or N3, M0	<5
	Any M1	<5
Primary Tumor (T)		
T1	Tumor >3 cm in diameter	
T2	Tumor <3 cm in diameter or with associated atelectasis–obstructive pneumonitis extending to the hilar region	
T3	Tumor with direct extension into the chest wall, diaphragm, mediastinum, pleura, or pericardium	
T4	Tumor invades the mediastinum, or presence of a malignant pleural effusion	
Regional Lymph Nodes (N)		
N0	No node involvement	
N1	Metastasis to lymph nodes in the peribronchial and ipsilateral (same side as the primary tumor) hilar regions	
N2	Metastasis to ipsilateral hilar and subcarinal (under the bifurcation of the trachea into the lungs) lymph nodes	
N3	Metastasis to contralateral mediastinal or hilar nodes or any nodes new to the clavicular (collar) bone	
Distance Metastasis (M)		
M0	No known metastasis	
M1	Distant metastasis present with site specified (e.g., brain, tumor)	

codes if required. One must follow all instructions, such as *see* Neoplasm, by site, benign, or *see also* Neoplasm, by site, malignant. It is important to follow all steps to ensure correct code assignment. The temptation to go directly to the Neoplasm Table should be avoided.

Morphology Codes

Morphology codes (M codes) identify the type of cell that has become neoplastic in its biological activity or behavior. Morphology codes may be required, and facility policy will determine whether these codes should be assigned. They are most often used in cancer registries and pathology departments. M codes are another means of collecting and reporting data on patients with cancer. M codes are not required for inpatient billing, so they have no effect on hospital reimbursement. If an encoder is used for code assignment, M codes may be automatically assigned to correspond with assignment of documented neoplasm codes.

Morphology codes consist of the letter M and five digits; the first four identify the **histologic type** of neoplasm or the type of tissue or cell in which the neoplasm occurs. The fifth digit identifies its behavior. Four-digit histologic types are listed in Appendix A of the ICD-9-CM code book, and the one-digit behavior codes are as follows:

- 0   Benign
- 1   Uncertain whether benign or malignant
  Borderline malignancy
- 2   Carcinoma in situ
  Intraepithelial
  Noninfiltrating
  Noninvasive

	Malignant			Benign	Uncertain Behavior	Unspecified
	Primary	Secondary	Ca in situ	Benign	Uncertain Behavior	Unspecified
Neoplasm, neoplastic	199.1	199.1	234.9	229.9	238.9	239.9

Notes — 1. The list below gives the code numbers for neoplasms by anatomical site. For each site there are six possible code numbers according to whether the neoplasm in question is malignant, benign, in situ, of uncertain behavior, or of unspecified nature. The description of the neoplasm will often indicate which of the six columns is appropriate; e.g., malignant melanoma of skin, benign fibroadenoma of breast, carcinoma in situ of cervix uteri.

Where such descriptors are not present, the remainder of the Index should be consulted where guidance is given to the appropriate column for each morphological (histological) variety listed; e.g., Mesonephroma — see Neoplasm, malignant; Embryoma — see also Neoplasm, uncertain behavior; Disease, Bowen's — see Neoplasm, skin, in situ. However, the guidance in the Index can be overridden if one of the descriptors mentioned above is present; e.g., malignant adenoma of colon is coded to 153.9 and not to 211.3 as the adjective "malignant" overrides the Index entry "Adenoma - see also Neoplasm, benign."

2. Sites marked with the sign * (e.g., face NEC*) should be classified to malignant neoplasm of skin of these sites if the variety of neoplasm is a squamous cell carcinoma or an epidermoid carcinoma and to benign neoplasm of skin of these sites if the variety of neoplasm is a papilloma (any type).

	Primary	Secondary	Ca in situ	Benign	Uncertain Behavior	Unspecified
abdomen, abdominal	195.2	198.89	234.8	229.8	238.8	239.8
cavity	195.2	198.89	234.8	229.8	238.8	239.8
organ	195.2	198.89	234.8	229.8	238.8	239.8
viscera	195.2	198.89	234.8	229.8	238.8	239.8
wall	173.50	198.2	232.5	216.5	238.2	239.2
basal cell carcinoma	173.51	—	—	—	—	—
specified type NEC	173.59	—	—	—	—	—
squamous cell carcinoma	173.52	—	—	—	—	—
connective tissue	171.5	198.89	—	215.5	238.1	239.2
abdominopelvic	195.8	198.89	234.8	229.8	238.8	239.8
accessory sinus - *see* Neoplasm, sinus						
acoustic nerve	192.0	198.4	—	225.1	237.9	239.7
acromion (process)	170.4	198.5	—	213.4	238.0	239.2
adenoid (pharynx) (tissue)	147.1	198.89	230.0	210.7	235.1	239.0
adipose tissue (*see also* Neoplasm, connective tissue)	171.9	198.89	—	215.9	238.1	239.2
adnexa (uterine)	183.9	198.82	233.3	221.8	236.3	239.5
adrenal (cortex) (gland) (medulla)	194.0	198.7	234.8	227.0	237.2	239.7
ala nasi (external)	173.30	198.2	232.3	216.3	238.2	239.2
alimentary canal or tract NEC	159.9	197.8	230.9	211.9	235.5	239.0
alveolar	143.9	198.89	230.0	210.4	235.1	239.0
mucosa	143.9	198.89	230.0	210.4	235.1	239.0
lower	143.1	198.89	230.0	210.4	235.1	239.0
upper	143.0	198.89	230.0	210.4	235.1	239.0
ridge or process	170.1	198.5	—	213.1	238.0	239.2

FIGURE 10-2. Excerpt from the Neoplasm Table.

- 3   Malignant, primary site
- 6   Malignant, metastatic site
  Secondary site
- 9   Malignant, uncertain whether primary or metastatic site

The Alphabetic Index will facilitate assignment of the appropriate M code. The Neoplasm Table does not contain M codes.

EXAMPLE   Adenocarcinoma of the prostate (primary site), 185, M8140/3 (C61, M8140/3).

As was discussed earlier in this chapter, malignant neoplasms that originate in epithelial glandular tissue are called *adenocarcinomas*. Look up "Adenocarcinoma" in the Alphabetic Index (Figure 10-3). No further description or classification is provided beyond adenocarcinoma, and no subterm is given for prostate, so the M code that is in parentheses after the main term "Adenocarcinoma" is assigned as M8140, with the fifth digit of 3 because this is a primary malignancy. To locate the ICD-9-CM code, follow the *see also* instruction and go to the Neoplasm Table to identify the neoplasm, by site, malignant.

EXAMPLE   Adenoma of the prostate, 600.20, M8140/0 (D29.1, M8140/0).

Adenocarcinoma (M8140/3) - *see also*
Neoplasm, by site, malignant

Note   The list of adjectival modifiers
below is not exhaustive. A description
of adenocarcinoma that does not appear in this list should be coded in
the same manner as carcinoma
with that description. Thus, "mixed
acidophil-basophil adenocarcinoma"
should be coded in the same manner as "mixed acidophil-basophil
carcinoma," which appears in the list
under "Carcinoma."

Except where otherwise indicated, the
morphological varieties of adenocarcinoma in the list below should
be coded by site as for "Neoplasm,
malignant."

with
    apocrine metaplasia (M8573/3)
    cartilaginous (and osseous) metapla-
        sia (M8571/3)
    osseous (and cartilaginous) metapla-
        sia (M8571/3)
    spindle cell metaplasia (M8572/3)
    squamous metaplasia (M8570/3)
acidophil (M8280/3)
    specified site - *see* Neoplasm, by site,
        malignant
    unspecified site 194.3
acinar (M8550/3)
acinic cell (M8550/3)
adrenal cortical (M8370/3) 194.0
alveolar (M8251/3)
    and
        epidermoid carcinoma, mixed
            (M8560/3)
        squamous cell carcinoma, mixed
            (M8560/3)
apocrine (M8401/3)
    breast - *see* Neoplasm, breast, malig-
        nant
    specified site NEC - *see* Neoplasm,
        skin, malignant
    unspecified site 173.99
basophil (M8300/3)
    specified site - *see* Neoplasm, by site,
        malignant
    unspecified site 194.3
bile duct type (M8160/3)
    liver 155.1
    specified site NEC - *see* Neoplasm, by
        site, malignant
    unspecified site 155.1
bronchiolar (M8250/3) - *see* Neoplasm,
    lung, malignant
ceruminous (M8420/3) 173.29
chromophobe (M8270/3)
    specified site - *see* Neoplasm, by site,
        malignant
    unspecified site 194.3
clear cell (mesonephroid type)
    (M8310/3)
colloid (M8480/3)
cylindroid type (M8200/3)
diffuse type (M8145/3)

Adenocarcinoma *(Continued)*
    specified site - *see* Neoplasm, by site,
        malignant
    unspecified site 151.9
    duct (infiltrating) (M8500/3)
        with Paget's disease (M8541/3) - *see*
            Neoplasm, breast, malignant
        specified site - *see* Neoplasm, by site,
            malignant
        unspecified site 174.9
    embryonal (M9070/3)
    endometrioid (M8380/3) - *see* Neo-
        plasm, by site, malignant
    eosinophil (M8280/3)
        specified site - *see* Neoplasm, by site,
            malignant
        unspecified site 194.3
    follicular (M8330/3)
        and papillary (M8340/3) 193
        moderately differentiated type
            (M8332/3) 193
        pure follicle type (M8331/3) 193
        specified site - *see* Neoplasm, by site,
            malignant
        trabecular type (M8332/3) 193
        unspecified type 193
        well differentiated type (M8331/3)
            193
    gelatinous (M8480/3)
    granular cell (M8320/3)
    Hürthle cell (M8290/3) 193
    in
        adenomatous
            polyp (M8210/3)
            polyposis coli (M8220/3) 153.9
        polypoid adenoma (M8210/3)
        tubular adenoma (M8210/3)
        villous adenoma (M8261/3)
    infiltrating duct (M8500/3)
        with Paget's disease (M8541/3) - *see*
            Neoplasm, breast, malignant
        specified site - *see* Neoplasm, by site,
            malignant
        unspecified site 174.9
    inflammatory (M8530/3)
        specified site - *see* Neoplasm, by site,
            malignant
        unspecified site 174.9
    in situ (M8140/2) - *see* Neoplasm, by
        site, in situ
    intestinal type (M8144/3)
        specified site - *see* Neoplasm, by site,
            malignant
        unspecified site 151.9
    intraductal (noninfiltrating) (M8500/2)
        papillary (M8503/2)
            specified site - *see* Neoplasm, by
                site, in situ
            unspecified site 233.0
        specified site - *see* Neoplasm, by site,
            in situ
        unspecified site 233.0
    islet cell (M8150/3)
        and exocrine, mixed (M8154/3)
            specified site - *see* Neoplasm, by
                site, malignant
            unspecified site 157.9
        pancreas 157.4
        specified site NEC - *see* Neoplasm, by

Adenocarcinoma *(Continued)*
    islet cell *(Continued)*
        site, malignant
        unspecified site 157.4
    lobular (M8520/3)
        specified site - *see* Neoplasm, by site,
            malignant
        unspecified site 174.9
    medullary (M8510/3)
    mesonephric (M9110/3)
    mixed cell (M8323/3)
    mucinous (M8480/3)
    mucin-producing (M8481/3)
    mucoid (M8480/3) - *see also* Neoplasm,
        by site, malignant
        cell (M8300/3)
            specified site - *see* Neoplasm, by
                site, malignant
            unspecified site 194.3
    nonencapsulated sclerosing (M8350/3)
        193
    oncocytic (M8290/3)
    oxyphilic (M8290/3)
    papillary (M8260/3)
        and follicular (M8340/3) 193
        intraductal (noninfiltrating)
            (M8503/2)
            specified site - *see* Neoplasm, by
                site, in situ
            unspecified site 233.0
        serous (M8460/3)
            specified site - *see* Neoplasm, by
                site, malignant
            unspecified site 183.0
    papillocystic (M8450/3)
        specified site - *see* Neoplasm, by site,
            malignant
        unspecified site 183.0
    pseudomucinous (M8470/3)
        specified site - *see* Neoplasm, by site,
            malignant
        unspecified site 183.0
    renal cell (M8312/3) 189.0
    sebaceous (M8410/3)
    serous (M8441/3) - *see also* Neoplasm,
        by site, malignant
        papillary
            specified site - *see* Neoplasm, by
                site, malignant
            unspecified site 183.0
    signet ring cell (M8490/3)
    superficial spreading (M8143/3)
    sweat gland (M8400/3) - *see* Neoplasm,
        skin, malignant
    trabecular (M8190/3)
    tubular (M8211/3)
    villous (M8262/3)
    water-clear cell (M8322/3) 194.1

FIGURE 10-3. Index entry for main term "Adenocarcinoma."

Note that the only difference in assignment of M codes for these two examples is the fifth digit assigned for behavior of the neoplasm. In this example, a subterm for prostate is provided, and instead of instructions to use the Neoplasm Table, assignment of code 600.20 is given.

In the following examples, a step-by-step explanation will be given for coding of neoplasms with the appropriate M code.

EXAMPLE

Basal cell carcinoma left cheek (primary site), 173.31, M8090/3.
1. Look up "Carcinoma" in Alphabetic Index.
2. Review subterms; "basal cell" is a subterm.
3. Note M code (M8090) is classified as a primary malignancy (3).
4. Follow instructions to *see also* Neoplasm, skin, malignant.
5. Go to the Neoplasm Table.
6. Locate the site—skin—and review subterms under "Skin."
7. Locate the subterm "cheek," and follow the instructional note to see also Neoplasm, skin, face. Find the code under the appropriate column, which, in this case, is a primary malignancy of the skin of the face, basal cell.
8. Assign codes 173.31 and M8090/3 (C44.39, M8090/3).

EXAMPLE

Squamous cell in situ carcinoma of the endocervix, 233.1, M8070/2.
1. Look up "Carcinoma" in the Alphabetic Index.
2. Review subterms; "squamous cell" is a subterm.
3. Note M code (M8070) is classified as squamous cell in situ (2).
4. Follow instructions, specified site—see Neoplasm, by site, in situ.
5. Go to the Neoplasm Table.
6. Locate the site—cervix—and review subterms under "Cervix."
7. Locate the subterm "endocervix," and find the code under the appropriate column, which, in this case, is a carcinoma in situ of the endocervix.
8. Assign codes 233.1 and M8070/2 (in situ) (D06.0, M8070/2).

EXERCISE 10-1

Assign only M codes for the following.

1. Squamous cell carcinoma, in situ neoplasm   _____
2. Cancer, secondary neoplasm   _____
3. Ewing's sarcoma, primary neoplasm   _____
4. Periosteal fibrosarcoma, primary neoplasm   _____
5. Melanoma, primary neoplasm   _____
6. Leukemia   _____
7. Lymphoma   _____
8. Adenoma, benign neoplasm   _____
9. Renal cell carcinoma, metastatic neoplasm   _____
10. Hürthle cell adenocarcinoma, primary neoplasm   _____

Primary and Secondary Neoplasms

Sometimes incomplete documentation makes it difficult to determine whether a neoplasm is primary or secondary. It is possible to have more than one primary cancer. At times, a secondary or metastatic cancer has been found, and the primary is unknown or has yet to be determined. Documentation in the health record may be incomplete and the terminology confusing.

As was described previously, a metastatic neoplasm is a secondary neoplasm that has spread from the original or primary site. The site of the metastasis may be close to the original site (e.g., breast spread to axillary lymph nodes) or to distant sites (e.g., lung spread to the brain). Neoplasms can metastasize to more than one site. If this is the case, codes are assigned to each metastatic site. Terminology used to describe metastatic sites varies greatly, depending on the documenting physician. For example, if a patient has a non–small cell primary lung carcinoma with secondary malignancy of the brain, it may be documented in the health record as follows:

EXAMPLE Lung cancer with metastasis to the brain, 162.9, 198.3 (C34.90, C79.31).

The code that would be assigned is primary lung cancer with a secondary code assigned for the metastatic brain malignancy.

EXAMPLE Lung cancer metastatic to the brain, 162.9, 198.3 (C34.90, C79.31).

The codes assigned are the same as in the preceding example.

EXAMPLE Brain cancer metastatic from the lung, 162.9, 198.3 (C34.90, C79.31).

The codes assigned are the same as in the preceding example.

EXAMPLE Non–small cell carcinoma of lung and brain, 162.9, 198.3 (C34.90, C79.31).

Non–small cell carcinoma is a malignancy that originates in the lung, so the lung is primary. If a cancer that originates in the lung has spread to the brain, that is a metastasis.

EXAMPLE Metastatic lung cancer, 162.9, 199.1 (C34.90, C79.9).

According to *Coding Clinic* (1985:M-J:p9-12),[4] if a morphology type is not stated, assign the site qualified as "metastatic" to the primary malignant code for that site. The code assigned is primary lung cancer (162.9 [C34.90]), with an unknown secondary malignancy site (199.1 [C79.9]) because the metastatic site was not documented in this example.

If the documentation in the health record only identifies one site and it is identified as metastatic, then a determination has to be made as to whether to code the site as a primary malignancy or secondary malignancy. The following steps are followed to make that determination:

1. If the morphology type is documented, refer to the morphology type in the Alphabetic Index and code to the primary condition of that site.

EXAMPLE Metastatic islet cell carcinoma of the pancreas, 157.4, 199.1 (C25.4, C79.9).

In the preceding example, the carcinoma is documented as metastatic. The first step is to locate the morphology type in the Alphabetic Index. There are subterms for islet cell of the pancreas with code, 157.4 (C25.4), so that code should be assigned. If no specific site is listed as a subterm, assign the code for primary neoplasm of an unspecified site (199.1 [C80.1]). When a primary site has been determined, a code must be assigned to identify a secondary (metastatic) site. If no metastatic site is specified, then the code 199.1 (C79.9), unknown site, secondary, is assigned.

2. If the process in step 1 leads to code 199.0 or 199.1 or if the morphology is not stated, the site should be coded as a primary malignancy, unless it is included in the following list of exceptions.

Malignant neoplasms of the following sites are exceptions, and instead of coding to an unknown primary or to the morphology, the following sites are always coded as secondary neoplasms of that site:

- Bone
- Brain
- Diaphragm
- Heart
- Liver
- Lymph nodes
- Mediastinum
- Meninges
- Peritoneum
- Pleura
- Retroperitoneum
- Spinal cord
- Sites classifiable to 195.0-8

EXAMPLE   Metastatic carcinoma of the breast, 174.9, 199.1 (C50.919, C79.9).

In the preceding example, there is no subterm for breast or unspecified site. In the Neoplasm Table, unspecified site, primary is coded to 199.1 (C80.1). When code 199.0 or 199.1 is obtained, then a review of the exception list is performed. Because breast is not on the list, it is assigned as the primary site, 174.9 (C50.919), and the code 199.1 (C79.9) is used to identify the unknown secondary.

EXAMPLE   Metastatic brain cancer, 199.1, 198.3 or 198.3, 199.1 (depending on the reason for the patient's admission) (C80.1, C79.31 or C79.31, C80.1).

In this example, the brain is on the list of secondary neoplasms, and the morphology type is not stated; therefore the code 198.3 (C79.31) is assigned for secondary neoplasm of the brain and 199.1 (C80.1) for unknown primary. Sequencing of the primary and secondary neoplasms would depend on the focus of treatment.

EXAMPLE   Renal cell carcinoma (RCC) with metastasis to the adrenal glands
        Primary neoplasm: Renal cell carcinoma
        Secondary neoplasm: Adrenal glands

EXAMPLE   Metastatic bone cancer
        Primary neoplasm: Unknown primary site
        Secondary neoplasm: Bones

Specific instructions are provided at the beginning of the "Neoplasm" chapter in the code book (Figure 10-4).

2. NEOPLASMS (140–239)

1. Content:

This chapter contains the following broad groups:

140–195 Malignant neoplasms, stated or presumed to be primary, of specified sites, except of lymphatic and hematopoietic tissue

196–198 Malignant neoplasms, stated or presumed to be secondary, of specified sites

199 Malignant neoplasms, without specification of site

200–208 Malignant neoplasms, stated or presumed to be primary, of lymphatic and hematopoietic tissue

210–229 Benign neoplasms

230–234 Carcinoma in situ

235–238 Neoplasms of uncertain behavior [see Note, at beginning of section 235–238]

239 Neoplasms of unspecified nature

2. Functional activity

All neoplasms are classified in this chapter, whether or not functionally active. An additional code from Chapter 3 may be used to identify such functional activity associated with any neoplasm, e.g.:

catecholamine-producing malignant pheochromocytoma of adrenal:

code 194.0, additional code 255.6

basophil adenoma of pituitary with Cushing's syndrome:

code 227.3, additional code 255.0

3. Morphology [Histology]

For those wishing to identify the histological type of neoplasms, a comprehensive coded nomenclature, which comprises the morphology rubrics of the ICD-Oncology, is given after the E-code chapter.

4. Malignant neoplasms overlapping site boundaries

Categories 140–195 are for the classification of primary malignant neoplasms according to their point of origin. A malignant neoplasm that overlaps two or more subcategories within a three-digit rubric and whose point of origin cannot be determined should be classified to the subcategory .8 "Other." For example, "carcinoma involving tip and ventral surface of tongue" should be assigned to 141.8. On the other hand, "carcinoma of tip of tongue, extending to involve the ventral surface" should be coded to 141.2, as the point of origin, the tip, is known. Three subcategories (149.8, 159.8, 165.8) have been provided for malignant neoplasms that overlap the boundaries of three-digit rubrics within certain systems. Overlapping malignant neoplasms that cannot be classified as indicated above should be assigned to the appropriate subdivision of category 195 (Malignant neoplasm of other and ill-defined sites).

FIGURE 10-4. Instructional notes at the beginning of the "Neoplasm" chapter in the Tabular List.

EXERCISE 10-2

Identify the following neoplasms in terms of primary or secondary, as in the earlier examples.

1. Colorectal adenocarcinoma with metastatic liver cancer
   Primary neoplasm _____
   Secondary neoplasm _____

2. Thyroid malignancy with mets to the lymph nodes of the neck
   Primary neoplasm _____
   Secondary neoplasm _____

3. Metastatic ovarian cancer
   Primary neoplasm _____
   Secondary neoplasm _____

4. Pancreatic cancer with extension into the liver
    Primary neoplasm _____
    Secondary neoplasm _____
5. Recurrence of cancer in the bladder
    Primary neoplasm _____
    Secondary neoplasm _____
6. Adenocarcinoma sigmoid colon with pericolic nodal involvement
    Primary neoplasm _____
    Secondary neoplasm _____
7. Inflammatory breast cancer with spread to the axillary lymph nodes
    Primary neoplasm _____
    Secondary neoplasm _____
8. Metastatic bone cancer from the prostate
    Primary neoplasm _____
    Secondary neoplasm _____
9. Endometrial adenocarcinoma with metastasis to the ovary
    Primary neoplasm _____
    Secondary neoplasm _____
10. Acinic cell carcinoma of the parotid gland
    Primary neoplasm _____
    Secondary neoplasm _____

Contiguous Sites

As is pointed out in the instructional note (Figure 10-4), a neoplasm can overlap two or more subcategories, and determination of the exact point of origin may be difficult. These would be assigned to subcategory 8, "Other."

It is important to code any alterations to the functional activity of an organ caused by the neoplasm. Neoplasms of the endocrine glands or organs that secrete hormones are more likely to have disturbances in their functional activity because hormone production may increase or decrease because of the neoplasm.

EXAMPLE   Malignant neoplasm of the thyroid with hyperthyroidism, 193, 242.80 (C73, E05.80).

DISEASE CONDITIONS

Neoplasms (140-239) are the topic of Chapter 2 in your ICD-9-CM code book; it is divided into the following categories:

CATEGORY	SECTION TITLES
140-149	Malignant Neoplasm of Lip, Oral Cavity, and Pharynx
150-159	Malignant Neoplasm of Digestive Organs and Peritoneum
160-165	Malignant Neoplasm of Respiratory and Intrathoracic Organs
170-176	Malignant Neoplasm of Bone, Connective Tissue, Skin, and Breast
179-189	Malignant Neoplasm of the Genitourinary Organs
190-199	Malignant Neoplasm of Other and Unspecified Sites
200-208	Malignant Neoplasm of Lymphatic and Hematopoietic Tissue
209	Neuroendocrine Tumors
210-229	Benign Neoplasms
230-234	Carcinoma In Situ
235-238	Neoplasms of Uncertain Behavior
239	Neoplasms of Unspecified Nature

Chapter 2 in the ICD-10-CM code book is divided into the following categories:

CATEGORY	SECTION TITLES
C00-C14	Malignant Neoplasm of Lip, Oral Cavity, and Pharynx
C15-C26	Malignant Neoplasm of Digestive Organs
C30-C39	Malignant Neoplasm of Respiratory and Intrathoracic Organs
C40-C41	Malignant Neoplasm of Bone and Articular Cartilage
C43-C44	Malignant Neoplasm of Skin
C45-C49	Malignant Neoplasm of Mesothelial and Soft Tissue
C50	Malignant Neoplasm of Breast
C51-C58	Malignant Neoplasm of Female Genital Organs
C60-C63	Malignant Neoplasm of Male Genital Organs
C64-C68	Malignant Neoplasm of Urinary Tract
C69-C72	Malignant Neoplasm of Eye, Brain, and Other Parts of the Central Nervous System
C73-C75	Malignant Neoplasm of Thyroid and Other Endocrine Glands
C76-C80	Malignant Neoplasm of Ill-Defined, Secondary, and Unspecified Sites
C81-C96	Malignant Neoplasm of Lymphoid, Hematopoietic, and Related Tissue
D00-D09	In Situ Neoplasms
D10-D36	Benign Neoplasms
D37-D48	Neoplasms of Uncertain Behavior
D49	Neoplasms of Unspecified Behavior

Malignant Neoplasm of Lip, Oral Cavity, and Pharynx

Several types of oral cancers have been identified; 90% of these are squamous cell carcinomas. Cancers are often discovered after they have already spread, usually to the lymph nodes of the neck. Smoking has been associated with about 70% to 80% of oral cancers. Also, heavy alcohol adds to the risk. The lips and tongue are most commonly affected (Figure 10-5).

EXAMPLE   The patient is being treated for squamous cell carcinoma of the hypopharynx, 148.9 (C13.9).

FIGURE 10-5. Squamous cell carcinoma of the mouth.

FIGURE 10-6. Adenocarcinoma distal rectum.

EXERCISE 10-3

Assign codes to the following conditions.

1. Squamous cell carcinoma, base of tongue   _____
2. Adenocarcinoma of parotid gland   _____
3. Biopsy-proven squamous cell carcinoma, right tonsil   _____
4. Cancer lower lip   _____

Malignant Neoplasm of Digestive Organs and Peritoneum

According to the Centers for Disease Control and Prevention (CDC), colorectal cancer (Figure 10-6) primarily affects men and women aged 50 years or older. For men, colorectal cancer is the third most common cancer after prostate cancer and lung cancer. For women, colorectal cancer is the third most common cancer after breast cancer and lung cancer. The best prevention is regular screening.

Hepatocellular carcinoma is a primary neoplasm of the liver (Figure 10-7). Patients who develop primary liver cancer often have some type of chronic liver disease such as cirrhosis. The liver is also a common site for metastasis.

EXAMPLE | The patient has adenocarcinoma of the rectosigmoid junction, 154.0 (C19).

Malignant ascites is a condition in which excess fluid, which contains malignant cells, accumulates in the abdomen or peritoneum. A diagnostic paracentesis can be performed to determine if cancer cells are present. Patients with breast, ovarian, uterine, colon, stomach, intestinal, or pancreatic cancers are more likely to develop malignant ascites. Ascites can be very uncomfortable for the patient, and a therapeutic paracentesis may be necessary to drain the fluid and provide symptom relief. There is an instructional note in the code book to code the responsible neoplasm first. As the code for malignant ascites is a symptom code from Chapter 16, there is a guideline that states that a code from this chapter, when associated with an existing primary or secondary malignancy site, cannot be used as a principal or first-listed diagnosis. In a patient with cancer and multiple metastatic sites, it may be necessary to query the physician as to which cancer site is causing the ascites.

FIGURE 10-7. Hepatocellular carcinoma.

EXAMPLE

Patient presented to the Emergency Room with shortness of breath due to extensive malignant ascites. She has inoperable ovarian cancer. A therapeutic percutaneous peritoneal cavity paracentesis was performed, 183.0, 789.51, 54.91 (C56.9, R18.0, 0W9G3ZZ).

EXERCISE 10-4

Assign codes to the following conditions.

1. Hepatocellular carcinoma _____
2. Adenocarcinoma, head of pancreas _____
3. Fibrosarcoma of spleen _____
4. Adenocarcinoma of the duodenum _____
5. Gastric adenocarcinoma _____
6. Cholangiocarcinoma of the extrahepatic bile ducts _____

Malignant Neoplasm of Respiratory and Intrathoracic

Lung cancer, which is one of the most common types of cancer, is classified into two main categories: small cell lung cancer (SCLC) and non-small cell lung cancer (NSCLC). More than 85% of lung cancers are caused by smoking. Bronchogenic carcinoma is the most common type of malignant lung cancer (Figure 10-8). The lung is frequently a site for metastasis. Benign tumors of the lung are rare.

EXAMPLE

The patient was diagnosed with adenocarcinoma, right lower lobe of lung, 162.5 (C34.31).

Malignant pleural effusion is a condition in which fluid accumulates in the pleural space and contains malignant cells. Malignant pleural effusions can result from lymphomas, breast cancer, and small cell lung cancer. Pleural effusions can be very uncomfortable for the patient, and a therapeutic thoracentesis may be necessary to drain the fluid and provide symptom relief. There is an instructional note in the code book to code first malignant neoplasm, if known. In the past, malignant pleural effusions were coded to secondary neoplasm of the pleura, but metastasis to the pleura is not always present in a patient with malignant pleural effusions.

FIGURE 10-8. Bronchogenic carcinoma. The tumor, a squamous cell carcinoma, appears gray-white and infiltrates the lung tissue.

EXAMPLE   Patient presented to the ER with shortness of breath due to right-sided malignant pleural effusion due to SCLC. A thoracentesis was performed. 162.9, 511.81, 34.91, (C34.91, J91.0, 0W993ZZ).

EXERCISE 10-5

Assign codes to the following conditions.

1. Malignant mesothelioma of the pleura   _____

2. Cancer of the larynx   _____

3. Oat cell cancer of right main bronchus   _____

4. Squamous cell carcinoma of thymus   _____

5. Cancer maxillary sinus   _____

Malignant Neoplasm of Bone, Connective Tissue, Skin, and Breast

One in eight women has or will develop breast cancer in her lifetime (Figure 10-9). The 5-year survival rate exceeds 95% if detected early. Infiltrating or invasive ductal carcinoma is the most common type of breast cancer. Cancers of the connective tissue develop in the muscles, fat, blood, lymph vessels, and nerves.

Osteosarcoma is the most common primary malignant cancer of the bone and usually occurs in young people between the ages of 10 and 30. These tumors develop most often in bones of the arms, legs, or pelvis.

EXAMPLE   The patient is being seen for fibrosarcoma distal femur 171.3 (C49.20).

FIGURE 10-9. Breast carcinoma.

EXERCISE 10-6

Assign codes to the following conditions,

1. Ewing's sarcoma 7th rib _____

2. Basal cell carcinoma right cheek _____

3. Kaposi's sarcoma skin in patient with acquired immunodeficiency syndrome (AIDS) _____

4. Upper outer quadrant malignancy of right breast _____

5. Osteosarcoma left humerus _____

6. Lentigo malignant melanoma sole of left foot _____

7. Malignant neoplasm male breast _____

Malignant Neoplasm of Genitourinary Organs

Malignancy can affect any organ in the genitourinary system. Many neoplasms are related to age; for example, Wilms' tumor is a common childhood tumor of the kidney. Testicular cancer usually affects young men, and the incidence of prostate cancer increases with age. Most kidney (Figure 10-10) and bladder (Figure 10-11) malignancies occur in adults between 60 and 70 years of age. As with many cancers, genetic, environmental, and behavioral risk factors may contribute to the cause.

EXAMPLE The patient is being treated for a malignancy of his right testis (descended), 186.9 (C62.11).

EXERCISE 10-7

Assign codes to the following conditions.

1. Endometrial carcinoma _____

2. Renal cell carcinoma _____

3. Tubo-ovarian cancer _____

4. Transitional cell carcinoma lower neck of bladder, causing urinary obstruction _____

5. Leiomyosarcoma of uterus _____

FIGURE 10-10. Renal cell carcinoma.

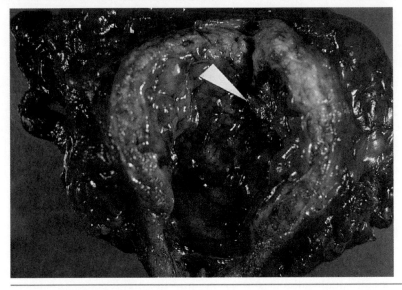

FIGURE 10-11. Bladder cancer.

Malignant Neoplasm of Other and Unspecified Sites

This section contains a variety of neoplasms, including those of the eye, brain, spinal cord, thyroid, and other endocrine glands. This is also where secondary or metastatic neoplasm codes are located. The 196 category is used to identify the spread of cancer to the lymph nodes; fourth-digit classifications identify the body region of the lymph nodes for specificity. In contrast, code 198.5 is the code assigned to metastasis to the bone, and in this case, specificity is not necessary for code assignment. It does not matter whether this is a vertebral bone, a pelvic bone, or the humerus.

EXAMPLE | The patient has metastatic lung cancer; no known primary, 199.1, 197.0 (C80.1, C78.00).

EXERCISE 10-8

Assign codes to the following conditions.

1. Seizure due to carcinoma of parietal lobe of the brain _____

2. Glioblastoma multiforme brain _____

3. Metastatic melanoma to the brain; melanoma skin lesion excised 5 years ago _____

4. Neuroblastoma left adrenal gland _____

5. Teratocarcinoma pineal gland _____

6. Left orbital rhabdomyosarcoma _____

7. Anaplastic astrocytoma spinal cord with metastasis to the vertebral bodies _____

8. Carcinomatosis _____

9. Metastasis to the mastectomy site; mastectomy performed 1 year ago _____

Malignant Neoplasm of Lymphatic and Hematopoietic Tissue

Lymphoma is cancer of the lymphatic system. Two main types have been identified: Hodgkin's disease (HD) (Figure 10-12) or lymphoma, and non-Hodgkin's lymphoma (NHL). The incidence of non-Hodgkin's is greater than that of Hodgkin's disease. The lymphatic system follows the blood vessels, and groups are located in areas of the neck, axillary, groin, abdomen, and pelvic regions. Some organs contain lymphatic tissue and may be affected. These organs include the spleen, thymus gland, bone marrow, tonsils, and adenoids. According to *Coding Clinic* (1992:2Q:p3-4),[5] although lymphoma may be present in different or multiple areas of the body, it is not considered metastatic. Lymphomas should not be confused with solid tumors (malignancies) that have metastasized to the lymph nodes.

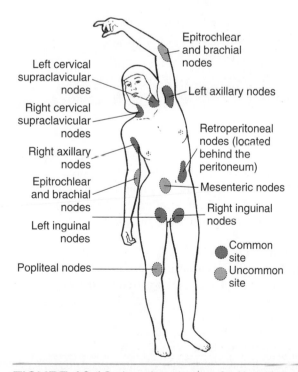

FIGURE 10-12. Lymph node sites for Hodgkin's disease.

FIGURE 10-13. Peripheral blood smears. **A,** Acute lymphoblastic leukemia. **B,** Chronic myelogenous leukemia. **C,** Chronic lymphocytic leukemia.

If a patient is in remission, he or she is considered to have lymphoma, and a code from categories 200-202 should be assigned. There are different classifications of remission. **Complete remission** means there are no signs or symptoms of the cancer. **Partial remission** means there are still a few signs and symptoms of the cancer and the cancer cells have significantly decreased. The remission fifth digit (if available) should only be assigned if documented by the physician as being in remission.

Leukemia is cancer of the white blood cells that begins in the blood-forming cells of the bone marrow. As the disease progresses, leukemic cells invade other parts of the body, such as the lymph nodes, spleen, liver, and central nervous system. Various types of leukemia have been identified (Figure 10-13). Some develop suddenly and are acute leukemias; others are of the chronic variety.

EXAMPLE   The patient was diagnosed with nodular sclerosis Hodgkin's, 201.50 (C81.10).

EXERCISE 10-9

Assign codes to the following conditions.

1. Acute lymphocytic leukemia (ALL), relapsed   _____
2. Primary central nervous system (brain) diffuse large B-cell   _____
    lymphoma (non-Hodgkin's)
3. Chronic myelogenous leukemia (CML)   _____
4. Lymphoma ileum   _____
5. Burkitt's lymphoma in remission   _____

Neuroendocrine Tumors

Code category 209 includes codes for benign and malignant carcinoid neoplasms. Neuroendocrine tumors can be benign and/or malignant neoplasms that arise in the endocrine or neuroendocrine cells throughout the body. These neoplasms are usually slow-growing. There are two groups of neuroendocrine neoplasms:

- Carcinoid
- Pancreatic endocrine

The most common sites for carcinoid neoplasms are the bronchi, stomach, small intestine, appendix, and rectum. They are classified according to the embryonic site of origin such as:

- **Foregut**—bronchi and stomach
- **Midgut**—small intestine and appendix
- **Hindgut**—colon and rectum

Benign tumors are usually very small. Malignant tumors are larger and do metastasize. The most common metastatic sites are the lymph nodes, liver, lung, bone, and skin.

EXAMPLE | Malignant carcinoid neoplasm of the appendix, 209.11 (C7a.020).

EXAMPLE | Benign carcinoid neoplasm of the rectum, 209.57 (D3a.026).

EXERCISE 10-10

Assign codes to the following conditions.

1. Malignant carcinoid tumor foregut _____
2. Benign carcinoid tumor, sigmoid colon _____
3. Carcinoid neoplasm, small intestine, malignant _____

Benign Neoplasms

A benign neoplasm or tumor is not malignant. It will not metastasize to other parts of the body, but it could continue to grow and may cause damage to neighboring organs and structures. It may be necessary to remove a benign neoplasm. Benign neoplasms may recur.

Lipoma is a growth of fat cells within a capsule that is usually found just below the skin. Lipomas are the most common benign soft tissue growths. For the most part, lipomas are small and movable, and they remain the same size and are not painful. It may be necessary to excise a lipoma if it becomes painful or infected, if it limits function or mobility, or if it increases in size.

Leiomyoma or uterine fibroids are tumors or growths within the walls of the uterus. These are the most common benign tumors in women of childbearing age. Not all fibroids cause symptoms. When fibroids become symptomatic, the following symptoms may be present:

- Heavy bleeding
- Painful periods
- Feeling of fullness in the pelvic region
- Urinary frequency
- Pain during sex
- Infertility, miscarriage, or early onset of labor

Treatment will depend on the severity of symptoms, the size and location of the fibroids, and the patient's age and desired fertility.

EXAMPLE | Patient is being seen because of a cavernous lymphangioma, 228.1 (D18.1).

EXERCISE 10-11

Assign codes to the following conditions.

1. Warthin's tumor _____
2. Adenoma of the pituitary gland _____
3. Chondromyxoid fibroma of the left tibia _____
4. Squamous papilloma soft palate _____
5. Osteoma proximal right femur _____
6. Enchondroma fifth metacarpal _____
7. Lipoma spermatic cord _____
8. Rhabdomyoma left ventricle of heart _____
9. Hemangioma of liver _____
10. Submucosal uterine fibroid _____

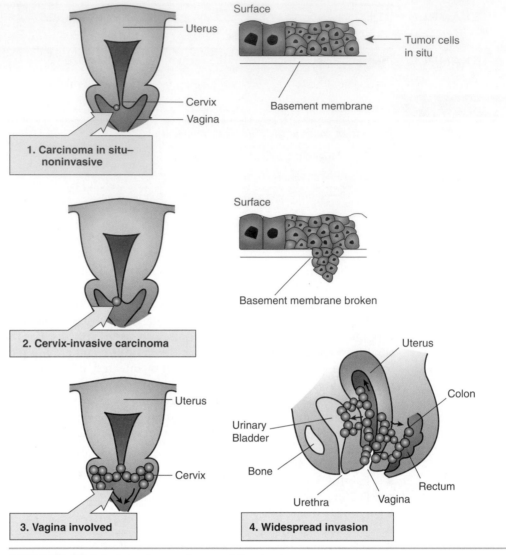

FIGURE 10-14. Invasive carcinoma of the cervix.

Carcinoma In Situ

Carcinoma in situ consists of malignant cells that remain within the original site with no spread or invasion to neighboring tissues (Figure 10-14). Usually, the physician or the pathology report will confirm that the condition is "in situ." These tumors are usually curable because they are at the earliest stage of development.

EXAMPLE   Patient has Bowen's disease, 232.9 (D04.9).

EXERCISE 10-12

Assign codes to the following conditions.

1.   Carcinoma in situ of the cervix   _____
2.   Carcinoma in situ of the urinary bladder   _____
3.   Cervical intraepithelial neoplasia III   _____
4.   Ductal carcinoma in situ (DCIS) left breast   _____

Neoplasms of Uncertain Behavior

Neoplasms that fall into the categories of uncertain behavior are neither malignant nor benign. On pathologic examination, the behavior cannot be determined or predicted. In some instances, progression to some type of malignancy may occur. For example, myelodysplastic syndrome has been known to progress to leukemia.

| EXAMPLE | Patient is seen in consultation because of type 2 neurofibromatosis, 237.72 (Q85.02). |

EXERCISE 10-13

Assign codes to the following conditions.

1. Myelodysplastic syndrome (MDS) _____
2. Polycythemia vera _____
3. Refractory anemia _____
4. Paraganglioma of carotid body _____

Neoplasms of Unspecified Behavior

This category is used when terms such as "growth," "neoplasm," or "tumor" are used to describe a medical finding. At times, this condition may require further investigation and testing. Sometimes, these findings are not investigated because the patient is elderly and has other chronic conditions, and aggressive treatment would not be pursued.

On occasion, a physician will document a patient as having a mass with no further specification other than site or location of the mass. Usually, this occurs when no pathology report is available when the physician is documenting details in the health record. According to *Coding Clinic* (2006:1Q:p4),[6] if the diagnosis is documented as "mass" or "lesion," it would be incorrect to select a code for neoplasm of unspecified behavior.

| EXAMPLE | Mass of the liver, 573.9 (R16.0). |

In this example, under the main term "mass," there is no subterm for liver. The *Coding Clinic* states if there is no index entry for a specific site, go to the main term "disease," liver.

If terms such as lump or lesion are used, the same logic is applied. If a subterm cannot be found under "lump," "lesion," or "mass," go to the main term "disease."

| EXAMPLE | Patient will need to follow up for definitive diagnosis of neoplasm sigmoid colon 239.0 (D49.0). |

EXERCISE 10-14

Assign codes to the following conditions.

1. Intracranial tumor _____
2. Neoplasm bladder _____
3. Growth left ovary _____
4. Mass right lung _____
5. Right breast lump _____
6. Lesion brain was identified by MRI _____

Coding and Sequencing of Neoplasms

In addition to assigning neoplasm codes, it is important to know how these codes are sequenced in accordance with the guidelines. The principal diagnosis is determined according to the reason the patient is admitted and the treatment provided. Documentation by physicians may be confusing in determining the principal diagnosis. They often will document the cancer as the reason for admission. Physicians may document cancers that have been previously removed. Physicians are not trained to document in accordance with coding guidelines. They may document the reason for admission as the cancer when the patient is receiving treatment for a complication of the cancer or of the cancer treatments.

Malignancy as Principal Diagnosis

When a patient is admitted for determination of whether a malignancy is present and a malignancy is found, the code for the primary malignancy is the principal diagnosis.

EXAMPLE | Patient was admitted for total thyroidectomy. Fine needle aspiration biopsy on an outpatient basis was inconclusive. Total thyroidectomy was performed, and a diagnosis of anaplastic cancer was determined, 193, 06.4 (C73, 0GTK0ZZ).

As in the previous example, during the course of determining whether a malignancy is present, a malignancy is found and a secondary malignancy is identified. The code for the primary neoplasm is the principal diagnosis, and the secondary malignancy is assigned as an additional code.

EXAMPLE | Patient has papillary thyroid cancer that has spread to the cervical lymph nodes, 193, 196.0 (C73, C77.0).

Recurrence of Primary Malignancy

If a primary malignancy was previously excised or eradicated but has now recurred, the malignancy is coded to a primary malignant neoplasm.

EXAMPLE | Recurrence of transitional cell bladder cancer, posterior wall, 188.4 (C67.4).

Physicians may document a malignancy as recurrent at a site where a malignancy and the organ has been previously excised. This cannot be an actual recurrent neoplasm if the organ is no longer present. It may be necessary to query the physician to determine the metastatic site(s).

EXAMPLE | Recurrent ovarian cancer. Patient had hysterectomy and bilateral salpingo-oophorectomy 3 years ago, 199.1, V10.43, V45.77 (may need to query the site of recurrence) (C79.9, Z85.43, Z90.722, Z90.710, Z90.79).

When a patient is admitted for removal of a known malignancy, the malignancy is the principal diagnosis. In some cases, a biopsy may have been performed previously that confirms the presence of a malignancy. The patient is readmitted for more definitive surgery. The pathology report following the surgery may report negative findings for malignancy. According to *Coding Clinic* (1985:M-J:p9-12),[4] if the physician documents the malignancy as shown on the biopsy, the malignancy is assigned as the principal diagnosis for the definitive surgery even though no further evidence of malignancy is seen on the pathology report.

EXAMPLE | Patient has a fine needle aspiration biopsy that shows Hürthle carcinoma of the left lobe of the thyroid. Patient is admitted for a partial thyroidectomy. The pathology report from the thyroidectomy shows no evidence of malignancy, 193, 06.39 (C73, 0GTG0ZZ).

When a patient is admitted with a sign or symptom (which codes to Chapter 16) related to a known primary or secondary malignancy, the primary or secondary malignancy code is the principal diagnosis.

EXAMPLE | Convulsion due to glioblastoma multiforme temporal lobe of brain, 191.2, 780.39 (the convulsion is coded as an additional code because convulsions are not integral to the brain neoplasm) (C71.2, R56.9).

When a patient is admitted with a primary neoplasm and a metastatic neoplasm and treatment is directed to the metastatic neoplasm, the metastatic neoplasm is the principal diagnosis.

EXAMPLE | Patient is admitted for wedge resection of metastatic liver cancer. Patient had a colorectal cancer removed 3 months ago and is undergoing treatment, 197.7, 154.0, 50.22 (C78.7, C19, 0FB00ZZ).

According to *Coding Clinic* (1988:1Q:p4-5),[7] when a patient is admitted to the hospital for treatment by brachytherapy, the principal diagnosis is the malignancy that is being treated (which could be either a primary or a secondary malignancy).

EXAMPLE | Patient was admitted for implantation of brachytherapy (high dose rate Iridium 192) for cancer of cervix, 180.9, 92.27 (C53.9, DU1198Z).

According to *Coding Clinic* (1997:2Q:p3),[8] when a patient is admitted with an obstruction due to a neoplasm (primary or secondary), the neoplasm is coded as the principal diagnosis. An additional code should be assigned to identify the obstruction.

EXAMPLE | Large bowel obstruction due to adenocarcinoma of the colon, 153.9, 560.9 (C18.9, in ICD-10-CM, intestinal obstruction due to a specified condition is coded to that condition).

Complications as Principal Diagnosis

Often, complications are associated with malignancies or the treatment of malignancies. When the complication is the reason for admission or treatment, the complication is the principal diagnosis. The guidelines address some of the most common examples such as anemia and dehydration.

EXAMPLE | Patient admitted for treatment of anemia due to gastric cancer with 2 units of packed red cells (percutaneously into peripheral vein), 285.22, 151.9, 99.04 (C16.9, D63.0, 30233N1).

EXAMPLE | Patient has become extremely dehydrated following last chemotherapy session for breast cancer. Patient is admitted for IV fluids, 276.51, 174.9 (E86.0, C50.919).

EXAMPLE | Neutropenic fever with neutropenia due to chemotherapy for acute lymphocytic leukemia, 288.03, 780.61, 204.00, E933.1 (T45.1x5A, D70.1, R50.81, C91.00).

Principal Diagnosis for Encounters for Chemotherapy/Immunotherapy and Radiation

When a patient is admitted solely for the administration of chemotherapy, chemoembolization, immunotherapy, and/or radiation, the principal diagnosis will be a V58.XX code. In cases where chemotherapy, chemoembolization, immunotherapy, or radiation is performed in conjunction with surgical removal of a neoplasm, the primary or secondary neoplasm code is the principal diagnosis, and no V58.XX code is assigned.

If a patient is admitted for both radiation and chemotherapy during the same encounter, either V code can be sequenced as the principal with the other V code used as a secondary diagnosis code.

If complications occur during an encounter for chemotherapy/immunotherapy/radiation treatment, codes to identify the complications are assigned as secondary diagnosis codes.

EXAMPLE

> Patient was admitted for chemotherapy (percutaneous central vein) for osteosarcoma of right humerus. Patient became dehydrated and was treated with additional IV fluids, V58.11, 170.4, 276.51, 99.25 (Z51.11, C40.01, E86.0, 3E04305).

EXAMPLE

> Patient is admitted for chemotherapy (percutaneous central vein) for Burkitt's lymphoma, V58.11, 200.20, 99.25 (Z51.11, C83.70, 3E04305).

EXAMPLE

> Patient is admitted for radiation therapy (heavy particle) for prostate cancer, V58.0, 185, 92.29 (Z51.0, C61, DV004ZZ).

Coding of Previously Excised Malignancies

If a primary malignancy has been previously excised and is no longer being treated, it is assigned a V code for history of personal malignancy.

EXAMPLE

> Patient had a mastectomy 5 years ago for breast cancer. She is not being actively treated, V10.3, V45.71 (Z85.3, Z90.10).

However, if a previously excised malignancy is still being treated actively, it is appropriate to assign the neoplasm code.

EXAMPLE

> Patient had a lobectomy for lung cancer 6 months ago. The patient will receive the fifth cycle of chemotherapy next week, 162.9, V45.76 (C34.90, Z90.2).

If a patient has a primary and an associated secondary malignancy that was previously excised and/or treated, only the V code for the history of the primary malignancy is assigned. No V codes are used to identify the personal history of a secondary malignancy. If a secondary malignancy has been completely excised or treated and is no longer active, no code is assigned.

EXAMPLE

> Patient had breast cancer with metastasis to axillary lymph nodes.
> Patient was treated with mastectomy and chemotherapy. There has been no recurrence of any disease, and she is no longer being actively treated, V10.3, V45.71 (Z85.3, Z90.10).

Neoplasm-Related Pain

When a patient has pain due to a previously identified neoplasm, code 338.3 is assigned. This code can be assigned as either principal or secondary, depending on the circumstances of the admission.

If a patient is admitted for pain management or pain control, the 338.3 code is assigned as the principal diagnosis, and the malignancy code(s) is assigned as a secondary code(s).

EXAMPLE

> Patient was admitted for control of back pain due to vertebral metastasis. Patient has a history of prostate cancer. After pain medications were adjusted and pain was controlled, he was discharged to hospice care, 338.3, 198.5, V10.46 (G89.3, C79.51, Z85.46).

If a patient is admitted for management of the malignancy and the pain associated with the malignancy, the malignancy code is assigned as the principal diagnosis with the 338.3 pain code assigned as a secondary diagnosis.

EXAMPLE

> Patient was admitted for back pain due to vertebral metastasis. An MRI indicates that the disease has progressed. Patient has a history of prostate cancer. Beam radiation with heavy particles was administered, 198.5, V10.46, 338.3, 92.29 (C79.51, G89.3, Z85.46, DP0C4ZZ).

EXERCISE 10-15

Complete the following exercises.

1. If a patient is admitted and treated for anemia due to a malignancy, the malignancy code is the principal diagnosis in ICD-9-CM.
   A. True
   B. False

2. If a patient has a complication during an encounter for chemotherapy, the complication code is the principal diagnosis.
   A. True
   B. False

3. If a malignancy of the bladder has been previously excised and now there is a recurrence of a malignancy within the bladder, the recurrence is coded as a primary malignancy.
   A. True
   B. False

4. A personal history V code is assigned for a history of a secondary malignancy.
   A. True
   B. False

5. The primary neoplasm is always principal even if the treatment is directed at the secondary neoplasm.
   A. True
   B. False

6. If a patient is admitted for treatment of dehydration due to a malignancy, the dehydration is the principal diagnosis.
   A. True
   B. False

7. When a patient is admitted for immunotherapy, the V58.11 is assigned as the principal diagnosis.
   A. True
   B. False

8. When a patient is admitted for brachytherapy, the V58.0 is assigned as the principal diagnosis.
   A. True
   B. False

FACTORS INFLUENCING HEALTH STATUS AND CONTACT WITH HEALTH SERVICES (V CODES/Z CODES)

In the past, V/Z codes have been considered primarily for use in the outpatient setting. This has changed with the addition of more V/Z codes each year. As was discussed in Chapter 8, it may be difficult to locate V/Z codes in the Index. Coders often say, "I did not know there was a V/Z code for that." Refer to Chapter 8 for a listing of common main terms used to locate V/Z codes.

Also in Chapter 8, it was pointed out that it may be easy to lose track of indentations in the Alphabetic Index for a personal and family history of neoplasms. Verification in the Tabular should alert the coder of a wrong code selection.

The Guidelines provide instructions for the use and sequencing of some important V/Z codes. If a patient is admitted solely for administration of chemotherapy, immunotherapy or radiation therapy, a code from category V58 should be the principal diagnosis followed by codes for the malignancies being treated. If they are admitted for more than one type of therapy, either code can be principal.

V/Z codes that may be used with neoplasms include the following:

V07.39	Other prophylactic chemotherapy
V07.51	Prophylactic use of selective estrogen receptor modulators (SERMs)
V07.52	Prophylactic use of aromatase inhibitors
V07.59	Prophylactic use of other agents affecting estrogen receptors and estrogen levels
V10.00	Personal history of malignant neoplasm—gastrointestinal tract, unspecified
V10.01	Personal history of malignant neoplasm—tongue
V10.02	Personal history of malignant neoplasm—other and unspecified oral cavity and pharynx
V10.03	Personal history of malignant neoplasm—esophagus
V10.04	Personal history of malignant neoplasm—stomach
V10.05	Personal history of malignant neoplasm—large intestine
V10.06	Personal history of malignant neoplasm—rectum, rectosigmoid junction, and anus
V10.07	Personal history of malignant neoplasm—liver
V10.09	Personal history of malignant neoplasm—other
V10.11	Personal history of malignant neoplasm—bronchus and lung
V10.12	Personal history of malignant neoplasm—trachea
V10.20	Personal history of malignant neoplasm—respiratory organ, unspecified
V10.21	Personal history of malignant neoplasm—larynx
V10.22	Personal history of malignant neoplasm—nasal cavities, middle ear, and accessory sinuses
V10.29	Personal history of malignant neoplasm—other respiratory and intrathoracic organs
V10.3	Personal history of malignant neoplasm—breast
V10.40	Personal history of malignant neoplasm—female genital organ, unspecified
V10.41	Personal history of malignant neoplasm—cervix uteri
V10.42	Personal history of malignant neoplasm—other parts of uterus
V10.43	Personal history of malignant neoplasm—ovary
V10.44	Personal history of malignant neoplasm—other female genital organs
V10.45	Personal history of malignant neoplasm—male genital organ, unspecified
V10.46	Personal history of malignant neoplasm—prostate
V10.47	Personal history of malignant neoplasm—testis
V10.48	Personal history of malignant neoplasm—epididymis
V10.49	Personal history of malignant neoplasm—other male genital organs
V10.50	Personal history of malignant neoplasm—urinary organ, unspecified
V10.51	Personal history of malignant neoplasm—bladder
V10.52	Personal history of malignant neoplasm—kidney
V10.53	Personal history of malignant neoplasm—renal pelvis
V10.59	Personal history of malignant neoplasm—other urinary organs
V10.60	Personal history of malignant neoplasm—leukemia, unspecified
V10.61	Personal history of malignant neoplasm—lymphoid leukemia
V10.62	Personal history of malignant neoplasm—myeloid leukemia
V10.63	Personal history of malignant neoplasm—monocytic leukemia
V10.69	Personal history of malignant neoplasm—other leukemia

V10.71	Personal history of malignant neoplasm—lymphosarcoma and reticulosarcoma
V10.72	Personal history of malignant neoplasm—Hodgkins disease
V10.79	Personal history of malignant neoplasm—other lymphatic and hematopoietic neoplasms
V10.81	Personal history of malignant neoplasm—bone
V10.82	Personal history of malignant neoplasm—malignant melanoma of skin
V10.83	Personal history of malignant neoplasm—other malignant neoplasm skin
V10.84	Personal history of malignant neoplasm—eye
V10.85	Personal history of malignant neoplasm—brain
V10.86	Personal history of malignant neoplasm—other parts of the nervous system
V10.87	Personal history of malignant neoplasm—thyroid
V10.88	Personal history of malignant neoplasm—other endocrine glands and related structures
V10.89	Personal history of malignant neoplasm—other
V10.9	Personal history of malignant neoplasm—unspecified
V12.41	Personal history of benign neoplasm of the brain
V12.72	Personal history of diseases of digestive system—colonic polyps
V16.0	Family history of malignant neoplasm—gastrointestinal tract
V16.1	Family history of malignant neoplasm—trachea, bronchus, and lung
V16.2	Family history of malignant neoplasm—other respiratory and intrathoracic organs
V16.3	Family history of malignant neoplasm—breast
V16.40	Family history of malignant neoplasm—genital organ, unspecified
V16.41	Family history of malignant neoplasm—ovary
V16.42	Family history of malignant neoplasm—prostate
V16.43	Family history of malignant neoplasm—testis
V16.49	Family history of malignant neoplasm—other genital organ
V16.51	Family history of malignant neoplasm—kidney
V16.52	Family history of malignant neoplasm—bladder
V16.59	Family history of malignant neoplasm—other urinary organ
V16.6	Family history of malignant neoplasm—leukemia
V16.7	Family history of malignant neoplasm—other lymphatic and hematopoietic neoplasms
V16.8	Family history of malignant neoplasm—other specified malignant neoplasm
V16.9	Family history—unspecified malignant neoplasm
V18.51	Family history of certain other specific conditions—digestive disorders, colonic polyps
V44.0	Artificial opening status—tracheostomy
V44.1	Artificial opening status—gastrostomy
V44.2	Artificial opening status—ileostomy
V44.3	Artificial opening status—colostomy
V44.4	Artificial opening status—other artificial opening of gastrointestinal tract
V44.50	Artificial opening status—cystostomy, unspecified
V44.51	Artificial opening status—cutaneous vesicostomy
V44.52	Artificial opening status—appendicovesicostomy
V44.59	Artificial opening status—other cystostomy
V44.6	Artificial opening status—other artificial opening of urinary tract
V44.7	Artificial opening status—vagina
V44.8	Artificial opening status—other artificial opening status
V44.9	Artificial opening status—unspecified artificial opening status
V45.71	Acquired absence of organ—breast and nipple
V45.72	Acquired absence of organ—intestine (large, small)
V45.73	Acquired absence of organ—kidney

V45.74	Acquired absence of organ—other parts of urinary tract
V45.75	Acquired absence of organ—stomach
V45.76	Acquired absence of organ—lung
V45.77	Acquired absence of organ—genital organs
V45.78	Acquired absence of organ—eye
V45.79	Acquired absence of organ—other acquired absence of organ
V45.87	Transplanted organ removal status
V50.41	Prophylactic organ removal—breast
V50.42	Prophylactic organ removal—ovary
V50.49	Prophylactic organ removal—other
V51.0	Encounter for breast reconstruction following mastectomy
V55.0	Attention to artificial openings—tracheostomy
V55.1	Attention to artificial openings—gastrostomy
V55.2	Attention to artificial openings—ileostomy
V55.3	Attention to artificial openings—colostomy
V55.4	Attention to artificial openings—other artificial opening of digestive tract
V55.5	Attention to artificial openings—cystostomy
V55.6	Attention to artificial openings—other artificial opening of urinary tract
V55.7	Attention to artificial openings—vagina
V55.8	Attention to artificial openings—other specified artificial opening
V55.9	Attention to artificial openings—unspecified artificial opening
V58.0	Encounter for radiotherapy
V58.11	Encounter for antineoplastic chemotherapy
V58.12	Encounter for antineoplastic immunotherapy
V58.42	Aftercare following surgery for neoplasm
V58.44	Aftercare following organ transplant
V71.1	Observation for suspected malignant neoplasm
V76.0	Special screening for malignant neoplasms—respiratory organs
V76.10	Special screening for malignant neoplasms—breast, unspecified
V76.11	Screening mammogram for high-risk patient
V76.12	Other screening mammogram
V76.19	Other screening breast examination
V76.2	Special screening for malignant neoplasms—cervix
V76.3	Special screening for malignant neoplasms—bladder
V76.41	Special screening for malignant neoplasms—rectum
V76.42	Special screening for malignant neoplasms—oral cavity
V76.43	Special screening for malignant neoplasms—skin
V76.44	Special screening for malignant neoplasms—prostate
V76.45	Special screening for malignant neoplasms—testis
V76.46	Special screening for malignant neoplasms—ovary
V76.47	Special screening for malignant neoplasms—vagina
V76.49	Special screening for malignant neoplasms—other sites
V76.50	Special screening for malignant neoplasms—intestine, unspecified
V76.51	Special screening for malignant neoplasms—colon
V76.52	Special screening for malignant neoplasms—small intestine
V76.81	Special screening for malignant neoplasms—nervous system
V76.89	Special screening for malignant neoplasms—other neoplasm
V84.01	Genetic susceptibility to malignant neoplasm—breast
V84.02	Genetic susceptibility to malignant neoplasm—ovary
V84.03	Genetic susceptibility to malignant neoplasm—prostate
V84.04	Genetic susceptibility to malignant neoplasm—endometrium

V84.09	Genetic susceptibility to malignant neoplasm—other malignant neoplasm
V87.41	Personal history of antineoplastic chemotherapy
V88.01	Acquired absence of both cervix and uterus
V88.02	Acquired absence of uterus with remaining cervical stump
V88.03	Acquired absence of cervix with remaining uterus

There are some important V/Z code categories related to neoplasms and the treatment and follow-up of neoplasms. First, there are a number of screening codes and codes for family history of malignancies. A screening examination occurs in the absence of any signs or symptoms. The patient is asymptomatic.

EXAMPLE

Screening for prostate cancer, V76.44 (Z12.5).

EXAMPLE

Patient has a family history of leukemia, V16.6 (Z80.6).

Other important V/Z code categories include aftercare and follow-up. Many of these services are performed in the outpatient setting. Aftercare codes are generally listed first and explain the reason for the encounter. Aftercare codes are used following the initial treatment of a disease and when the patient requires continued care during the healing and recovery stages or because of the long-term effects of the disease.

EXAMPLE

Patient admitted to a long-term care facility to recover from major surgery for colon cancer. Patient will undergo chemotherapy after discharge, V58.42, 153.9 (Z48.3, C18.9).

Even after a patient has been successfully treated for a malignancy, periodic, routine follow-up examinations may be necessary to determine if there has been any recurrence of the cancer. When there is no evidence of any type of recurrence, a code from the V67.X follow-up examination should be assigned. A code from the V10 category should also be assigned as an additional code to show the reason for the follow-up examination. If there is any evidence of recurrence at the primary site and/or metastasis to a secondary site, the appropriate neoplasm codes are assigned and code from category V67 is not assigned.

EXAMPLE

Patient had a surveillance cystoscopy done because of previous bladder cancer, which was surgically removed. No evidence of recurrence was found. The patient will follow up in 3 months, V67.09, V10.51, 57.32 (Z08, Z85.51, 0TJB8ZZ).

EXAMPLE

Patient had a surveillance cystoscopy (transurethral) done because of previous bladder cancer. A recurrence of the cancer was excised from the posterior bladder wall, 188.4, 57.49 (C67.4, 0TBB8ZZ).

EXERCISE 10-16

Assign codes to the following conditions.

1. History of adenocarcinoma of the prostate _____

2. Screening mammogram for patient with strong family history _____
   of breast cancer

3. Personal history of benign brain neoplasm previously removed _____

4. Admission for takedown of colostomy; previous colon _____
   resection for malignancy

COMMON TREATMENTS

Cancer is treated by various modalities (i.e., surgery, chemotherapy, radiation, immunotherapy, or other methods). The type of treatment will depend on the location, grading and stage of the neoplasm, and the health of the patient. Chemotherapy destroys cancer cells, but it may also target fast-growing healthy tissue. Often chemotherapy drugs are used in combinations because the drugs work better together than separately. Immunotherapy agents stimulate the immune system's response against tumors. Radiation therapy uses ionizing radiation to destroy cancer cells and shrink tumors. It is administered externally by external beam therapy or internally via brachytherapy.

CONDITION	MEDICATION/TREATMENT
Malignancies	Chemotherapy drugs are often given in combination with other chemotherapy drugs or hormonal therapy. The treatment will depend on the type of cancer. Some common drugs include carboplatin (Paraplatin), cisplatin (Platinol), cyclophosphamide (Cytoxan, Neosar), docetaxel (Taxotere), doxorubicin (Adriamycin), erlotinib (Tarceva), etoposide (VePesid, Toposar, Etopophos), fluorouracil (5-FU), gemcitabine (Gemzar), ifosfamide (Ifex), imatinib mesylate (Gleevec), irinotecan (Camptosar), methotrexate (Folex, Mexate, Amethopterin), mitomycin (Mitomycin-C), paclitaxel (Taxol, Abraxane), rituximab (Rituxan), sorafenib (Nexavar), sunitinib (Sutent), topotecan (Hycantin), vinblastine (Velban), vincristine (Oncovin, Vincasar PFS).
Melanoma and kidney cancer	Immunotherapy with interleukin and interferon
Superficial bladder cancer	Intravesical Bacillus Calmette-Guerin (BCG) immunotherapy
Certain types of breast or colon cancer	Capecitabine (Xeloda)—interferes with cancer cell growth and reproduction
Certain types of breast cancer	Tamoxifen (Nolvadex)—interferes with estrogen activity
Advanced prostate cancer in men and uterine fibroid tumors in women	Leuprolide acetate for depot suspension (Lupron Depot)
Certain types of leukemia (CML) and certain gastrointestinal stromal tumors	Imatinib (Gleevec) prevents the growth of cancer cells
Neutropenia due to chemotherapy	Pegfilgrastim (Neulasta) or filgrastim (Neupogen) builds up or stimulates white cell counts
Anemia due to malignancy	Epoetin alfa (Procrit, Epogen), darbepoetin alfa (Aranesp)
Symptoms of malignancy and treatment	Pain medications (narcotics), antiemetics to suppress nausea and vomiting
Human papilloma virus	Vaccination for prevention

PROCEDURES

Neoplasms can affect any body system, so ICD-9-CM codes can be located in all of the chapters of the Procedure Tabular. The same is true for ICD-10-PCS; any of the tables in the Medical and Surgical section may be used. There may also be procedures that can be located in the Radiation Oncology, Placement, and Administration sections.

Chemotherapy/Immunotherapy/Radiation

Operative procedures are often performed to biopsy and resect or excise areas or organs that are affected by neoplastic conditions. At times, a neoplasm is considered unresectable, and other treatments are necessary. Sometimes, patients will receive chemotherapy or radiation therapy to shrink the tumor before surgery is performed. **Chemotherapy** consists of administration of drugs or medications to treat disease. In cancer patients, antineoplastic drugs are used. These drugs can be given intravenously, orally, subcutaneously, intramuscularly, or intrathecally. The introduction of chemotherapy is found in the Administration section of ICD-10-PCS. **Chemoembolization** is the intra-arterial administration of chemotherapy with collagen particles to enhance the delivery of chemotherapy to the targeted area. According to *Coding Clinic* (1995:4Q:p67-68),[9] this should be treated as an encounter for chemotherapy, and V58.11 (Z51.11) should be assigned as the principal diagnosis. Procedure code 99.25 (3E04305) includes chemoembolization. An additional diagnosis code is assigned for the malignancy. **Radiation** treatment involves the use of high-energy radiation to treat patients with cancer. **Brachytherapy** is the placement of radioactive material directly into or near the cancer. The radiation is delivered by needles, wires, or catheters and may be in the form of seeds. According to *Coding Clinic* (1988:1Q:p4-5),[7] "when the purpose of a hospital admission is for the treatment of a malignancy by implantation or insertion of radioactive elements, the principal diagnosis is the neoplastic condition (malignancy) being treated with the radioactive element." Radiation and brachytherapy are found under the Radiation Oncology section of ICD-10-PCS. **Immunotherapy** is the administration of agents that stimulate the immune system's response against tumors. **Biological response modifiers (BRMs)** are a type of immunotherapy and are used to fight certain cancers and even conditions such as rheumatoid arthritis. They can destroy cancer cells, stimulate the immune system to destroy cancer cells, or change cancer cells to normal cells. Immunotherapy is found in the Administration section of ICD-10-PCS.

The Guidelines provide instructions for the use and sequencing of some important V codes. If a patient is admitted solely for administration of chemotherapy, immunotherapy, or radiation therapy, a code from category V58 should be the principal diagnosis followed by codes for the malignancies being treated. If they are admitted for more than one type of therapy, either code can be principal.

EXAMPLE

Patient was admitted for the administration of chemotherapy (percutaneous central vein) for osteosarcoma of upper end of the tibia, V58.11, 170.7, 99.25 (Z51.11, C40.20, 3E04305).

EXAMPLE

Radioactive seeds were implanted within Iodine 125 at high dose rate for treatment of prostate cancer, 185, 92.27 (C61, DV1099Z).

EXAMPLE

Patient is admitted for chemoembolization of hepatocellular carcinoma, V58.11, 155.0, 99.25 (Z51.11, C22.0, 3E063GC).

Palliative procedures may be performed to correct a condition that is causing problems or pain for the patient. It is not meant to cure. Palliative surgery may be performed to relieve an obstruction caused by a tumor. Sometimes radiation is administered for palliative treatment.

Biopsy

Biopsy specimens can be obtained in several ways. The approach used varies with the location of the mass, the age of the patient, and the availability of technology. A **biopsy** consists of removal of a representative sample of a tumor mass for pathologic examination and diagnosis. An **excisional biopsy** is the total removal of local small masses or growths (Figure 10-15). The root operation for a biopsy is excision.

- **Incisional biopsy:** This is the removal of a small piece of tumor. Sometimes, nearby lymph nodes may also be removed and tested for metastasis.
- **Core biopsy:** This procedure is less invasive than surgical biopsy. A large needle is used to extract a core sample. Usually, a smaller sample of tissue is provided, and the cancerous tissue may be missed. Occasionally, a new sample must be obtained.

FIGURE 10-15. Excision of lesion. **A,** Location of lesion. **B,** Surgical margins. **C,** Lesion excised. **D,** Closure of surgical site.

- **Fine needle aspiration (FNA):** This method, which requires use of a very small needle, works best for masses that are superficial or easily accessible. The specimen is small, and sometimes, findings are inconclusive.
- **Endoscopic biopsy:** This is a biopsy that is performed during an endoscopic examination. After a biopsy is performed, a more definitive surgical procedure may be necessary.

EXAMPLE

Patient had an FNA biopsy of a thyroid mass last week; this confirmed papillary thyroid cancer. Patient underwent total thyroidectomy, 193, 06.4 (C73, 0GTK0ZZ).

Occasionally, a biopsy will be performed during the same operative episode as a more definitive treatment. In these cases, sequencing of the procedures would follow the Uniform Hospital Discharge Data Set (UHDDS) guidelines for selection of a principal procedure, and the procedure that is performed for definitive treatment is the principal procedure.

EXAMPLE

Patient (female) was taken to the operating room for an open biopsy of a breast mass in the right upper outer quadrant. Frozen section showed invasive ductal carcinoma; a simple mastectomy with removal of three axillary lymph nodes was performed during the same operative episode. Nodes were negative for malignancy, 174.4, 85.43, 85.12 (C50.411, 0HTT0ZZ, 07B50ZZ, 0HBT0ZX).

Surgery

Endoscopic procedures are minimally invasive procedures during which a scope is used to examine the inside of the body. It is also possible for the clinician to perform a biopsy, remove a small polyp or foreign body, or control bleeding with the use of an endoscope.

Preventive or prophylactic surgery is performed to remove tissue that has the potential to become cancerous. A woman may have a prophylactic mastectomy as the result of a strong family history of breast cancer and/or a positive breast cancer gene (*BRCA1* or *BRCA2*). The principal or first-listed diagnosis should be a code from subcategory V50.4X, prophylactic organ removal. The appropriate V codes to identify the reason for the removal should also be assigned. If a patient has a malignancy of the breast and decides to have the other breast removed, also as a prophylactic measure, the malignancy code should be assigned first with a V50.41 code for the prophylactic removal of the other breast. **Staging surgeries** are performed to determine the extent of the disease and are generally more accurate than laboratory and imaging tests. **Debulking** procedures are performed when it is impossible to remove the tumor entirely. In many of these cases a number of organs may be involved and may also have to be removed. The tumor is removed to as great an extent as possible, and adjunctive treatment such as chemotherapy or radiation may be used to treat the remaining disease. **Restorative or reconstruction** surgery is performed to restore function and enhance aesthetic appearance after surgery. Breast reconstruction is commonly performed after a mastectomy. Breast reconstruction procedures will be covered in Chapter 20.

EXAMPLE

> Patient was admitted for prophylactic removal of ovaries due to genetic susceptibility and positive family history with laparoscopic removal, V50.42, V16.41, V84.02, 65.53 (Z40.02, Z80.41, Z15.02, OUT24ZZ).

EXERCISE 10-17

Assign codes for all diagnoses and procedures.

1. Refractory aplastic anemia with excess blasts (RAEB-2) for bone marrow transplant (BMT); donor is the patient's sister _____

2. Transitional cell carcinoma of the bladder with transurethral resection of tumor _____

3. Renal cell cancer of the right kidney with right laparoscopic nephrectomy _____

4. Vaginal brachytherapy to the cervix with high dose rate Iridium 192 for endometrial carcinoma _____

5. Acoustic neuroma with hearing loss; craniotomy for removal of tumor _____

6. Wide excision of melanoma, right shoulder with skin grafting; split-thickness graft taken from thigh _____

7. Diagnostic percutaneous biopsy of intrathoracic lymph node showed non-Hodgkin's lymphoma in patient who has had a kidney transplant _____

8. Admission for chemotherapy; patient has a malignancy of the esophagus _____

9. Classic Whipple for carcinoma of the head of pancreas _____

10. Ascending colon cancer with right hemicolectomy _____

DOCUMENTATION/REIMBURSEMENT/MS-DRGS

Often, coding difficulties are due to lack of documentation. Sometimes pathology and other test results are not available at the time of discharge or when the physician is dictating the discharge summary or is reporting the final diagnoses.

The physician may document the cancer as if it is the principal diagnosis because it is the most serious and can be a life-threatening condition. However, the cancer may not fit the definition of a principal diagnosis or may not follow the neoplasm guidelines. Physicians will sometimes document metastatic breast carcinoma, and further into the record, it may be noted that the patient has had a mastectomy and has received a combination of chemotherapy and radiation therapy. In this case, it is most likely a primary breast cancer that has spread to an undocumented secondary site.

It is difficult to pinpoint any particular codes that may be frequently missed complications/comorbidities from this chapter. There are numerous primary and secondary neoplasms on the CC listing. There are no neoplasm codes on the MCC listing. It is important to code all current primary and secondary neoplasms, even when this is not the main reason for a patient's admission to the hospital.

Assign All Procedure Codes

It is very important to assign all procedure codes because this could make the difference between a medical MS-DRG and a surgical MS-DRG. Likewise, it is also important to follow the guidelines for selection of the appropriate principal diagnosis.

EXAMPLE

DIAGNOSES	CODES	MS-DRG	RW
Malignant neoplasm brain with craniotomy with excision of tumor	191.9 (C71.9) 01.59 (00B00ZZ)	027	2.1307
Malignant neoplasm brain with craniotomy with excision of tumor (in the body of the operative report is documentation of chemo wafers implanted on the brain)	191.9 (C71.9) 01.59 (00B00ZZ) 00.10 (3E0Q705)	023	5.0883

MS-DRG With and Without MCC/CC

EXAMPLE

DIAGNOSES	CODES	MS-DRG	RW
Hodgkin's lymphoma, multiple sites, patient is cachectic	201.98 (C81.98) 799.4 (R64)	841	1.6376
Hodgkin's lymphoma, multiple sites	201.98 (C81.98)	842	1.0389

The presence of a CC can make a difference in reimbursement depending on the principal diagnosis and the MS-DRG assigned. The code for cachexia (799.4[R64]) is a CC.

CHAPTER REVIEW EXERCISE

Assign codes for all diagnoses and procedures.

1. Adenocarcinoma of the prostate with radical retropubic excision and regional pelvic lymph nodes _____

2. Adenocarcinoma of the distal esophagus; patient is status post-laparoscopic jejunostomy prior to radiation treatments _____

3. Chronic lymphocytic leukemia (CLL) _____

4. Splenectomy showed non-Hodgkin's lymphoma of the spleen _____

5. Von Recklinghausen's disease

6. Hydrocephalus due to malignant ependymoma fourth ventricle; the patient was admitted for ventriculoperitoneal shunt placement

7. Diagnostic laparoscopic needle biopsy of the right adrenal gland; physician documented pheochromocytoma

8. Fibrosarcoma of the soft tissue of left thigh with mets to brain

9. Malignant melanoma left thigh previously excised; patient admitted for immunotherapy with high-dose interleukin-2 via central venous infusion because of spread to inguinal lymph nodes

10. Intraperitoneal metastatic carcinoma; unknown primary; treatment focused on determining primary source

11. Left hemiplegia due to tumor right frontal lobe

12. Primary central nervous system (spinal cord) lymphoma; admitted for chemotherapy

13. Admission for red blood cell transfusion (peripheral venous) due to anemia caused by renal cell carcinoma

14. Dehydration due to chemotherapy in patient with carcinoma of breast with metastasis to axillary lymph nodes

15. Recurrent seizures due to metastasis to brain from lung cancer

16. Cerebral meningioma

17. Choroidal melanoma

18. Admission for chemoembolization of hepatocellular carcinoma (HCC)

19. Neutropenic fever in a patient who is undergoing treatment for leukemia; patient is anemic due to chemotherapy

20. Intestinal obstruction due to peritoneal metastasis from inoperable colorectal cancer

21. Impending hip fracture due to metastasis to bone; patient has a previous history of breast cancer treated with mastectomy; internal fixation of upper right femur

22. Patient's myelodysplastic syndrome has progressed to acute myelogenous leukemia

23. Prophylactic removal of both breasts due to positive genetic susceptibility and positive family history; a bilateral modified radical mastectomy was performed

24. Chronic myeloproliferative disease

25. Falx cerebri meningioma surgically removed

26. Basophil adenoma of the pituitary gland causing Cushing's syndrome

27. Carcinoma of the breast in the right upper and lower quadrant

28. Metastatic ovarian cancer; admitted for pain control

29. Cancer head of pancreas with spread to the liver

30. Endometrial adenocarcinoma with mets to ovary

31. Parotidectomy for Warthin's tumor of the left parotid gland

32. Adenocarcinoma of the upper stomach with spread to the lower esophagus and lungs

Write the correct answer(s) in the blank(s) provided.

33. If a hospital's base payment rate was $4,000.00, what would be the hospital payment for MS-DRG 023? _____

34. At the hospital in #33, what would the payment rate be for MS-DRG 027? _____

35. If a coder missed the procedure code for the chemo wafer, how much reimbursement would be lost? _____

CHAPTER GLOSSARY

Adenocarcinomas: malignancies of epithelial glandular tissue such as those found in the breast, prostate, and colon.

Benign: neoplasm or tumor; means that it is not malignant.

Biological response modifier (BRM): immunotherapy that can destroy cancer cells, stimulate the immune system to destroy cancer cells, or change cancer cells to normal cells.

Biopsy: removal of a representative sample for pathologic examination and diagnosis.

Brachytherapy: placement of radioactive material directly into or near the cancer.

Carcinomas: malignant tumors originating from epithelial tissue (e.g., in the skin, bronchi, and stomach).

Carcinoma in situ: malignant cells that remain within the original site with no spread or invasion into neighboring tissue.

Chemoembolization: intra-arterial administration of chemotherapy with collagen particles to enhance the delivery of chemotherapy to the targeted area.

Chemotherapy: the use of drugs or medications to treat disease.

Complete remission: there are no signs or symptoms of the cancer.

Core biopsy: procedure in which a large needle is used to extract a core sample.

Debulking: procedures performed when it is impossible to remove the tumor entirely.

Endoscopic biopsy: biopsy that is performed during endoscopic examination.

Excisional biopsy: total removal of local small masses or growths.

Fibromas: neoplasms of fibrous connective tissue.

Fine needle aspiration: procedure in which a very small needle is used; works best for masses that are superficial or easily accessible.

Foregut: bronchi and stomach (sites of carcinoid neoplasms).

Grading: pathologic examination of tumor cells. Degree of cell abnormality determines the grade of cancer.

Hindgut: colon and rectum (sites of carcinoid neoplasms).

Histologic type: type of tissue or cell in which the neoplasm occurs.

Immunotherapy: administration of agents that stimulate the immune system's response against tumors.

Incisional biopsy: procedure in which a representative sample of a tumor mass is removed to permit pathologic examination.

Leiomyoma: tumor or growth within the walls of the uterus. Also called *uterine fibroid.*

Leukemia: cancer of the white blood cells that begins in the blood-forming cells of the bone marrow.

Lipoma: growth of fat cells within a capsule that is usually found just below the skin.

Lymphoma: cancer of the lymphatic system.

Malignancy: neoplasm that has the ability to invade adjacent structures and spread to distant sites.

Malignant ascites: excess fluid that contains malignant cells that accumulates in the abdomen or peritoneum.

Malignant pleural effusion: fluid accumulates in the pleural space and contains malignant cells.

Melanomas: malignant changes of melanin cells.

Metastasis: spread of a cancer from one part of the body to another, as in the appearance of neoplasms in parts of the body separate from the site of the primary tumor.

Midgut: small intestine and appendix (sites of carcinoid neoplasms).

Morphology codes (M codes): codes that identify the type of cell that has become neoplastic and its biological activity or behavior.

Myeloma: malignancy that originates in the bone marrow.

Neoplasm: abnormal growth.

Palliative: procedure performed to correct a condition that is causing problems for the patient.

Partial remission: there are still a few signs and symptoms of the cancer, and the cancer cells have significantly decreased.

Preventive or prophylactic surgery: procedure performed to remove tissue that has the potential to become cancerous.

Primary site: site at which the neoplasm begins or originates.

Radiation: use of high-energy radiation to treat cancer.

Restorative or reconstructive: surgery performed to restore function and enhance aesthetic appearance after surgery.

Sarcomas: malignant growths of connective tissue (e.g., muscle, cartilage, lymph tissue, and bone).

Staging: means of categorizing a particular cancer that assists in determination of a patient's treatment plan and the need for further therapy.

Staging surgeries: procedures performed to help the clinician determine the extent of disease; these are generally more accurate than laboratory and imaging tests.

Undifferentiated: tumor cells that are highly abnormal (e.g., immature, primitive).

Well-differentiated: tumor cells that closely resemble mature, specialized cells.

REFERENCES

1. Chabner D. The Language of Medicine, 8th ed. St. Louis, Saunders, 2007, Table 19-2, p 776.
2. Chabner D. The Language of Medicine, 8th ed. St. Louis, Saunders, 2007, Table 19-3, p 777.
3. Modified from Harrison's Manual of Medicine, 15th ed. New York, McGraw-Hill Professional, 2002, p 284.
4. American Hospital Association. *Coding Clinic for ICD-9-CM* 1985:M-J:p9-12. Neoplasm coding—Guidelines.
5. American Hospital Association. *Coding Clinic for ICD-9-CM* 1992:2Q:p3-4.
   Lymphoma involvement in bone, metastatic vs primary.
6. American Hospital Association. *Coding Clinic for ICD-9-CM* 2006:1Q:p4. Correct coding of mass or lesion.
7. American Hospital Association. *Coding Clinic for ICD-9-CM* 1988:1Q:p4-5. Implantation or insertion of radioactive elements.
8. American Hospital Association. *Coding Clinic for ICD-9-CM* 1997:2Q:p3. Small bowel obstruction due to abdominal carcinomatosis.
9. American Hospital Association. *Coding Clinic for ICD-9-CM* 1995:4Q:p67-68. Chemoembolization with chemotherapy.

11

Diseases of the Blood and Blood-Forming Organs

(ICD-9-CM Chapter 4, Codes 280-289, and ICD-10-CM Chapter 3, Codes D50-D89)

CHAPTER OUTLINE

ICD-9-CM Official Guidelines for Coding and Reporting

ICD-10-CM Official Guidelines for Coding and Reporting

Guideline Differences Between ICD-9-CM and ICD-10-CM

Major Differences Between ICD-9-CM and ICD-10-CM

Anatomy and Physiology

Disease Conditions

- Deficiency Anemias
- Hemolytic Anemias
- Aplastic Anemias
- Other and Unspecified Anemias
- Coagulation Disorders
- Purpura and Other Hemorrhagic Conditions
- Diseases of the White Blood Cells
- Other Diseases of Blood and Blood-Forming Organs

Factors Influencing Health Status and Contact with Health Services (V Codes/Z Codes)

Common Treatments

Procedures

Documentation/Reimbursement/MS-DRGs

- MS-DRG With and Without MCC/CC
- Correct Procedure Code

Chapter Review Exercise

Chapter Glossary

References

LEARNING OBJECTIVES

1. Apply and assign the correct ICD-9-CM and ICD-10-CM codes in accordance with Official Guidelines for Coding and Reporting
2. Identify major differences between ICD-9-CM and ICD-10-CM related to the blood-forming organs
3. Identify pertinent anatomy and physiology of the blood and blood-forming organs
4. Identify diseases of the blood and blood-forming organs
5. Assign the correct V/Z codes and procedure codes related to the blood-forming organs
6. Identify laboratory values and diagnostic tests
7. Explain the importance of documentation in relation to MS-DRGs for reimbursement

ABBREVIATIONS/ ACRONYMS

ASA aspirin

CBC complete blood count

CKD chronic kidney disease

DIC disseminated intravascular coagulation

ESRD end-stage renal disease

Hct hematocrit

Hgb hemoglobin

HIV human immunodeficiency virus

ICD-9-CM *International Classification of Diseases, 9th Revision, Clinical Modification*

ICD-10-CM *International Classification of Diseases, 10th Revision, Clinical Modification*

ICD-10-PCS *International Classification of Diseases, 10th Revision, Procedure Classification System*

ITP idiopathic thrombocytopenic purpura

MS-DRG Medicare Severity diagnosis-related group

PT prothrombin time

PTT partial thromboplastin time

WBC white blood cell

ICD-9-CM

Official Guidelines for Coding and Reporting

Please refer to the companion Evolve website for the most current guidelines.

Chapter 4: Diseases of Blood and Blood Forming Organs (280-289)

a. Anemia of chronic disease

Subcategory 285.2, Anemia in chronic illness, has codes for anemia in chronic kidney disease, code 285.21; anemia in neoplastic disease, code 285.22; and anemia in other chronic illness, code 285.29. These codes can be used as the principal/first listed code if the reason for the encounter is to treat the anemia. They may also be used as secondary codes if treatment of the anemia is a component of an encounter, but not the primary reason for the encounter. When using a code from subcategory 285 it is also necessary to use the code for the chronic condition causing the anemia.

1) Anemia in chronic kidney disease

When assigning code 285.21, Anemia in chronic kidney disease, it is also necessary to assign a code from category 585, Chronic kidney disease, to indicate the stage of chronic kidney disease.

See I.C.10.a. Chronic kidney disease (CKD).

EXAMPLE

Anemia due to end-stage renal disease (ESRD), 285.21, 585.6 (N18.6, D63.1, ICD-10-CM instructs to code the underlying renal disease first).

---

2) Anemia in neoplastic disease

When assigning code 285.22, Anemia in neoplastic disease, it is also necessary to assign the neoplasm code that is responsible for the anemia. Code 285.22 is for use for anemia that is due to the malignancy, not for anemia due to antineoplastic chemotherapy drugs. Assign code 285.3 for anemia due to antineoplastic chemotherapy.

See I.C.2.c.1 Anemia associated with malignancy.
See I.C.2.c.2 Anemia associated with chemotherapy, immunotherapy and radiation therapy.

EXAMPLE

Anemia due to metastatic bone cancer. The patient has a history of primary breast cancer that was treated with mastectomy 4 years ago, 285.22, 198.5, V10.3, V45.71 (C79.51, D63.0, Z85.3, Z90.10, ICD-10-CM instructs to code the neoplasm first).

EXAMPLE

Patient is being treated for anemia due to chemotherapy. The patient has primary rectal cancer, 285.3, 154.1 (T45.1x5A, C20, D64.81).

Coding Clinic (2009:4Q:p80-82)[1] states that it is not necessary to assign an E code to identify the adverse effect because that information is included in the code title 285.3, Antineoplastic chemotherapy-induced anemia.

Apply the General Coding Guidelines as found in Chapter 5 and the Procedural Guidelines as found in Chapter 6.

ICD-10-CM **Official Guidelines for Coding and Reporting**	Please refer to the companion Evolve website for the most current guidelines. **3. Chapter 3: Disease of the blood and blood-forming organs and certain disorders involving the immune mechanism (D50-D89)** Reserved for future guideline expansion.

Apply the General Coding Guidelines as found in Chapter 5 and the Procedural Guidelines as found in Chapter 7.

GUIDELINE DIFFERENCES BETWEEN ICD-9-CM AND ICD-10-CM

There are no official guidelines in ICD-10-CM at this time regarding diseases of the blood and blood-forming organs. However, there is a change in how anemia due to a neoplastic disease is sequenced if the patient is being treated primarily for anemia. There is an ICD-9-CM guideline concerning this in the neoplasm chapter. However, in the ICD-10-CM Tabular, there is an instructional notation under code D63.0, Anemia in neoplastic disease, to first code the neoplasm (C00 to D49). This could make a difference in the assignment of a principal diagnosis when a patient is being treated only for anemia.

In ICD-10-CM, there are also instructions in the Tabular to *"code first the underlying disease"* when the anemia is due to chronic kidney disease (CKD) or some other specified chronic disease.

MAJOR DIFFERENCES BETWEEN ICD-9-CM AND ICD-10-CM

Most of the codes from ICD-9-CM Chapter 4 are included in ICD-10-CM Chapter 3. In ICD-10-CM, there are some codes from ICD-9-CM, Chapter 1, Infectious and Parasitic Diseases (e.g., D86 sarcoidosis), and Chapter 3, Endocrine, Nutritional, and Metabolic Diseases and Immunity Disorders.

■ In ICD-10-CM, many conditions or diseases can be coded with greater specificity.
■ Procedural complications affecting the spleen are included in Chapter 3 of ICD-10-CM.

ANATOMY AND PHYSIOLOGY

Blood is a viscous fluid that circulates through the vessels of the circulatory system as a result of the pumping action of the heart. Blood has three major functions. First, it transports oxygen, nutrients, hormones, enzymes, waste products, and carbon dioxide to and from cells. Second, blood promotes homeostasis and regulates body temperature. **Homeostasis** means balance or equilibrium. It is the ability of an organism or cell to maintain internal equilibrium by adjusting its physiologic processes. Third, blood provides a protective mechanism that combats foreign materials and assists in the body's defense against disease. Blood loss is prevented by clotting mechanisms within the body.

Blood is composed of plasma and formed elements or corpuscles. Corpuscles include erythrocytes (red blood cells), leukocytes (white blood cells), and platelets or thrombocytes.

TABLE 11-1 NORMAL LABORATORY VALUES[2]

WBC 5000-10,000 mm³ or μL

Differential	
Segs (polyps)	54%-62%
Lymphs	20%-40%
Eos	1%-3%
Baso	0%-1%
Mono	3%-7%
RBC	(M) 4.5-6.0 million per mm³ or μL
	(F) 4.0-5.5 million per mm³ or μL
Hct	(M) 40%-50%
	(F) 37%-47%
HGB	(M) 14-16 g/dL
	(F) 12-14 g/dL
Platelets	150,000-350,000/mm³ or μL

Baso, Basophils; *Eos*, eosinophils; *Hct*, hematocrit; *HGB*, hemoglobin; *Lymphs*, lymphocytes; *Mono*, monocytes; *RBC*, red blood cell; *Segs*, segments; *WBC*, white blood cell.

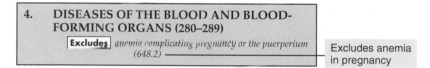

4. DISEASES OF THE BLOOD AND BLOOD-FORMING ORGANS (280–289)

Excludes *anemia complicating pregnancy or the puerperium (648.2)* ———— Excludes anemia in pregnancy

FIGURE 11-1. Excludes note that affects the entire chapter.

All of these components differ in terms of appearance, structure and type, function, life span, number, and means of production. **Erythrocytes**, or red blood cells, are made within the marrow of the bones; their main responsibility is to carry oxygen throughout the body and remove carbon dioxide. These are the cells that give blood its red color. **Leukocytes**, or white blood cells, increase in number to battle infection, inflammation, and other diseases. Five different types of white blood cells have been identified, and each has a role in fighting infection. White cells include neutrophils, monocytes, lymphocytes, eosinophils, and basophils. **Platelets** or **thrombocytes** circulate in the blood and assist in the clotting process.

Complete blood count (CBC) is a blood test that is commonly used to evaluate a patient's overall health; it detects a variety of disorders such as anemia, infection, and leukemia. This test measures the following:

- Hemoglobin (Hgb), a protein in red blood cells that carries oxygen to body tissues
- Hematocrit (Hct), the percentage of blood volume made up of red blood cells
- White blood cells (WBCs), which fight infection
- Platelets, which are essential to blood clotting

See Table 11-1 for normal values.

DISEASE CONDITIONS

Chapter 4 in the ICD-9-CM code book focuses on Diseases of the Blood and Blood-Forming Organs (280-289). This relatively small chapter is the only chapter that is not divided into sections. Of interest is an Excludes note that appears at the very beginning of the chapter. This signifies that the instructions given in the note pertain to the entire chapter. The Excludes note shown in Figure 11-1 instructs the coder to refer to code 648.2 for anemia complicating pregnancy or the puerperium. Because anemia is a condition that is commonly associated with pregnancy and the puerperium, this topic will be covered in Chapter 16, Complications of Pregnancy, Childbirth, and the Puerperium.

Excludes
note

FIGURE 11-2. The Excludes note under code 282.0, hereditary spherocytosis, excludes hemolytic anemia of newborn (773.0-773.5).

Neoplastic diseases of the blood, such as leukemia, are discussed in Chapter 15, Neoplasms; hematologic disorders involving newborns are addressed in Chapter 17, Congenital Anomalies and Perinatal Conditions. The Excludes note under code 282.0, hereditary spherocytosis, excludes hemolytic anemia of the newborn (773.0-773.5), as is illustrated in Figure 11-2.

Although ICD-9-CM is not divided into sections, ICD-10-CM is divided into the following categories:

CATEGORY	SECTION TITLES
D50-D53	Nutritional Anemias
D55-D59	Hemolytic Anemias
D60-D64	Aplastic and Other Anemias and Other Bone Marrow Failure Syndromes
D65-D69	Coagulation Defects, Purpura, and Other Hemorrhagic Conditions
D70-D77	Other Disorders of Blood and Blood-forming Organs
D78	Intraoperative and Postprocedural Complications of Spleen
D80-D89	Certain Disorders Involving the Immune Mechanism

Deficiency Anemias

Anemia occurs when hemoglobin drops, which interrupts the transport of oxygen throughout the body. The most common type of anemia is iron-deficiency anemia. In women, this condition is often due to heavy blood loss during menstrual periods. In older men and women, it may be an indication of gastrointestinal blood loss. Pregnant women and children need more iron, so a deficiency is likely due to insufficient iron in the diet. Testing may be necessary to determine a cause.

If a particular cause were determined, it would be appropriate to code the underlying condition. The sequencing of diagnoses would be determined by the coding guidelines for ICD-9-CM. Some of the reasons for iron deficiency include the following:

- Inadequate intake of iron in the diet
- Chronic blood loss
- Impaired absorption during digestion
- Liver disease
- Infection
- Cancers (neoplasms)

Numerous symptoms can indicate anemia; these include pallor, fatigue, lethargy, cold intolerance, irritability, stomatitis, headache, loss of appetite, numbness and tingling sensations, brittle hair, spoon-shaped and brittle nails, and edema, especially of the ankles. Severe anemia can result in tachycardia, palpitations, dyspnea (difficulty breathing), and syncope (fainting). Treatment depends on the cause, but the approach may be as simple as eating iron-rich foods or taking an iron supplement such as ferrous sulfate or ferrous gluconate. Blood transfusions may be necessary.

Look up the main term "Anemia" in the Index, and see the many subterms for the various types of anemia. "Deficiency" is also a subterm with many subterms, as is shown in Figure 11-3. At the subterm "in," entries are found for anemia in chronic illness, anemia in

Anemia *(Continued)*
   congenital *(Continued)*
      pernicious 281.0
      spherocytic (*see also* Spherocytosis)
        282.0
   Cooley's (erythroblastic) 282.49
   crescent - *see* Disease, sickle-cell
   cytogenic 281.0
   Dacie's (nonspherocytic)
      type I 282.2
      type II 282.3
   Davidson's (refractory) 284.9
   deficiency 281.9 ────────── Subterm "deficiency"
      2,3 diphosphoglycurate mutase
        282.3
      2,3 PG 282.3
      6-PGD 282.2
      6-phosphogluronic dehydrogenase
        282.2
      amino acid 281.4
      combined B_{12} and folate 281.3
      enzyme, drug-induced (hemolytic)
        282.2
      erythrocytic glutathione 282.2
      folate 281.2
        dietary 281.2
        drug-induced 281.2
      folic acid 281.2
        dietary 281.2
        drug-induced 281.2

FIGURE 11-3. Alphabetic Index entry for "anemia" and the subterm "deficiency."

Anemia *(Continued)*
   in
      chronic illness NEC 285.29
      chronic kidney disease 285.21
      end-stage renal disease 285.21
      neoplastic disease 285.22

FIGURE 11-4. Anemia due to chronic diseases.

end-stage renal disease/chronic kidney disease, and anemia in neoplastic disease. The term *chronic anemia* is not equated to "chronic simple anemia" or "anemia in chronic disease" (Figure 11-4). Chronic anemia is coded to 285.9 (D64.9) because no specific subterm is available for chronic, so the default code for anemia (285.9) code is assigned.

EXAMPLE   Patient is being treated as an outpatient for anemia due to inadequate dietary iron intake, 280.1 (D50.8).

EXAMPLE   Patient is being treated for folate deficiency anemia, 281.2 (D52.9).

EXERCISE 11-1

Assign codes to the following conditions.

1. Iron deficiency anemia due to chronic blood loss   _____
2. Vitamin B_{12} deficiency anemia   _____
3. Megaloblastic anemia   _____

Hemolytic Anemias

The hemolytic anemias are assigned to hereditary and acquired code categories (Figure 11-5). **Hemolytic anemia** results from abnormal or excessive destruction of red blood cells. **Sickle cell anemia** is one of the more common types of hereditary hemolytic anemia; it is found often in the African American population and among people living in Africa, the Mediterranean, Arabia, and South Asia. Red blood cells change from a disc shape to a crescent or "sickle" shape. This causes obstruction of the small blood vessels and eventual damage from thrombus formation, repeated organ infarctions, and tissue necrosis throughout the body. Varying degrees of disease severity and symptoms have been reported. Reported symptoms include severe anemia, hyperbilirubinemia or jaundice, splenomegaly, delayed and impaired growth and development, vascular occlusion, and infarctions, which can result in permanent damage, pain, frequent infection, and congestive heart failure. Most treatment is supportive in nature. A drug called Hydrea (hydroxyurea) has reduced the number of crises.

Look up "Sickle cell" in the Index; both subterms of anemia and disease instruct the coder to *see also* Disease, sickle cell. When looking up "Anemia," under the subterm "Sickle cell," the coder is instructed to *see also* Disease, sickle cell (Figure 11-6). Under the main term "Disease" and the subterm "Sickle cell," code selections are more detailed (Figure 11-7). Remember to follow these cross-references for identification of the code that best describes the patient's condition. Code 282.5 (D57.3) for sickle cell trait is assigned when a patient is a carrier and the disease has remained asymptomatic. When both sickle cell trait and sickle cell anemia are present, only sickle cell anemia is coded. Codes under the subcategory 282.6X have an additional fifth digit that relates to the absence or presence of a "crisis." The crisis may include additional conditions such as an infarction, acute chest syndrome, and

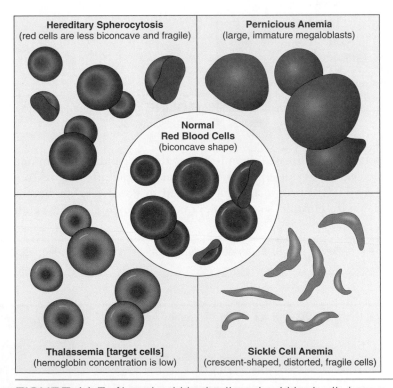

Hereditary Spherocytosis
(red cells are less biconcave and fragile)

Pernicious Anemia
(large, immature megaloblasts)

**Normal
Red Blood Cells**
(biconcave shape)

Thalassemia [target cells]
(hemoglobin concentration is low)

Sickle Cell Anemia
(crescent-shaped, distorted, fragile cells)

FIGURE 11-5. Normal red blood cells and red blood cells in several types of anemia.

Anemia (*Continued*)
  sickle-cell (*see also* Disease, sickle-cell)
    282.60

see also
instruction

FIGURE 11-6. *See also* Disease, sickle-cell.

Disease, diseased *(Continued)*
  sickle-cell 282.60
    with
      crisis 282.62
      Hb-S disease 282.61
      other abnormal hemoglobin
          (Hb-D) (Hb-E) (Hb-G) (Hb-J)
          (Hb-K) (Hb-O) (Hb-P) (high fe-
          tal gene) (without crisis) 282.68
        with crisis 282.69
    elliptocytosis 282.60
    Hb-C (without crisis) 282.63
      with
        crisis 282.64
        vaso-occlusive pain 282.64
    Hb-S 282.61
      with
        crisis 282.62
        Hb-C (without crisis) 282.63
          with
            crisis 282.64
            vaso-occlusive pain 282.64
        other abnormal hemoglobin (Hb-
            D) (Hb-E) (Hb-G) (Hb-J)
            (Hb-K) (Hb-O) (Hb-P) (high
            fetal gene) (without crisis)
            282.68
          with crisis 282.69
    spherocytosis 282.60
    thalassemia (without crisis) 282.41
      with
        crisis 282.42
        vaso-occlusive pain 282.42

FIGURE 11-7. Code selections are more detailed under the main terms "Disease" and subterm "sickle-cell."

splenic sequestration. These conditions would be coded additionally, and the sequencing of the codes depends on the reason for admission and the coding guidelines.

EXAMPLE   Patient was admitted with sickle cell crisis with acute chest syndrome. Patient has Hb-SS disease, 282.62, 517.3 (D57.01).

Another hereditary disease that is prevalent among people from Greece and Italy (Mediterranean countries), the Middle East, South Asia, and Africa is **thalassemia**. Similar to sickle cell anemia, the disease manifests in varying degrees. Cooley's anemia is another name that is used to describe the beta thalassemias. Frequent blood transfusions are administered, along with treatment with an iron chelation drug, which helps the body get rid of excess iron resulting from repeated transfusions. Occasionally, bone marrow transplant is performed, but this is a risky procedure, and a suitable donor is required.

EXAMPLE   Patient admitted with sickle cell thalassemia with vaso-occlusive pain crisis, 282.42 (D57.419).

EXERCISE 11-2

Assign codes to the following conditions.

1. Cooley's anemia   _____
2. Sickle cell trait with sickle cell anemia   _____
3. Acholuric jaundice   _____
4. Sickle cell Hb-C with vaso-occlusive crisis   _____
5. Sickle cell thalassemia   _____

Aplastic Anemias

Aplastic anemia is characterized by a reduction in new blood cells due to impairment or failure of bone marrow function. Decreased production of erythrocytes, leukocytes, and thrombocytes, also defined as pancytopenia, can lead to many complications. In 50% of cases, the cause of aplastic anemia is unknown or **idiopathic** in nature. Some drugs, industrial agents, chemicals, or radiation can affect the bone marrow. If these are the cause, an additional E code is required. If the causative factor can be identified and eliminated, the bone marrow possibly can recover. Viruses such as hepatitis C may also cause aplastic anemia.

If a patient has the following three conditions—neutropenia, thrombocytopenia, and anemia, also known as **pancytopenia**—the code 284.1X would be assigned. According to *Coding Clinic* (2005:3Q:p11-12),[3] an exception occurs when a patient is admitted with neutropenic fever and is also pancytopenic; in this case, it is acceptable to assign the neutropenia code (288.00 [D70.9]) as the principal diagnosis, with an additional code 284.1X (D61.81) used to describe the pancytopenia and 780.61 (R50.81) for the fever.

When a patient is admitted for neutropenic fever, investigations for any infectious source(s) are performed. Blood, sputum, and urine, and other sites may be cultured to try to identify an infection. The patient will be started on antibiotics, blood counts will be monitored, and neutropenic precautions will be implemented. If an infectious source is identified, treatment will be adjusted for that infection, and the infection should be the principal diagnosis.

EXAMPLE
Patient was admitted with neutropenic fever. Patient is currently being treated for diffuse large B-cell lymphoma. Broad-spectrum antibiotics were started. The urine culture and chest x-ray were negative. The blood cultures from the Hickman catheter and peripheral vein site were positive for *Staphylococcus aureus*. Vancomycin therapy was increased to 1 g every 12 hours. Patient had a MSSA bacteremia due to central line infection, 999.32, 790.7, 041.11, 202.80, E879.8 (T80.21xA, R78.81, C83.30, B95.6, Y84.8).

EXAMPLE
Patient has pancytopenia due to oral methotrexate which is taken for treatment of rheumatoid arthritis, initial encounter, 284.12, 714.0, E933.2 (T45.1x5A, D61.1, M06.9).

EXAMPLE
Infant with congenital aplastic anemia 284.01 (D61.09).

EXERCISE 11-3

Assign codes to the following conditions.

1. Aplastic anemia due to hepatitis C _____
2. Idiopathic aplastic anemia _____
3. Fanconi's anemia _____
4. Neutropenic fever. No infectious source found _____
5. Pancytopenia in patient with aplastic anemia _____

Other and Unspecified Anemias

This category includes acute posthemorrhagic anemia or anemia due to acute blood loss. Confusion arises regarding anemia related to blood loss and whether blood loss is acute or chronic and/or both. Sometimes, blood loss is well-documented, but the resultant anemia may not be documented by the physician. Whenever doubt occurs, the coder should query the physician. If acute and chronic blood loss anemias are present, both are coded, and acute blood loss anemia is sequenced first.

EXAMPLE

Patient has anemia due to gastric cancer, 285.22, 151.9 (C16.9, D63.0).

EXAMPLE

Patient treated for anemia due to acute blood loss 285.1 (D62).

EXERCISE 11-4

Assign codes to the following conditions.

1. Anemia due to end-stage renal disease (ESRD) _____
2. Normocytic anemia _____
3. Sideroblastic anemia _____
4. Anemia due to chronic disease _____

Coagulation Disorders

Excessive bleeding that occurs after a minor injury may be a sign of a **coagulation defect**, which is a breakdown in the blood clotting process. Multiple reasons may account for excessive bleeding:

■ Acute viral infection in children
■ Autoimmune reactions in adults
■ End-stage renal failure
■ Ingestion of aspirin (acetylsalicylic acid [ASA])
■ Vitamin K deficiency
■ Liver disease
■ Inherited disorders
■ Hemorrhagic fever viruses

Multiple warning signs may indicate a coagulation defect; these include bleeding from gums or repeated nosebleeds, petechiae (Figure 11-8), ecchymoses (bruises), hemarthroses (bleeding into a joint), hemoptysis (coughing up blood), hematemesis (vomiting blood), melena (blood in feces), anemia, feeling faint and anxious, low blood pressure, and increased pulse. Blood tests that involve bleeding time, prothrombin time (PT), or partial thromboplastin time (PTT) can measure the coagulation of blood. Occasionally, patients who take anticoagulants such as warfarin (Coumadin) will have complications. Some common complications include gastrointestinal bleeding, epistaxis, hematuria, or hemorrhage from any tissue. Their coagulation laboratory test results may be abnormal, but this does not mean that they have a coagulopathy, and the condition should not be coded as such. It should be coded to abnormal coagulation profile, 790.92, (R79.1) which can be located in the Alphabetic Index under the main term "Findings, abnormal, without diagnosis." It is a common mistake to assign code 286.59 (D68.9) (coagulopathy) when a patient is taking an anticoagulant. Per *Coding Clinic* (2006:2Q:p17),[4] a code from category 286, coagulation defects, is not appropriate for patients on anticoagulant therapy. The V code V58.61 (Z79.01) is assigned to identify the long-term use of anticoagulant medication such as Coumadin, which is located in the Alphabetic Index under the main term "Long-term drug use." A code would also be assigned for the diagnosis for which the patient is on anticoagulation therapy.

EXAMPLE

Patient is taking Coumadin for previous history of pulmonary embolism, V12.55, V58.61 (Z86.71, Z79.01).

FIGURE 11-8. Petechiae.

Hemophilia is an inherited clotting disorder. **Hemophilia A**, the most common form, is a deficiency or abnormality of clotting factor VIII. **Hemophilia B** (Christmas disease) is the result of a deficiency of factor IX, and **Hemophilia C** is a mild form characterized by a decrease in factor XI. As with some of the other diseases of the blood, varying degrees of severity are reported. A common treatment consists of replacement therapy for factor VIII with cryoprecipitate. Unfortunately, transmission of viruses such as hepatitis and human immunodeficiency virus (HIV) has resulted from this treatment. Currently, blood products are treated in an effort to destroy known viruses, but risk of unknown infection or immune reaction is still present.

Disseminated intravascular coagulation (DIC) is a disorder that causes depletion of clotting factors in the blood. Risk factors include recent sepsis, severe injury or trauma, recent surgery and anesthesia, complications of labor and delivery, cancer, transfusion reaction, and liver disease. Treatment may include transfusion of coagulation factors with fresh frozen plasma; the underlying cause must be determined so the appropriate treatment can be provided.

EXAMPLE   Patient was treated for coagulopathy due to chronic liver disease, 286.7, 571.9 (D68.4, K76.9).

EXERCISE 11-5

Assign codes to the following conditions.

1. Rosenthal's hemophilia   _____
2. Classic hemophilia   _____
3. Christmas disease   _____
4. DIC   _____
5. von Willebrand's disease   _____

Purpura and Other Hemorrhagic Conditions

Purpura is characterized by ecchymoses or small hemorrhages in the skin, mucous membranes, or serosal surfaces that are due to blood disorders, vascular abnormalities, or trauma. A patient with idiopathic thrombocytopenic purpura (ITP) experiences a decrease in the number of platelets with no identifiable cause. Following laboratory testing, a bone marrow biopsy may be necessary. Treatments may include corticosteroids, immunosuppressive therapy, and possibly splenectomy.

Secondary thrombocytopenia is characterized by a decrease in the number of platelets; it is due to specific diseases such as congestive splenomegaly, Felty's syndrome, tuberculosis, sarcoidosis, lupus erythematosus, and chronic alcoholism. Some external causes include drugs, blood transfusions, and overhydration.

EXAMPLE	Thrombocytopenia due to chronic alcoholism, 287.49, 303.90 (D69.59, F10.20).

EXAMPLE	Patient admitted with idiopathic thrombocytopenic purpura, 287.31 (D69.3).

EXERCISE 11-6

Assign codes to the following conditions.

1. Idiopathic nonthrombocytopenic purpura   _____
2. Thrombocytopenia due to systemic lupus erythematosus   _____
3. Schönlein-Henoch purpura   _____
4. Low platelets   _____

Diseases of the White Blood Cells

Leukocytosis (neutrophilia or granulocytosis) is characterized by an increase in the number of white cells in the blood. Usually, no treatment is required. If leukocytosis persists, investigation to rule out a neoplastic process or infection may become necessary. Leukocytosis may also be related to certain drugs or may occur in response to stress. The most common white blood cell condition is agranulocytosis, or **neutropenia**, which is an abnormal decrease in granular leukocytes in the blood. Radiation therapy, drugs used for chemotherapy, and other chemicals may cause neutropenia. With severe neutropenia, a patient may become immunocompromised; his or her ability to fight infection may be hampered, and treatment often consists of antibiotics. Testing may be necessary to determine cause and select appropriate treatment.

EXAMPLE	Infant is being treated for congenital agranulocytosis, 288.01 (D70.0).

Other Diseases of Blood and Blood-Forming Organs

This includes conditions of the spleen, lymphatic system, and bone marrow. The spleen serves as a blood reservoir, filters the blood and removes old or defective blood cells, and serves as part of the immune system by helping to fight infection. The spleen can become enlarged (**splenomegaly**) due to infections or other diseases. A swollen spleen is at risk for rupturing, which could result in significant blood loss. **Lymphadenitis** is the inflammation of a lymph node that is typically caused by a bacterial infection and can easily be treated with antibiotics.

EXAMPLE | Ultrasound exam showed that the patient has a splenic infarction, 289.59 (D73.5).

EXERCISE 11-7

Assign codes to the following conditions.

1. Neutropenic fever   _____
2. Leukocytosis   _____
3. Eosinophilia   _____
4. Leukopenia   _____
5. Factor V Leiden mutation   _____
6. Mesenteric lymphadenitis   _____

FACTORS INFLUENCING HEALTH STATUS AND CONTACT WITH HEALTH SERVICES (V CODES/Z CODES)

In the past, V/Z codes were primarily considered for use in the outpatient setting. This has changed with the addition of more V/Z codes each year. As was discussed in Chapter 8, it may be difficult to locate V/Z codes in the Index. Coders often say, "I did not know there was a V/Z code for that." Refer to Chapter 8 for a listing of common main terms used to locate V/Z codes.

A review of the Tabular reveals that some V/Z codes pertain to diseases of the blood and blood-forming organs:

V12.3	Personal history of diseases of blood and blood-forming organs
V18.2	Family history of anemia
V18.3	Family history of other blood disorders
V42.81	Organ or tissue replaced by transplant—bone marrow
V42.82	Organ or tissue replaced by transplant—peripheral stem cells
V58.2	Blood transfusion without reported diagnosis
V58.61	Long-term (current) use of anticoagulants
V58.63	Long-term (current) use of antiplatelets/antithrombotics
V58.66	Long-term (current) use of aspirin
V59.01	Donor whole blood
V59.02	Donor stem cells
V59.09	Donor, other
V59.3	Donor bone marrow
V72.86	Encounter for blood typing
V78.0	Special screening for iron deficiency anemia
V78.1	Special screening for other and unspecified deficiency anemia
V78.2	Special screening sickle cell disease or trait
V78.3	Special screening, other hemoglobinopathies
V78.8	Special screening, other disorders of blood and blood-forming organs
V78.9	Special screening, unspecified disorder of blood and blood-forming organs
V83.01	Asymptomatic hemophilia A carrier
V83.02	Symptomatic hemophilia A carrier

Some V codes describe the long-term use of a particular type of medication such as anticoagulants or antiplatelets/antithrombotics. **Anticoagulants** are medications that are used to prevent venous thrombi. They can be administered parenterally with heparin, or warfarin (Coumadin) can be taken orally. **Parenteral** drug administration is when medications are administered other than through the digestive tract, such as by intravenous or intramuscular injections. **Antiplatelet** drugs are used to prevent clumping of platelets or formation of an arterial thrombus. Medications that are used as antiplatelet therapy include clopidogrel (Plavix), ticlopidine (Ticlid), dipyridamole (Persantin), and aspirin (ASA).

EXAMPLE	Screening for iron deficiency anemia, V78.0 (Z13.0).

EXAMPLE	Long-term use of ASA due to family history of stroke, V58.66, V17.1 (Z79.82, Z82.3).

EXERCISE 11-8

Assign codes to the following conditions.

1. Bone marrow donor _____
2. Long-term use of Coumadin _____
3. Screening for sickle cell disease _____
4. Long-term use of Plavix _____

COMMON TREATMENTS

CONDITION	MEDICATION/TREATMENT
Anemia	Treatment depends on the cause
Anemia due to chronic kidney disease	Epoetin alfa (Epogen, Procrit)
Iron-deficiency anemia	Iron supplements, ferrous sulfate (FeoSol)
Pernicious anemia	B_{12} injections
Anemia of chronic disease	Treatment of the underlying cause/disease
Sickle cell anemia	Hydroxyurea (Droxia, Hydrea)
Hemophilia A	Desmopressin acetate (DDAVP), recombinant or plasma concentrate factor VIII, cryoprecipitate
Neutropenia	Filgrastim (Neupogen)

PROCEDURES

Procedures that may be related to disease of the blood and blood-forming organs can be located in the following ICD-9-CM chapters of the Procedure Tabular:

8. Operations on the Hemic and Lymphatic System (40-21)
16. Miscellaneous Diagnostic and Therapeutic Procedures (87-99)

Procedures related to the blood and blood-forming organs in ICD-10-PCS can be located in the following tables:

072-07Y	Lymphatic and Hemic Systems
302-3EI	Administration
4A0-4B0	Measuring and Monitoring

Blood transfusion, which can be performed for many reasons, is the administration of donor blood cells into a patient. The root operation in ICD-10-PCS for transfusion is transfusion. The most common types of transfusions consist of red blood cells, plasma, and platelets. Sometimes, before undergoing an elective surgery, a patient will donate his or her own blood to be used in the event a transfusion is needed. This is known as an **autologous transfusion**.

1. Stem cells from the donor's circulating blood are collected in a transfer bag or marrow cells are aspirated from the donor's hip bone (ilium).

2. Stem cells or marrow cells are mixed with an anticlotting agent and strained to remove bits of bone and fat.

3. Stem cells or marrow cells are given intravenously via a catheter implanted in the upper chest and leading to a central vein.

DONOR

PATIENT

FIGURE 11-9. Peripheral stem cell and bone marrow transplants.

Apheresis is a procedure that separates the different components of the blood and removes a certain part of the blood, such as occurs in leukapheresis, plateletpheresis, and plasmapheresis. A therapeutic plasmapheresis or plasma exchange occurs when the plasma is removed and is replaced with fresh plasma. The root operation in ICD-10-PCS for therapeutic plasmaphersis is pheresis.

Bone marrow biopsy and/or aspiration is a diagnostic procedure that can be used to identify types of blood disorders. The root operation in ICD-10-PCS for bone marrow biopsy is extraction. The root operation in ICD-10-PCS for bone marrow aspiration is drainage. It may also be performed to evaluate the patient's response to treatment.

Peripheral stem cell and bone marrow transplants (Figure 11-9) are used to treat patients with certain leukemias and cancers, bone marrow failure syndromes, and genetic disease. Prior to transplant, the patient is prepared with radiation and/or chemotherapy to get rid of the defective or malignant cells and reduce the body's immunity so it will not reject the transplanted cells.

EXERCISE 11-9

Assign codes for all diagnoses and procedures.

1. Patient with profound pancytopenia had a diagnostic percutaneous bone marrow biopsy iliac crest _____

2. Thrombocytopenia was treated with transfusion of platelets (nonautologous infusion in peripheral vein) _____

3. Therapeutic single plasmapheresis performed on patient with thrombotic thrombocytopenic purpura _____

4. DIC with transfusion of fresh frozen plasma (percutaneous infusion, central vein, nonautologous) _____

5. Postoperative blood loss anemia with autologous transfusion of red blood cells _____

DOCUMENTATION/REIMBURSEMENT/MS-DRGS

Often, coding difficulties are due to lack of documentation. Sometimes pathology and other test results are not available at the time of discharge or when the physician is dictating the discharge summary or is reporting the final diagnoses.

Documentation difficulties include lack of documentation regarding various types of anemia and the relationship of anemia to other chronic illnesses and diseases such as ESRD and neoplastic disease. Sometimes, acute and/or chronic blood loss is documented, but in the record, no mention of associated anemia is made by the physician.

Frequently missed complications/comorbidities from this chapter include:

- Acute post-hemorrhagic anemia
- Aplastic anemia
- DIC
- Pancytopenia

MS-DRG With and Without MCC/CC

EXAMPLE A patient had a total abdominal hysterectomy for fibroid uterus. The patient was symptomatic with menorrhagia. Patient has von Willebrand's disease.

DIAGNOSES	CODES	MS-DRG	RW
Fibroid uterus with menorrhagia and von Willebrand's disease	218.9, 626.2, 286.4 (D25.9, N92.0, D68.0)	742	1.3883
Total abdominal hysterectomy	68.49 (0UT90ZZ)		
Fibroid uterus with menorrhagia	218.9, 626.2 (D25.9, N92.0)	743	0.9079
Total abdominal hysterectomy	68.49 (0UT90ZZ)		

In this case, von Willebrand's disease is a CC, and this affects reimbursement.

Correct Procedure Code

It is important to assign all procedure codes. A surgical MS-DRG is likely to have a higher relative weight than a medical MS-DRG. Reimbursement may be lost if the appropriate procedure codes are not assigned.

EXAMPLE A patient is being admitted for a total splenectomy for treatment of idiopathic thrombocytopenic purpura (ITP).

DIAGNOSES	CODES	MS-DRG	RW
ITP with splenectomy	287.31 (D69.3)	801	1.5586
	41.5 (07TP0ZZ)		
ITP	287.31 (D69.3)	813	1.4372

In this case, the total splenectomy affects the MS-DRG assignment.

CHAPTER REVIEW EXERCISE

Assign codes for all diagnoses and procedures.

1. Vitamin K deficiency _____
2. Pernicious anemia _____
3. Coagulopathy indicated by abnormal coagulation profile due to Coumadin taken for atrial fibrillation. Patient has been on Coumadin for 1 year. _____
4. Hemophilia A carrier _____
5. Pseudocholinesterase deficiency _____
6. Polycythemia, benign _____
7. Severe congenital aplastic anemia treated with bone marrow transplant, allogeneic from related donor (percutaneous central vein) _____
8. Sickle cell Hb-SS disease with crisis _____
9. Anemia due to AIDS _____
10. Anemia due to acute and chronic blood loss treated with transfusion of 2 units of packed red blood cells (percutaneous peripheral vein, nonautologous) _____
11. Coagulopathy due to cirrhosis _____
12. History of bone marrow transplant _____
13. Chronic agranulocytosis _____
14. Chronic lymphadenitis _____
15. Hypersplenism _____
16. Congestive splenomegaly _____
17. Hemochromatosis _____
18. Lymphocytic leukemoid reaction _____
19. Lupus anticoagulant _____
20. Neutropenia due to infection _____

Write the correct answer(s) in the space(s) provided.

21. Which blood component is essential for clotting?

    _____

22. Describe apheresis.

    _____

23. List two warning signs of a coagulation disorder.

    _____

24. Which cells fight infection, inflammation, and other diseases?

    _____

25. Define idiopathic.

    _____

CHAPTER GLOSSARY

Anemia: occurs when hemoglobin drops, which interrupts the transport of oxygen throughout the body.

Anticoagulant medications: medications that are used to prevent venous thrombi.

Antiplatelet medications: medications that are used to prevent clumping of platelets or formation of an arterial thrombus.

Apheresis: procedure that separates different components of blood and removes a certain part of the blood, such as occurs in leukapheresis, plateletpheresis, and plasmapheresis.

Aplastic anemia: reduction in new blood cells due to impairment or failure of bone marrow function.

Autologous transfusion: transfusion of a patient's own blood. Blood may have been donated prior to an elective procedure.

Blood: viscous fluid that circulates through the vessels of the circulatory system as a result of the pumping action of the heart.

Bone marrow biopsy: diagnostic procedure that is used to identify types of anemia and cell deficiencies and to detect leukemia.

Coagulation defect: breakdown in the clotting process of the blood.

Disseminated intravascular coagulation: disorder that results in depletion of clotting factors in the blood.

Erythrocytes: another name for red blood cells that are made in the marrow of bones; their main responsibility is to carry oxygen around the body and remove carbon dioxide. These are the cells that give blood its red color.

Hemolytic anemias: result from abnormal or excessive destruction of red blood cells.

Hemophilia A: most common type of hemophilia; deficiency or abnormality in clotting factor VIII.

Hemophilia B: another name for Christmas disease, which results from a deficiency of factor IX.

Hemophilia C: mild form of hemophilia with decreased factor XI.

Homeostasis: the ability of an organism or cell to maintain internal equilibrium by adjusting its physiologic processes.

Idiopathic: causative factor is unknown.

Leukocytes: white blood cells increase in number to battle infection, inflammation, and other diseases.

Leukocytosis: increase in the number of white cells in the blood; it may be a sign of infection or may indicate stress on the body.

Lymphadenitis: inflammation of a lymph node that is usually caused by a bacterial infection.

Neutropenia: abnormal decrease in granular leukocytes in the blood.

Pancytopenia: decrease in production of erythrocytes (red blood cells), leukocytes (white blood cells), and thrombocytes (platelets).

Parenteral: when medications are administered other than through the digestive tract, such as by intravenous or intramuscular injection.

Platelets: another name for thrombocytes. Platelets circulate in the blood and assist in the clotting process.

Purpura: ecchymoses or small hemorrhages in the skin, mucous membranes, or serosal surfaces due to blood disorders, vascular abnormalities, or trauma.

Secondary thrombocytopenia: decrease in the number of platelets due to specific diseases or external causes, such as drugs, blood transfusions, and overhydration.

Sickle cell anemia: one of the most common hemolytic anemias, in which the shape of the red blood cell changes from a disc to a crescent or "sickle," causing obstruction of small blood vessels and eventual damage throughout the body.

Splenomegaly: enlarged spleen.

Thalassemia: hereditary disease that is similar to sickle cell anemia and occurs in varying degrees.

Thrombocytes: another name for platelets. Thrombocytes circulate in the blood and assist in the clotting process.

REFERENCES

1. American Hospital Association. *Coding Clinic for ICD-9-CM* 2009:4Q:80-82. Antineoplastic chemotherapy-induced anemia.
2. Chabner D. The Language of Medicine, 8th ed. St. Louis, Saunders, 2007, p 506
3. American Hospital Association. *Coding Clinic for ICD-9-CM* 2005:3Q:p11-12. Neutropenic fever with pancytopenia.
4. American Hospital Association. *Coding Clinic for ICD-9-CM* 2006:2Q:p17. Hemoptysis and GI bleeding due to anticoagulants.

12

Endocrine, Nutritional, and Metabolic Diseases, and Immunity Disorders

(ICD-9-CM Chapter 3, Codes 240-279, and ICD-10-CM Chapter 4, Codes E00-E89)

CHAPTER OUTLINE

ICD-9-CM Official Guidelines for Coding and Reporting
ICD-10-CM Official Guidelines for Coding and Reporting
Guideline Differences Between ICD-9-CM and ICD-10-CM
Major Differences Between ICD-9-CM and ICD-10-CM
Anatomy and Physiology
Disease Conditions
    Disorders of Thyroid Gland
    Disorders of Other Endocrine Glands
    Nutritional Deficiencies
    Other Metabolic and Immunity Disorders
Factors Influencing Health Status and Contact with Health Services (V Codes/Z Codes)
Common Treatments
Procedures
    Bariatric Procedures
    Insulin Pumps
Documentation/Reimbursement/MS-DRGs
    MS-DRG With and Without MCC/CC
    Two Diagnoses That Equally Meet the Definition for Principal Diagnosis
    Diabetic Manifestation Versus Not Related to Diabetes
Chapter Review Exercise
Chapter Glossary
References

LEARNING OBJECTIVES

1. Apply and assign the correct ICD-9-CM and ICD-10-CM codes in accordance with Official Guidelines for Coding and Reporting
2. Identify major differences between ICD-9-CM and ICD-10-CM related to the endocrine, nutritional, and metabolic diseases and immunity disorders
3. Identify pertinent anatomy and physiology of the endocrine, nutritional, and metabolic diseases and immunity disorders
4. Identify endocrine, nutritional, and metabolic diseases and immunity disorders

5. Assign the correct V/Z codes and procedure codes related to the endocrine, nutritional, and metabolic diseases and immunity disorders
6. Identify common treatments, medications, laboratory values, and diagnostic tests
7. Explain the importance of documentation in relation to MS-DRGs for reimbursement

ABBREVIATIONS/ ACRONYMS

AIDS acquired immunodeficiency syndrome

AML acute myeloid leukemia

BMI body mass index

BPD biliopancreatic diversion

CC complication/comorbidity

CDC Centers for Disease Control and Prevention

CF cystic fibrosis

DI diabetes insipidus

DM diabetes mellitus

GVHD graft-versus-host disease

hGH human growth hormone

ICD-9-CM *International Classification of Diseases,*

9th Revision, Clinical Modification

ICD-10-CM *International Classification of Diseases, 10th Revision, Clinical Modification*

ICD-10-PCS *International Classification of Diseases, 10th Revision, Procedure Coding System*

IDDM insulin-dependent diabetes mellitus

IV intravenous

MEN multiple endocrine neoplasia

MS-DRG Medicare Severity diagnosis-related group

NIDDM non–insulin-dependent diabetes mellitus

OIG Office of the Inspector General

PKU phenylketonuria

SCID severe combined immunodeficiency

SIADH syndrome of inappropriate antidiuretic hormone secretion

TLS tumor lysis syndrome

TPN total parenteral nutrition

TSH thyroid-stimulating hormone

UTI urinary tract infection

VBG vertical banded gastroplasty

ICD-9-CM

Official Guidelines for Coding and Reporting

Please refer to the companion Evolve website for the most current guidelines.

3. Chapter 3: Endocrine, Nutritional, and Metabolic Diseases and Immunity Disorders (240-279)

a. Diabetes mellitus

Codes under category 250, Diabetes mellitus, identify complications/manifestations associated with diabetes mellitus. A fifth-digit is required for all category 250 codes to identify the type of diabetes mellitus and whether the diabetes is controlled or uncontrolled.

See I.C.3.a.7 for secondary diagnosis.

1) Fifth-digits for category 250:

The following are the fifth-digits for the codes under category 250:

0 type II or unspecified type, not stated as uncontrolled
1 type I, [juvenile type], not stated as uncontrolled
2 type II or unspecified type, uncontrolled
3 type I, [juvenile type], uncontrolled

The age of a patient is not the sole determining factor, though most type I diabetics develop the condition before reaching puberty. For this reason type I diabetes mellitus is also referred to as juvenile diabetes.

EXAMPLE Juvenile diabetes, 250.01 (E10.9).

EXAMPLE The patient is a 16-year-old with obesity and diabetes mellitus, type II, uncontrolled, 250.02, 278.00 (E11.65, E66.9).

---

2) Type of diabetes mellitus not documented

If the type of diabetes mellitus is not documented in the medical record the default is type II.

EXAMPLE ┃ The patient takes daily insulin for diabetes, 250.00, V58.67 (E11.9, Z79.4).

3) Diabetes mellitus and the use of insulin

All type I diabetics must use insulin to replace what their bodies do not produce. However, the use of insulin does not mean that a patient is a type I diabetic. Some patients with type II diabetes mellitus are unable to control their blood sugar through diet and oral medication alone and do require insulin. If the documentation in a medical record does not indicate the type of diabetes but does indicate that the patient uses insulin, the appropriate fifth-digit for type II must be used. For type II patients who routinely use insulin, code V58.67, Long-term (current) use of insulin, should also be assigned to indicate that the patient uses insulin. Code V58.67 should not be assigned if insulin is given temporarily to bring a type II patient's blood sugar under control during an encounter.

EXAMPLE ┃ A patient with type II diabetes has been undergoing changes to daily insulin dosages. The patient's diabetes is uncontrolled, 250.02, V58.67 (E11.65, Z79.4).

4) Assigning and sequencing diabetes codes and associated conditions

When assigning codes for diabetes and its associated conditions, the code(s) from category 250 must be sequenced before the codes for the associated conditions. The diabetes codes and the secondary codes that correspond to them are paired codes that follow the etiology/manifestation convention of the classification. *(See Section I.A.6., Etiology/manifestation convention).* Assign as many codes from category 250 as needed to identify all of the associated conditions that the patient has. The corresponding secondary codes are listed under each of the diabetes codes (Figure 12-1).

EXAMPLE ┃ The patient was admitted for care of a diabetic left midfoot ulcer. The patient also had chronic kidney disease due to type II diabetes, 250.80, 707.14, 250.40, 585.9 (E11.621, L97.429, E11.22, N18.9).

(a) Diabetic retinopathy/diabetic macular edema

Diabetic macular edema, code 362.07, is only present with diabetic retinopathy. Another code from subcategory 362.0, Diabetic retinopathy, must be used with code 362.07. Codes under subcategory 362.0 are diabetes manifestation codes, so they must be used following the appropriate diabetes code.

5) Diabetes mellitus in pregnancy and gestational diabetes

(a) For diabetes mellitus complicating pregnancy, see Section I.C.11.f., Diabetes mellitus in pregnancy.

(b) For gestational diabetes, see Section I.C.11.g., Gestational diabetes.

6) Insulin pump malfunction

(a) Underdose of insulin due to insulin pump failure

An underdose of insulin due to an insulin pump failure should be assigned 996.57, Mechanical complication due to insulin pump, as the principal or first listed code, followed by the appropriate diabetes mellitus code based on documentation.

(b) Overdose of insulin due to insulin pump failure

The principal or first listed code for an encounter due to an insulin pump malfunction resulting in an overdose of insulin, should also be 996.57, Mechanical complication due to insulin pump, followed by code 962.3, Poisoning

● **250.4 Diabetes with renal manifestations**

    Use additional code to identify manifestation, as:
        chronic kidney disease (585.1–585.9) diabetic:
            nephropathy NOS (583.81)
            nephrosis (581.81)
        intercapillary glomerulosclerosis (581.81)
        Kimmelstiel-Wilson syndrome (581.81)

● **250.5 Diabetes with ophthalmic manifestations**

    Use additional code to identify manifestation, as:
        diabetic:
            blindness (369.00–369.9)
            cataract (366.41)
            glaucoma (365.44)
            macular edema (362.07)
            retinal edema (362.07)
            retinopathy (362.01–362.07)

● **250.6 Diabetes with neurological manifestations**

    Use additional code to identify manifestation, as:
        diabetic:
            amyotrophy (358.1)
            gastroparalysis (536.3)
            gastroparesis (536.3)
            mononeuropathy (354.0–355.9)
            neurogenic arthropathy (713.5)
            peripheral autonomic neuropathy (337.1)
            polyneuropathy (357.2)

● **250.7 Diabetes with peripheral circulatory disorders**

    Use additional code to identify manifestation, as:
        diabetic:
            gangrene (785.4)
            peripheral angiopathy (443.81)

● □ **250.8 Diabetes with other specified manifestations**
    Diabetic hypoglycemia
    Hypoglycemic shock

    Use additional code to identify manifestation, as:
        any associated ulceration (707.10–707.9)
        diabetic bone changes (731.8)

    Use additional E code to identify cause, if drug-
        induced

FIGURE 12-1. Tabular entry for diabetes mellitus.

    by insulins and antidiabetic agents, and the appropriate diabetes mellitus code based on documentation.

7) Secondary Diabetes Mellitus

    Codes under category 249, Secondary diabetes mellitus, identify complications/manifestations associated with secondary diabetes mellitus. Secondary diabetes is always caused by another condition or event (e.g., cystic fibrosis, malignant neoplasm of pancreas, pancreatectomy, adverse effect of drug, or poisoning).

(a) Fifth-digits for category 249:

    A fifth-digit is required for all category 249 codes to identify whether the diabetes is controlled or uncontrolled.

(b) Secondary diabetes mellitus and the use of insulin

    For patients who routinely use insulin, code V58.67, Long-term (current) use of insulin, should also be assigned. Code V58.67 should not be assigned if insulin is given temporarily to bring a patient's blood sugar under control during an encounter.

(c) Assigning and sequencing secondary diabetes codes and associated conditions

When assigning codes for secondary diabetes and its associated conditions (e.g. renal manifestations), the code(s) from category 249 must be sequenced before the codes for the associated conditions. The secondary diabetes codes and the diabetic manifestation codes that correspond to them are paired codes that follow the etiology/manifestation convention of the classification. Assign as many codes from category 249 as needed to identify all of the associated conditions that the patient has. The corresponding codes for the associated conditions are listed under each of the secondary diabetes codes. For example, secondary diabetes with diabetic nephrosis is assigned to code 249.40, followed by 581.81.

(d) Assigning and sequencing secondary diabetes codes and its causes

The sequencing of the secondary diabetes codes in relationship to codes for the cause of the diabetes is based on the reason for the encounter, applicable ICD-9-CM sequencing conventions, and chapter-specific guidelines.

If a patient is seen for treatment of the secondary diabetes or one of its associated conditions, a code from category 249 is sequenced as the principal or first-listed diagnosis, with the cause of the secondary diabetes (e.g. cystic fibrosis) sequenced as an additional diagnosis.

EXAMPLE

Uncontrolled diabetes mellitus due to Cushing's syndrome. Patient has been on insulin for the last year. 249.01, 255.0, V58.67 (E24.9, E08.65, Z79.4).

If, however, the patient is seen for the treatment of the condition causing the secondary diabetes (e.g., malignant neoplasm of pancreas), the code for the cause of the secondary diabetes should be sequenced as the principal or first-listed diagnosis followed by a code from category 249.

(i) Secondary diabetes mellitus due to pancreatectomy

For postpancreatectomy diabetes mellitus (lack of insulin due to the surgical removal of all or part of the pancreas), assign code 251.3, Postsurgical hypoinsulinemia. Assign a code from subcategory 249, **Secondary diabetes mellitus and a code from subcategory V88.1, Acquired absence of pancreas** as additional codes. Code also any diabetic manifestations (e.g. diabetic nephrosis 581.81).

(ii) Secondary diabetes due to drugs

Secondary diabetes may be caused by an adverse effect of correctly administered medications, poisoning or late effect of poisoning.

See section I.C.17.e for coding of adverse effects and poisoning, and section I.C.19 for E code reporting.

Apply the General Coding Guidelines as found in Chapter 5 and the Procedural Guidelines as found in Chapter 6.

ICD-10-CM

Official Guidelines for Coding and Reporting

Please refer to the companion Evolve website for the most current guidelines.

4. Chapter 4: Endocrine, Nutritional, and Metabolic Diseases (E00-*E89*)

a. Diabetes mellitus

The diabetes mellitus codes are combination codes that include the type of **diabetes mellitus**, the body system affected, and the complications affecting that body system. As many codes within a particular category as are necessary to describe all of the complications of the disease may be used. They should be sequenced based on the reason for a particular encounter. Assign as many codes from categories E08 – E13 as needed to identify all of the associated conditions that the patient has.

1) **Type of diabetes**

   The age of a patient is not the sole determining factor, though most type 1 diabetics develop the condition before reaching puberty. For this reason type 1 diabetes mellitus is also referred to as juvenile diabetes.

2) **Type of diabetes mellitus not documented**

   If the type of diabetes mellitus is not documented in the medical record the default is E11.-, Type 2 diabetes mellitus.

3) **Diabetes mellitus and the use of insulin**

   If the documentation in a medical record does not indicate the type of diabetes but does indicate that the patient uses insulin, code E11, Type 2 diabetes mellitus, should be assigned. **Code** Z79.4, Long-term (current) use of insulin, should also be assigned to indicate that the patient uses insulin. Code Z79.4 should not be assigned if insulin is given temporarily to bring a type 2 patient's blood sugar under control during an encounter.

4) **Diabetes mellitus in pregnancy and gestational diabetes**

   See Section I.C.15. Diabetes mellitus in pregnancy.

   See Section I.C.15. Gestational (pregnancy induced) diabetes

5) **Complications due to insulin pump malfunction**

   (a) **Underdose of insulin due *to* insulin pump failure**

   An underdose of insulin due to an insulin pump failure should be assigned to a code from subcategory T85.6, Mechanical complication of other specified internal and external prosthetic devices, implants and grafts, that specifies the type of pump malfunction, as the principal or **first-listed** code, followed by code T38.3x6-, Underdosing of insulin and oral hypoglycemic [antidiabetic] drugs. Additional codes for the type of diabetes mellitus and any associated complications due to the underdosing should also be assigned.

   (b) **Overdose of insulin due to insulin pump failure**

   The principal or **first-listed** code for an encounter due to an insulin pump malfunction resulting in an overdose of insulin, should also be T85.6-, Mechanical complication of other specified internal and external prosthetic devices, implants and grafts, followed by code T38.3x1-, Poisoning by insulin and oral hypoglycemic [antidiabetic] drugs, accidental (unintentional).

6) **Secondary Diabetes Mellitus**

   Codes under **categories** E08, Diabetes mellitus due to underlying condition, and E09, Drug or chemical induced diabetes mellitus, identify complications/manifestations associated with secondary diabetes mellitus. Secondary diabetes is always caused by another condition or event (e.g., cystic fibrosis, malignant neoplasm of pancreas, pancreatectomy, adverse effect of drug, or poisoning).

   (a) **Secondary diabetes mellitus and the use of insulin**

   For patients who routinely use insulin, code Z79.4, Long-term (current) use of insulin, should also be assigned. Code Z79.4 should not be assigned if insulin is given temporarily to bring a patient's blood sugar under control during an encounter.

   (b) **Assigning and sequencing secondary diabetes codes and its causes**

   The sequencing of the secondary diabetes codes in relationship to codes for the cause of the diabetes is based on the **Tabular List** instructions for categories E08 and E09. For example, for category E08, Diabetes mellitus due to underlying condition, code first the underlying condition; for category E09, Drug or chemical induced diabetes mellitus, code first the drug or chemical (T36-T65).

   (i) **Secondary diabetes mellitus due to pancreatectomy**

   For postpancreatectomy diabetes mellitus (lack of insulin due to the surgical removal of all or part of the pancreas), assign code E89.1, **Postprocedural hypoinsulinemia.** Assign a code from category **E13** and a code **from subcategory Z90.41-, Acquired absence of pancreas,** as additional codes.

   (ii) **Secondary diabetes due to drugs**

   Secondary diabetes may be caused by an adverse effect of correctly administered medications, poisoning or late effect of poisoning.

   See section I.C.19.e for coding of adverse effects and poisoning, and section I.C.20 for external cause code reporting.

Apply the General Coding Guidelines as found in Chapter 5 and the Procedural Guidelines as found in chapter 7.

GUIDELINE DIFFERENCES BETWEEN ICD-9-CM AND ICD-10-CM

There are no major guideline differences between the ICD-9-CM and ICD-10-CM.

MAJOR DIFFERENCES BETWEEN ICD-9-CM AND ICD-10-CM

- In ICD-10-CM, there are five category codes for diabetes mellitus:

E08	Diabetes mellitus due to underlying condition
E09	Drug or chemical induced diabetes mellitus
E10	Type I diabetes mellitus
E11	Type II diabetes mellitus
E13	Other specified diabetes mellitus

- In ICD-10-CM, if a condition such as diabetes mellitus is drug-induced, there is an instructional Code first (T36-T65) note to identify the drug or chemical involved.
- In ICD-9-CM, there are fifth digits to identify whether a patient's diabetes is controlled, uncontrolled, or unspecified. In ICD-10-CM, there are Alphabetic Index entries for "out of control" and "poorly controlled" diabetes that state to code to diabetes by type, with hyperglycemia.
- In ICD-9-CM there is no specific code to identify hyperglycemia with diabetes. In ICD-10-CM, there are codes to identify both hyperglycemia and hypoglycemia in a diabetic patient.
- Procedural complications affecting the endocrine system and metabolic complications are included in Chapter 4 of ICD-10-CM. Some of the complications include:
  - Hypofunction of various endocrine glands following surgery
  - Postoperative hemorrhage and hematoma

ANATOMY AND PHYSIOLOGY

The **endocrine system** (Figure 12-2) works with the nervous system to maintain body functions and homeostasis and to respond to stress. The endocrine system is composed of many glands that are located throughout the body. These glands secrete **hormones** that can regulate bodily functions such as urinary output, cellular metabolic rate, growth, and development.

Major endocrine glands include the following:
- Anterior pituitary
- Posterior pituitary
- Thyroid
- Parathyroid
- Adrenal cortex
- Adrenal medulla
- Pancreas
- Ovaries
- Testes
- Thymus
- Pineal gland

See Table 12-1 for a listing of the glands, corresponding hormones, and expected hormonal response.

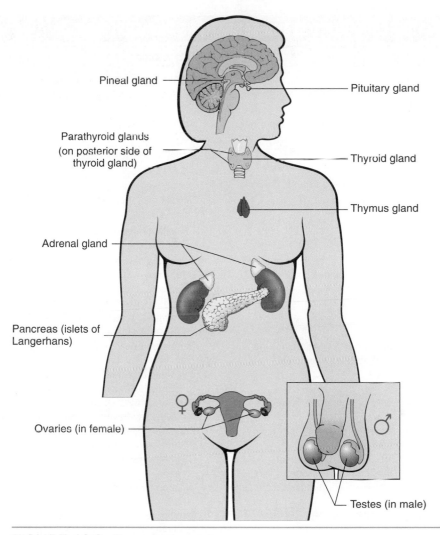

FIGURE 12-2. The endocrine system.

Endocrine diseases may result from an abnormal decrease or increase in hormone production. Changes in the size of a gland can alter hormone production. If the gland becomes larger, this is called **hyperplasia** and/or **hypertrophy**. If the gland becomes smaller, this is called **hypoplasia** and/or **atrophy**. Infection, inflammation, radiation, trauma, and surgical procedures can produce changes in the gland and hormonal dysfunction.

Some common mental and physical symptoms include the following:

- Growth abnormalities
- Emotional disturbances
- Skin, hair, and nail changes
- Edema
- Hypertension or hypotension
- Cardiac arrhythmias
- Changes in urine output
- Muscle weakness or atrophy
- Menstrual irregularities
- Impotence
- Changes in libido
- Infertility
- Fatigue

TABLE 12-1 MAJOR ENDOCRINE GLAND SECRETIONS AND FUNCTIONS[1]

Endocrine Gland	Hormone	Target Action
Anterior pituitary	Growth hormone (GH)	Promotes bone and tissue growth
	Thyrotropin (thyroid-stimulating hormone [TSH])	Stimulates thyroid gland and production of thyroxine
	Corticotropin (adrenocorticotropic hormone [ACTH])	Stimulates adrenal cortex to produce glucocorticoids
	Gonadotropin	Initiates growth of eggs in ovaries; stimulates spermatogenesis in testes
	Follicle-stimulating hormone (FSH)	
	Luteinizing hormone (LH)	Causes ovulation; stimulates ovaries to produce estrogen and progesterone; stimulates testosterone production
	Prolactin	Stimulates breast development and formation of milk during pregnancy and after delivery
	Melanocyte-stimulating hormone (MSH)	Regulates skin pigmentation
Posterior pituitary	Vasopressin (antidiuretic hormone [ADH])	Stimulates water resorption by renal tubules; has antidiuretic effect
	Oxytocin	Stimulates uterine contractions; stimulates ejection of milk in mammary glands; causes ejection of secretions in male prostate gland
Thyroid	Thyroxine (T_4) and triiodothyronine (T_3)—thyroid hormone (TH)	Regulates rate of cellular metabolism (catabolic phase)
	Calcitonin	Promotes retention of calcium and phosphorus in bone; opposes effect of parathyroid hormone
Parathyroid	Parathyroid hormone (parathormone, PTH)	Regulates metabolism of calcium; elevates serum calcium levels by drawing calcium from bones
Adrenal cortex	Mineralocorticoids (MCs), primarily aldosterone	Promote retention of sodium by kidneys; regulate electrolyte and fluid homeostasis
	Glucocorticoids (GCs): cortisol, corticosterone, cortisone	Regulate metabolism of carbohydrates, proteins, and fats in cells
	Gonadocorticoids: androgens, estrogens, progestins	Govern secondary sex characteristics and masculinization
Adrenal medulla	Catecholamines: epinephrine and norepinephrine	Produce quick-acting "fight or flight" response during stress; increase blood pressure, heart rate, and blood glucose level; dilate bronchioles
Pancreas	Insulin	Regulates metabolism of glucose in body cells; maintains proper blood glucose level
	Glucagon	Increases concentration of glucose in blood by causing conversion of glycogen to glucose
Ovaries	Estrogens	Cause development of female secondary sex characteristics
	Progesterone	Prepares and maintains endometrium for implantation and pregnancy
Testes	Testosterone	Stimulates and promotes growth of male secondary sex characteristics and is essential for erections
Thymus	Thymosin	Promotes development of immune cells (gland atrophies during adulthood)
Pineal gland	Melatonin	Regulates daily patterns of sleep and wakefulness; inhibits hormones that affect ovaries; other functions unknown

DISEASE CONDITIONS

Diseases of the Endocrine, Nutritional and Metabolic Disease, and Immunity Disorders (240-279), Chapter 3 in the ICD-9-CM code book, is divided into the following categories:

CATEGORY	SECTION TITLES
240-246	Disorders of Thyroid Gland
249-259	Diseases of Other Endocrine Glands
260-269	Nutritional Deficiencies
270-279	Other Metabolic and Immunity Disorders

Diseases of the endocrine system and nutritional and metabolic disorders (E00 to E89), covered in Chapter 4 of the ICD-10-CM code book, are divided into the following categories:

CATEGORY	SECTION TITLES
E00-E07	Disorders of the Thyroid Gland
E08-E13	Diabetes Mellitus
E15-E16	Other of Glucose Regulation and Pancreatic Internal Secretion
E20-E35	Disorders of Other Endocrine Glands
E36	Intraoperative Complications of Endocrine System
E40-E46	Malnutrition
E50-E64	Other Nutritional Deficiencies
E65-E68	Overweight, Obesity, and Other Hyperalimentation
E70-E88	Metabolic Disorders
E89	Postprocedural Endocrine and Metabolic Complications and Disorders, Not Elsewhere Classified

Disorders of Thyroid Gland

Goiter

Goiter is an enlargement of the thyroid gland (Figure 12-3). This enlargement may be uniform throughout the gland or diffuse. Enlargement may also occur in the form of nodules or nodular goiter. A goiter can cause difficulties in swallowing and/or breathing and may or may not be associated with hormonal disturbances. The most common cause is lack of iodine in the diet. Goiters due to iodine deficiency are rare in the United States since the introduction of iodized salt.

FIGURE 12-3. Goiter. Note the enlarged neck due to enlargement of the thyroid gland.

FIGURE 12-4. Myxedema.

EXAMPLE   Patient has a multinodular goiter, 241.1 (E04.2).

Hypothyroidism

Hypothyroidism is diminished production of thyroid hormone, manifested by low metabolic rate, tendency toward weight gain, somnolence, and sometimes myxedema. **Myxedema** is a skin and tissue disorder that is usually due to severe, prolonged hypothyroidism (Figure 12-4). Symptoms include dull, puffy, yellowed skin; coarse, sparse hair; and periorbital edema and prominent tongue.

EXAMPLE   Patient has hypothyroidism, 244.9 (E03.9).

Hashimoto's disease is an inflammation of the thyroid gland that often results in hypothyroidism. It is most common in women and individuals who have a family history of thyroid disease. Onset of Hashimoto's is slow, and it may not be detected for years. The most common signs and symptoms of Hashimoto's disease include the following:

- Intolerance to cold
- Weight gain
- Fatigue
- Constipation
- Goiter
- Dry skin
- Hair loss
- Heavy or irregular menses
- Difficulty with concentration

EXAMPLE   Patient has constipation and fatigue due to autoimmune thyroiditis, 245.2, 564.00 (the fatigue code comes from the symptom chapter) (E06.3, K59.00).

Hyperthyroidism/Graves' Disease

Hyperthyroidism (Figure 12-5) is an abnormality of the thyroid gland in which secretion of thyroid hormone is usually increased and is no longer under the regulatory control of hypothalamic-pituitary centers.

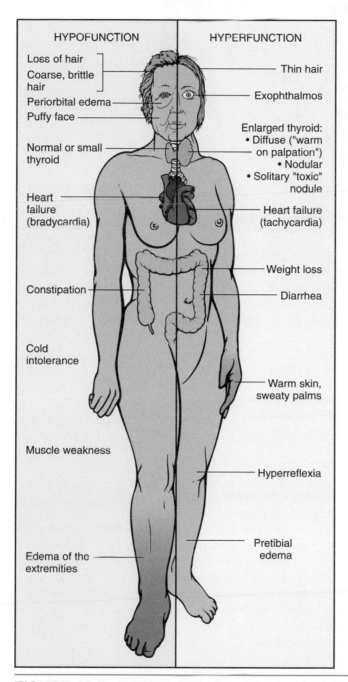

HYPOFUNCTION

- Loss of hair
- Coarse, brittle hair
- Periorbital edema
- Puffy face
- Normal or small thyroid
- Heart failure (bradycardia)
- Constipation
- Cold intolerance
- Muscle weakness
- Edema of the extremities

HYPERFUNCTION

- Thin hair
- Exophthalmos
- Enlarged thyroid:
  - Diffuse ("warm on palpation")
  - Nodular
  - Solitary "toxic" nodule
- Heart failure (tachycardia)
- Weight loss
- Diarrhea
- Warm skin, sweaty palms
- Hyperreflexia
- Pretibial edema

FIGURE 12-5. Comparison of hypothyroidism and hyperthyroidism.

FIGURE 12-6. Exophthalmos in Graves' disease.

Graves' disease, the most common form of hyperthyroidism, occurs as the result of an autoimmune response that attacks the thyroid gland, resulting in overproduction of the thyroid hormone thyroxine. Graves' disease is most common among women between 20 and 40 years of age. The most common signs and symptoms include the following:

- Anxiety
- Irritability
- Difficulty sleeping
- Rapid or irregular heartbeat
- Tremor of hands or fingers
- Increased perspiration
- Sensitivity to heat
- Weight loss
- Brittle hair
- Goiter
- Light menstrual periods
- Frequent bowel movements

Graves' ophthalmopathy is also fairly common and may result in **exophthalmos**, or bulging eyes (Figure 12-6). A complication of hyperthyroidism is **thyrotoxic crisis or storm**. This is a sudden intensification of symptoms combined with fever, rapid pulse, and delirium. Medical attention is required when a crisis episode occurs.

Common causes of a thyrotoxic storm or crisis include a medical illness or infection. Other causes include the following:

- Emotional stress
- Diabetic ketoacidosis
- Hypoglycemia
- Cerebrovascular accident
- Pulmonary embolism
- Bowel infarction
- Trauma
- Increase in thyroid hormone from surgery, radioiodine therapy, or iodinated contrast dye

EXAMPLE   Weight loss due to Graves' disease, 242.00 (E05.00).

EXAMPLE | Patient with history of hyperthyroidism and is status post thyroidectomy. Patient is treated for hypothyroidism with Synthroid, 244.0 (E89.0).

EXERCISE 12-1

Assign codes to the following conditions.

1. Thyroid nodule   _____

2. Hypothyroidism following radiation treatments for Graves'   _____
   disease

3. Graves' disease with thyrotoxic crisis   _____

4. Hashimoto's disease   _____

5. Congenital hypothyroidism   _____

Disorders of Other Endocrine Glands

Diabetes Mellitus

Diabetes mellitus is a chronic syndrome of impaired carbohydrate, protein, and fat metabolism caused by insufficient production of insulin by the pancreas or faulty utilization of insulin by the cells. The coding of diabetes mellitus (DM) may be complicated because various manifestations are associated with the disease.

There are two major types of diabetes mellitus: type I and type II. These types vary in origin, pathology, genetics, age of onset, and treatment (Table 12-2). Patients with type I diabetes are insulin-dependent; this condition usually develops early in life. The pancreas produces insulin in very small amounts or not at all. Type II diabetes usually is of adult-onset. The pancreas continues to produce insulin, but it is not properly metabolized. Occasionally, patients with type II diabetes must be treated with insulin so that acceptable glucose levels are maintained; the fact that they are taking insulin does not mean that they are dependent on insulin or that they have type I diabetes. Type II diabetes is much more common than type I; 90% to 95% of diabetic patients have type II diabetes. Type II diabetes in adolescents and children is a relatively new phenomenon, and statistics are still being collected. Sometimes, diabetes is documented as insulin-dependent diabetes mellitus (IDDM) or non–insulin-dependent diabetes mellitus (NIDDM). Documentation of insulin dependence does not determine appropriate fifth-digit assignment because a patient with type II diabetes may be on insulin. If only IDDM is documented, and type I or type II is not specified, according to coding guidelines, the appropriate fifth-digit code should be assigned for type II diabetes.

According to *Coding Clinic* (1991:3Q:p6),[3] "Two types of complications may occur with diabetes mellitus. One of these is the acute metabolic complication that is part of diabetes

---

TABLE 12-2 COMPARISON OF TYPE I AND TYPE II DIABETES MELLITUS[2]

	Type I	Type II
Features	Usually occurs before age 30	Usually occurs after age 30
	Abrupt, rapid onset	Gradual onset; asymptomatic
	Little or no insulin production	Insulin usually present
	Thin or normal body weight at onset	85% are obese
	Ketoacidosis often occurs	Ketoacidosis seldom occurs
Symptoms	Polyuria (glycosuria promotes loss of water)	Polyuria sometimes seen
	Polydipsia (dehydration causes thirst)	Polydipsia sometimes seen
	Polyphagia (tissue breakdown causes hunger)	Polyphagia sometimes seen
Treatment	Insulin	Diet; oral hypoglycemics or insulin

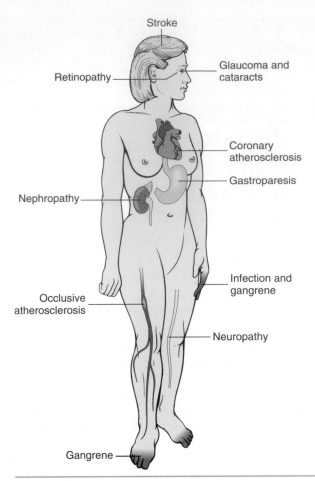

FIGURE 12-7. Possible manifestations/complications of diabetes mellitus.

itself and does not require an additional code. The other is the late effect or chronic effect that occurs in another body system due to the diabetes and requires a code from the 250.4X to 250.8X series with an additional code for the manifestation" (Figure 12-7).

EXAMPLE

The patient is treated for diabetic ketoacidosis. Patient has type I DM, 250.13 (E10.10).
    Acidosis would not be coded as an additional code in a diabetic patient with ketoacidosis, per the Excludes note under code 276.2 (E87.2).

Category 250.0X (E11.9), Diabetes mellitus without mention of complication, would have no additional diabetic subcategory codes or manifestation codes (i.e., 205.4X, Diabetes with renal manifestation codes) (Figure 12-8).

There are subcategories for metabolic complications that require no additional manifestation code (Figure 12-9). Subcategories are available for the following diabetic complications and manifestations (Figure 12-10).

Subcategory 250.9X (E11.8) is reserved for diabetes with unspecified complication (Figure 12-11). In the inpatient setting, it may be beneficial to query the physician for specific documentation regarding any diabetic complications and/or manifestations.

The appropriate diabetes and manifestation codes as documented in the health record, as well as the correct fifth digits must be assigned. See Figure 12-12 for fifth-digit subclassifications for use with category 250.

According to *Coding Clinic* (2002:2Q:p13),[4] the coder must query the physician if diabetes has been documented as "poorly controlled" or "poor control," to verify whether "uncontrolled" is meant so that the fifth digit can be assigned. There may be conflicting

● **250.0 Diabetes mellitus without mention of complication**
    Diabetes mellitus without mention of complication
       or manifestation classifiable to 250.1–250.9
    Diabetes (mellitus) NOS

FIGURE 12-8. Diabetes mellitus without complications.

● **250.1 Diabetes with ketoacidosis**
    Diabetic:
        acidosis without mention of coma
        ketosis without mention of coma
● **250.2 Diabetes with hyperosmolarity**
    Hyperosmolar (nonketotic) coma
● **250.3 Diabetes with other coma**
    Diabetic coma (with ketoacidosis)
    Diabetic hypoglycemic coma
    Insulin coma NOS
    Excludes *diabetes with hyperosmolar coma (250.2)*

FIGURE 12-9. Diabetes with metabolic complication subcategories.

● **250.4 Diabetes with renal manifestations**

Use additional code to identify manifestation, as:
    chronic kidney disease (585.1–585.9) diabetic:
        nephropathy NOS (583.81)
        nephrosis (581.81)
        intercapillary glomerulosclerosis (581.81)
        Kimmelstiel-Wilson syndrome (581.81)

● **250.5 Diabetes with ophthalmic manifestations**

Use additional code to identify manifestation, as:
    diabetic:
        blindness (369.00–369.9)
        cataract (366.41)
        glaucoma (365.44)
        macular edema (362.07)
        retinal edema (362.07)
        retinopathy (362.01–362.07)

● **250.6 Diabetes with neurological manifestations**

Use additional code to identify manifestation, as:
    diabetic:
        amyotrophy (358.1)
        gastroparalysis (536.3)
        gastroparesis (536.3)
        mononeuropathy (354.0–355.9)
        neurogenic arthropathy (713.5)
        peripheral autonomic neuropathy (337.1)
        polyneuropathy (357.2)

● **250.7 Diabetes with peripheral circulatory disorders**

Use additional code to identify manifestation, as:
    diabetic:
        gangrene (785.4)
        peripheral angiopathy (443.81)

● □ **250.8 Diabetes with other specified manifestations**
    Diabetic hypoglycemia
    Hypoglycemic shock

Use additional code to identify manifestation, as:
    any associated ulceration (707.10–707.9)
    diabetic bone changes (731.8)

Use additional E code to identify cause, if drug-
    induced

FIGURE 12-10. Diabetes with complications/manifestations.

> ●❑ **250.9 Diabetes with unspecified complication**

FIGURE 12-11. Diabetes with unspecified complication.

> ● **250 Diabetes mellitus**
>
> | Excludes | *gestational diabetes (648.8)*
> *hyperglycemia NOS (790.6)*
> *neonatal diabetes mellitus (775.1)*
> *nonclinical diabetes (790.29)*
>
> The following fifth-digit subclassification is for use with category 250:
>
> 0 **type II or unspecified type, not stated as uncontrolled**
>   Fifth-digit 0 is for use for type II patients, even if the patient requires insulin
>   Use additional code, if applicable, for associated long-term (current) insulin use V58.67
> 1 **type I [juvenile type], not stated as uncontrolled**
> 2 **type II or unspecified type, uncontrolled**
>   Fifth-digit 2 is for use for type II patients, even if the patient requires insulin
>   Use additional code, if applicable, for associated long-term (current) insulin use V58.67
> 3 **type I [juvenile type], uncontrolled**

FIGURE 12-12. Fifth-digit subclassification for use with category 250.

information regarding which diabetes code should be used for a patient with uncontrolled diabetes, type I or type II. According to *Coding Clinic* (1997:4Q:p33),[5] the correct code for a patient with uncontrolled diabetes mellitus, adult-onset type, requiring insulin is 250.02.

Sometimes a physician will document that a patient's diabetes is "out of control." According to the Alphabetic Index, out of control is coded as uncontrolled diabetes. When documentation is unclear about the cause of the diabetes, the default is type II diabetes mellitus.

It is possible for a diabetic patient to have more than one complication and/or manifestation of diabetes, so it is necessary for the coder to use as many codes as necessary to completely describe the patient's diabetic conditions. The 250.4X to 250.8X codes should be sequenced before the associated manifestation codes. It is very important to follow the guidelines with regard to coding and sequencing of manifestation codes.

EXAMPLE

A patient is admitted with diabetic gangrene of the left little toe. The toe was completely amputated. The patient has uncontrolled type I diabetes, 250.73, 785.4, 84.11 (E10.52, E10.65, 0Y6Y0Z0).

EXAMPLE

Patient is admitted with diabetic ketoacidosis. Patient also has diabetic gastroparesis (type I), 250.13, 250.63, 536.3 (E10.10, E10.43).

Before a diagnosis can be coded as a diabetic manifestation, a direct cause-and-effect relationship must be established. The manifestation must be documented as diabetic or due to diabetes. For a patient who has diabetes and a cataract, diabetic cataract may not be assigned without documentation linking the cataract to the diabetes.

EXAMPLE

Patient has diabetes and senile cataracts bilaterally, 250.00, 366.10 (E11.9, H25.9).

EXAMPLE

Patient has cataracts due to diabetes, 250.50, 366.41 (E11.36).

Diabetes, diabetic (brittle) (congenital)
(familial) (mellitus) (severe) (slight)
(without complication) 250.0

> Note   Use the following fifth-digit
> subclassification with category 250:
>
> 0   type II or unspecified type, not
>   stated as uncontrolled
>
>   Fifth-digit 0 is for use for type
>   II patients, even if the patient
>   requires insulin
>
> 1   type I [juvenile type], not stated
>   as uncontrolled
> 2   type II or unspecified type,
>   uncontrolled
>
>   Fifth-digit 2 is for use for type
>   II patients, even if the patient
>   requires insulin
>
> 3   type I [juvenile type], uncon-
>   trolled

→ with
    coma (with ketoacidosis) 250.3
    hyperosmolar (nonketotic) 250.2
    complication NEC 250.9
    specified NEC 250.8
    gangrene 250.7 [785.4]
    hyperosmolarity 250.2
    ketosis, ketoacidosis 250.1
    osteomyelitis 250.8 [731.8]
    specified manifestations NEC 250.8

FIGURE 12-13. Alphabetic Index of "Diabetes with …"

A couple of exceptions to this rule should be noted. See Figure 12-13 for Index terms under the main term "Diabetes." Note the term "with" and the selections underneath that term. If a patient has diabetes, and if that patient also has osteomyelitis, a cause-and-effect relationship may be assumed, unless it is documented as unrelated. This is supported by *Coding Clinic* (2004:1Q:p14-15):[6] "If the physician indicates diabetic osteomyelitis, or the patient has both diabetes and acute osteomyelitis and no other cause of the osteomyelitis is documented, it would be appropriate to assign codes 250.80, Diabetes with other specified manifestations, Type II, or unspecified type, not stated as uncontrolled, 731.8, Other bone involvement in diseases classified elsewhere, and 730.0X, Acute osteomyelitis. ICD-9-CM assumes a relationship between diabetes and osteomyelitis when both conditions are present, unless the physician has indicated in the medical record that the acute osteomyelitis is totally unrelated to the diabetes."

EXAMPLE   Acute osteomyelitis right calcaneus in patient with type I diabetes that is poorly controlled, 250.81, 731.8, 730.07 (M86.171, E10.65; the Alphabetic Index entry in ICD-10 does not include a subterm entry of "with osteomyelitis" under diabetes). The physician would have to be queried about whether "poorly controlled" meant "uncontrolled" for assignment of code 250.83.

Secondary Diabetes

Secondary diabetes mellitus is a form of the disease that develops as a result of another disease or condition. Secondary diabetes can be caused by any condition that damages or interferes with the function of the pancreas. Common conditions that may cause secondary diabetes include pancreatitis, tumor of the pancreas, cystic fibrosis, hemochromatosis, acromegaly, Cushing's syndrome, pheochromocytoma, and drug usage (e.g., corticosteroids). If the underlying cause can be successfully treated, insulin production may improve or return to normal.

The codes for secondary diabetes are similar to the 250.XX diabetes codes. There are fourth-digit subcategory codes for metabolic complications and manifestations. There are also fifth-digit subclassification codes to indicate whether the secondary diabetes is controlled or not. A fifth digit of 0 stands for "not stated as uncontrolled, or unspecified," and a fifth digit of 1 stands for "uncontrolled."

EXAMPLE   Patient has uncontrolled diabetic nephropathy. Diabetes is due to chronic pancreatitis, 249.41, 583.81, 577.1 (K86.1, E08.65).

Steroid-induced diabetes is diabetes that results from the use of steroids. Steroids enhance insulin resistance, making insulin less effective. If the pancreas cannot make enough insulin to keep blood glucose within a normal range and the patient is on steroids, this could be steroid-induced diabetes. Steroid-induced diabetes may go away when steroids are discontinued. If the patient has a condition that requires long-term treatment with steroids, diabetes may remain. An episode of steroid-induced diabetes may be an indicator that the patient is at risk for developing diabetes later in life.

EXAMPLE   Patient with steroid-induced diabetes due to long-term use of prednisone taken for rheumatoid arthritis. 249.00, 714.0, V58.65, E932.0 (T38.0x5S, E09.9, M06.9, Z79.52).

Hypoglycemia

Hypoglycemia occurs when glucose or blood sugar becomes abnormally low. This is a relatively common occurrence in a diabetic patient. Hypoglycemia can also occur in patients who do not have diabetes mellitus. Normal fasting blood glucose levels range from 70 to 99 mg/dL.

EXAMPLE   Patient with hypoglycemia, 251.2 (E16.2).

EXAMPLE   Patient who has type II diabetes with hypoglycemia, 250.80 (E11.649).

Hyperglycemia

Hyperglycemia occurs when glucose or blood sugar becomes abnormally high. This also is a relatively common occurrence in a diabetic patient. In contrast to hypoglycemia, hyperglycemia is not assigned to a different fourth-digit subcategory. Patients who do not have diabetes may have episodes of hyperglycemia. Sometimes, medication such as steroids can cause hyperglycemia.

EXAMPLE   Patient with diabetes and hyperglycemia, 250.00 (E11.65).

EXAMPLE   Patient with hyperglycemia due to long-term use of prednisone taken for rheumatoid arthritis, 790.29, 714.0, V58.65, E932.0 (T38.0x5S, R73.9, M06.9, Z79.52).

Gestational Diabetes

Gestational diabetes is discussed in Chapter 21, Complications of Pregnancy, Childbirth, and the Puerperium.

FIGURE 12-14. Effects of growth hormone. **A,** Comparison of gigantism, normal growth, and dwarfism. **B,** Hands with clinical signs of acromegaly. **C,** Face with clinical signs of acromegaly.

Hyperpituitarism

Hyperpituitarism results from increased production of pituitary hormones, particularly of human growth hormone (hGH). **Gigantism** or **acromegaly** may occur, depending on the time of life when hormonal dysfunction begins (Figure 12-14).

Gigantism occurs when hypersecretion of hGH occurs before puberty, along with proportionate overgrowth of all body tissues, especially of the long bones. Often, a pituitary adenoma results from oversecretion of hGH. Acromegaly results when hypersecretion of hGH occurs after puberty, along with overgrowth of the face, hands, feet, and soft tissues. Pituitary adenoma is often the cause.

EXAMPLE | Patient has hypersecretion of growth hormone, 253.0 (E22.0).

Hypopituitarism

Hypopituitarism is a condition that is caused by low levels of pituitary hormones. Hormones secreted by the pituitary gland may affect the function of other glands. Lack of thyroid-stimulating hormone (TSH) affects the function of the thyroid gland. Hypopituitarism may be caused by a variety of conditions, such as the following:

- Tumor
- Head trauma
- Brain surgery
- Stroke
- Infections of brain

Occasionally, immune system or metabolic disease such as sarcoidosis, histiocytosis X, and hemochromatosis can cause hypopituitarism. The code 253.7 is used to identify hypopituitarism that is hormone-induced, hypophysectomy-induced, radiotherapy-induced, or post-ablative in nature.

EXAMPLE | The patient has hypopituitarism due to pituitary adenoma, 227.3, 253.2 (D35.2, E23.0).

EXAMPLE | The patient has hypopituitarism due to abscess of the brain, 324.0, 253.2 (G06.0, E23.0).

Diabetes Insipidus

Diabetes insipidus (DI) or water diabetes is a deficiency in the release of vasopressin by the posterior pituitary gland. The patient excretes volumes of dilute urine and experiences excessive thirst, fatigue, and dehydration. The underlying cause needs to be identified and treated.

Underlying causes of DI include the following:

- Stroke
- Neoplasm
- Polycystic kidney disease
- Neurosurgery

Although DI and DM both include the term *diabetes* in their names, the two conditions are not related.

EXAMPLE | The patient suffers from diabetes insipidus, 253.5 (E23.2).

Hyperparathyroidism

Hyperparathyroidism results from an overactive parathyroid gland that secretes excessive parathyroid hormone, causing increased levels of circulating calcium due to loss of calcium in the bone.

Hyperparathyroidism may be primary or secondary. In most cases, primary hyperparathyroidism is caused by a parathyroid adenoma. Secondary hyperparathyroidism is often related to chronic kidney disease.

EXAMPLE | The patient was treated for hyperplasia of the parathyroid. The patient was hypercalcemic, 252.01 (E21.0). Note the Excludes note under 275.4, Disorders of calcium metabolism (Figure 12-15). Hypercalcemia or hypocalcemia would not be coded as an additional code with any parathyroid disorder codes (252.00-252.9).

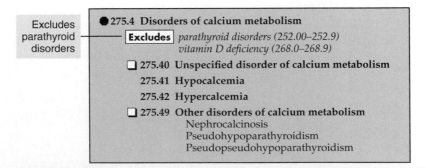

FIGURE 12-15. Disorders of calcium metabolism Excludes note.

FIGURE 12-16. Cushingoid features—moon face, obesity, and cutaneous striae.

Hypoparathyroidism

Hypoparathyroidism is caused by an underactive parathyroid gland that results in decreased levels of circulating calcium. The primary manifestation is **tetany**, a continuous muscle spasm. Vitamin D and calcium supplements are often used to treat this condition.

EXAMPLE

The patient had tetany due to hypoparathyroidism. The patient is hypocalcemic and is treated with calcium supplements, 252.1 (E20.9).

Cushing's Syndrome

Cushing's syndrome is a condition that results in excessive circulating cortisol levels due to chronic hypersecretion of the adrenal cortex. Common signs and symptoms include the following:

■ Fatigue
■ Muscle weakness
■ Changes in body appearance with fat deposits in the scapular and abdominal areas
■ Moon face
■ Hypertension
■ Edema

Other complications include hyperlipidemia, osteoporosis, diabetes, excessive hair growth, amenorrhea, impotence, and psychiatric disturbances (Figure 12-16). The skin becomes thin and bruises easily, and red or purple stretch marks develop.

Administration of glucocorticoids (steroids) to treat other diseases can result in **iatrogenic** (treatment-induced) Cushing's. The patient's appearance may be described as "cushingoid" (Figure 12-16).

EXAMPLE

Patient has Cushing's syndrome and hyperlipidemia, 255.0, 272.4 (E24.9, E78.5).

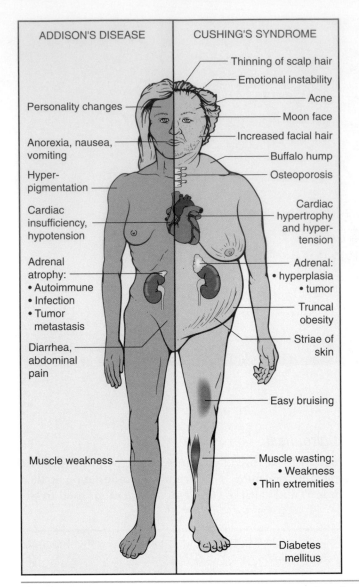

FIGURE 12-17. Comparison of adrenocortical hypofunction and hyperfunction.

Addison's Disease

Addison's disease is an adrenocortical insufficiency that may be caused by neoplasms, surgical removal of the adrenal gland, autoimmune processes, tuberculosis, hemorrhage, and/or infection. Addison's is characterized by the following symptoms:

- Hypotension
- Weight loss
- Anorexia
- Weakness
- Bronze skin coloring

Other complications include cardiovascular problems such as irregular pulse, reduced cardiac output, and orthostatic hypotension (Figure 12-17). Emotional disturbances such as depression and anxiety are common. When dehydration and electrolyte imbalances occur, medical attention is required to prevent a life-threatening situation.

EXAMPLE   Patient was admitted to the hospital for treatment of dehydration and for prevention of Addison's crisis, 276.51, 255.41 (E86.0, E27.1).

EXERCISE 12-2

Assign codes to the following conditions.

1. Diabetic with episode of hypoglycemia _____

2. Diabetic retinopathy, DM type II _____

3. Diabetic hyperosmolar coma _____

4. Hyperparathyroidism _____

5. Syndrome of inappropriate antidiuretic hormone secretion (SIADH) _____

6. Vasopressin deficiency _____

7. Diabetic gangrene, left big toe _____

8. Diabetes type II, uncontrolled; peripheral vascular disease _____

9. Steroid-induced diabetes; patient has been on long-term steroids for Crohn's disease _____

10. Multiple endocrine neoplasia, type I _____

11. Charcot's arthropathy right foot due to diabetes, type I uncontrolled _____

12. Hypoglycemic shock in type I diabetes _____

13. Overactive bladder due to diabetes _____

14. Diabetic patient with hyperglycemia treated with insulin. Patient is normally on oral medication for diabetes. _____

15. Syncope caused by autonomic neuropathy due to diabetes mellitus. The patient has type II diabetes. _____

Nutritional Deficiencies

Malnutrition

Malnutrition is a nutritional disorder that is caused by primary deprivation of protein energy as the result of poverty, self-imposed starvation, or in relation to deficiency diseases such as cancer (Figure 12-18). Signs and symptoms of malnutrition include the following:

- Loss of energy
- Diarrhea
- Drastic weight change (loss or gain)
- Skin lesions
- Loss of hair
- Poor nails
- Edema
- Delayed healing
- Greasy stools due to loss of body fat

Other complications, such as muscle wasting, enlarged glands, and hepatomegaly, may occur as malnutrition progresses. Blood and urine tests show many abnormalities. Treatment is based on the underlying cause and the severity of malnutrition.

EXAMPLE The patient was found to have severe malnutrition, 261 (E43).

Vitamin Deficiencies

Vitamin deficiencies may be caused by many different factors, such as poor nutrient absorption, digestive tract disorders, lifestyle issues (e.g., alcohol, smoking, medications,

FIGURE 12-18. Malnourishment.

FIGURE 12-19. Rickets. The bowing of legs in a toddler due to formation of poorly mineralized bones.

over-exercising), chronic illness, age, and many other factors. Applicable codes are included in the following code categories:

264 (E50)	Vitamin A deficiency
265 (E51-E52)	Thiamine and niacin deficiency states
266 (E53)	Deficiency of B complex components
267 (E54)	Ascorbic acid deficiency
268 (E55)	Vitamin D deficiency
269 (E63)	Other nutritional deficiencies

The deficiency anemias are located in the "Blood and Blood-Forming Organs" chapter. A diagnosis can be stated as a vitamin deficiency or a specific name may be used for that particular deficiency (Figure 12-19). Another name for vitamin C deficiency is scurvy.

EXAMPLE Rickets due to vitamin D deficiency, 268.0 (E55.0).

EXERCISE 12-3

Assign codes to the following conditions.

1. Emaciation _____
2. Vitamin B$_{12}$ deficiency _____
3. Night blindness due to vitamin A deficiency _____
4. Severe protein calorie malnutrition _____

Other Metabolic and Immunity Disorders

Disorders of Fluid, Electrolyte, and Acid–Base Balance

Fluid balance occurs when the amount of fluid taken in is equal to the amount that is lost from the body. **Euvolemia** is the state of normal body fluid volume. A patient's fluid balance provides important information about their hydration, renal, and cardiovascular function. **Fluid overload** or **hypervolemia** occurs when there is too much fluid in the body. Fluid overload may be the result of too much sodium intake, due to IVs or blood transfusions, or a side effect of medication. Some conditions of the heart, kidney, and liver can affect fluid balance. The chief cause of fluid overload is heart failure. When fluid overload is due to congestive heart failure, it is not coded separately. Fluids can build up in various parts of the body causing edema. Peripheral edema is swelling that occurs in the lower extremities. Fluid can also build up in the lungs causing pulmonary edema or in the abdomen causing ascites.

EXAMPLE

Patient has volume overload due to noncompliance with dialysis for end-stage renal disease, 276.69, 585.6, V45.12 (E87.79, N18.6, Z91.15).

Hypovolemia occurs due to decreased plasma volume. **Dehydration** is when the body does not have enough water or fluids as it should. Dehydration can be caused by losing too much fluid (e.g., vomiting or diarrhea), not drinking enough water or fluids, or both. **Volume depletion** may be the result of either dehydration or hypovolemia.

EXAMPLE

Patient was seen in the Emergency Room and treated with IV fluids due to dehydration from gastroenteritis, 276.51, 558.9 (E86.0, K52.9).

Dehydration occurs frequently as the result of other medical conditions and principal diagnosis selection, and sequencing may be confusing. According to the neoplasm guidelines, if an admission occurs for the management of dehydration due to malignancy or therapy for the malignancy, or a combination of both, and only dehydration is being treated, then dehydration is designated as the principal diagnosis, followed by the code(s) for malignancy. According to *Coding Clinic* (2002:3Q:p21-22; 2003:1Q:p22),[7-8] in admissions in which severe dehydration causes acute renal failure, acute renal failure is the principal diagnosis.

Hypernatremia or hyponatremia with dehydration is coded only to the hypernatremia or hyponatremia code; the dehydration code is not assigned. It is clear in the Index under the main term "Dehydration," that hypernatremia/hyponatremia with dehydration requires only one code (Figure 12-20). This is not as clear in the Index under "Hypernatremia" or "Hyponatremia." Hypernatremia includes a subterm "with water depletion." Hyponatremia has no subterm, so if a coder does not look up "Dehydration," the fact that this is a single code assignment could be overlooked.

Dehydration (cachexia) 276.51
with
hypernatremia 276.0
hyponatremia 276.1
newborn 775.5

Hypernatremia 276.0
with water depletion 276.0

Hyponasality 784.49
Hyponatremia 276.1
Hypo-ovarianism 256.39

FIGURE 12-20. Alphabetic Index entries for "dehydration," "hypernatremia," and "hyponatremia."

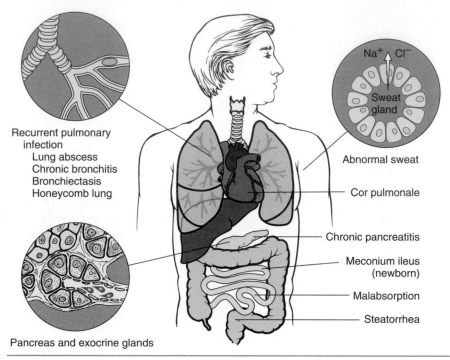

Recurrent pulmonary
infection
Lung abscess
Chronic bronchitis
Bronchiectasis
Honeycomb lung

Pancreas and exocrine glands

Abnormal sweat

Cor pulmonale

Chronic pancreatitis

Meconium ileus
(newborn)

Malabsorption

Steatorrhea

FIGURE 12-21. Abnormal chloride transport associated with cystic fibrosis affects the secretions of all exocrine glands, especially the pancreas, intestine, and bronchi.

EXAMPLE Patient was admitted for dehydration and was hypernatremic with a sodium level of 146, 276.0 (E87.0).

Cystic Fibrosis

Cystic fibrosis (CF) or mucoviscidosis is a **genetic** (inherited) condition that affects the cells that produce mucus, sweat, saliva, and digestive juices (Figure 12-21). Instead of being thin and slippery, these secretions are thick and sticky, plugging up tubes, ducts, and passageways, especially in the pancreas and lungs. No cure is available, and treatment is directed at the complications and manifestations of the disease. The most frequent complications are respiratory infections such as pneumonia, bronchitis, and bronchiectasis. Asthma may also develop. Although the organism *Pseudomonas aeruginosa* does not cause problems in a healthy person, it is a common infective organism in the patient with CF. Presence of *Pseudomonas* organism in the patient's sputum does not necessarily indicate that the patient has pneumonia due to *Pseudomonas*.

According to *Coding Clinic* (1990:4Q:p17),[9] when a patient is admitted for a complication of CF, the complication is the principal diagnosis, and CF is a secondary diagnosis. The codes 277.02, cystic fibrosis with pulmonary manifestations, and 277.03, cystic fibrosis with gastrointestinal manifestations, identify the two major systems that are affected by the disease. If the patient has both respiratory and digestive manifestations, both cystic fibrosis codes are used.

EXAMPLE Patient who suffers from CF is admitted because of acute bronchitis. Patient also has pancreatic insufficiency due to CF, 466.0, 277.02, 277.03, 577.8 (J20.9, E84.0, E84.8, K86.8).

Dysmetabolic Syndrome X

Dysmetabolic Syndrome X is characterized by abdominal obesity, insulin resistance, dyslipidemia, and elevated blood pressure or hypertension. Patients with these conditions are considered to be at greater risk for type II diabetes, cardiovascular disease, and stroke. Other names for dysmetabolic syndrome X include metabolic syndrome, syndrome X, insulin resistance syndrome, obesity syndrome, and Reaven's syndrome. In the ICD-9-CM code book, there is an instructional note to use additional codes for any associated manifestations such as cardiovascular disease or obesity.

EXAMPLE Patient was seen in the clinic for dietary counseling for dysmetabolic syndrome X. Patient is obese with a BMI of 35, has hypertriglyceridemia and hypertension, V65.3, 277.7, 278.00, V85.35, 272.1, 401.9 (Z71.3, E88.81, E66.9, Z68.35, E78.1, I10).

Obesity

Obesity is defined as an increase in body weight beyond the limitations of skeletal and physical requirements as a result of excessive accumulation of fat in the body. In the United States, obesity has reached epidemic proportions, with two thirds of American adults being overweight and one in three considered obese. **Body mass index** (BMI) uses weight and height to estimate body fat.

According to the Centers for Disease Control and Prevention (CDC), for adults, body mass index (BMI) is defined as follows:

Below 18.5	Underweight
Between 18.5 and 24.9	Healthy weight or normal
Between 25.0 and 29.0	Overweight
30.0 and above	Obese

V/Z codes should be used in combination with overweight and obesity codes to indicate a patient's BMI, if documented. According to General Coding Guidelines, it is acceptable to assign a body mass index (BMI) code based on medical record documentation from clinicians who are not the patient's provider. BMI is often documented in nurse's or dietitian's notes. There are different BMI codes for pediatric and adult patients. The pediatric BMI codes are for use for persons between 2 and 20 years of age. The adult BMI codes are for use for persons 21 years of age and older.

EXAMPLE Patient is obese with a BMI of 31, 278.00, V85.31 (E66.9, Z68.31).

Morbid obesity is the term that applies to patients who are 100 pounds overweight or over 50% above their ideal body weight. A BMI of 40 or higher defines morbid obesity. Many complications may be related to obesity, including the following:
- Diabetes
- Hypertension
- Heart disease
- Stroke
- Certain cancers such as breast and colon
- Depression
- Osteoarthritis

EXAMPLE | Patient is morbidly obese with a BMI of 41 and suffers from DM, 278.01, 250.00, V85.41 (E66.01, E11.9, Z68.41).

Hypervitaminosis

Hypervitaminosis is toxicity that results from an excess of any vitamin but especially fat-soluble vitamins such as A, D, and K. If toxicity occurs because of an overdose, a poisoning code would be assigned. Poisonings are discussed in Chapter 24.

EXAMPLE | Hypervitaminosis (vitamin D), 278.4 (E67.3).

Tumor Lysis Syndrome

Tumor lysis syndrome (TLS) is the development of electrolyte and metabolic disturbances that can occur after treatment of cancer, usually lymphoma and leukemia, and sometimes even without treatment. Patients with pre-existing kidney disease are at increased risk for developing TLS. Tumor lysis syndrome is caused by the breakdown of dying cancer cells and includes hyperkalemia, hyperphosphatemia, hyperuricemia and hyperuricosuria, and hypocalcemia. Acute renal failure and acute uric acid nephropathy can develop as a result of these electrolyte and metabolic disturbances. Although a patient may not have any symptoms in the early stages, as it progresses, symptoms include nausea and vomiting, shortness of breath, irregular heartbeat, lethargy, cloudy urine, and/or joint discomfort. Preventative measures can be taken before and during treatment that include IV hydration and medications such as allopurinol or rasburicase and alkalinization of urine with sodium bicarbonate. If TLS is untreated or it progresses, it can cause acute kidney failure, cardiac arrhythmias, seizures, loss of muscle control, and death.

EXAMPLE | Patient was admitted to the hospital due to possible acute myeloid leukemia. After confirmation of his AML, it was decided to administer chemotherapy. His labs were followed and showed tumor lysis syndrome due to the chemo, 205.00, 277.88, E933.1, 99.25 (C92.00, T45.1x5A, E88.3, 3E04305).

Immunity Disorders

The **immune system**, the body's major defense mechanism, responds to invasion of the body by foreign substances. The immune system consists of lymphoid tissues such as thymus, bone marrow, tonsils, adenoids, spleen, and appendix. When the immune system malfunctions and homeostasis is interrupted, the response may be classified as one of the following:

- Hyperactive responses (such as allergies)
- Immunodeficiency in which the response is inadequate (such as acquired immunodeficiency syndrome [AIDS])
- Autoimmune disorders in which the immune response is misdirected (such as systemic lupus erythematosus)
- Attacks on beneficial foreign tissues (such as transplants or blood transfusion)

Disorders that are coded in this section include acquired hypogammaglobulinemia, selective immunoglobulin A deficiency, X-linked agammaglobulinemia, severe combined immunodeficiency (SCID), thymic hypoplasia or DiGeorge's syndrome, and graft-versus-host disease.

Patients may become immunocompromised by medications; this is seen when patients undergo transplantation and are taking antirejection drugs or when a patient undergoes chemotherapy treatment for cancer. A patient may also be in an immunocompromised state that is associated with a disease process. According to *Coding Clinic* (1992:3Q:p13-14),[10] an expected side effect for transplant patients or chemotherapy patients is a compromised immune system, and codes should not be assigned for the immunocompromised state. However, if the cause of that state is not identified, code 279.9, Unspecified disorder of immune mechanism, should be assigned.

EXAMPLE   Patient has a diagnosis of Wiskott-Aldrich syndrome, 279.12 (D82.0).

Graft-versus-host disease

Graft-versus-host disease (GVHD) is a common complication that can occur after a stem cell or bone marrow transplant in which the newly transplanted material attacks the transplant recipient's body. GVHD can sometimes occur following a blood transfusion or any organ transplant where white blood cells are present. There is less risk for graft-versus-host disease when the match between donor and recipient is optimal. The greater the mismatch, the greater the risk of GVHD.

There are two types of graft-versus-host disease:
- Acute—usually occurs during the first 3 months following a transplant.
- Chronic—usually occurs after the third month following a transplant.

It is possible to develop acute on chronic graft-versus-host disease.

Symptoms in acute GVHD include:
- Abdominal pain and cramps
- Diarrhea
- Fever
- Jaundice
- Skin rash and/or desquamation
- Vomiting
- Weight loss

Symptoms in chronic GVHD include:
- Dry eye and dry mouth
- Hair loss
- Hepatitis
- Lung and digestive tract disorders
- Skin rash
- Skin thickening

In both acute and chronic GVHD, the patient is more susceptible to infections. Treatment includes corticosteroids, immunosuppressants, antibiotics, and immunoglobulins.

EXAMPLE   Patient was seen in the clinic for desquamation of skin. He had a bone marrow transplant 2 months ago. The physician is treating him for acute GVHD, 996.85, 279.51, 695.89, E878.0 (T86.09, D89.810, R23.4, Y83.0).

EXERCISE 12-4

Assign codes to the following conditions.

1. Hypocalcemia _____
2. Hypovolemia _____
3. Alpha 1-antitrypsin deficiency _____
4. Severe obesity with BMI of 40 _____
5. Metabolic acidosis _____

FACTORS INFLUENCING HEALTH STATUS AND CONTACT WITH HEALTH SERVICES (V CODES/Z CODES)

In the past, V/Z codes have been considered for use primarily in the outpatient setting. This has changed with the addition of more V/Z codes each year. As was discussed in Chapter 8, it is difficult to locate V/Z codes in the Index. Coders will often say, "I did not know there was a V/Z code for that."

Refer to Chapter 8 for a listing of common main terms to locate V/Z codes. V/Z codes that may be used with diseases of the endocrine glands, nutritional and metabolic diseases, and immunity disorders include the following:

V07.4	Hormone replacement therapy (postmenopausal)
V10.87	Personal history of malignant neoplasm—thyroid
V10.88	Personal history of malignant neoplasm—other endocrine glands and related structures
V12.1	Personal history of nutritional deficiency
V12.21	Personal history of gestational diabetes
V12.29	Personal history of other endocrine, metabolic, and immunity disorders
V16.8	Family history of other specified malignant neoplasm
V18.0	Family history of diabetes mellitus
V18.11	Family history of multiple endocrine neoplasia (MEN) syndrome
V18.19	Family history of other endocrine and metabolic disease
V42.82	Organ or tissue replaced by transplant—pancreas
V45.86	Bariatric surgery status
V45.79	Acquired absence of organ—other acquired absence of an organ
V45.85	Insulin pump status
V51.0	Encounter for breast reconstruction following mastectomy
V53.91	Fitting and adjustment of insulin pump
V58.67	Long-term (current) use of insulin
V65.3	Dietary surveillance and counseling
V65.46	Encounter for insulin pump training
V76.49	Special screening for malignant neoplasms—other sites
V76.89	Special screening for malignant neoplasms—other neoplasm
V77.0	Special screening for thyroid disorders
V77.1	Special screening for diabetes mellitus
V77.2	Special screening for malnutrition
V77.3	Special screening for phenylketonuria (PKU)
V77.4	Special screening for galactosemia
V77.5	Special screening for gout
V77.6	Special screening for cystic fibrosis
V77.7	Special screening for other inborn errors of metabolism
V77.8	Special screening for obesity
V77.91	Special screening for lipid disorders
V77.99	Special screening for other and unspecified endocrine, nutritional, metabolic, and immunity disorders
V83.81	Cystic fibrosis gene carrier
V84.81	Genetic susceptibility to multiple endocrine neoplasia (MEN)
V85.0	Body mass index (BMI) less than 19, adult
V85.1	Body mass index (BMI) 19-24, adult
V85.21	Body mass index (BMI) 25.0-25.9, adult
V85.22	Body mass index (BMI) 26.0-26.9, adult
V85.23	Body mass index (BMI) 27.0-27.9, adult

V85.24	Body mass index (BMI) 28.0-28.9, adult
V85.25	Body mass index (BMI) 29.0-29.9, adult
V85.30	Body mass index (BMI) 30.0-30.9, adult
V85.31	Body mass index (BMI) 31.0-31.9, adult
V85.32	Body mass index (BMI) 32.0-32.9, adult
V85.33	Body mass index (BMI) 33.0-33.9, adult
V85.34	Body mass index (BMI) 34.0-34.9, adult
V85.35	Body mass index (BMI) 35.0-35.9, adult
V85.36	Body mass index (BMI) 36.0-36.9, adult
V85.37	Body mass index (BMI) 37.0-37.9, adult
V85.38	Body mass index (BMI) 38.0-38.9, adult
V85.39	Body mass index (BMI) 39.0-39.9, adult
V85.41	Body Mass Index 40.0-44.9, adult
V85.42	Body Mass Index 45.0-49.9, adult
V85.43	Body Mass Index 50.0-49.9, adult
V85.44	Body Mass Index 60.0-69.9, adult
V85.45	Body Mass Index 70 and over, adult
V85.51	Body mass index, pediatric, less than 5th percentile for age
V85.52	Body mass index, pediatric, 5th percentile to less than 85th percentile for age
V85.53	Body mass index, pediatric, 85th percentile to less than 95th percentile for age
V85.54	Body mass index, pediatric, greater than or equal to 95th percentile for age

EXAMPLE Patient has a family history of diabetes, V18.0 (Z83.3).

EXAMPLE Patient is a type II diabetic who has been treated with insulin, 250.00, V58.67 (E11.9, Z79.4).

EXERCISE 12-5

Assign codes to the following conditions.

1. Status post pancreas transplant   _____
2. Dietary counseling for patient with new diagnosis of DM   _____
3. Personal history of malignant thyroid neoplasm   _____
4. Family history of Graves' disease   _____
5. History of rickets as a child   _____

COMMON TREATMENTS

CONDITION	MEDICATION/TREATMENT
Goiter	Small doses of iodine if due to iodine deficiency; otherwise, radioactive iodine or surgical treatment if symptomatic
Hypothyroidism/Hashimoto's disease	Levothyroxine (levothroid and synthroid) which is the most common thyroid hormone replacement medication
Hyperthyroidism/Graves' disease	Antithyroid medications such as Tapazole; radioactive iodine or surgery
Diabetes	Diet, monitoring of blood sugars, and insulins such as Regular, Lente, Humalog, NPH; oral medications such as Glyburide, Micronase, Diabeta, Glucophage, etc.
Hyperpituitarism	Decrease the amount of hormone secreted, usually with radiation or surgery

CONDITION	MEDICATION/TREATMENT
Hypopituitarism	Removal of tumor if that is the cause, or hormone replacement therapy
Diabetes insipidus	Depending on cause, vasopressin medication
Hyperparathyroidism	Treatment depends on the cause.
Hypoparathyroidism	Replacement therapy with calcium and vitamin D
Cushing's syndrome	Removal of tumor if that is the cause, or medication to suppress the production of cortisol
Addison's disease	Replacement therapy with corticosteroids
Malnutrition	Treat symptoms and/or underlying cause; nutritional supplements; replace missing nutrients, possibly with TPN (total parenteral nutrition).
Vitamin deficiencies	Treat symptoms and/or underlying cause; replace missing vitamins.
Hypokalemia	Replace with potassium supplement, such as K-Dur, K-Lyte, K-Tab, K-Lor, Micro-K.
Hyperkalemia	Remove potassium from body with Kayexalate, diuretics, sodium bicarbonate, intravenous calcium, glucose, or insulin.
Cystic fibrosis	Postural drainage and chest percussion treatments, pancreatic enzymes and vitamins, antibiotics for infection, and possibly lung transplant
Obesity	Diet, exercise, behavior modification, and bariatric surgery
Hypervitaminosis	Stop taking specific vitamin.
Graft-versus-host disease	Corticosteroids, immunosuppressants, antibiotics, and immunoglobulins

PROCEDURES

Some of the procedures that may be related to diseases of the endocrine, nutritional, and metabolic diseases, and immunity disorders may be located in the following chapters of the Procedure Tabular:

2. Operations on the Endocrine System (06-07)

Procedures discussed in Chapter 2 include incisional, excisional, and many diagnostic and exploratory procedures such as biopsies on various glands of the endocrine system.

Procedures related to the endocrine system in ICD-10-PCS can be located in the following tables:

0F1-0FY	Gastrointestinal System
0F1-0FY	Hepatobiliary System and Pancreas
0G2-0GW	Endocrine System

EXAMPLE | Goiter with complete thyroidectomy, 240.9, 06.4 (E04.9, 0GTK0ZZ).

EXAMPLE | Conn's syndrome due to adenoma of right adrenal gland with diagnostic percutaneous biopsy of adrenal gland 227.0, 255.12, 07.11 (D35.01, E26.01, 0GB33ZX).

Bariatric Procedures

Bariatrics is the branch of medicine that is concerned with the management (prevention or control) of obesity and allied diseases. In some cases, bariatric surgery may be necessary to treat obesity and to control and/or prevent the secondary complications associated with obesity.

Two main types of bariatric surgery are performed: restrictive and malabsorptive gastric procedures that are performed for weight loss. Malabsorptive procedures tend to be more

FIGURE 12-22. Insulin pump.

successful for long-term weight loss. Some examples of malabsorptive procedures include the following:

■ Roux-en-Y gastric bypass
■ Biliopancreatic diversion (BPD)
■ "Duodenal switch" procedure
    Some examples of restrictive procedures include the following:
■ Gastric banding
■ Vertical banded gastroplasty (VBG)
    The root operation for the gastric bypass procedures is bypass, and the root operation for the banding procedures is restriction.

EXAMPLE	Morbidly obese patient (BMI 42) with diabetes mellitus. A laparoscopic gastric banding was performed 278.01, 250.00, V85.41, 44.95 (E66.01, E11.9, Z68.41, 0DV64CZ).

Insulin Pumps

An insulin pump is a small, computerized device that is attached to the body and delivers insulin via a catheter (Figure 12-22). This pump provides a continuous drip of insulin throughout the day. The patient may also administer a bolus of insulin by pushing a button. The code for subcutaneous implantation of the pump is 86.06; 38.91 is used for any associated catheterization, and 99.17 signifies infusion of insulin. The root operation for insulin pump implantation is insertion.

EXAMPLE	Patient has brittle Type I diabetes and is admitted for implantation (percutaneous) of insulin pump (subcutaneous infusion device implanted in abdomen), 250.01, 86.06, 99.17 (E10.9, 0JH83VZ).

EXERCISE 12-6

Assign codes for all diagnoses and procedures.

1. Multinodular goiter, which is symptomatic for dysphagia; total thyroidectomy was performed _____

2. Biopsy of pituitary gland: pituitary adenoma (transsphenoidal approach) _____

3. Diabetes type I with insertion of insulin pump with arterial catheterization _____

4. Pheochromocytoma with laparoscopic excision right adrenal gland _____

5. Morbid obesity with BMI of 40; laparoscopic VBG was performed _____

DOCUMENTATION/REIMBURSEMENT/MS-DRGs

Often, coding difficulties are due to lack of documentation. Sometimes pathology and other test results are not available at the time of discharge or when the physician is dictating the discharge summary or is reporting the final diagnoses.

Malnutrition may not be well-documented by the physician. Nutritional consults or dietitian notes should be reviewed. A physician query would be needed to confirm any diagnoses based on a dietitian's assessment.

Many of the conditions and diseases related to nutritional and metabolic disorders are supported by laboratory tests. Coders should not assign a diagnosis code on the basis of abnormal laboratory findings alone. A laboratory value may be higher or lower than the normal range, but this does not necessarily indicate a disorder. If abnormal laboratory value(s) is noted and treatment is given or documentation supports monitoring, it would be appropriate to query the physician regarding the abnormal laboratory value(s). An abnormal finding must be clinically significant to be coded, per *Coding Clinic* (1990:2Q:p15-16).[11]

Frequently missed complications/comorbidities from this chapter include the following:

- Acidosis
- Alkalosis
- Hypernatremia
- Hyponatremia
- Malnutrition

MS-DRG With and Without MCC/CC

EXAMPLE
Patient was admitted with Addison's crisis, and sodium on admission was 115 (normal, 135-148 mEq/L).
Patient treated with hypertonic saline IVs. The physician documents in the discharge summary that the patient's sodium levels improved dramatically before discharge.

DIAGNOSES	CODES	MS-DRG	RW
Addison's crisis with hyponatremia	255.41, 276.1 (E27.2, E87.1)	644	1.0655
Addison's crisis without hyponatremia	255.41 (E27.2)	645	0.7198

The presence of a complication or comorbidity can make a difference in reimbursement, depending on the principal diagnosis and the MS-DRG assigned. The code for hyponatremia is a complication/comorbidity. In this case, it would be necessary to query the physician regarding the low sodium levels and treatment with hypertonic saline IV before the hyponatremia code is assigned.

Two Diagnoses That Equally Meet the Definition for Principal Diagnosis

Dehydration may cause confusion when selecting a principal diagnosis because dehydration is often caused by other conditions. If two or more conditions are present on admission and meet the definition for principal diagnosis, either one could be selected as principal.

EXAMPLE
A patient was admitted with urinary tract infection (UTI) and moderate dehydration. The dehydration was treated aggressively with intravenous fluids, and the UTI was treated with intravenous (IV) antibiotics.

DIAGNOSES	CODES	MS-DRG	RW
Dehydration and UTI	276.51, 599.0 (E86.0, N39.0)	641	0.6916
UTI and dehydration	599.0, 276.51 (N39.0, E86.0)	690	0.7864

In this case, both UTI and dehydration were treated by measures that would require inpatient admission, so it would be possible to sequence either diagnosis as the principal diagnosis. If the patient had been treated with IV fluids for dehydration and oral antibiotics for the UTI, dehydration should be the principal because oral antibiotics would not typically require inpatient hospitalization.

Diabetic Manifestation Versus Not Related to Diabetes

Documentation with regard to diabetes can be conflicting and/or may need clarification. Sometimes documentation is inconsistent, and diabetes has been documented as both type I and type II within the record. A patient is either type I or type II, and it is necessary to query the physician to determine which type is correct. It is also important to make sure that any manifestations are documented as related to diabetes. In addition, when a principal diagnosis is selected, the diabetes codes must be sequenced before any manifestation code. This can make a significant difference in MS-DRG assignment and reimbursement.

EXAMPLE

DIAGNOSES	CODES	MS-DRG	RW
Diabetic ulcer left toe	250.80, 707.15 (E11.621, L97.529)	639	0.5544
Ulcer left toe, diabetes	707.15, 250.00 (L97.529, E11.9)	594	0.7591

CHAPTER REVIEW EXERCISE

Assign codes for all diagnoses and procedures.

1. Homocystinemia _____
2. Conn's syndrome _____
3. Myxedema _____
4. Idiopathic Cushing's syndrome _____
5. Testicular hypogonadism _____
6. Overproduction of growth hormone _____
7. Hyponatremia due to dehydration _____
8. Gouty arthritis _____
9. Monoclonal gammopathy _____
10. Respiratory acidosis with metabolic alkalosis _____
11. Overweight with BMI of 26.0 _____
12. Volume depletion _____
13. Patient with cystic fibrosis admitted with exacerbation of respiratory symptoms _____
14. Hyperthyroidism with exophthalmos _____
15. Poorly controlled diabetes (type II) with diabetic gastroparesis; patient is on insulin _____
16. Albinism _____
17. Amyloidosis _____
18. Proliferative retinopathy due to DM, type II, out of control _____
19. Diabetes due to prednisone (adverse effect) _____
20. Hyperlipidemia due to Cushing's syndrome _____
21. Thiamine deficiency due to chronic alcoholism _____
22. Phenylketonuria (PKU) _____
23. Chronic kidney disease due to diabetic nephropathy; juvenile-onset diabetes, stage III _____

24. Severe obesity with BMI 43 and obstructive sleep apnea; patient had Roux-en-Y gastric bypass to jejunum   _____

25. Erectile dysfunction due to diabetes mellitus, type 2   _____

26. Inanition   _____

27. Patient is immunocompromised because of medications taken for pancreas transplant   _____

Write the correct answer(s) in the space(s) provided.

28. List a couple of conditions that qualify a person as morbidly obese.

_____
_____

29. What type of diabetes is the most common?

_____

30. What organism may cause complications for a patient with cystic fibrosis?

_____

CHAPTER GLOSSARY

Acromegaly: condition that results when hypersecretion of hGH occurs after puberty, along with overgrowth of the face, hands, feet, and soft tissues.

Addison's disease: adrenocortical insufficiency that may be caused by neoplasms, surgical removal of the adrenal gland, autoimmune processes, tuberculosis, hemorrhage, and/or infection.

Atrophy: when a gland becomes smaller.

Bariatrics: branch of medicine that is concerned with the management (prevention or control) of obesity and allied diseases.

Body mass index: uses weight and height to estimate body fat.

Cushing's syndrome: condition that results in excessive circulating cortisol levels caused by chronic hypersecretion of the adrenal cortex.

Cystic fibrosis: genetic (inherited) condition that affects the cells that produce mucus, sweat, saliva, and digestive juices. Instead of being thin and slippery, these secretions are thick and sticky, plugging up tubes, ducts, and passageways, especially in the pancreas and lungs.

Dehydration: occurs when the body does not have enough water or fluids as it should.

Diabetes insipidus: deficiency in the release of vasopressin by the posterior pituitary gland.

Diabetes mellitus: chronic syndrome of impaired carbohydrate, protein, and fat metabolism caused by insufficient production of insulin by the pancreas or faulty utilization of insulin by the cells.

Dysmetabolic Syndrome X: characterized by abdominal obesity, insulin resistance, dyslipidemia, and elevated blood pressure or hypertension.

Endocrine system: body system composed of many glands that secrete hormones that regulate bodily functions; it works with the nervous system to maintain body activities and homeostasis and to respond to stress.

Exophthalmos: bulging of the eyes.

Euvolemia: state of normal body fluid volume.

Fluid overload: occurs when there is too much fluid in the body.

Genetic: inherited.

Gigantism: condition that occurs when hypersecretion of hGH occurs before puberty, along with proportionate overgrowth of all bodily tissues, especially the long bones.

Goiter: enlargement of the thyroid gland.

Graft-versus-host disease (GVHD): common complication that can occur after a stem cell or bone marrow transplant in which the newly transplanted material attacks the transplant recipient's body.

Graves' disease: the most common form of hyperthyroidism; it occurs through an autoimmune response that attacks the thyroid gland, resulting in overproduction of the thyroid hormone thyroxine.

Hashimoto's disease: inflammation of the thyroid gland that often results in hypothyroidism.

Hormones: substances secreted by glands that can regulate bodily functions, such as urinary output, cellular metabolic rate, and growth and development.

Hyperglycemia: condition that results when glucose or blood sugar becomes abnormally high. This is a relatively common event in patients with diabetes.

Hyperparathyroidism: condition that results when an overactive parathyroid gland secretes excessive parathyroid hormone, causing increased levels of circulating calcium associated with loss of calcium in the bone.

Hyperpituitarism: increased production of the pituitary hormones, particularly hGH.

Hyperplasia: enlargement of a gland.

Hyperthyroidism: abnormality of the thyroid gland in which secretion of thyroid hormone is usually increased and is no longer under the regulatory control of hypothalamic-pituitary centers.

Hypertrophy: enlargement of a gland.

Hypervitaminosis: toxicity resulting from an excess of any vitamin, especially fat-soluble vitamins such as A, D, and K.

Hypervolemia: occurs when there is too much fluid in the body.

Hypoglycemia: condition that results when glucose or blood sugar becomes abnormally low.

Hypoparathyroidism: underactive parathyroid gland that results in decreased levels of circulating calcium.

Hypopituitarism: condition caused by low levels of pituitary hormones. Hormones secreted by the pituitary gland can affect the functions of other glands.

Hypoplasia: atrophy; condition that results when a gland becomes smaller.

Hypothyroidism: condition caused by low levels of pituitary hormones. Hormones secreted by the pituitary gland can affect the functions of other glands.

Hypovolemia: occurs due to decreased plasma volume.

Iatrogenic: caused by medical treatment.

Immune system: the body's major defense mechanism that responds to invasion of the body by foreign substances.

Malnutrition: nutrition disorder caused by primary deprivation of protein energy caused by poverty or self-imposed starvation, or associated with deficiency diseases such as cancer.

Morbid obesity: applies to patients who are 50% to 100% or 100 pounds above their ideal body weight. A BMI of 40 or higher defines morbid obesity.

Myxedema: skin and tissue disorder that is usually due to severe prolonged hypothyroidism.

Obesity: condition defined as an increase in body weight beyond the limitation of skeletal and physical requirements, caused by excessive accumulation of fat in the body.

Secondary diabetes mellitus: form of the disease that develops as a result of another disease or condition.

Steroid-induced diabetes: diabetes that is caused by the use of steroids.

Tetany: a continuous muscle spasm.

Thyrotoxic crisis or storm: complication of hyperthyroidism associated with a sudden intensification of symptoms combined with fever, rapid pulse, and delirium.

Tumor lysis syndrome (TLS): development of electrolyte and metabolic disturbances that can occur after treatment of cancer, usually lymphoma and leukemia, and sometimes even without treatment.

Vitamin deficiency: condition caused by many different factors, such as poor nutrient absorption, digestive tract disorders, lifestyle issues (e.g., alcohol, smoking, medication, overexercising), chronic illness, age, and many other factors.

Volume depletion: may be the result of either dehydration or hypovolemia.

REFERENCES

1. Frazier ME, Drzymkowski JW. Essentials of Human Diseases and Conditions, 3rd ed. St. Louis, Saunders, 2004, Table 4-1, pp 150-151.
2. Chabner D. The Language of Medicine, 7th ed. St. Louis, Saunders, 2004, Table 18-13, p 745.
3. American Hospital Association. *Coding Clinic for ICD-9-CM* 1991:3Q:p6. Diabetes mellitus complications.
4. American Hospital Association. *Coding Clinic for ICD-9-CM* 2002:2Q:p13. Poorly controlled diabetes.
5. American Hospital Association. *Coding Clinic for ICD-9-CM* 1997:4Q:p33. Adult-onset uncontrolled diabetes requiring insulin.
6. American Hospital Association. *Coding Clinic for ICD-9-CM* 2004:1Q:p14-15. Ulcer, diabetic vs decubitus, with osteomyelitis.
7. American Hospital Association. *Coding Clinic for ICD-9-CM* 2002:3Q:p21-22. ARF due to dehydration and treated with IV hydration only.
8. American Hospital Association. *Coding Clinic for ICD-9 CM* 2003:1Q:p22. Clarification— Renal failure due to dehydration with IV hydration.
9. American Hospital Association. *Coding Clinic for ICD-9-CM* 1990:4Q:p17. Cystic fibrosis sequencing—Guidelines.
10. American Hospital Association. *Coding Clinic for ICD-9-CM* 1992:3Q:p13-14. Immunocompromised state due to medication.
11. American Hospital Association. *Coding Clinic for ICD-9-CM* 1990:2Q:p15-16. Abnormal findings—Guidelines.

13

Mental, Behavioral, and Neurodevelopmental Disorders

(ICD-9-CM Chapter 5, Codes 290-319, and ICD-10-CM Chapter 5, Codes F01-F99)

LEARNING OBJECTIVES

1. Apply and assign the correct ICD-9-CM and ICD-10-CM codes in accordance with Official Guidelines for Coding and Reporting
2. Identify major differences between ICD-9-CM and ICD-10-CM related to mental, behavioral, and neurodevelopmental disorders
3. Identify pertinent anatomy and physiology of mental, behavioral, and neurodevelopmental disorders
4. Identify various mental, behavioral, and neurodevelopmental disorders
5. Assign the correct V/Z codes and procedure codes related to mental, behavioral, and neurodevelopmental disorders
6. Identify common treatments and medications
7. Explain the importance of documentation in relation to MS-DRGs for reimbursement

ABBREVIATIONS/ ACRONYMS

ADD attention deficit disorder

ADHD attention deficit hyperactivity disorder

CC complication/comorbidity

DSM-IV-TR *Diagnostic and Statistical Manual of Mental Disorders, Fourth Edition, Text Revision*

DTs delirium tremens

ECT electroconvulsive therapy

ICD-9-CM *International Classification of Diseases,*

9th Revision, Clinical Modification

ICD-10-CM *International Classification of Diseases, 10th Revision, Clinical Modification*

ICD-10-PCS *International Classification of Diseases, 10th Revision, Procedure Coding System*

IQ intelligence quotient

LD learning disability/difficulty

MR mental retardation

MRCP mental retardation, cerebral palsy

MS-DRG Medicare Severity diagnosis-related group

OBS organic brain syndrome

OIG Office of the Inspector General

PKU phenylketonuria

PTSD posttraumatic stress disorder

ICD-9-CM Official Guidelines for Coding and Reporting	Please refer to the companion Evolve website for the most current guidelines. **5. Chapter 5: Mental Disorders (290-319)** Reserved for future guideline expansion

There are no specific official ICD-9-CM coding and reporting guidelines for Chapter 5, Mental, Behavioral, and Neurodevelopmental Disorders (290-319).

Apply General Coding Guidelines as found in Chapter 5 and the Procedural Guidelines as found in Chapter 6.

ICD-10-CM Official Guidelines for Coding and Reporting	Please refer to the companion Evolve website for the most current guidelines. **5. Chapter 5: Mental and behavioral disorders (F01-F99)** **a. Pain disorders related to psychological factors** Assign code F45.41, for pain that is exclusively psychological. Code F45.41, Pain disorder **exclusively** related **to** psychological factors, should be used following the appropriate code from category G89, Pain, not elsewhere classified, if there is documentation of a psychological component for a patient with acute or chronic pain. *See Section I.C.6. Pain*

Apply General Coding Guidelines as found in Chapter 5 and the Procedural Guidelines as found in Chapter 7.

The *Diagnostic and Statistical Manual of Mental Disorders, Fourth Edition* (DSM-IV), is used by healthcare professionals to diagnose mental disorders on the basis of specific criteria. A multiaxial assessment system is used to assess clinical disorders, personality disorders and mental retardation, medical conditions that may affect psychological condition, psychosocial and environmental factors (stressors such as homelessness or unemployment), and global assessment of functioning.

The DSM-IV-TR, or a text revision (TR), was published in 1996. It includes ICD-9-CM codes that should be assigned to all mental disorders and conditions. Many healthcare professionals use these ICD-9-CM codes within their documentation. These professionals may be taking the codes from the DSM-IV-TR, so it is always recommended to verify codes with the ICD-9-CM code book, to ensure accurate code assignment.

The DSM-5 is currently in development. A draft has been released for comment with an expected final publication in May 2013.

GUIDELINE DIFFERENCES BETWEEN ICD-9-CM AND ICD-10-CM

Because there are no official ICD-9-CM guidelines at this time regarding mental disorders, there are no guideline differences. There is an ICD-10-CM guideline for pain disorders related to psychological factors.

MAJOR DIFFERENCES BETWEEN ICD-9-CM AND ICD-10-CM

- ICD-10-CM does not have codes for history of drug and alcohol dependence. In ICD-10-CM, past history of drug and alcohol dependence are assigned codes for "in remission."
- There is a notation under category F10 in ICD-10-CM to use an additional code for blood alcohol level, if applicable (Y90.-).
- ICD-10-CM has expanded the nicotine abuse codes to identify the type of nicotine product (e.g., cigarettes, chewing tobacco, or other tobacco product).
- The fifth digits used to identify drug and type of alcohol usage (continuous, episodic, and unspecified) in ICD-9-CM are not applicable in ICD-10-CM.

ANATOMY AND PHYSIOLOGY

No one body system is known to cause or be affected by mental disorders because the causes of mental illness are not always known. Stress can be a contributing factor in mental disorders. Psychological issues can and do affect one's physical health.

DISEASE CONDITIONS

Mental Disorders (290-319), which is Chapter 5 in your ICD-9-CM code book, is divided into the following categories:

CATEGORY	SECTION TITLES
290-294	Organic Psychotic Conditions
295-299	Other Psychoses
300-316	Neurotic Disorders, Personality Disorders, and Other Nonpsychotic Mental Disorders
317-319	Intellectual Disabilities

Mental Disorders, found in Chapter 5 in the ICD-10-CM code book, are divided into the following categories:

CATEGORY	SECTION TITLES
F01-F09	Mental Disorders Due to Known Physiological Conditions
F10-F19	Mental and Behavioral Disorders Due to Psychoactive Substance Abuse
F20-F29	Schizophrenia, Schizotypal and Delusional, and Other Non-Mood Psychotic Disorders
F30-F39	Mood (Affective) Disorders
F40-F48	Anxiety, Dissociative, Stress-Related, Somatoform, and Other Nonpsychotic Mental Disorders
F50-F59	Behavioral Syndromes Associated with Physiological Disturbances and Physical Factors
F60-F69	Disorders of Adult Personality and Behavior
F70-F79	Mental Retardation
F80-F89	Pervasive and Specific Developmental Disorders
F90-F98	Behavioral and Emotional Disorders with Onset Usually Occurring in Childhood and Adolescence
F99	Unspecified Mental Disorder

Organic Psychotic Conditions

Organic psychosis occurs as the result of deterioration in the brain. It is usually progressive and irreversible, as in senile dementia and Alzheimer's disease. Organic brain damage may be produced by a variety of conditions, including arteriosclerosis, thrombi, metabolic conditions, infection, toxins, tumors, alcohol, and drugs. The onset and severity of damage depend on the cause. **Organic brain syndrome** (OBS) or disease is a general term that is used to describe the decrease in mental function caused by other physical disease(s).

Dementia

Dementia is a progressive deterioration of mental faculties that is characterized by impairment of memory and one or more cognitive impairments in areas such as language, reasoning, judgment, calculation, and problem-solving abilities. **Cognitive impairment** is a decline in mental activities associated with thinking, learning, and memory. Dementia can occur at any age but is more prevalent in the elderly. Disease processes that may be associated with dementia include the following:

■ Alzheimer's disease
■ Lewy body disease
■ Alcoholism
■ AIDS
■ Parkinson's disease
■ Normal pressure hydrocephalus with dementia
■ Genetic or metabolic disease (e.g., thyroid)
■ Toxic or traumatic injury
■ Malignant disease and treatment

Although the term "senile" may be associated with those who are 65 years of age or older, it should not be assumed that because a patient is older than 65, a condition is due to senility. The physician must document within the health record the specific type of dementia. For many of the dementia codes, code assignment may depend on the presence of behavioral disturbances such as aggressiveness, combativeness, violence, or wandering off.

EXAMPLE | Patient is 70 years old and has dementia, 294.20 (F03).

EXAMPLE | Patient is 60 years old and has senile dementia, 290.0 (F03).

Alcohol/Drug Psychoses

Psychosis is an impairment in mental state by which one's perception of reality becomes distorted. It may include visual or auditory hallucinations, paranoia or delusions, personality changes, and disorganized thinking. The use of alcohol or drugs could lead to alcohol- or drug-related psychosis. Psychotic episodes vary from person to person.

Alcohol withdrawal symptoms vary in severity from mild shakiness and sweating to the worst form, **delirium tremens** (DTs). Delirium tremens may involve severe mental or neurologic changes such as delirium and/or hallucinations. This is a life-threatening condition. People who have gone through withdrawal once are more likely to have withdrawal symptoms again when they stop drinking. Seizures are also a common form of withdrawal. Three codes are specific to alcohol withdrawal:

291.0 (F10.231)   Alcohol withdrawal delirium
291.3 (F10.251)   Alcohol withdrawal hallucinosis
291.81 (F10.239)   Alcohol withdrawal

"Only one code should be assigned to describe alcohol withdrawal. Code 291.0 takes precedence over the other two codes, and 291.3 takes precedence over the 291.81 code," according to *Coding Clinic* (1991:2Q:p11-12)[1] (Figure 13-1). If a patient is experiencing

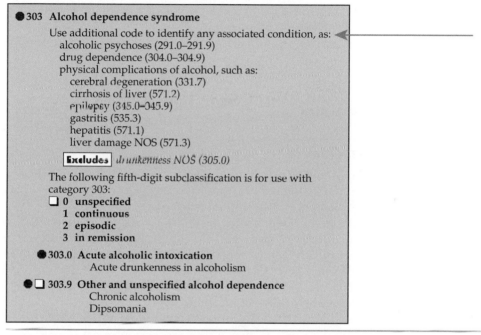

● 291.8 **Other specified alcohol-induced mental disorders**
   291.81 **Alcohol withdrawal**
      Alcohol:
         abstinence syndrome or symptoms
         withdrawal syndrome or symptoms
      Excludes | *alcohol withdrawal:*
         delirium (291.0)
         hallucinosis (291.3)
         delirium tremens (291.0)

FIGURE 13-1. Excludes note for alcohol withdrawal.

● 303 **Alcohol dependence syndrome**
   Use additional code to identify any associated condition, as:
      alcoholic psychoses (291.0–291.9)
      drug dependence (304.0–304.9)
      physical complications of alcohol, such as:
         cerebral degeneration (331.7)
         cirrhosis of liver (571.2)
         epilepsy (345.0–345.9)
         gastritis (535.3)
         hepatitis (571.1)
         liver damage NOS (571.3)
      Excludes | *drunkenness NOS (305.0)*
   The following fifth-digit subclassification is for use with
   category 303:
   ☐ 0 **unspecified**
      1 **continuous**
      2 **episodic**
      3 **in remission**
● 303.0 **Acute alcoholic intoxication**
      Acute drunkenness in alcoholism
● ☐ 303.9 **Other and unspecified alcohol dependence**
      Chronic alcoholism
      Dipsomania

FIGURE 13-2. Use additional code for category 303.

symptoms of withdrawal, the alcohol dependence category 303 instructs the use of an additional code for alcoholic psychoses (withdrawal), drug dependence, and/or any physical complications related to alcohol (Figure 13-2). When a patient is admitted for withdrawal symptoms, the withdrawal code is assigned as the principal diagnosis.

EXAMPLE Seizure due to alcohol withdrawal. Patient is an alcoholic who usually drinks every day but hasn't had a drink in 2 days, 291.81, 780.39, 303.91 (F10.239, R56.9).

EXAMPLE Wernicke-Korsakoff syndrome. Patient is an alcoholic who has not had a drink in 2 years, 291.1, 303.93 (F10.26, F10.21).

Admissions to the hospital for drug psychosis are on the rise. A number of drugs can induce psychosis; cocaine and methamphetamine are the most common.

EXAMPLE Paranoia due to methamphetamine (meth). Patient is dependent on meth, continuous use, 292.11, 304.41 (F15.259).

EXERCISE 13-1

Assign codes to the following conditions.

1. Delirium tremens due to chronic alcoholism, continuous   _____
2. Pre-senile dementia with depression   _____
3. Morphine-induced delirium (adverse effect)   _____
4. Organic brain syndrome   _____
5. Dementia due to neurosyphilis with behavioral disturbances   _____
6. Dementia due to malnutrition   _____
7. Normal pressure hydrocephalus with dementia   _____
8. Creutzfeldt-Jacob disease with dementia with behavioral disturbance   _____
9. AIDS-related dementia   _____
10. Binswanger's disease   _____

Other Psychoses

Schizophrenia

Schizophrenia is a disorder of the brain. A person with schizophrenia may have trouble differentiating between real and unreal experiences and may not demonstrate logical thinking, normal emotional responses to others, and appropriate behavior in social situations. A genetic component is associated with the disease in that people who have family members with the disease are more likely to exhibit the disease themselves. Schizophrenia usually has its onset during young adulthood, and it affects men and women equally. Five types of schizophrenia have been identified:

- Catatonic—withdrawn, in own world
- Paranoid—suspicious of others
- Disorganized—disorganized thought process, unable to communicate coherently
- Undifferentiated—mixed types of schizophrenia
- Residual—has milder symptoms that come and go

EXAMPLE   The patient has been in a chronic catatonic state of schizophrenia, 295.22 (F20.2).

Mood Disorders

Mood disorders occur when a change in mood has been present for a prolonged time. The two most common mood disorders (**affective disorders**) are major depression and bipolar disorder (manic-depressive illness). Mood disorders can be triggered by a life event or by a chemical imbalance. The type of depression that is included in category 296 is different than depression, not otherwise specified (311). **Bipolar disorder** is characterized by mood swings. Onset of symptoms is most likely to occur in early adulthood. A person with bipolar disorder can have four main types of mood "episodes":

1. **Depression**—a feeling of sadness that can go on for a long period of time; lack of enjoyment of the things one would normally do
2. **Mania**—the other side of depression, in which a person feels so good it is like a "high"; may do risky things
3. **Hypomania**—milder form of mania, but this "feel good" mood can change to depression or mania
4. **Mixed mood**—alternating between mania and depression, very quickly

Major depressive disorder is characterized by one or more major depressive episodes with a history of mania, hypomania, or mixed episodes. In major depression, more numerous symptoms of depression may be present, and usually, the symptoms are more severe. Major depression is most likely to occur in persons between the ages of 25 and 44; an episode may last from 6 to 9 months.

EXAMPLE

> The patient was diagnosed with major depressive disorder of moderate severity, single episode, 296.22 (F32.1).

EXAMPLE

> The patient is in a severe manic phase of bipolar I disorder, 296.43 (F31.13).

EXERCISE 13-2

> *Assign codes to the following conditions.*
>
> 1. Bipolar disorder, currently depressed _____
> 2. Autism _____
> 3. Major depressive disorder, recurrent _____
> 4. Paranoid schizophrenia _____
> 5. Delusional disorder _____

Neurotic Disorders, Personality Disorders, and Other Nonpsychotic Mental Disorders

Anxiety Disorders

Following is a breakdown of the different types of anxiety disorders:
- Generalized anxiety disorder
- Panic disorder
- Phobias
- Posttraumatic stress disorder

Most people experience mild anxiety and nervousness at various times during their lives, such as during a job interview, a business presentation, or social events.

Generalized anxiety disorder refers to chronic, exaggerated worry, tension, and irritability that may occur without cause or may be more intense than is warranted by the situation. Physical symptoms include restlessness, sleeping problems, headache, trembling, twitching, muscle tension, and sweating.

Panic disorder is a terrifying experience that occurs suddenly without warning. Physical symptoms include pounding heart, chest pains, dizziness, nausea, shortness of breath, trembling, choking, fear of dying, sweating, feelings of unreality, numbness, hot flashes or chills, and a feeling of going out of control or "crazy." Because panic attacks are unpredictable, many people live in fear of when the next one will occur.

Phobias are irrational anxieties or fears that can interfere with one's everyday life or daily routine. For example, if fear of heights would keep a person from visiting relatives who live on the 13th floor of an apartment building, the fear is excessive and disproportionate to the situation. A person without a phobia but with a fear of heights would still be able to go to visit the relatives. If situations are avoided because of fear, or if fear prevents one from enjoying life or preoccupies one's thinking, hindering ability to work, sleep, or do other things, then it becomes irrational.

Posttraumatic stress disorder (PTSD) is an anxiety disorder that is triggered by memories of a traumatic event. This disorder commonly affects survivors of traumatic events, such as sexual or physical assault, war, torture, a natural disaster, an automobile accident, or an airplane crash. In addition, PTSD can affect rescue workers at the site of an airplane crash or a mass shooting or someone who witnessed a tragic accident.

Anxiety (neurosis) (reaction) (state)
  300.00
  alcohol-induced 291.89
  depression 300.4
  drug-induced 292.89
  due to or associated with physical
      condition 293.84
  generalized 300.02
  hysteria 300.20
  in
      acute stress reaction 308.0
      transient adjustment reaction 309.24
  panic type 300.01
  separation, abnormal 309.21
  syndrome (organic) (transient) 293.84

FIGURE 13-3. Index entry for the main term "Anxiety."

Depression 311
  acute (*see also* Psychosis, affective) 296.2
      recurrent episode 296.3
      single episode 296.2
  agitated (*see also* Psychosis, affective)
      296.2
      recurrent episode 296.3
      single episode 296.2
  anaclitic 309.21
  anxiety 300.4
  arches 734
      congenital 754.61

FIGURE 13-4. Index entry for the main term "Depression."

300.4 Dysthymic disorder
      Anxiety depression
      Depression with anxiety
      Depressive reaction
      Neurotic depressive state
      Reactive depression

  Excludes *adjustment reaction with depressive symptoms*
          (309.0–309.1)
          depression NOS (311)
          manic-depressive psychosis, depressed type
          (296.2–296.3)
          reactive depressive psychosis (298.0)

FIGURE 13-5. Tabular entry for "Depression with anxiety."

EXAMPLE The patient suffers from agoraphobia, 300.22 (F40.00).

EXAMPLE The patient has generalized anxiety, 300.02 (F41.1).

Coding diagnoses of depression and anxiety may be confusing. As illustrated in Figure 13-3, under the main term "Anxiety" is a subterm for "Depression (300.4)"; under the main term "Depression" is a subterm for "Anxiety (300.4)," as shown in Figure 13-4. Verification of code selection in the Tabular (Figure 13-5) reveals the terminology "Depression with anxiety." The Tabular makes the code assignment of 300.4 for a patient with depression and anxiety understandable.

Personality Disorders

A **personality disorder** is a pattern of behavior that can disrupt many aspects of a person's life. Personality disorders range from mild to severe and are often exacerbated during times of stress or external pressure. If a personality disorder is associated with neuroses, psychosis, or a physical condition, this should be coded. Personality disorders are divided into three clusters:

1. Cluster A—patients appear odd or eccentric, socially awkward
   * Paranoid—are suspicious of and do not trust others
   * Schizoid—loners who lack or do not show emotion
   * Schizotypal—seek isolation
2. Cluster B—patients appear dramatic, emotional, or erratic
   * Antisocial—disregard and tend to violate the rights of others, fail to conform to societal norms
   * Borderline—have difficulty coping with minor stress, have unstable relationships, and are self-destructive
   * Histrionic—are overly dramatic with a need to be the center of attention
   * Narcissistic—have an inflated sense of self-importance
3. Cluster C—patients appear anxious and fearful
   * Avoidant—avoid social situations because of fear of criticism, disapproval, or rejection; view themselves as inferior
   * Dependent—rely on others to make decisions for them; fear losing the support and approval of others
   * Obsessive-compulsive—are excessively preoccupied with orderliness, perfection, and mental and interpersonal control

EXAMPLE   Patient has an obsessive-compulsive personality disorder, 301.4 (F60.5).

EXAMPLE   Patient has a passive-aggressive personality, 301.84 (F60.89).

Sexual Disorders

Sexual activities that are not practiced by the majority of the population have been characterized as "deviant" or "variant" behavior. Although some may experiment with a variety of sexual behaviors, it is not until a person begins to rely on the deviant behavior as a means of sexual gratification that it becomes a more permanent trait. "Unconventional" sexual behaviors or paraphilias are coded to category 302 and include some of the following:

Transvestism—assuming the appearance, manner, or roles traditionally associated with members of the opposite sex (cross-dressing)

Exhibitionism—recurrent intense sexual urges and fantasies of exposing the genitals to an unsuspecting stranger

Fetishism—recurrent intense sexual urges and fantasies of using inanimate objects for sexual arousal or orgasm. Objects commonly used include female clothing such as shoes, earrings, or undergarments

Voyeurism—recurrent intense sexual urges and fantasies involving observing unsuspecting people who are naked, disrobing, or engaging in sexual activity

Sadism—the act or sense of gaining pleasure from inflicting physical or psychological pain on another

Masochism—the act or sense of gaining pleasure from experiencing physical or psychological pain

EXAMPLE   Patient is an exhibitionist, 302.4 (F65.2).

Sexual Problems

Sexual problems may be due to organic or medical conditions or to psychological dysfunction. Alcohol and drug use can also affect sexual function. After medical problems have been ruled out, a psychological cause can be explored.

EXAMPLE | Patient is treated for impotence due to psychogenic cause, 302.72 (F52.21).

EXAMPLE | Patient treated for erectile dysfunction, 607.84 (N52.9).

If a patient has erectile dysfunction, it has to be specified as due to psychogenic causes to be coded to 302.72 (F52.21).

EXAMPLE | Patient is being seen for psychogenic dyspareunia, 302.76 (F52.6).

EXAMPLE | Patient is being seen for dyspareunia, 625.0 (N94.1).

Alcohol/Drug Dependence and Abuse

Alcohol dependence, or alcoholism, is a chronic disease that is characterized by a strong compulsion to drink, increasing tolerance, the inability to stop drinking once the person has started, and physical dependence and withdrawal symptoms.

If alcohol dependence is associated with alcoholic psychosis, drug dependence or abuse, or physical complications, all diagnoses should be coded. Under category 303 are instructions on how to code those associated conditions (see Figure 13-2). Code 303.0X, Alcohol dependence syndrome, acute alcoholic intoxication is assigned when a patient is intoxicated and there is documentation of alcohol dependence. Code 303.0X includes both the acute intoxication and the chronic alcoholism. Code 303.0X should not be assigned with code 303.9X. Review the documentation in the record to determine the correct code.

Drug dependence or addiction is similar to dependence on alcohol. It includes a compulsion to take the drug, increased tolerance, an inability to stop using, and physical withdrawal if the person does not have the drug.

It may be difficult for a healthcare provider to determine whether a patient is actually dependent on alcohol or drugs, so abuse codes tend to be used more often. It is possible that a patient is dependent on one drug and is abusing another drug or alcohol. Abuse and dependence codes of different substances can be used for the same patient.

According to *Coding Clinics* (1991:2Q:p10; 1986:M-A:p12),[2,3] the coder is instructed to use combination codes when dependent on more than one drug; these include the following:

■ Combination of opioid-type drug dependence with any other drug dependence
■ Combinations of drug dependence that exclude an opioid-type drug dependence

A healthcare provider may document polysubstance abuse without mentioning which substances are being abused. As this is not documented as dependence, it is coded to 305.9X. Sometimes a patient is dependent on one drug and abuses another.

Dependence is not limited to illegal substances and can occur with prescription drugs. Because drugs have generic and brand names and because these are used interchangeably, it may be difficult to determine which category is assigned for a particular drug dependence. A drug reference book or an Internet search can be used to determine the generic name or category of the drug.

EXAMPLE | Alcoholic gastritis, 535.30, 303.90 (K29.20, F10.20). Upon verification of the 535.30 code in the Tabular, no instructions about coding for alcoholism are provided; because this code is specific to alcoholic gastritis, it would appear that both conditions are covered by the single code. However, it is necessary to code 303.90 for alcohol dependence.

Fifth-digit subclassifications are used in drug and alcohol abuse and dependence categories 303, 304, and 305.0, 305.2-305.9. The pattern of usage must be documented by the physician and/or provider who is legally responsible for establishing the patient's diagnosis. According to *Coding Clinic* (2010:1Q:p21),[1] when the documentation is not specific or is unclear regarding the pattern of abuse or dependence, assign the fifth digit "0" to indicate unspecified.

When a patient is admitted for a medical condition, they may have a comorbidity of alcohol dependence. Along with treating the medical condition, the patient's alcohol dependence may need to be stabilized with drugs to prevent withdrawal. Because they are treating to prevent withdrawal does not mean that the patient is experiencing withdrawal and therefore withdrawal is not coded.

Drug or alcohol abuse indicates a problem with the substance that occurs without craving and physical dependence. However, it is likely that substance abuse can still cause problems with work, school, and home responsibilities and can interfere with relationships.

Particularly in the Emergency Room setting, physicians may document that the patient is a "drug seeker" or has "drug-seeking behavior." According to *Coding Clinic* (1999:3Q:p20),[5] "the appropriate codes are 305.90, unspecified drug abuse, and V65.2, person feigning illness."

EXAMPLE | Patient is being treated for withdrawal due to dependence on Valium, 292.0, 304.10 (F13.239).

Attention Deficit Disorder

Attention deficit disorder (ADD) and **attention deficit hyperactivity disorder** (ADHD) are common childhood disorders. ADHD and ADD are not learning disabilities, but they are characterized by inattention, hyperactivity, and impulsivity. Three subtypes of ADHD have been identified:
1. Hyperactive/impulsive type—patient does not show significant inattention
2. Inattentive type—patient does not show significant hyperactive-impulsive behavior; sometimes called ADD
3. Combined type—patient displays both inattentive and hyperactive-impulsive symptoms

Other disorders that sometimes accompany ADHD include Tourette's syndrome, oppositional defiant disorder, conduct disorder, anxiety and depression, and bipolar disorder. Attention deficit hyperactivity disorder continues into adulthood in about 50% of persons with childhood ADHD.

Oppositional Defiant Disorder

Oppositional defiant disorder is defined as a pattern of uncooperative, defiant, and hostile behavior toward authority figures that does not involve major antisocial violations, is not normal for the patient's developmental stage, and results in significant functional impairment. A certain level of oppositional behavior is common in children and adolescents. It should be considered a disorder only when behaviors are more frequent and intense than in unaffected peers and when they cause dysfunction in social, academic, or work-related arenas.

Learning Disorders

Learning disabilities or differences (LDs) affect a person's ability to understand or use spoken or written language (**dyslexia**), to do mathematical calculations (**dyscalculia**), to coordinate movements such as writing (**dysgraphia**), or to direct attention. Although LDs may occur in very young children, these disorders usually are not recognized until the child reaches school age.

EXERCISE 13-3

Assign codes to the following conditions.

1. Obsessive-compulsive disorder   _____
2. Borderline personality   _____
3. Attention deficit disorder with overactivity   _____
4. Postconcussion syndrome due to previous head trauma   _____
5. Addiction to heroin and OxyContin   _____
6. Cirrhosis due to chronic alcoholism   _____
7. Dyslexia, developmental   _____
8. Pedophile   _____
9. Posttraumatic stress syndrome   _____
10. Panic attack   _____

Intellectual Disabilities

Mental retardation (MR) is a disorder in which a person's overall intellectual functioning is well below average and intelligence quotient (IQ) is around 70 or less. Individuals with MR also may have a significantly impaired ability to cope with common life demands and lack some of the daily living skills that are expected of people in their age group and culture. Impairment may interfere with learning, communication, self-care, independent living, social interaction, play, work, and safety. MR appears in childhood before age 18. There are a variety of causes for mental retardation or intellectual disability; however, often the cause is not documented. Causes of mental retardation are discussed in the following paragraphs.

Genetic Causes

- Defective genes, as in Fragile X syndrome, which is the most common inherited cause of mental retardation
- Chromosomal disorders such as Down's syndrome that are characterized by an abnormal number of chromosomes
- Congenital hypothyroidism, which can result in MR and stunted growth if the patient is not treated with thyroid replacement
- Inborn errors of metabolism may result in MR. More than 300 gene disorders involve inborn errors of metabolism. These include the following:
  - Phenylketonuria (PKU)
  - Tay-Sachs disease
  - Galactosemia
  - Homocystinuria
  - Maple syrup urine disease
  - Biotinidase deficiency

External Causes

- During pregnancy, the following factors can result in MR:
  - Malnutrition
  - Mother's use of alcohol and drugs
  - Environmental toxins such as lead and mercury
  - Viral infections such as rubella and cytomegalovirus
  - Untreated diabetes mellitus
- During birth, the following conditions can result in MR:
  - Low birth weight
  - Premature birth
  - Deprivation of oxygen

■ After birth, the following conditions can result in MR:
  • Complications from infectious diseases such as measles, chickenpox, and whooping cough
  • Exposure to lead and mercury
  • Accidental injury to the brain
  • Severe child abuse
  • Poverty

At the beginning of this section, instructions state an additional code(s) should be assigned to identify any associated psychiatric or physical condition(s). A number of congenital syndromes may have some form of associated MR. The most common severity level is mild intellectual disability; 85% of those affected have the mild type.

ICD-9-CM codes for intellectual disability are classified by IQ, as follows:

IQ 50-70	Mild intellectual disabilities
IQ 35-49	Moderate intellectual disabilities
IQ 20-34	Severe intellectual disabilities
IQ less than 20	Profound intellectual disabilities

Documentation of intellectual disability in the health record may not include the IQ, but the condition often is described by severity.

EXAMPLE Fragile X syndrome with mild intellectual disability, 759.83, 317 (Q99.2, F70).

EXAMPLE MRCP with IQ of 37, 343.9, 318.0 (G80.9, F71).

EXERCISE 13-4

Assign codes to the following conditions.

1. Shaken baby syndrome with profound intellectual disability; _____
   injury happened 2 years ago
2. Trisomy 21 with moderate intellectual disability _____
3. Severe mental retardation due to Angelman's syndrome _____
4. Mild mental retardation due to Lesch-Nyhan syndrome _____
5. Cerebral palsy with intellectual disability _____

FACTORS INFLUENCING HEALTH STATUS AND CONTACT WITH HEALTH SERVICES (V CODES/Z CODES)

In the past, V/Z codes have been considered primarily for use in the outpatient setting. This has changed with the addition of more V/Z codes each year. As discussed in Chapter 8, it may be difficult for the coder to locate V/Z codes in the Index. Coders often say, "I did not know there was a V/Z code for that." Refer to Chapter 8 for a listing of common main terms used to locate V/Z codes.

There is a V/Z code for personal history of alcoholism (V11.3), but this code is not usually assigned. Code 303.93 for alcohol dependence in remission is a more appropriate code because no cure is known for alcoholism and it is still present, although the patient may no longer drink alcohol.

V11.0	Personal history of schizophrenia
V11.1	Personal history of affective disorders
V11.2	Personal history of neurosis
V11.3	Personal history of alcoholism

V11.8	Personal history of other mental disorders
V11.9	Personal history of unspecified mental disorder
V15.41	History of physical abuse
V15.42	History of emotional abuse
V15.49	Psychological trauma—other
V15.82	Personal history of tobacco use
V18.4	Family history of intellectual disabilities
V40.0	Problems with learning
V40.1	Problems with communication, including speech
V40.2	Other mental problems
V40.31	Wandering in diseases classified elsewhere
V40.39	Other specified behavior problem
V40.9	Unspecified mental or behavioral problems
V41.7	Problems with sexual function
V58.69	Long-term (current) use of other medications
V58.83	Encounter for therapeutic drug monitoring
V60.0	Lack of housing
V60.1	Inadequate housing
V60.2	Inadequate material resources
V60.81	Foster care (status)
V60.89	Other specified housing or economic circumstances
V61.01	Family disruption due to family member on military deployment
V61.02	Family disruption due to return of family member from military deployment
V61.03	Family disruption due to divorce or legal separation
V61.04	Family disruption due to parent-child estrangement
V61.05	Family disruption due to child in welfare custody
V61.06	Family disruption due to child in foster care or in care of nonparental family member
V61.07	Family disruption due to death of family member
V61.08	Family disruption due to other extended absence of family member
V61.09	Other family disruption
V61.10	Counseling for marital and partner problems, unspecified
V61.11	Counseling for victim of spousal and partner abuse
V61.12	Counseling for perpetrator of spousal and partner abuse
V61.20	Counseling for parent–child problem, unspecified
V61.21	Counseling for victim of child abuse
V61.22	Counseling for perpetrator of parental child abuse
V61.23	Counseling for parent–biological child problem
V61.24	Counseling for parent–adopted child problem
V61.25	Counseling for parent (guardian)–foster child problem
V61.26	Substance abuse in family
V61.29	Other parent–child problems
V61.3	Problems with aged parents or in-laws
V61.41	Problems with alcoholism in family
V62.0	Unemployment
V62.1	Adverse effects of work environment
V62.21	Personal current military deployment status
V62.22	Personal history of return from military deployment
V62.29	Other occupational circumstances or maladjustment
V62.3	Educational circumstances
V62.4	Social maladjustment
V62.5	Legal circumstances

V62.81	Interpersonal problems, not elsewhere classified
V62.82	Bereavement, uncomplicated
V62.83	Counseling for perpetrator of physical/sexual abuse
V62.84	Suicidal ideation
V62.89	Other psychosocial circumstances
V62.9	Unspecified psychosocial circumstances
V65.2	Person feigning illness
V65.42	Counseling on substance use and abuse
V65.5	Person with feared complaint in whom no diagnosis was made
V66.3	Convalescence and palliative care following psychotherapy and other treatment for mental disorder
V67.3	Follow-up examination following psychotherapy and other treatment for mental disorder
V68.1	Issue of repeat prescriptions
V69.2	Problems related to high-risk sexual behavior
V69.3	Problems related to gambling and betting
V69.8	Other problems related to lifestyle
V69.9	Problems related to lifestyle, unspecified
V70.1	General psychiatric examination, requested by the authority
V70.2	General psychiatric examination, other and unspecified
V70.4	Examination for medicolegal reasons
V71.01	Observation for suspected adult antisocial behavior
V71.02	Observation for childhood or adolescent antisocial behavior
V71.5	Observation following alleged rape or seduction
V71.81	Observation and evaluation for abuse and neglect
V71.9	Observation for other suspected mental condition
V79.0	Special screening for depression
V79.1	Special screening for alcoholism
V79.2	Special screening for intellectual disabilities
V79.3	Special screening for developmental handicaps in early childhood
V79.8	Special screening for other specified mental disorders and developmental handicaps
V79.9	Special screening for unspecified mental disorder and developmental handicap

EXAMPLE Adjustment disorder with depressed mood due to unemployment, 309.0, V62.0 (F43.21, Z56.0).

EXAMPLE Counseling regarding marital problems, V61.10 (Z71.89).

EXERCISE 13-5

Assign codes to the following conditions.

1. Screening for depression _____
2. Malingerer _____
3. Examination for blood alcohol test _____
4. Counseling for mother and son due to son's ADD _____
5. Laboratory testing (liver function tests) on patient who takes Cognex for Alzheimer's disease with dementia _____

COMMON TREATMENTS

Many of the mental disorders can be treated with psychotherapy. Often, a combination of psychotherapy and medication is necessary for effective treatment.

CONDITION	MEDICATIONS
Dementia	Depends on type of dementia
Alcohol withdrawal	Benzodiazepam, such as diazepam (Valium) or chlordiazepoxide (Librium or Libritabs), may be used to reduce anxiety
	Multivitamin; thiamine and folate
	Beta blockers such as propranolol (Inderal) or atenolol (Tenormin) reduce heart rate and tremors
	Phenytoin (Dilantin), carbamazepine (Tegretol), and divalproex sodium (Depakote) are antiseizure medications that can be used to treat or prevent seizures
Drug withdrawal	Treatment depends on the drug
Schizophrenia	Often requires a combination of antipsychotic, antidepressant, and antianxiety medications such as haloperidol (Haldol), chlorpromazine (Thorazine), thioridazine (Mellaril), fluphenazine (Prolixin), Serentil, Seroquel, Clozaril, and Zyprexa
Depression	Antidepressants such as fluoxetine (Prozac), paroxetine (Paxil), sertraline hydrochloride (Zoloft), citalopram hydrobromide (Celexa), nefazodone (Serzone), mirtazapine (Remeron), venlafaxine (Effexor), and bupropion hydrochloride (Wellbutrin)
Bipolar disorder	Medications include lithium; anticonvulsants such as carbamazepine (Tegretol), divalproex sodium (Depakote), gabapentin (Neurontin), and lamotrigine (Lamictal); antidepressants such as bupropion hydrochloride (Wellbutrin) or sertraline hydrochloride (Zoloft); neuroleptics (e.g., Haldol); and benzodiazepines (e.g., lorazepam)
Anxiety	Diazepam (Valium), lorazepam (Ativan), clorazepate (Tranxene), alprazolam (Xanax), paroxetine (Paxil), buspirone (Buspar)
Panic disorder	Alprazolam (Xanax), paroxetine (Paxil)
Phobias	Amitriptyline (Elavil), desipramine (Norpramin), imipramine (Tofranil), nortriptyline (Pamelor), phenelzine (Nardil)
PTSD	Medications to reduce anxiety, depression, and insomnia associated with PTSD
ADD/ADHD	Methylphenidate (Ritalin, Concerta), amphetamine dextroamphetamine (Adderall), pemoline (Cylert), atomoxetine (Strattera)

PROCEDURES

Procedures that are possibly related to mental disorders may be located in the following chapters of the Procedure Tabular:

Chapter 16, Miscellaneous Diagnostic and Therapeutic Procedures (87-99)

Procedures related to mental disorders in ICD-10-PCS can be located in the following tables:

GZ1-GZJ	Mental Health
HZ2-HZ9	Substance Abuse

This chapter covers a wide variety of diagnostic and therapeutic procedures. Some procedures would be appropriate for mental disorders such as detoxification and/or rehabilitation for alcohol and drug abuse. Sometimes, a patient's medical condition is stabilized in a hospital setting, and then the patient is transferred to a facility that is better equipped to offer specialized mental health care. Facility policy may determine which procedures are coded or provided by the facility.

Electroconvulsive Therapy

Electroconvulsive therapy (ECT) is a treatment in which electricity is used to induce seizures. The procedure root type is electroconvulsive therapy. ECT is usually only considered when patients have not responded well to drug therapies. It is primarily used to treat severe depression and other disorders such as schizophrenia, mania, or catatonia. A course of treatments usually consists of 6 to 12 treatments, but may be more or may be less.

Detoxification and Rehabilitation

Detoxification is the active management of withdrawal symptoms in a patient who is physically dependent on alcohol or drugs. The procedure root type for detoxification is detoxification services. It consists of evaluation, observation, and monitoring, along with administration of thiamine, multivitamins, and other medications as needed. Detoxification for alcohol may require a 4- to 5-day period; depending on the drug, it may go on for days or months.

Rehabilitation is a structured program with the goal to stop and recover from the use of alcohol and/or drugs. The procedure root type for rehabilitation is counseling and/or psychotherapy. Many different types of programs are available in a variety of settings; these include inpatient, outpatient, day treatment, residential treatment, half-way houses, and so forth.

Facility policy will determine the coding of these procedures. In the hospital setting, a patient may be treated to prevent alcohol and drug withdrawal or to alleviate symptoms of withdrawal, but this may not constitute true detoxification.

EXERCISE 13-6

Assign codes for all diagnoses and procedures.

1. Electroconvulsive therapy for schizophrenia _____

2. Detoxification and rehabilitation (12-step group counseling) _____
   for chronic alcoholism, continuous

3. Detoxification for heroin dependence, daily use _____

DOCUMENTATION/REIMBURSEMENT/MS-DRGs

Often, coding difficulties are due to lack of documentation. Sometimes test results are not available at the time of discharge or when the physician is dictating the discharge summary or is reporting the final diagnoses.

In the inpatient setting, mental health disorders are often secondary to a more acute medical condition. Many physicians are vague in their descriptions of mental disorders. They may not say that a patient is dependent on drugs or alcohol and may document the condition as drug and/or alcohol abuse. In the health record, information may also be limited for determination of whether usage is continuous, episodic, or in remission. Often, the unspecified fifth digit will need to be assigned. A number of patients are being treated for depression and are on medications. The 311 depression code is often used because of insufficient documentation regarding whether this is an adjustment disorder, a single episode, recurrent, and/or a mood disorder. If they are available, the coder should review consultation reports from the psychologist or the psychiatrist for more specific diagnoses. The coder may need to query the physician to get needed documentation and assign the most appropriate diagnosis code. The presence of an MCC (major complication/comorbidity) or CC (complication/comorbidity) can make a difference in reimbursement, depending on the principal diagnosis and the MS-DRG assigned.

Frequently missed complications/comorbidities from this chapter include the following:

- Alcohol withdrawal
- Drug withdrawal
- Major depressive disorder
- Autism
- Drug dependence with continuous use

Detoxification and Rehabilitation

EXAMPLE

The patient is admitted for detoxification and rehabilitation (Group 12-step) of heroin and alcohol dependence. The patient uses $30 of heroin per day and drinks 1 quart of wine every day. No IV drug use.

DIAGNOSES	CODES	MS-DRG	RW
Heroin and alcohol dependence Detox/Rehab	304.01 (F11.20) 303.91 (F10.20) 94.69 (HZ2ZZZZ, HZ43ZZ)	895	1.0275
Heroin and alcohol dependence Detox only	304.01 (F11.20) 303.91 (F10.20) 94.68 (HZ2ZZZZ)	897	0.6513

It is important to code the appropriate procedure code to include both the detoxification and rehabilitation if performed as it may affect MS-DRG assignment.

CHAPTER REVIEW EXERCISE

Assign codes for all diagnoses and procedures.

1. Dysthymic disorder _____
2. Panic disorder with agoraphobia _____
3. Fragile X syndrome with IQ of 25; family history of mental retardation _____
4. Inhalant abuse _____
5. Tourette's syndrome _____
6. Malnutrition due to anorexia nervosa _____
7. History of alcoholism with 1 year of sobriety _____
8. Mental retardation due to chickenpox 2 years ago _____
9. Alcoholic cardiomyopathy _____
10. Holiday heart syndrome with atrial fibrillation; patient had a drinking binge over Labor Day weekend; history of alcohol abuse _____
11. Depression with anxiety _____
12. Social phobia _____
13. Dementia due to multiple sclerosis _____
14. Adjustment disorder with conduct disturbance due to parents' divorce _____
15. Hypochondria _____
16. Gambling addiction _____
17. Psychogenic asthma _____
18. Pica in an adult patient _____
19. Enuresis, psychogenic _____
20. Fear of flying _____
21. History of emotional abuse _____

22. Parkinson's disease with dementia and related behavioral disturbances _____

23. Suicidal ideation _____

24. Unable to tolerate CT scan due to claustrophobia _____

Write the correct answer(s) in the space(s) provided.

25. Which procedure code groups into the higher paying MS-DRG in the Detoxification and Rehabilitation example?

_____

26. List four types of Cluster B personality disorders.

_____

_____

_____

_____

27. When are learning disabilities usually recognized?

_____

28. List four causes of mental retardation.

_____

_____

_____

_____

CHAPTER GLOSSARY

Affective disorders: a category of mental health problems that include major depressive disorders and bipolar disorders.

Attention deficit disorder: a common childhood disorder characterized by inattention and impulsivity.

Attention deficit hyperactivity disorder: a common childhood disorder characterized by inattention, hyperactivity, and impulsivity.

Bipolar disorder: brain disorder that causes unusual shifts in a person's mood, energy, and ability to function; different from the normal ups and downs that everyone goes through; symptoms of bipolar disorder can be severe.

Cognitive impairment: a decline in mental activities associated with thinking, learning, and memory.

Delirium tremens: life-threatening condition that may involve severe mental or neurologic changes such as delirium and/or hallucinations.

Dementia: progressive deterioration of mental faculties characterized by impairment of memory and one or more cognitive impairments such as language, reasoning and judgment, and calculation and problem-solving abilities.

Depression: affective disorder that is characterized by sadness, lack of interest in everyday activities and events, and a sense of worthlessness.

Detoxification: active management of withdrawal symptoms in a patient who is physically dependent on alcohol or drugs.

Dyscalculia: learning disability that affects a child's ability to do mathematical calculations.

Dysgraphia: learning disability that affects a child's ability to coordinate movements such as writing.

Dyslexia: learning disability that affects a child's ability to understand or use spoken or written language.

Electroconvulsive therapy: psychiatric treatment in which electricity is used to induce seizures.

Exhibitionism: recurrent intense sexual urges and fantasies of exposing the genitals to an unsuspecting stranger.

Fetishism: recurrent intense sexual urges and fantasies of using inanimate objects for sexual arousal or orgasm. Objects commonly used include female clothing such as shoes, earrings, or undergarments.

Generalized anxiety disorder: chronic, exaggerated worry, tension, and irritability that may be without cause or may be more intense than the situation warrants.

Hypomania: milder form of mania, but this "feel good" mood can change to depression or mania.

Major depressive disorder: characterized by one or more major depressive episodes with a history of mania, hypomania, or mixed episodes.

Mania: the other side of depression, in which a person feels so good it is like a "high"; may do risky things.

Masochism: the act or sense of gaining pleasure from experiencing physical or psychological pain.

Mental retardation: disorder in which a person's overall intellectual functioning is well below average, with an intelligence quotient (IQ) around 70 or less.

Mixed mood: alternating between mania and depression, very quickly.

Mood disorder: condition that occurs with a change in mood over a prolonged period.

Oppositional defiant disorder: pattern of uncooperative, defiant, and hostile behavior toward authority figures that does not involve major antisocial violations, is not accounted for by the child's developmental stage, and results in significant functional impairment.

Organic brain syndrome: general term used to describe a decrease in mental function due to other physical disease(s).

Panic disorder: terrifying experience that occurs suddenly without warning. Physical symptoms include pounding heart, chest pains, dizziness, nausea, shortness of breath, trembling, choking, fear of dying, sweating, feelings of unreality, numbness, hot flashes or chills, and a feeling of going out of control or "crazy."

Personality disorder: a pattern of behavior that can disrupt many aspects of a person's life.

Phobia: irrational anxiety or fear that can interfere with one's everyday life or daily routine.

Posttraumatic stress disorder: anxiety disorder that is triggered by memories of a traumatic event.

Psychosis: impairment in mental state in which perception of reality has become distorted.

Rehabilitation: structured program with the goal of stopping and recovering from the use of alcohol and/or drugs.

Sadism: the act or sense of gaining pleasure from inflicting physical or psychological pain on another.

Schizophrenia: disorder of the brain characterized by trouble differentiating between real and unreal experiences, along with problems with logical thinking, normal emotional responses to others, and appropriate behavior in social situations.

Transvestism: assuming the appearance, manner, or roles traditionally associated with members of the opposite sex (cross-dressing).

Voyeurism: recurrent intense sexual urges and fantasies involving observing unsuspecting people who are naked, disrobing, or engaging in sexual activity.

REFERENCES

1. American Hospital Association. *Coding Clinic for ICD-9-CM* 1991:2Q:p11-12. Psychoactive substance–induced organic mental syndromes.
2. American Hospital Association. *Coding Clinic for ICD-9-CM* 1991:2Q:p10. Dependence of drug.
3. American Hospital Association. *Coding Clinic for ICD-9-CM* 1986:M-A:p12. Polydrug addict.
4. American Hospital Association. *Coding Clinic for ICD-9-CM* 2010:1Q:p21. Fifth digits for pattern of use for alcohol and drug abuse/dependence.
5. American Hospital Association. *Coding Clinic for ICD-9-CM* 1999:3Q:p20. Drug-seeking behavior.

14

Diseases of the Nervous System and Sense Organs

(ICD-9-CM Chapter 6, Codes 320-389, and ICD-10-CM Chapter 6, Codes G00-G99, Chapter 7, Codes H00-H59, and Chapter 8, Codes H60-H95)

LEARNING OBJECTIVES

1. Apply and assign the correct ICD-9-CM and ICD-10-CM codes in accordance with Official Guidelines for Coding and Reporting
2. Identify major differences between ICD-9-CM and ICD-10-CM related to the nervous system and sense organs
3. Identify pertinent anatomy and physiology of the nervous system and sense organs
4. Identify diseases of the nervous system and sense organs
5. Assign the correct V/Z codes and procedure codes related to the nervous system and sense organs
6. Identify common treatments, medications, laboratory values, and diagnostic tests
7. Explain the importance of documentation in relation to MS-DRGs for reimbursement

ABBREVIATIONS/ ACRONYMS

CNS central nervous system

CPAP continuous positive airway pressure

CSF cerebrospinal fluid

CVA cerebrovascular accident

DBS deep brain stimulation

EEG electroencephalogram

EMG electromyelogram

ICD-9-CM *International Classification of Diseases, 9th Revision, Clinical Modification*

ICD-10-CM *International Classification of Diseases, 10th Revision, Clinical Modification*

ICD-10-PCS *International Classification of Diseases, 10th Revision, Procedure Coding System*

IOL intraocular lens

IOP intraocular pressure

IV intravenous

LP lumbar puncture

MRI magnetic resonance imaging

MS-DRG Medicare Severity diagnosis-related group

NPH normal pressure hydrocephalus

OM otitis media

OSA obstructive sleep apnea

PDT photodynamic therapy

SIRS systemic inflammatory response syndrome

SOM serous otitis media

SZ seizure

VPS ventriculoperitoneal shunt

ICD-9-CM

Official Guidelines for Coding and Reporting

Please refer to the companion Evolve website for the most current guidelines.

6. **Chapter 6: Diseases of Nervous System and Sense Organs (320-389)**
   a. **Pain—Category 338**
      1) **General coding information**

Codes in category 338 may be used in conjunction with codes from other categories and chapters to provide more detail about acute or chronic pain and neoplasm-related pain, unless otherwise indicated below.

If the pain is not specified as acute or chronic, do not assign codes from category 338, except for post-thoracotomy pain, postoperative pain, neoplasm related pain, or central pain syndrome.

A code from subcategories 338.1 and 338.2 should not be assigned if the underlying (definitive) diagnosis is known, unless the reason for the encounter is pain control/management and not management of the underlying condition.

EXAMPLE

The patient is admitted with acute chest pain due to pneumonia, 486 (J18.9). Only the code for pneumonia would be assigned.

EXAMPLE

The patient is admitted for acute pain control after falling off a ladder and suffering two broken ribs. The patient was admitted for pain control, 338.11, 807.02, E881.0 (G89.11, S22.49xA, W11.xxxA).

(a) **Category 338 Codes as Principal or First-Listed Diagnosis**

Category 338 codes are acceptable as principal diagnosis or the first-listed code:
• When pain control or pain management is the reason for the admission/ encounter (e.g., a patient with displaced intervertebral disc, nerve impingement

and severe back pain presents for injection of steroid into the spinal canal). The underlying cause of the pain should be reported as an additional diagnosis, if known.

- When an admission or encounter is for a procedure aimed at treating the underlying condition (e.g., spinal fusion, kyphoplasty), a code for the underlying condition (e.g., vertebral fracture, spinal stenosis) should be assigned as the principal diagnosis. No code from category 338 should be assigned.

EXAMPLE The patient is having acute pain due to a headache and is admitted for pain control, 338.19, 784.0 (R51).

- When a patient is admitted for the insertion of a neurostimulator for pain control, assign the appropriate pain code as the principal or first-listed diagnosis. When an admission or encounter is for a procedure aimed at treating the underlying condition, and a neurostimulator is inserted for pain control during the same admission/encounter, a code for the underlying condition should be assigned as the principal diagnosis, and the appropriate pain code should be assigned as a secondary diagnosis.

(b) **Use of Category 338 Codes in Conjunction With Site Specific Pain Codes**

(i) **Assigning Category 338 Codes and Site-Specific Pain Codes**

Codes from category 338 may be used in conjunction with codes that identify the site of pain (including codes from chapter 16) if the category 338 code provides additional information. For example, if the code describes the site of the pain, but does not fully describe whether the pain is acute or chronic, then both codes should be assigned.

(ii) **Sequencing of Category 338 Codes with Site-Specific Pain Codes**

The sequencing of category 338 codes with site-specific pain codes (including chapter 16 codes) is dependent on the circumstances of the encounter/admission as follows:

- If the encounter is for pain control or pain management, assign the code from category 338 followed by the code identifying the specific site of pain (e.g., encounter for pain management for acute neck pain from trauma is assigned code 338.11, Acute pain due to trauma, followed by code 723.1, Cervicalgia, to identify the site of pain).

- If the encounter is for any other reason except pain control or pain management, and a related definitive diagnosis has not been established (confirmed) by the provider, assign the code for the specific site of pain first, followed by the appropriate code from category 338.

2) **Pain due to devices, implants and grafts**

Pain associated with devices, implants or grafts left in a surgical site (for example painful hip prosthesis) is assigned to the appropriate code(s) found in Chapter 17, Injury and Poisoning. Use additional code(s) from category 338 to identify acute or chronic pain due to presence of the device, implant or graft (338.18-338.19 or 338.28-338.29).

EXAMPLE Acute pain secondary to painful right knee prosthesis, 996.77, 719.46, 338.18, E878.1 (T84.84xA, M25.561, G89.18, Y83.1)

3) **Postoperative Pain**

Post-thoracotomy pain and other postoperative pain are classified to subcategories 338.1 and 338.2, depending on whether the pain is acute or chronic. The default for post-thoracotomy and other postoperative pain not specified as acute or chronic is the code for the acute form.

Routine or expected postoperative pain immediately after surgery should not be coded.

(a) **Postoperative pain not associated with specific postoperative complication**
Postoperative pain not associated with a specific postoperative complication is assigned to the appropriate postoperative pain code in category 338.

(b) **Postoperative pain associated with specific postoperative complication**
Postoperative pain associated with a specific postoperative complication (such as painful wire sutures) is assigned to the appropriate code(s) found in Chapter 17, Injury and Poisoning. If appropriate, use additional code(s) from category 338 to identify acute or chronic pain (338.18 or 338.28). If pain control/management is the reason for the encounter, a code from category 338 should be assigned as the principal or first-listed diagnosis in accordance with *Section I.C.6.a.1.a above.*

(c) **Postoperative pain as principal or first-listed diagnosis**
Postoperative pain may be reported as the principal or first-listed diagnosis when the stated reason for the admission/encounter is documented as postoperative pain control/management.

(d) **Postoperative pain as secondary diagnosis**
Postoperative pain may be reported as a secondary diagnosis code when a patient presents for outpatient surgery and develops an unusual or inordinate amount of postoperative pain.

The provider's documentation should be used to guide the coding of postoperative pain, as well *as Section III. Reporting Additional Diagnoses and Section IV. Diagnostic Coding and Reporting in the Outpatient Setting.*

See Section II.1.2 for information on sequencing of diagnoses for patients admitted to hospital inpatient care following post-operative observation.

See Section II.J for information on sequencing of diagnoses for patients admitted to hospital inpatient care from outpatient surgery.

See Section IV.A.2 for information on sequencing of diagnoses for patients admitted for observation.

4) **Chronic pain**
Chronic pain is classified to subcategory 338.2. There is no time frame defining when pain becomes chronic pain. The provider's documentation should be used to guide use of these codes.

5) **Neoplasm Related Pain**
Code 338.3 is assigned to pain documented as being related, associated or due to cancer, primary or secondary malignancy, or tumor. This code is assigned regardless of whether the pain is acute or chronic.

This code may be assigned as the principal or first-listed code when the stated reason for the admission/encounter is documented as pain control/pain management. The underlying neoplasm should be reported as an additional diagnosis.

EXAMPLE

Patient is admitted for pain control due to metastatic bone cancer. Patient has a past history of primary breast cancer, 338.3, 198.5, V10.3 (G89.3, C79.51, Z85.3).

When the reason for the admission/encounter is management of the neoplasm and the pain associated with the neoplasm is also documented, code 338.3 may be assigned as an additional diagnosis.

See Section I.C.2 for instructions on the sequencing of neoplasms for all other stated reasons for the admission/encounter (except for pain control/pain management).

EXAMPLE

Patient was admitted for back pain due to vertebral metastasis. An MRI indicates that the disease has progressed. Patient has a history of prostate cancer. Radiation was administered prior to discharge of the patient, 198.5, V10.46, 338.3, 92.29 (C79.51, G89.3, Z85.46; radiation is delivered by external beam radiation via a linear accelerator using electrons, DPOC3ZZ).

6) **Chronic pain syndrome**
This condition is different from that described by the term "chronic pain," and therefore this code should be used only when the provider has specifically documented this condition.

Apply the General Coding Guidelines as found in Chapter 5 and the Procedural Guidelines as found in Chapter 6.

ICD-10-CM

Official Guidelines for Coding and Reporting

Please refer to the companion Evolve website for the most current guidelines.
6. **Chapter 6: Diseases of Nervous System and Sense Organs (G00-G99)**
   a. **Dominant/nondominant side**
      Codes from category G81, Hemiplegia and hemiparesis, and subcategories, G83.1, Monoplegia of lower limb, G83.2, Monoplegia of upper limb, and G83.3, Monoplegia, unspecified, identify whether the dominant or nondominant side is affected. Should **the affected site be documented, but not specified as dominant or nondominant**, and the classification system does not indicate a default, **code selection is as follows:**
      • For ambidextrous patients, the default should be dominant.
      • **If the left side is affected, the default is non-dominant.**
      • **If the right side is affected, the default is dominant.**
   b. **Pain—Category G89**
      1) **General coding information**
         Codes in category G89, Pain, not elsewhere classified, may be used in conjunction with codes from other categories and chapters to provide more detail about acute or chronic pain and neoplasm-related pain, unless otherwise indicated below.
            If the pain is not specified as acute or chronic, post-thoracotomy, postprocedural, or neoplasm-related, do not assign codes from category G89.
            A code from category G89 should not be assigned if the underlying (definitive) diagnosis is known, unless the reason for the encounter is pain control/management and not management of the underlying condition.
            When an admission or encounter is for a procedure aimed at treating the underlying condition (e.g., spinal fusion, kyphoplasty), a code for the underlying condition (e.g., vertebral fracture, spinal stenosis) should be assigned as the principal diagnosis. No code from category G89 should be assigned.
         (a) **Category G89 Codes as Principal or First-Listed Diagnosis**
            Category G89 codes are acceptable as principal diagnosis or the first-listed code:
            • When pain control or pain management is the reason for the admission/encounter (e.g., a patient with displaced intervertebral disc, nerve impingement and severe back pain presents for injection of steroid into the spinal canal). The underlying cause of the pain should be reported as an additional diagnosis, if known.
            • When a patient is admitted for the insertion of a neurostimulator for pain control, assign the appropriate pain code as the principal or **first-listed** diagnosis. When an admission or encounter is for a procedure aimed at treating the underlying condition and a neurostimulator is inserted for pain control during the same admission/encounter, a code for the underlying condition should be assigned as the principal diagnosis and the appropriate pain code should be assigned as a secondary diagnosis.
         (b) **Use of Category G89 Codes in Conjunction with Site Specific Pain Codes**
            (i) **Assigning Category G89 and Site-Specific Pain Codes**
               Codes from category G89 may be used in conjunction with codes that identify the site of pain (including codes from chapter 18) if the category G89 code provides additional information. For example, if the code describes the site of the pain, but does not fully describe whether the pain is acute or chronic, then both codes should be assigned.

(ii) Sequencing of Category G89 Codes with Site-Specific Pain Codes
The sequencing of category G89 codes with site-specific pain codes (including chapter 18 codes), is dependent on the circumstances of the encounter/admission as follows:

- If the encounter is for pain control or pain management, assign the code from category G89 followed by the code identifying the specific site of pain (e.g., encounter for pain management for acute neck pain from trauma is assigned code G89.11, Acute pain due to trauma, followed by code M54.2, Cervicalgia, to identify the site of pain).
- If the encounter is for any other reason except pain control or pain management, and a related definitive diagnosis has not been established (confirmed) by the provider, assign the code for the specific site of pain first, followed by the appropriate code from category G89.

2) Pain due to devices, implants and grafts
See Section I.C.19. Pain due to medical devices

3) Postoperative Pain
The provider's documentation should be used to guide the coding of postoperative pain, as well as *Section III. Reporting Additional Diagnoses* and *Section IV. Diagnostic Coding and Reporting in the Outpatient Setting.*

The default for post-thoracotomy and other postoperative pain not specified as acute or chronic is the code for the acute form.

Routine or expected postoperative pain immediately after surgery should not be coded.

(a) Postoperative pain not associated with specific postoperative complication
Postoperative pain not associated with a specific postoperative complication is assigned to the appropriate postoperative pain code in category G89.

(b) Postoperative pain associated with specific postoperative complication
Postoperative pain associated with a specific postoperative complication (such as painful wire sutures) is assigned to the appropriate code(s) found in Chapter 19, Injury, poisoning, and certain other consequences of external causes. If appropriate, use additional code(s) from category G89 to identify acute or chronic pain (G89.18 or G89.28).

4) Chronic pain
Chronic pain is classified to subcategory G89.2. There is no time frame defining when pain becomes chronic pain. The provider's documentation should be used to guide use of these codes.

5) Neoplasm Related Pain
Code G89.3 is assigned to pain documented as being related, associated or due to cancer, primary or secondary malignancy, or tumor. This code is assigned regardless of whether the pain is acute or chronic.

This code may be assigned as the principal or first-listed code when the stated reason for the admission/encounter is documented as pain control/pain management. The underlying neoplasm should be reported as an additional diagnosis.

When the reason for the admission/encounter is management of the neoplasm and the pain associated with the neoplasm is also documented, code G89.3 may be assigned as an additional diagnosis. It is not necessary to assign an additional code for the site of the pain.

See Section I.C.2 for instructions on the sequencing of neoplasms for all other stated reasons for the admission/encounter (except for pain control/pain management).

6) Chronic pain syndrome
Central pain syndrome (G89.0) and chronic pain syndrome (G89.4) are different than the term "chronic pain," and therefore codes should only be used when the provider has specifically documented this condition.

See Section I.C.5. Pain disorders related to psychological factors

7. Chapter 7: Diseases of Eye and Adnexa (H00-H59)
Reserved for future guideline expansion

8. Chapter 8: Diseases of Ear and Mastoid Process (H60-H95)
Reserved for future guideline expansion

Apply the General Coding Guidelines as found in Chapter 5 and the Procedural Guidelines as found in Chapter 7.

GUIDELINE DIFFERENCES BETWEEN ICD-9-CM AND ICD-10-CM

- Codes for hemiplegia and monoplegia identify whether the dominant or nondominant side is affected. If the information is not available, the default is Dominant. The default for ambidextrous people is also Dominant.
- There are currently no guidelines in ICD-10-CM for diseases of eye and adnexa and diseases of the ear and mastoid process.

MAJOR DIFFERENCES BETWEEN ICD-9-CM AND ICD-10-CM

- Codes for TIA are now included in the nervous system chapter in ICD-10-CM.
- Codes for migraine have been expanded to fifth and sixth characters to indicate whether the migraine is intractable and to reflect additional specificity.
- Codes for secondary parkinsonism have been expanded at the fourth or fifth characters for more specificity.

ANATOMY AND PHYSIOLOGY

The nervous system is composed of specialized tissue that controls the actions and reactions of the body and the way it adjusts to changes that occur inside and outside the body. The nervous system is divided into two main systems: the central nervous system and the peripheral nervous system (Figures 14-1 and 14-2). The central nervous system and the peripheral nervous system are each further divided into two parts. The central nervous system is made up of the brain and the spinal cord, and the peripheral nervous system is made up of the somatic nervous system and the autonomic nervous system.

Central Nervous System

Different areas of the brain are in control of different functions of the body (Figure 14-3). For example, the cerebral cortex controls thought, language, and reasoning; the brain stem is in control of breathing and blood pressure; and the hippocampus is in control of memory and learning. The spinal cord serves as a pathway for information passing from the brain to the peripheral nervous system. Both the brain and the spinal cord are covered by bone— the brain by the skull, and the spinal cord by the vertebral column; both are covered by membranes called the meninges. The meninges (Figure 14-4) are made up of three layers: dura, arachnoid, and pia. In the spinal column, the dura is not attached to the vertebrae but is separated from them by the epidural space. The purpose of these membranes is to protect the brain and the spinal cord.

The spinal cord, which is located in the vertebral foramen, consists of 31 segments, each of which has a pair of spinal nerves that exit from the segment. The purpose of the spinal cord is to conduct nerve impulses and spinal reflexes.

Peripheral Nervous System

The peripheral nervous system connects the central nervous system to other parts of the body. It may be broken down into two parts: the somatic nervous system and the autonomic nervous system. The **somatic nervous system** sends sensory information (taste, hearing, smell, and vision) to the central nervous system (CNS) and motor nerve impulses to the skeletal muscles.

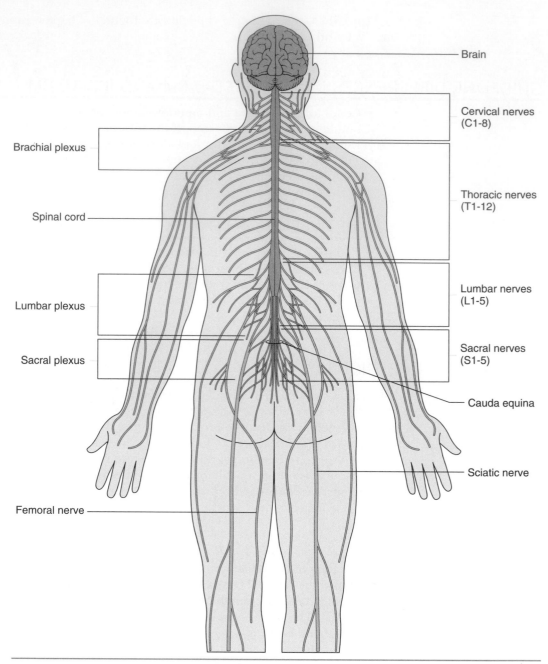

FIGURE 14-1. The brain and the spinal cord, spinal nerves, and spinal plexuses.

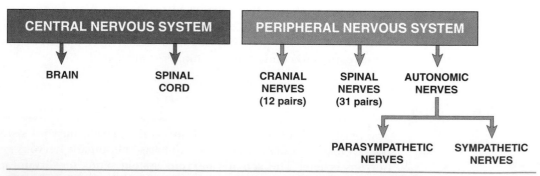

FIGURE 14-2. Divisions of the central nervous system (CNS) and peripheral nervous system (PNS). The autonomic nervous system is a part of the peripheral nervous system.

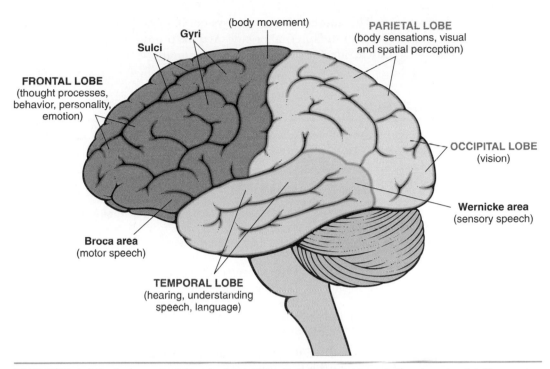

FIGURE 14-3. Left cerebral hemisphere (lateral view). Gyri (convolutions) and sulci (fissures) are indicated. Note the lobes of the cerebrum and the functional centers that control speech, vision, movement, hearing, thinking, and other processes.

FIGURE 14-4. Meninges, frontal view.

The **autonomic nervous system** has both sensory and motor functions that involve the CNS and the internal organs. Actions produced by this system, such as beating of the heart muscle, are for the most part involuntary.

DISEASE CONDITIONS

Diseases of the Nervous System and Sense Organs (320-389), Chapter 6 in the ICD-9-CM code book, is divided into the following categories:

CATEGORY	SECTION TITLES
320-326	Inflammatory Diseases of the Central Nervous System
327	Organic Sleep Disorders
330-337	Hereditary and Degenerative Diseases of the Central Nervous System
338	Pain
340-349	Other Disorders of the Central Nervous System
350-359	Disorder of the Peripheral Nervous System
360-379	Disorders of the Eye and Adnexa
380-389	Diseases of the Ear and Mastoid Process

Diseases of the Nervous System (G00-G99), Chapter 6 in the ICD-10-CM code book, Diseases of the Eye and Adnexa (H00-H59), Chapter 7 in the ICD-10-CM code book, and Diseases of the Ear and Mastoid Process (H60-95), Chapter 8 in the ICD-10-CM code book, are divided into the following categories:

CATEGORY	SECTION TITLES
G00-G009	Inflammatory Disease of the Central Nervous System
G10-G13	Systemic Atrophies Primarily Affecting the Central Nervous System
G20-G26	Extrapyramidal and Movement Disorders
G30-G32	Other Degenerative Diseases of the Nervous System
G35-G37	Demyelinating Diseases of the Central Nervous System
G40-G47	Episodic and Paroxysmal Disorders
G50-G59	Nerve, Nerve Root, and Plexus Disorders
G60-G64	Polyneuropathies and Other Disorders of the Peripheral Nervous System
G70-G73	Diseases of Myoneural Junction and Muscle
G80-G83	Cerebral Palsy and Other Paralytic Syndromes
G89-G99	Other Disorders of the Nervous System
H00-H05	Disorders of Eyelid, Lacrimal System, and Orbit
H10-H11	Disorders of the Conjunctiva
H15-H21	Disorders of Sclera, Cornea, Iris, and Ciliary Body
H25-H28	Disorders of the Lens
H30-H36	Disorders of the Choroid and Retina
H40-H42	Glaucoma
H43-H44	Disorders of the Vitreous Body and Globe
H46-H47	Disorders of the Optic Nerve and Visual Pathways
H49-H52	Disorders of Ocular Muscles, Binocular Movement, Accommodation, and Refraction
H53-H54	Visual Disturbances and Blindness
H55-H57	Other Disorders of Eye and Adnexa
H59	Intraoperative and Postprocedural Complications and Disorders of Eye and Adnexa, Not Elsewhere Classified
H60-H62	Diseases of External Ear
H65-H75	Diseases of Middle Ear and Mastoid
H80-H83	Diseases of the Inner Ear
H90-H94	Other Disorders of Ear
H95	Intraoperative and Postprocedural Complications and Disorders of Ear and Mastoid Process, Not Elsewhere Classified

Inflammatory Diseases of the Central Nervous System

Meningitis is an infection or inflammation of the meninges. Meningitis is caused by a viral or bacterial organism and may be treated with antibiotics. Vaccines are available to prevent meningitis that is due to *Streptococcus pneumoniae*. It should be noted that often, coding of meningitis requires two codes, and in most cases, the Tabular List instructs to code the underlying condition first. For more information on coding guidelines for underlying conditions, refer to Chapter 5 in this text, General Coding Guidelines.

EXAMPLE The patient was treated for meningitis due to Lyme disease, 088.81, 320.7 (A69.21).

The signs and symptoms of meningitis include high fever, headache, and stiff neck. Other symptoms that may be present are nausea, vomiting, sleepiness, and sensitivity to bright lights. To diagnose meningitis, physicians perform a lumbar puncture (Figure 14-5) to obtain spinal fluid and to look for organisms that may be present. Bacterial meningitis is treated with antibiotics, and the treatment for viral meningitis (aseptic) is usually limited to treating the symptoms.

EXAMPLE Patient admitted for meningitis due to sarcoidosis, 135, 321.4 (D86.81).

EXAMPLE Patient is being treated for *Pseudomonas* meningitis, 320.82 (G00.8, B96.5).

Additional disease conditions found in the section on Inflammatory Diseases of the Central Nervous System often require the use of two codes and include the instruction to code first the underlying condition. It is also important to follow the Excludes notes for further instruction (Figure 14-6).

EXAMPLE Patient is being treated for encephalitis due to infectious mononucleosis, 075, 323.01 (B27.92).

EXAMPLE The patient was admitted with herpes encephalitis, 054.3 (B00.4).

Site of needle puncture

Dura mater and arachnoid membrane

Distal end of spinal cord

L3 L4

Subarachnoid space containing CSF

FIGURE 14-5. Lumbar (spinal) puncture. The patient lies laterally, with the knees drawn up to the abdomen and the chin brought down to the chest. This position increases the spaces between the vertebrae. The lumbar puncture needle is inserted between the third and fourth (or fourth and fifth) lumbar vertebrae, and it enters the subarachnoid space.

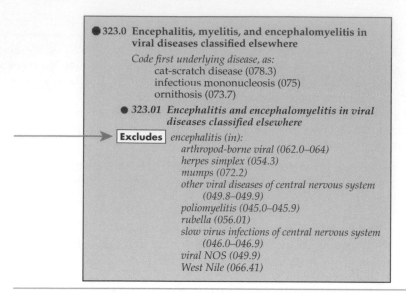

● 323.0 **Encephalitis, myelitis, and encephalomyelitis in viral diseases classified elsewhere**

Code first underlying disease, as:
        cat-scratch disease (078.3)
        infectious mononucleosis (075)
        ornithosis (073.7)

    ● **323.01 Encephalitis and encephalomyelitis in viral diseases classified elsewhere**

    Excludes *encephalitis (in):*
        arthropod-borne viral (062.0–064)
        herpes simplex (054.3)
        mumps (072.2)
        other viral diseases of central nervous system (049.8–049.9)
        poliomyelitis (045.0–045.9)
        rubella (056.01)
        slow virus infections of central nervous system (046.0–046.9)
        viral NOS (049.9)
        West Nile (066.41)

FIGURE 14-6. Refer to the Excludes notes for further instruction if an underlying disease is causing encephalitis, myelitis, and encephalomyelitis.

EXERCISE 14-1

Assign codes to the following conditions.

1. Meningitis due to *Salmonella*   _____
2. *Klebsiella pneumoniae* meningitis   _____
3. Gram-negative meningitis   _____
4. Spinal meningitis   _____
5. Encephalitis following chickenpox   _____

Organic Sleep Disorders

Some typical sleep problems include **insomnia**, (difficulty falling asleep, staying asleep, wakefulness, and early morning awakening) and **hypersomnia** (excessive sleep). These problems are classified in this section when they are caused by a physiologic condition.

EXAMPLE   The patient is being treated for insomnia due to anxiety, 307.42 (F51.05, F41.9).

Sleep apnea is a disorder that is characterized by breathing interruption during sleep. These patients awaken many times during the night to regain their breathing. This disorder results in sleep deprivation and can be life-threatening. Sleep apnea can result in a drop in the oxygen saturation of blood and is a cause of daytime **somnolence** (sleepiness). A person is more likely to have obstructive sleep apnea (OSA) if they are overweight, snore loudly, are hypertensive, or have a family history of sleep apnea. This obstruction occurs when there is a blockage in the airway. Obstructive sleep apnea is diagnosed by a sleep study or polysomnogram. Patients are treated with a CPAP (continuous positive airway pressure) mask. This mask helps push air into the breathing pathway. There are also surgical procedures to correct the obstruction.

Central sleep apnea occurs when the brain does not signal the muscles to breath. This might occur in a stroke victim that has nervous system dysfunction or in patients that have neurodegenerative illnesses such as Lou Gehrig's disease.

EXAMPLE Patient has obstructive sleep apnea, 327.23 (G47.33).

Hereditary and Degenerative Diseases of the Central Nervous System

Alzheimer's disease (Figure 14-7) is a disorder of the brain that causes a progressive decline in mental and physical function. This disease is the most common cause of mental deterioration, and medications are available now and others are in development to assist in the treatment of this disease. When a physician documents the condition as Alzheimer's dementia, it is necessary to use two codes, with Alzheimer's disease sequenced first. For many of the dementia codes, code assignment may depend on the presence of behavioral disturbances such as aggressiveness, combativeness, violence, or wandering off.

EXAMPLE Patient has Alzheimer's dementia without behavioral disturbance, 331.0, 294.10 (G30.9, F02.80).

Hydrocephalus is essentially excessive water (cerebrospinal fluid) on the brain. Cerebrospinal fluid (CSF) surrounds the brain and the spinal cord, and when this fluid accumulates on the brain, it causes pressure on brain tissue. Hydrocephalus may be acquired or congenital and communicating or obstructive. In communicating hydrocephalus, CSF can flow between ventricles of the brain, but it is blocked upon exit of the ventricle, as opposed to obstructive hydrocephalus, in which the flow between ventricles is blocked. In

FIGURE 14-7. Degenerative diseases of the brain preferentially involve various parts of the brain. Alzheimer's disease causes atrophy of the frontal and occipital cortical gyri. Huntington's disease affects the frontal cortex and basal ganglia. Parkinson's disease is marked by changes in the substantia nigra. Amyotrophic lateral sclerosis affects the motor neurons in the anterior horn of the spinal cord, brain stem, and frontal cortex of the brain.

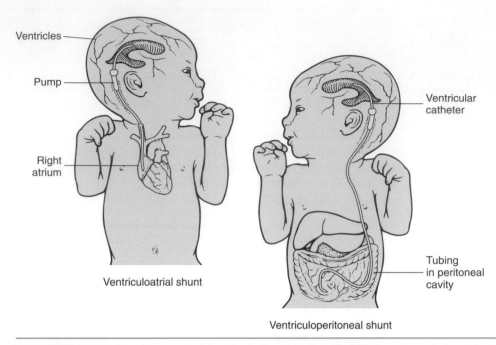

Ventricles

Pump

Right
atrium

Ventriculoatrial shunt

Ventricular
catheter

Tubing
in peritoneal
cavity

Ventriculoperitoneal shunt

FIGURE 14-8. Shunting procedures for hydrocephalus. Ventriculoperitoneal shunt is the preferred procedure.

addition, a condition known as normal pressure hydrocephalus (NPH) occurs in the elderly population and often occurs with dementia. Hydrocephalus is most often treated with a ventricular shunt (Figure 14-8). Hydrocephalus that is left untreated is a fatal condition.

EXAMPLE The patient has a shunt for noncommunicating hydrocephalus, 331.4, V45.2 (G91.1, Z98.2).

Parkinson's disease (Figure 14-9) is a progressive and chronic motor system disorder. Symptoms may include tremor, rigidity, and impaired balance or coordination. It is usually treated with drugs such as L-dopa and sometimes with implantation of an intracranial neurostimulator.

EXAMPLE Patient with Parkinson's disease, 332.0 (G20).

EXAMPLE Patient is being treated for parkinsonism in Huntington's disease, 333.4 (G10).

EXAMPLE Patient has parkinsonism due to Risperdal, 332.1, E939.3 (T43.595A, G21.11).

Pain

To use codes from this category, the pain must be specified as acute or chronic, with exceptions being made for the following:

- Post-thoracotomy pain
- Postoperative pain
- Neoplasm-related pain
- Central pain syndrome

FIGURE 14-9. Typical shuffling gait and posture of patients with Parkinson's disease.

If the cause of the pain (i.e., the underlying diagnosis) is known, then a code from 338.1 and 338.2 should **NOT** be used unless the purpose of the encounter is pain control.

EXAMPLE
> Patient is admitted from the Emergency Room with acute chest pain due to pneumonia, 486 (J18.9).
> The cause of the acute chest pain is known; therefore, no pain code is necessary.

EXAMPLE
> Patient presents to the ER in acute pain after falling off a horse at riding camp. Patient is admitted for acute pain control because of two broken ribs, 338.11, 807.02, E828.2, E849.4, E006.1, (G89.11, S22.49xA, V80.018A, Y93.52, Y92.39).
> Although there is a definitive diagnosis for the pain, the reason for admission is for pain control, not treatment of the broken ribs.

Pain is the principal diagnosis or first-listed diagnosis:
- When no definitive diagnosis has been established or;
- When admitted for pain management or control with the underlying cause as a secondary diagnosis including site-specific pain codes or;
- When admitted for postoperative pain control or;
- When admitted for pain control of neoplasm-related pain.

EXAMPLE
> Patient is having acute head pain caused by a headache and is admitted for pain control, 338.19 (Other acute pain) and 784.0 (head pain) (R51).

Pain is **NOT** the principal diagnosis or first-listed diagnosis:
- When a definitive diagnosis is known or;
- When site-specific pain is known and patient is admitted for workup of pain or;
- When the pain is due to a device.

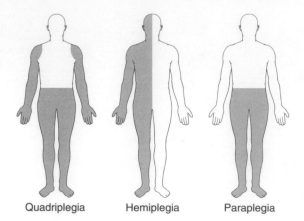

Quadriplegia   Hemiplegia   Paraplegia   **FIGURE 14-10.** Types of paralysis.

Other Disorders of the Central Nervous System

Hemiplegia and hemiparesis (Figure 14-10) describe paralysis of the body that could have a number of causes. One of the most common causes of hemiplegia is a cerebrovascular accident (CVA) (Figure 14-11). When a patient is admitted with an acute CVA and has hemiplegia at discharge, it is appropriate to code this condition. These codes have fifth digits that represent the side of the body that has been affected. If the patient is right-handed and the right side is affected, then the fifth digit 1 for the dominant side would be selected. *Coding Clinic* (1994:4Q:p36)[1] instructs the coder to select fifth digit 0 if no mention of dominant side is made in the record.

EXAMPLE | Patient has right-sided dominant spastic hemiparesis, 342.11 (G81.11).

Epilepsy is a disorder of the brain that is characterized by abnormal electrical discharges from the brain cells. Recurrent seizures are the main symptom of epilepsy. Two major types of seizures can occur: generalized and partial. Seizures may present in a variety of forms; patients may lose consciousness, their arms and legs may jerk, they may become incontinent, or they may stare blankly, unaware of their surroundings. A seizure disorder is coded to 345.9X (G40.–). If patient has recurrent seizures, this is also coded to 345.9X (G40.–). When it is documented as a convulsion or a single seizure then 780.39 (R56.9) is assigned.

Epilepsy has many causes; however, in approximately half of the cases, the cause is unknown. Epilepsy may be inherited, or it may be caused by injury to the brain, metabolic disturbances, alcohol and drug abuse, brain tumor, infection, stroke, fever, or it may occur in pregnancy. Epilepsy is generally treated with anticonvulsants such as Dilantin or Depakote, although in severe uncontrolled cases, surgery may be performed on the brain to remove the area of the brain where seizures originate. The most common diagnostic test for epilepsy is an electroencephalogram (EEG).

A fifth-digit subclassification for category 345 allows the identification of intractable epilepsy, **intractable** meaning "unable to control." The coder should be aware that the physician must document epilepsy as intractable, pharmacoresistant, poorly controlled, refractory, or treatment resistant before the fifth digit of 1 can be assigned. If this is not documented and the record suggests intractable, it may be necessary to query the physician.

EXAMPLE | Patient was admitted for intractable epilepsy, 345.91 (G40.919).

EXAMPLE | Patient is being treated for progressive myoclonic epilepsy, 345.10 (G40.309).

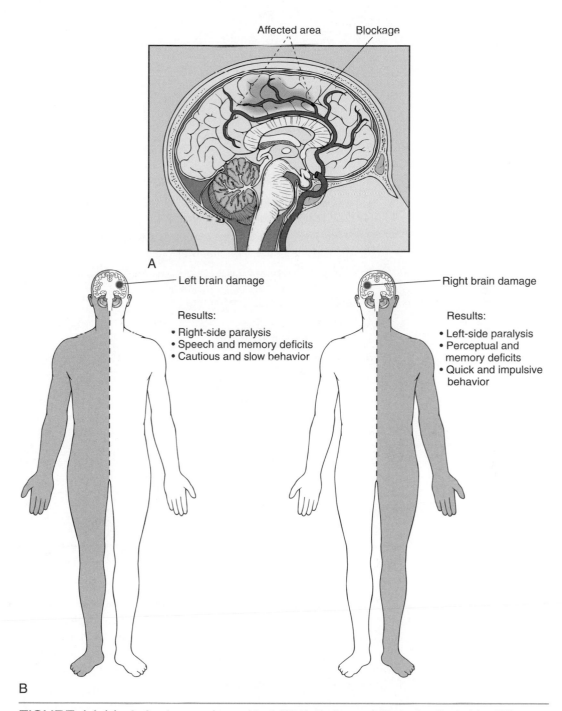

FIGURE 14-11. **A**, Cerebrovascular accident (CVA). **B**, Areas of the body affected by CVA.

EXERCISE 14-2

Assign codes to the following conditions.

1. Parkinson's dementia _____
2. Chronic hydrocephalus _____
3. Seizure disorder _____
4. Partial epilepsy, visual type _____
5. Uncontrolled grand mal epilepsy _____
6. Status epilepticus _____
7. Organic hypersomnia _____
8. Febrile seizures _____
9. Patient has hemiplegia, which is a late effect of a CVA _____
10. Patient is left-handed and has hemiparesis affecting his or her nondominant side _____
11. Patient is admitted for pain control with acute abdominal pain related to pancreatic cancer _____
12. Patient is admitted with back pain for intravenous (IV) pain management after a fall down the stairs _____
13. Patient is admitted for acute neck pain after an automobile accident; attending plans magnetic resonance imaging (MRI) of the neck to rule out fracture _____
14. Patient is readmitted for postoperative pain control after emergency appendectomy _____
15. Patient is admitted for narcotics to treat chronic pain syndrome _____

Disorders of the Peripheral Nervous System

Many of the codes in this chapter require the coder to apply the General Coding Guideline Rules for Multiple Coding. The "Code First" underlying condition applies often in this chapter. The coder must remember that the underlying condition is coded first; this is followed by the code for the manifestation.

EXAMPLE Patient has polyneuropathy in type II diabetes, 250.60, 357.2 (E11.42).

Myasthenia gravis is a chronic **autoimmune disorder** that manifests as muscle weakness of varying degrees. The most frequently affected muscles are those that control the eye, eyelid, face, and swallowing. Myasthenia gravis may be treated with medication, thymectomy, and/or plasmapheresis. Patients who present in crisis may have difficulty breathing and require a ventilator to assist with breathing. These crises may be brought on by many different events, such as infection, stress, or fever.

EXAMPLE Patient was admitted for an acute exacerbation of myasthenia gravis, 358.01 (G70.01).

Muscular dystrophy is a type of myopathy. **Myopathies** are general disorders that affect muscles and usually result in muscle weakening or atrophy. Many disease processes involve myopathies.

EXAMPLE Patient has Graves' myopathy, 242.90, 359.5 (E05.90, G73.7).

Critical illness polyneuropathy and myopathy are diseases of the nerves and muscles that occur as a complication of severe trauma or infection. These conditions are often diagnosed when there is an unexplained difficulty in weaning the patient from mechanical ventilation. These conditions are often associated with sepsis and are thought to be a manifestation of the systemic inflammatory response syndrome (SIRS).

EXAMPLE Patient is diagnosed with critical illness polyneuropathy, 357.82 (G62.81).

Disorders of the Eye and Adnexa

Many eye disorders are treated in the outpatient setting. Some of the conditions commonly found in inpatient records involve injuries to the eye (Figure 14-12), glaucoma, cataracts, macular degeneration, and visual impairment such as blindness. Injuries to the eye are covered in Chapter 19.

Macular degeneration (Figure 14-13) is the leading cause of vision loss in the United States. Persons affected by this disease tend to be elderly; vision is lost in the central portion of the eye, leaving the patient with peripheral vision or low vision. Two common types of this disease have been identified: dry and wet. The dry form is more common and is less aggressive than the wet type.

EXAMPLE Patient has exudative macular degeneration, 362.52 (H35.32).

Glaucoma (Figure 14-14) is a disorder of the optic nerve that may result in vision loss. The most common form is primary open angle glaucoma, in which the drainage canals of the eye become clogged over time and cause intraocular pressure (IOP) to rise; this damages the optic nerve. Glaucoma is most often treated with medicines in the form of eye drops. Surgical procedures, such as trabeculoplasty and trabeculectomy, may assist in the treatment of glaucoma. It is important to note that there is a specific code for borderline glaucoma or glaucoma suspect.

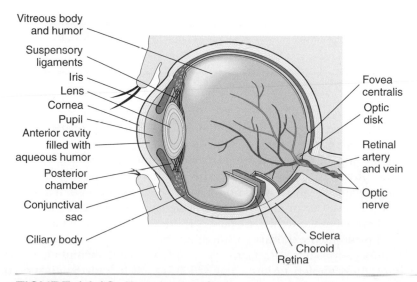

FIGURE 14-12. Normal eye anatomy.

FIGURE 14-13. Macular degeneration. **A**, Wet, atrophic, age-related macular degeneration. **B**, Dry, atrophic, age-related macular degeneration.

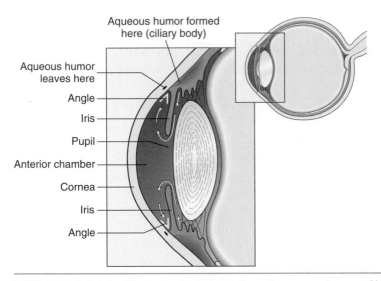

FIGURE 14-14. Glaucoma and circulation of aqueous humor. Circulation is impaired in glaucoma so that aqueous fluid builds up in the anterior chamber.

EXAMPLE | Patient is treated for open angle glaucoma, early stage, 365.10, 365.71 (H40.10).

EXAMPLE | Patient has glaucoma with Sturge-Weber syndrome, 759.6, 365.44 (Q85.8, H42).

Cataract (Figure 14-15) is a clouding of the lens of the eye that can cause obstructed vision. Most cataracts are related to the aging process; however, *Coding Clinic* (1985: Sept-Oct:p10)[2] advises not to use the code for senile cataract just because of a patient's age. The physician must document the type of cataract the patient has. *Coding Clinic* (1985: Sept-Oct:p11)[3] also advises not to make the assumption that a patient has a diabetic cataract just because he or she has both diabetes and a cataract. The physician must document diabetic cataract. Other risk factors for development of cataracts include smoking, diabetes, and prolonged exposure to sunlight. Cataracts are most often treated by surgery. Possible complications of cataract surgery include retinal detachment, anterior capsule contracture, and aftercataract. *Coding Clinic* (2000:1Q:p9-10)[4] advises to use code 996.53 for anterior capsule contracture.

FIGURE 14-15. Cataract. The lens appears cloudy.

Classification		Levels of Visual Impairment	Additional Descriptors Which May Be Encountered
"Legal"	WHO	Visual Acuity and/or Visual Field Limitation (Whichever Is Worse)	
	(Near-) normal vision	Range of Normal Vision 20/10 20/13 20/16 20/20 20/25 2.0 1.6 1.25 1.0 0.8	
		Near-Normal Vision 20/30 20/40 20/50 20/60 0.7 0.6 0.5 0.4 0.3	
	Low vision	Moderate Visual Impairment 20/70 20/80 20/100 20/125 20/160 0.25 0.20 0.16 0.12	Moderate low vision
Legal Blindness (U.S.A.) both eyes	Blindness (WHO) one or both eyes	Severe Visual Impairment 20/200 20/250 20/320 20/400 0.10 0.08 0.06 0.05 Visual field: 20 degrees or less	Severe low vision, "Legal" blindness
		Profound Visual Impairment 20/500 20/630 20/800 20/1000 0.04 0.03 0.025 0.02 Count fingers at: less than 3 m (10 ft) Visual field: 10 degrees or less	Profound low vision, Moderate blindness
		Near-Total Visual Impairment Visual acuity: less than 0.02 (20/1000) Count fingers: 1 m (3 ft) or less Hand movements: 5 m (15 ft) or less Light projection, light perception Visual field: 5 degrees or less	Severe blindness, Near-total blindness
		Total Visual Impairment No light perception (NLP)	Total blindness

Visual acuity refers to best achievable acuity with correction.
Non-listed Snellen fractions may be classified by converting to the nearest decimal equivalent, e.g., 10/200 = 0.05, 6/30 = 0.20.
CF (count fingers) without designation of distance, may be classified to profound impairment.
HM (hand motion) without designation of distance, may be classified to near-total impairment.
Visual field measurements refer to the largest field diameter for a 1/100 white test object.

FIGURE 14-16. Blindness and low vision table.

EXAMPLE   Patient has a mature senile cataract, 366.17 (H25.89).

Blindness and Low Vision

In the United States, **legal blindness** (Figure 14-16) is defined as severe or profound impairment in both eyes. ICD-9-CM always codes the better eye impairment first and the lesser eye disorder second.

> **EXAMPLE** Patient with better eye severe impairment; lesser eye profound impairment, 369.14. (To code in ICD-10-CM, the visual impairment category is needed.)

> **EXAMPLE** A patient is blind in right eye and had normal vision in the other eye, 369.63 (H54.41).

Diseases of the Ear and Mastoid Process

As with eye conditions, many disorders of the ear (Figure 14-17) are treated in the outpatient setting. At times, inpatient coders see patients with the diagnoses of otitis media, mastoiditis, vertigo, and cholesteatoma, and of course, patients with hearing loss.

Otitis media (OM) is a middle ear infection. It is the most common illness among children and babies. OM often occurs after another illness such as a cold. If the physician describes OM as suppurative, it is purulent or is expressing pus.

> **EXAMPLE** Patient has acute allergic serous otitis media, right ear, 381.04 (H65.111).

Mastoiditis is an infection of the mastoid bone of the skull. It is often the consequence of untreated OM and may be difficult to treat. Treatment usually consists of antibiotics and, as a last resort, a mastoidectomy to drain and remove the mastoid.

> **EXAMPLE** Patient is being treated for chronic recurrent mastoiditis in left ear, 383.1 (H70.12).

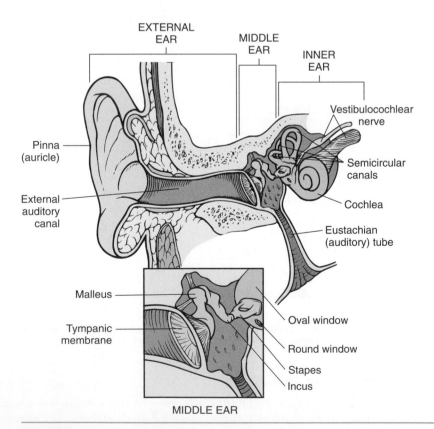

FIGURE 14-17. Normal ear.

A **cholesteatoma** is a growth in the middle ear that usually results from repeated ear infections. Cholesteatomas may cause hearing loss or dizziness and may require surgery.

EXAMPLE | Patient was diagnosed with an attic right cholesteatoma, 385.31 (H71.01).

EXERCISE 14-3

Assign codes to the following conditions.

1. Malignant neoplasm of the thyroid with myasthenia syndrome _____
2. Myasthenia gravis _____
3. Hereditary muscular dystrophy _____
4. Myopathy due to critical illness _____
5. What is the leading cause of vision loss in the United States? _____
6. An 80-year-old gentleman has cataracts and diabetes _____
7. Patient is blind by USA standards _____
8. SOM (serous otitis media) _____
9. Acute and chronic mastoiditis _____

FACTORS INFLUENCING HEALTH STATUS AND CONTACT WITH HEALTH SERVICES (V CODES/Z CODES)

In the past, V/Z codes have been considered for use primarily in the outpatient setting. This has changed with the addition of more V/Z codes each year. As was discussed in Chapter 8, it is difficult to locate V/Z codes in the Index. Coders will often say, "I did not know there was a V/Z code for that."

Refer to Chapter 8 for a listing of common main terms used to locate V/Z codes. V/Z codes that may be used with Nervous System and Sense Organ conditions include the following:

V12.40	Personal history of unspecified disorder of the nervous system and sense organs
V12.41	Personal history of benign neoplasm of the brain
V15.29	Personal history of surgery to other major organs that presents hazards to health
V17.1	Family history of stroke
V19.0	Family history of blindness or visual loss
V19.11	Family history of glaucoma
V19.19	Family history of other eye disorders
V19.2	Family history of deafness or hearing loss
V19.3	Family history of other ear disorders
V42.5	Cornea replaced by transplant
V43.0	Eye globe replaced by other means
V43.1	Lens replaced by other means
V45.2	Presence of cerebrospinal fluid drainage device
V45.61	Postprocedural state following cataract surgery
V45.69	Postprocedural state following surgery of eye and adnexa
V45.78	Acquired absence of eye

V52.2	Fitting and adjustment of artificial eye
V53.01	Fitting and adjustment of cerebral ventricular shunt
V53.02	Fitting and adjustment of neuropacemaker (brain, peripheral nerve, spinal cord)
V53.09	Fitting and adjustment of other devices related to nervous system and special senses
V53.1	Fitting and adjustment of spectacles and contact lens
V53.2	Fitting and adjustment of hearing aid
V58.71	Aftercare following surgery of the sense organs, NEC
V58.72	Aftercare following surgery of the nervous system, NEC
V72.11	Encounter for hearing exam following failed hearing screening
V72.12	Encounter for hearing conservation and treatment
V72.19	Encounter for other exam of ears and hearing
V80.09 (no translation screening for neurologic conditions in ICD-10)	Screening for other neurologic conditions
V80.1	Screening for glaucoma
V80.2	Screening for other eye conditions
V80.3	Screening for ear diseases

EXAMPLE Patient with previous cornea transplant, V42.5 (Z94.7).

EXERCISE 14-4

Assign codes to the following conditions.

1. Encounter for fitting of glasses _____

2. Patient is status cataract removal and has a history of cornea transplant _____

3. Patient previously had enucleation of right eye _____

4. Patient was screened for glaucoma _____

COMMON TREATMENTS

CONDITION	MEDICATION/TREATMENT
Alzheimer's	Tacrine (Cognex), donepezil hydrochloride (Aricept), rivastigmine tartrate (Exelon), galantamine (Reminyl), memantine HCl (Namenda)
Parkinson's	Entacapone (Comtan), pramipexole dihydrochloride (Mirapex), ropinirole hydrochloride (Requip), Carbidopa-Levodopa (Sinemet)
Epilepsy	Carbamazepine (Tegretol), clonazepam (Klonopin), phenytoin (Dilantin), sodium valproate and valproic acid (Depakote), levetiracetam (Keppra), topiramate (Topamax).
Myasthenia gravis	Neostigmine bromide—oral (Prostigmin), pyridostigmine (Regonol, Mestinon)
Muscular dystrophy	Phenytoin (Dilantin), phenytoin (Phenytek), Deltasone
Macular degeneration	Vitamins/photodynamic surgery
Glaucoma	Eye drops such as Xalatan (prostaglandins), Iopidine (adrenergics), Carbachol (miotic), Timoptic (beta blocker), and Diamox (carbonic anhydrase inhibitors)

PROCEDURES

Some procedures that may be related to diseases of the nervous system and sense organs may be located in the following ICD-9-CM chapters of the Procedure Tabular:

Chapter 1   Operations of the Nervous System (01-05)
Chapter 3   Operations of the Eye (08-16)
Chapter 4   Operations of the Ear (18-20)

Procedures related to the nervous system and sense organs in ICD-10-PCS may be found in the following tables:

Central Nervous System   001-00X
Peripheral Nervous System   012-01X
Eye   080-08Y
Ear, Nose, Sinus   090-09W

Lumbar Puncture

Lumbar puncture (LP), also known as spinal tap or spinal puncture, is used both diagnostically and therapeutically. The root operation in ICD-10-PCS for a lumbar puncture is drainage of the spinal canal. When LP is performed for diagnosis, the cerebrospinal fluid (CSF) is analyzed for infection, inflammatory diseases such as multiple sclerosis, subarachnoid hemorrhage, and certain types of carcinoma. When LP is done therapeutically, it may be done to decrease spinal fluid pressure in conditions such as normal pressure hydrocephalus, benign intracranial hypertension, or pseudotumor cerebri. When LP is done therapeutically, the coder will find this code listed in the ICD-9-CM Index under "Drainage, spinal."

EXAMPLE   Patient presents to the ER with high fever and neck pain. The physician performs a lumbar puncture to rule out meningitis, 780.60, 723.1, 03.31 (R50.9, M54.2, 009U3ZX).

Deep Brain Stimulation

A brain stimulator, also known as an intracranial neurostimulator, a **deep brain stimulator** (DBS), or a thalamic stimulator, is used to control tremors in patients with Parkinson's and in those who have the condition of essential tremor. The root operations in ICD-10-PCS for insertion of a neurostimulator are insertion of a stimulator and insertion of an electrode. An electrode is implanted, usually into the thalamus, and then is connected by a wire under the skin to a pulse generator implanted in the chest. Electrical impulses are sent to the thalamus, which in turn, controls tremors. For further information on this procedure, refer to *Coding Clinic* (1997:4Q;p57-58).[5] This code is indexed under "Implant, neurostimulator, electrodes, brain."

Ventricular Shunting

Shunting treatment of hydrocephalus is done to drain fluid from the brain to relieve pressure. The most common type of shunting (ventriculoperitoneal shunt) occurs between the ventricles of the brain and the abdominal cavity. The root operation in ICD-10-PCS for insertion of a ventricular shunt is bypass cerebral ventricle. In this case, the excess fluid is drained from the ventricles into the peritoneal cavity, where it is reabsorbed. When looking up this procedure in the Index under "Shunt, ventricular," it should be noted that the ventricle can also drain into other body areas. Sometimes, complications can occur in either the ventricular or the peritoneal part of the shunt. It may be necessary to perform surgery only at the site with the complication. This is a shunt revision. In these cases, the coder is directed to the Index under "Revision, shunt." The code will be determined by the site that is revised. It is important to review the operative record to determine which site (peritoneal or ventricular) is being revised.

When coding these cases, it is important to look in the Index under "Complication, mechanical, shunt, ventricular" for the appropriate diagnosis code, per *Coding Clinic* (1987:Sept-Oct:p10).[6]

EXAMPLE Patient admitted for insertion of ventriculoatrial shunt (synthetic substitute) for communicating hydrocephalus, 331.3, 02.32 (G91.0; 00160J2).

Electromyelogram

An **electromyelogram** (EMG) is a diagnostic test that measures electrical activity in muscles and nerves. The root operation in ICD-10-PCS for an EMG is measurement of musculoskeletal contractility. It is used to determine whether a patient has a disease that is damaging muscles, such as myasthenia gravis, or nerves, such as amyotrophic lateral sclerosis.

Hemispherectomy

Surgery for epilepsy currently consists of four basic types: amygdalohippocampectomy, lobectomy (temporal), hemispherectomy, and corpus callosotomy. The root operation in ICD-10-PCS for a hemispherectomy is resection of cerebral hemisphere. Surgery is not the norm for treatment of epilepsy, but it is used in the most severe cases when medications have failed to control seizures. Many tests must be performed before a person is considered a candidate for surgery and prior to the surgery itself.

Prior to surgery, in-depth electrodes may be placed along with a grid to record the brain's electrical activity. During this procedure, the surgeon makes small holes in the skull. Per *Coding Clinic* (1991:2Q:p14),[7] this procedure should be assigned code 01.24. This procedure is indexed under "Craniotomy." If a patient also is having video and radio EEG monitoring, an additional code is assigned.

Lobectomy, usually in the temporal region, is performed for partial seizures; during this surgery, the seizure focus is removed. During hemispherectomy, approximately half of the brain is removed. This procedure is usually performed on children.

EXAMPLE A patient with intractable epilepsy is admitted for a temporal lobectomy, 345.91, 01.53 (G40.919; 00B70ZZ).

Vagal Nerve Stimulation

A **vagal nerve stimulator** is a device that is used to treat intractable epilepsy. The root operation in ICD-10-PCS for a vagal nerve stimulator is insertion of a device and insertion of a stimulate lead. This device, which is similar to a heart pacemaker, is inserted into the upper chest and sends electrical currents to the vagus nerve in the neck, which in turn travels to the brain and reduces or controls seizures. According to *Coding Clinic* (1996:3Q:p12),[8] this code is indexed under "Implantation," "Neurostimulator," "Electrodes," and "Pulse generator implantation," codes 86.94-86.98.

EXAMPLE A patient with intractable epilepsy presents for implantation of a single array neurostimulator pulse generator with leads, 345.91, 04.92, 86.94 (G40.919, 0JH60M6, 00HE3MZ).

Photodynamic Therapy

Photodynamic therapy (PDT) is used in treatment of the wet form of macular degeneration. The root operation in ICD-10-PCS for PDT for macular degeneration is destruction of the retina. According to *Coding Clinic* (1991:2Q:p17),[9] no additional code is assigned for the

FIGURE 14-18. Phacoemulsification of a cataractous lens through a small, self-sealing, scleral tunnel incision.

drug (Visudyne) used in this treatment; the code for PDT can be located under "Destruction, lesion, retina by laser."

Cataract Extraction

Cataract extraction is usually performed by **phacoemulsification** (Figure 14-18), wherein an incision is made on the side of the cornea and the lens material is softened, broken, and suctioned out. Usually after the lens is removed, an artificial lens is inserted (intraocular lens [IOL]). The root operation in ICD-10-PCS for cataract removal is extraction, and the root operation for lens insertion is replacement. The codes for this procedure are indexed under "Extraction, cataract, phacoemulsification," and "Insertion, lens, with cataract extraction, one stage."

EXAMPLE

Patient is admitted for a mature senile cataract in the right eye to be removed by phacoemulsification with IOL replacement, 366.17, 13.41, 13.71 (H25.89, 08RJ3JZ, 08DJ3ZZ).

It is important to remember that when bilateral procedures are coded, the procedure code should be coded twice, unless a code is classified as bilateral. This follows the coding guideline from Chapter 6.

EXERCISE 14-5

Answer the following questions, and code all diagnoses and procedures as appropriate.

1. What is the name of the test used to measure electrical activity in muscles? _____

2. Name one reason a surgeon may perform a hemispherectomy. _____

3. What is PDT used to treat? _____

4. Patient with pseudotumor cerebri is treated with a therapeutic spinal tap. _____

5. Patient presents with malfunctioning ventriculoperitoneal shunt, and revision of the shunt is performed at the peritoneal site. _____

6. Patient with Parkinson's disease is admitted for insertion of a thalamic stimulator. _____

7. Patient admitted with nuclear senile cataract and an extracapsular cataract extraction with Yag laser with lens implant was performed. _____

8. A patient who had a cornea transplant on his right eye now has glaucoma in his left eye. He is admitted for a trabeculectomy ab externo. _____

DOCUMENTATION/REIMBURSEMENT/MS-DRGs

Often, coding difficulties are due to lack of documentation. Sometimes pathology and other test results are not available at the time of discharge or when the physician is dictating the discharge summary or is reporting the final diagnoses.

When coding meningitis, the causative organism may affect MS-DRG assignment.

Frequently missed complications/comorbidities from this chapter include the following:

- Seizure, petit mal, with intractable epilepsy
- Communicating hydrocephalus
- Secondary parkinsonism
- Reflex sympathetic dystrophy
- Cauda equina syndrome
- Leukodystrophy
- Progressive muscular dystrophy
- Idiopathic transverse myelitis
- Quadraplegia

Causative Organism

EXAMPLE

DIAGNOSES	CODE	MS-DRG	RW
Viral meningitis	047.9 (A87.9)	076	0.9051
Salmonella meningitis	003.21 (A02.21)	096	1.9247

Shunt Revision

EXAMPLE

DIAGNOSES/PROCEDURES	CODE	MS-DRG	RW
Hydrocephalus	331.4 (G91.9, 00W000Z)	033	1.3626
Revision ventriculoperitoneal shunt (revision of ventricular site)	02.42		
Hydrocephalus	331.4	042	1.6905
Revision ventriculoperitoneal shunt (revision peritoneal site)	54.95 (0DWW00Z)		

CHAPTER REVIEW EXERCISE

Answer the following questions and where applicable, assign codes for diagnoses, procedures, V/Z codes, and external cause codes.

1. Candidal meningitis _____

2. Meningitis with a headache due to herpes zoster virus _____

3. Meningitis due to whooping cough _____

4. Normal pressure hydrocephalus treated with a ventriculocisternal shunt _____

5. Acquired hydrocephalus _____

6. Parkinsonism in Shy-Drager syndrome _____

7. Benign essential tremor _____

8. Lou Gehrig's disease _____

9. Hemiplegia of the right side _____

10. Recurrent seizures   _____

11. History of seizures   _____

12. Jacksonian seizure   _____

13. Intractable epileptic convulsions   _____

14. Addison's disease with myopathy   _____

15. Intensive care unit myopathy   _____

16. Glaucoma suspect   _____

17. Aftercataract obscuring vision   _____

18. One eye blind, the other with near normal vision   _____

19. Lumbar puncture performed on a patient with probable diagnosis of _____ multiple sclerosis

Write the correct answer(s) in the space(s) provided.

20. What procedure would a surgeon use to treat tremors in Parkinson's disease?

_____

21. A patient with macular degeneration has the drug Visudyne injected, and then a laser is used. What is this procedure known as?

_____

22. What is the most common diagnostic test for epilepsy?

_____

23. If a surgeon performed a trabeculectomy, what would he or she be treating?

_____

CHAPTER GLOSSARY

Alzheimer's disease: disorder of the brain that causes a progressive decline in mental and physical function.

Autoimmune disorder: disorder that occurs when the immune system attacks itself inappropriately.

Autonomic nervous system: consists of both sensory and motor functions that involve the central nervous system and internal organs.

Cataract: clouding of the lens of the eye causing obstructed vision.

Cholesteatoma: growth in the middle ear that usually results from repeated ear infections.

Deep brain stimulator: a device implanted to control tremors.

Electromyelogram: test that measures electrical activity in muscles and nerves.

Epilepsy: disorder of the brain that is characterized by abnormal electrical discharges from the brain cells.

Glaucoma: disorder of the optic nerve that may result in vision loss.

Hemiplegia: paralysis of half of the body.

Hydrocephalus: cerebrospinal fluid collection in the skull.

Hypersomnia: excessive sleep.

Insomnia: difficulty falling asleep, wakefulness, and early morning awakening.

Intractable: not manageable.

Legal blindness: severe or profound impairment in both eyes.

Macular degeneration: vision loss in the central portion of the eye, leaving the patient with peripheral vision or low vision.

Mastoiditis: infection of the mastoid bone of the skull.

Meningitis: infection or inflammation of the meninges.

Muscular dystrophy: type of myopathy.

Myasthenia gravis: chronic autoimmune disorder that manifests as muscle weakness of varying degrees.

Myopathy: disorder that affects muscles, usually resulting in weakness or atrophy.

Otitis media: middle ear infection.

Parkinson's disease: progressive and chronic motor system disorder.

Phacoemulsification: incision is made on the side of the cornea and the lens material is softened, broken, and suctioned out.

Shunting: procedure to drain fluid from the brain to relieve pressure.

Sleep apnea: disorder characterized by breathing interruption during sleep.

Somatic nervous system: sends sensory (taste, hearing, smell) information to the central nervous system.

Somnolence: sleepiness.

Vagal nerve stimulator: a device to control seizures.

REFERENCES

1. American Hospital Association. *Coding Clinic for ICD-9-CM* 1994:4Q:p36. Hemiplegia and quadriplegia.
2. American Hospital Association. *Coding Clinic for ICD-9-CM* 1985:Sept-Oct:p10. Senile vs unspecified cataract in elderly patients.
3. American Hospital Association. *Coding Clinic for ICD-9-CM* 1985:Sept-Oct:p11. Diabetic cataract.
4. American Hospital Association. *Coding Clinic for ICD-9-CM* 2000:1Q:p9-10. Anterior capsule following cataract extraction.
5. American Hospital Association. *Coding Clinic for ICD-9-CM* 1997:4Q:p57-58. Thalamic stimulation.
6. American Hospital Association. *Coding Clinic for ICD-9-CM* 1987:Sept-Oct:p10. Malfunctioning ventriculoperitoneal shunt.
7. American Hospital Association. *Coding Clinic for ICD-9-CM* 1991:2Q:p14. Placement of in-depth electrodes through burr holes into brain.
8. American Hospital Association. *Coding Clinic for ICD-9-CM* 1996:3Q:p12. Placement of vagal nerve stimulator via carotid sheath.
9. American Hospital Association. *Coding Clinic for ICD-9-CM* 1991:2Q:p17. Photodynamic therapy.

15

Diseases of the Circulatory System

(ICD-9-CM Chapter 7, Codes 390-459, and ICD-10-CM Chapter 9, Codes I00-I99)

LEARNING OBJECTIVES

1. Apply and assign the correct ICD-9-CM and ICD-10-CM codes in accordance with Official Guidelines for Coding and Reporting
2. Identify major differences between ICD-9-CM and ICD-10-CM related to diseases of the circulatory system
3. Identify pertinent anatomy and physiology of the circulatory system
4. Identify diseases of the circulatory system
5. Assign the correct V/Z codes and procedure codes related to the circulatory system
6. Identify common treatments, medications, laboratory values, and diagnostic tests
7. Explain the importance of documentation in relation to MS-DRGs for reimbursement

ABBREVIATIONS/ ACRONYMS

ACS acute coronary syndrome

AF atrial fibrillation

AICD automatic implantable cardioverter-defibrillator

AIDS acquired immunodeficiency syndrome

AMI acute myocardial infarction

AV atrioventricular

AVM arteriovenous malformation

AVR aortic valve replacement

BNP brain natriuretic peptide

BP blood pressure

CAB coronary artery bypass

CABG coronary artery bypass graft

CAD coronary artery disease

CAT computerized axial tomography

CCU coronary care unit

CHB complete heart block

CHF congestive heart failure

CKD chronic kidney disease

COPD chronic obstructive pulmonary disease

CPK creatine phosphokinase

CPK-MB creatine phosphokinase, isoenzyme MB

CRT cardiac resynchronization therapy

CRT-D cardiac resynchronization treatment defibrillator

CRT-P cardiac resynchronization treatment pacemaker

CT computerized tomography

CVA cerebrovascular accident

CVL central venous line

CXR chest x-ray

DES drug-eluting stent

DOE dyspnea on exertion

DM diabetes mellitus

DVT deep vein thrombosis

EKG/ECG electrocardiogram

EP electrophysiologic

ER Emergency Room

HCVD hypertensive cardiovascular disease

HTN hypertension

ICD internal cardiac defibrillator

ICD-9-CM *International Classification of Diseases, 9th Revision, Clinical Modification*

ICD-10-CM *International Classification of Diseases, 10th Revision, Clinical Modification*

ICD-10-PCS *International Classification of Diseases, 10th Revision, Procedure Coding System*

ICV implantable cardioverter

IV intravenous

IVDU intravenous drug user

LAD left anterior descending

LCA left coronary artery

MI myocardial infarction

MRI magnetic resonance imaging

MS-DRG Medicare Severity diagnosis-related group

MUGA multiple-gated acquisition

MVR mitral valve replacement

NQMI non–Q wave myocardial infarction

NSTEMI non–ST elevation myocardial infarction

OM obtuse marginal

OSA obstructive sleep apnea

PCI percutaneous coronary intervention

PDA posterior descending artery

PHT pulmonary hypertension

PICC peripherally inserted central catheter

PPH primary pulmonary hypertension

PTCA percutaneous transluminal coronary angioplasty

RA right atrium

RBBB right bundle branch block

RCA right coronary artery

RFA radiofrequency ablation

RHD rheumatic heart disease

RW relative weight

SOB shortness of breath

SSS sick sinus syndrome

STEMI ST elevation myocardial infarction

SVT supraventricular tachycardia

TIA transient ischemic attack

TPA tissue plasminogen activator

TPN total parenteral nutrition

USA unstable angina

ICD-9-CM	Please refer to the companion Evolve website for the most current guidelines.

Official Guidelines for Coding and Reporting

7. Chapter 7: Diseases of Circulatory System (390-459)

a. Hypertension

Hypertension Table

The Hypertension Table (Figure 15-1), found under the main term, "Hypertension", in the Alphabetic Index, contains a complete listing of all conditions due to or associated with hypertension and classifies them according to malignant, benign, and unspecified.

1) Hypertension, Essential, or NOS

Assign hypertension (arterial) (essential) (primary) (systemic) (NOS) to category code 401 with the appropriate fourth digit to indicate malignant (.0), benign (.1), or unspecified (.9). Do not use either .0 malignant or .1 benign unless medical record documentation supports such a designation.

EXAMPLE Hypertension, 401.9 (I10).

EXAMPLE Malignant hypertension, 401.0 (I10).

EXAMPLE Benign hypertension, 401.1 (I10).

2) Hypertension with Heart Disease

Heart conditions (425.8, 429.0-429.3, 429.8, 429.9) are assigned to a code from category 402 when a causal relationship is stated (due to hypertension) or implied (hypertensive). Use an additional code from category 428 to identify the type of heart failure in those patients with heart failure. More than one code from category 428 may be assigned if the patient has systolic or diastolic failure and congestive heart failure.

The same heart conditions (425.8, 429.0-429.3, 429.8, 429.9) with hypertension, but without a stated causal relationship, are coded separately. Sequence according to the circumstances of the admission/encounter.

EXAMPLE Congestive heart failure due to hypertensive heart disease, 402.91, 428.0 (I11.0, I50.9).

EXAMPLE Congestive heart failure in a patient with hypertension, 428.0, 401.9 (I50.9, I10).

3) Hypertensive Chronic Kidney Disease

Assign codes from category 403, Hypertensive chronic kidney disease, when conditions classified to category 585 **or code 587** are present **with hypertension**. Unlike hypertension with heart disease, ICD-9-CM presumes a cause-and-effect relationship and classifies chronic kidney disease (CKD) with hypertension as hypertensive chronic kidney disease.

Fifth digits for category 403 should be assigned as follows:
- 0 with CKD stage I through stage IV, or unspecified.
- 1 with CKD stage V or end stage renal disease.

The appropriate code from category 585, Chronic kidney disease, should be used as a secondary code with a code from category 403 to identify the stage of chronic kidney disease.

See Section I.C.10.a for information on the coding of chronic kidney disease.

SECTION I INDEX TO DISEASES / Hypertension, hypertensive

	Malignant	Benign	Unspecified
Hypertension, hypertensive (arterial) (arteriolar) (crisis) (degeneration) (disease) (essential) (fluctuating) (idiopathic) (intermittent) (labile) (low renin) (orthostatic) (paroxysmal) (primary) (systemic) (uncontrolled) (vascular)	401.0	401.1	401.9
with			
chronic kidney disease	-	-	-
stage I through stage IV, or unspecified	403.00	403.10	403.90
stage V or end stage renal disease	403.01	403.11	403.91
heart involvement (conditions classifiable to 429.0–429.3, 429.8, 429.9 due to hypertension) (see also Hypertension, heart)	402.00	402.10	402.90
with kidney involvement - see Hypertension, cardiorenal			
renal involvement (only conditions classifiable to 585, 586, 587) (excludes conditions classifiable to 584) (see also Hypertension, kidney)	403.00	403.10	403.90
with heart involvement - see Hypertension, cardiorenal			
failure (and sclerosis) (see also Hypertension, kidney)	403.01	403.11	403.91
sclerosis without failure (see also Hypertension, kidney)	403.00	403.10	403.90
accelerated (see also Hypertension, by type, malignant)	401.0	-	-
antepartum - see Hypertension, complicating pregnancy, childbirth, or the puerperium			
cardiorenal (disease)	404.00	404.10	404.90
with			
chronic kidney disease	-	-	-
stage I through stage IV, or unspecified	404.00	404.10	404.90
and heart failure	404.01	404.11	404.91
stage V or end stage renal disease	404.02	404.12	404.92
and heart failure	404.03	404.13	404.93
heart failure	404.01	404.11	404.91
and chronic kidney disease	404.02	404.12	404.92
stage I through stage IV or unspecified	404.02	404.12	404.92
stage V or end stage renal disease	404.03	404.13	404.93
cardiovascular disease (arteriosclerotic) (sclerotic)	402.00	402.10	402.90
with			
heart failure	402.01	402.11	402.91
renal involvement (conditions classifiable to 403) (see also Hypertension, cardiorenal)	404.00	404.10	404.90
cardiovascular renal (disease) (sclerosis) (see also Hypertension, cardiorenal)	404.00	404.10	404.90
cerebrovascular disease NEC	437.2	437.2	437.2
complicating pregnancy, childbirth, or the puerperium	642.2	642.0	642.9
with			
albuminuria (and edema) (mild)	-	-	642.4
severe	-	-	642.5
chronic kidney disease	642.2	642.2	642.2
and heart disease	642.2	642.2	642.2
edema (mild)	-	-	642.4
severe	-	-	642.5
heart disease	642.2	642.2	642.2
and chronic kidney disease	642.2	642.2	642.2
renal disease	642.2	642.2	642.2
and heart disease	642.2	642.2	642.2
chronic	642.2	642.0	642.0
with pre-eclampsia or eclampsia	642.7	642.7	642.7
fetus or newborn	760.0	760.0	760.0
essential	-	642.0	642.0
with pre-eclampsia or eclampsia	-	642.7	642.7
fetus or newborn	760.0	760.0	760.0
fetus or newborn	760.0	760.0	760.0
gestational	-	-	642.3
pre-existing	642.2	642.0	642.0
with pre-eclampsia or eclampsia	642.7	642.7	642.7
fetus or newborn	760.0	760.0	760.0
secondary to renal disease	642.1	642.1	642.1
with pre-eclampsia or eclampsia	642.7	642.7	642.7
fetus or newborn	760.0	760.0	760.0
transient	-	-	642.3
due to			
aldosteronism, primary	405.09	405.19	405.99
brain tumor	405.09	405.19	405.99
bulbar poliomyelitis	405.09	405.19	405.99
calculus			
kidney	405.09	405.19	405.99
ureter	405.09	405.19	405.99
coarctation, aorta	405.09	405.19	405.99
Cushing's disease	405.09	405.19	405.99
glomerulosclerosis (see also Hypertension, kidney)	403.00	403.10	403.90
periarteritis nodosa	405.09	405.19	405.99
pheochromocytoma	405.09	405.19	405.99
polycystic kidney(s)	405.09	405.19	405.99
polycythemia	405.09	405.19	405.99
porphyria	405.09	405.19	405.99
pyelonephritis	405.09	405.19	405.99
renal (artery)			
aneurysm	405.01	405.11	405.91
anomaly	405.01	405.11	405.91
embolism	405.01	405.11	405.91

FIGURE 15-1. Hypertension table in Alphabetic Index.

EXAMPLE The patient was admitted with acute renal failure. The patient was given secondary diagnoses of benign hypertension and chronic kidney disease, stage III, 584.9, 403.10, 585.3 (N17.9, I12.9, N18.3).

4) Hypertensive Heart and Chronic Kidney Disease

Assign codes from combination category 404, Hypertensive heart and chronic kidney disease, when both hypertensive kidney disease and hypertensive heart disease are stated in the diagnosis. Assume a relationship between the hypertension and the chronic kidney disease, whether or not the condition is so designated. Assign an additional code from category 428, to identify the type of heart failure. More than one code from category 428 may be assigned if the patient has systolic or diastolic failure and congestive heart failure.

Fifth digits for category 404 should be assigned as follows:

- 0 without heart failure and with chronic kidney disease (CKD) stage I through stage IV, or unspecified
- 1 with heart failure and with CKD stage I through stage IV, or unspecified
- 2 without heart failure and with CKD stage V or end stage renal disease
- 3 with heart failure and with CKD stage V or end stage renal disease

The appropriate code from category 585, Chronic kidney disease, should be used as a secondary code with a code from category 404 to identify the stage of kidney disease.

See Section I.C.10.a for information on the coding of chronic kidney disease.

5) Hypertensive Cerebrovascular Disease

First assign codes from 430-438, Cerebrovascular disease, then the appropriate hypertension code from categories 401-405.

EXAMPLE Cerebrovascular accident in a patient with malignant hypertension, 434.91, 401.0 (I63.9, I10).

6) Hypertensive Retinopathy

Two codes are necessary to identify the condition. First assign the code from subcategory 362.11, Hypertensive retinopathy, then the appropriate code from categories 401-405 to indicate the type of hypertension.

EXAMPLE The patient is being treated for retinopathy due to labile hypertension, 362.11, 401.9 (H35.039, I10).

7) Hypertension, Secondary

Two codes are required: one to identify the underlying etiology and one from category 405 to identify the hypertension. Sequencing of codes is determined by the reason for admission/encounter.

EXAMPLE Hypertension due to periarteritis nodosa, 446.0, 405.99 (M30.0, I15.8).

8) Hypertension, Transient

Assign code 796.2, Elevated blood pressure reading without diagnosis of hypertension, unless patient has an established diagnosis of hypertension.
Assign code 642.3x for transient hypertension of pregnancy.

EXAMPLE
> The patient has an elevated blood pressure caused by the stress of being in an MVA, 796.2 (R03.0).

9) Hypertension, Controlled
Assign appropriate code from categories 401-405. This diagnostic statement usually refers to an existing state of hypertension under control by therapy.

EXAMPLE
> The patient's benign hypertension has been well controlled since the patient lost 20 pounds and started a regular exercise program, 401.1 (I10).

10) Hypertension, Uncontrolled
Uncontrolled hypertension may refer to untreated hypertension or hypertension not responding to current therapeutic regimen. In either case, assign the appropriate code from categories 401-405 to designate the stage and type of hypertension. Code to the type of hypertension.

EXAMPLE
> The patient's hypertension has been uncontrolled for the past 2 months in spite of changes in medication, 401.9 (I10).

11) Elevated Blood Pressure
For a statement of elevated blood pressure without further specificity, assign code 796.2, Elevated blood pressure reading without diagnosis of hypertension, rather than a code from category 401.

EXAMPLE
> The patient has high blood pressure; will recheck at next clinic visit. No medications were given, 796.2 (R03.0).

b. Cerebral infarction/stroke/cerebrovascular accident (CVA)
The terms stroke and CVA are often used interchangeably to refer to a cerebral infarction. The terms stroke, CVA, and cerebral infarction NOS are all indexed to the default code 434.91, Cerebral artery occlusion, unspecified, with infarction.
Additional code(s) should be assigned for any neurologic deficits associated with the acute CVA, regardless of whether or not the neurologic deficit resolves prior to discharge.
See Section I.C.18.d.3 for information on coding status post administration of tPA in a different facility within the last 24 hours.

c. Postoperative cerebrovascular accident
A cerebrovascular hemorrhage or infarction that occurs as a result of medical intervention is coded to 997.02, Iatrogenic cerebrovascular infarction or hemorrhage. Medical record documentation should clearly specify the cause-and-effect relationship between the medical intervention and the cerebrovascular accident in order to assign this code. A secondary code from the code range 430-432 or from a code from subcategories 433 or 434 with a fifth digit of "1" should also be used to identify the type of hemorrhage or infarct.
This guideline conforms to the use additional code note instruction at category 997. Code 436, Acute, but ill-defined, cerebrovascular disease, should not be used as a secondary code with code 997.02.

EXAMPLE | The patient had a postoperative cerebrovascular accident, which was embolic in nature. The patient had initially been admitted for treatment of coronary artery arteriosclerosis with CABG (left internal mammary artery and two saphenous vein grafts were used). Cardiopulmonary bypass was used during the surgery, 414.01, 997.02, 434.11, E878.2, E849.7, 36.12, 36.15, 39.61 (I25.10, I97.820, I63.40, 021109W, 02100A9, 5A1221Z).

d. Late Effects of Cerebrovascular Disease
1) Category 438, Late Effects of Cerebrovascular Disease
Category 438 is used to indicate conditions classifiable to categories 430-437 as the causes of late effects (neurologic deficits), themselves classified elsewhere. These "late effects" include neurologic deficits that persist after initial onset of conditions classifiable to 430-437. The neurologic deficits caused by cerebrovascular disease may be present from the onset or may arise at any time after the onset of the condition classifiable to 430-437.

Codes in category 438 are only for use for late effects of cerebrovascular disease, not for neurologic deficits associated with an acute CVA.

EXAMPLE | Aphasia due to cerebrovascular accident 3 months ago, 438.11 (I69.320).

EXAMPLE | The patient was admitted with left-sided hemiparesis due to a cerebrovascular accident. The patient has a history of previous CVA with residual facial droop, 434.91, 342.90, 438.83 (I63.9, G81.94, I69.392).

2) Codes from category 438 with codes from 430-437
Codes from category 438 may be assigned on a healthcare record with codes from 430-437, if the patient has a current cerebrovascular accident (CVA) and deficits from an old CVA.
3) Code V12.54
Assign code V12.54, Transient ischemic attack (TIA), and cerebral infarction without residual deficits (and not a code from category 438) as an additional code for history of cerebrovascular disease when no neurologic deficits are present.

EXAMPLE | The patient had a CVA in 2002 with no residuals, V12.54 (Z86.73).

e. Acute myocardial infarction (AMI)
1) ST elevation myocardial infarction (STEMI) and non ST elevation myocardial infarction (NSTEMI)
The ICD-9-CM codes for acute myocardial infarction (AMI) identify the site, such as anterolateral wall or true posterior wall. Subcategories 410.0-410.6 and 410.8 are used for ST elevation myocardial infarction (STEMI). Subcategory 410.7, Subendocardial infarction, is used for non ST elevation myocardial infarction (NSTEMI) and nontransmural MIs (Figure 15-2).
2) Acute myocardial infarction, unspecified
Subcategory 410.9 is the default for the unspecified term acute myocardial infarction. If only STEMI or transmural MI without the site is documented, query the provider as to the site, or assign a code from subcategory 410.9.
3) AMI documented as nontransmural or subendocardial but site provided
If an AMI is documented as nontransmural or subendocardial, but the site is provided, it is still coded as a subendocardial AMI. If NSTEMI evolves to STEMI, assign the STEMI code. If STEMI converts to NSTEMI due to thrombolytic therapy, it is still coded as STEMI.

● 410 **Acute myocardial infarction**
Includes: cardiac infarction
coronary (artery):
embolism
occlusion
rupture
thrombosis
infarction of heart, myocardium, or ventricle
rupture of heart, myocardium, or ventricle
ST elevation (STEMI) and non-ST elevation
(NSTEMI) myocardial infarction
any condition classifiable to 414.1-414.9
specified as acute or with a stated duration
of 8 weeks or less

The following fifth-digit subclassification is for use with
category 410:
☐ 0 **episode of care unspecified**
Use when the source document does not contain
sufficient information for the assignment of
fifth-digit 1 or 2.
1 **initial episode of care**
Use fifth-digit 1 to designate the first episode of
care (regardless of facility site) for a newly
diagnosed myocardial infarction. The fifth-
digit 1 is assigned regardless of the number of
times a patient may be transferred during the
initial episode of care.
2 **subsequent episode of care**
Use fifth-digit 2 to designate an episode of care
following the initial episode when the patient
is admitted for further observation, evaluation,
or treatment for a myocardial infarction that
has received initial treatment, but is still less
than 8 weeks old.

● 410.0 **Of anterolateral wall**
ST elevation myocardial infarction (STEMI) of
anterolateral wall
● ☐ 410.1 **Of other anterior wall**
Infarction:
anterior (wall) NOS (with contiguous portion of
intraventricular septum)
anteroapical (with contiguous portion of
intraventricular septum)
anteroseptal (with contiguous portion of
intraventricular septum)
ST elevation myocardial infarction (STEMI) of other
anterior wall

● 410.2 **Of inferolateral wall**
ST elevation myocardial infarction (STEMI) of
inferolateral wall

● 410.3 **Of inferoposterior wall**
ST elevation myocardial infarction (STEMI) of
inferoposterior wall

● ☐ 410.4 **Of other inferior wall**
Infarction:
diaphragmatic wall NOS (with contiguous
portion of intraventricular septum)
inferior (wall) NOS (with contiguous portion of
intraventricular septum)
ST elevation myocardial infarction (STEMI) of other
inferior wall

● ☐ 410.5 **Of other lateral wall**
Infarction:
apical-lateral
basal-lateral
high lateral
posterolateral
ST elevation myocardial infarction (STEMI) of other
lateral wall

● 410.6 **True posterior wall infarction**
Infarction:
posterobasal
strictly posterior
ST elevation myocardial infarction (STEMI) of true
posterior wall

● 410.7 **Subendocardial infarction**
Nontransmural infarction
Non-ST elevation myocardial infarction (NSTEMI)

● ☐ 410.8 **Of other specified sites**
Infarction of:
atrium
papillary muscle
septum alone
ST elevation myocardial infarction (STEMI) of other
specified sites

● ☐ 410.9 **Unspecified site**
Acute myocardial infarction NOS
Coronary occlusion NOS
Myocardial infarction NOS

FIGURE 15-2. Tabular entry for 410, Acute myocardial infarction.

EXAMPLE The patient was admitted with NSTEMI, 410.71 (I21.4).

EXAMPLE The patient was admitted with anterolateral wall STEMI, 410.01 (I21.09).

Apply the General Coding Guidelines as found in Chapter 5 and the Procedural Guidelines as found in Chapter 6.

ICD-10-CM	Please refer to the companion Evolve website for the most current guidelines.
Official Guidelines for Coding and Reporting	**9. Chapter 9: Diseases of Circulatory System (I00-I99)** **a. Hypertension** **1) Hypertension with Heart Disease** Heart conditions classified to I50.- or I51.4-I51.9, are assigned to, a code from category I11, Hypertensive heart disease, when a causal relationship is stated (due to hypertension) or implied (hypertensive). Use an additional code from category I50, Heart failure, to identify the type of heart failure in those patients with heart failure.

The same heart conditions (I50.-, I51.4-I51.9) with hypertension, but without a stated causal relationship, are coded separately. Sequence according to the circumstances of the admission/encounter.

2) Hypertensive Chronic Kidney Disease

Assign codes from category I12, Hypertensive chronic kidney disease, when both hypertension and a condition classifiable to category N18, Chronic kidney disease (CKD), are present. Unlike hypertension with heart disease, ICD-10-CM presumes a cause-and-effect relationship and classifies chronic kidney disease with hypertension as hypertensive chronic kidney disease.

The appropriate code from category N18 should be used as a secondary code with a code from category I12 to identify the stage of chronic kidney disease.

See Section I.C.14. Chronic kidney disease.

If a patient has hypertensive chronic kidney disease and acute renal failure, an additional code for the acute renal failure is required.

3) Hypertensive Heart and Chronic Kidney Disease

Assign codes from combination category I13, Hypertensive heart and chronic kidney disease, when both hypertensive kidney disease and hypertensive heart disease are stated in the diagnosis. Assume a relationship between the hypertension and the chronic kidney disease, whether or not the condition is so designated. If heart failure is present, assign an additional code from category I50 to identify the type of heart failure.

The appropriate code from category N18, Chronic kidney disease, should be used as a secondary code with a code from category I13 to identify the stage of chronic kidney disease.

See Section I.C.14. Chronic kidney disease.

The codes in category I13, Hypertensive heart and chronic kidney disease, are combination codes that include hypertension, heart disease and chronic kidney disease. The Includes note at I13 specifies that the conditions included at I11 and I12 are included together in I13. If a patient has hypertension, heart disease and chronic kidney disease then a code from I13 should be used, not individual codes for hypertension, heart disease and chronic kidney disease, or codes from I11 or I12.

For patients with both acute renal failure and chronic kidney disease an additional code for acute renal failure is required.

4) Hypertensive Cerebrovascular Disease

For hypertensive cerebrovascular disease, first assign the appropriate code from categories I60-I69, followed by the appropriate hypertension code.

5) Hypertensive Retinopathy

Subcategory H35.0, **Background retinopathy and retinal vascular changes**, should be used with code I10, Essential (primary) hypertension, to include the systemic hypertension. The sequencing is based on the reason for the encounter.

6) Hypertension, Secondary

Secondary hypertension is due to an underlying condition. Two codes are required: one to identify the underlying etiology and one from category I15 to identify the hypertension. Sequencing of codes is determined by the reason for admission/ encounter.

7) Hypertension, Transient

Assign code R03.0, Elevated blood pressure reading without diagnosis of hypertension, unless patient has an established diagnosis of hypertension. Assign code O13.-, Gestational [pregnancy-induced] hypertension without significant proteinuria, or O14.-, **Pre-eclampsia**, for transient hypertension of pregnancy.

8) Hypertension, Controlled

This diagnostic statement usually refers to an existing state of hypertension under control by therapy. Assign **the appropriate** code **from categories I10-I15, Hypertensive diseases**.

9) Hypertension, Uncontrolled

Uncontrolled hypertension may refer to untreated hypertension or hypertension not responding to current therapeutic regimen. In either case, assign **the appropriate** code **from categories I10-I15, Hypertensive diseases**.

b. Atherosclerotic *Coronary Artery Disease* **and** *Angina*

ICD-10-CM has combination codes for atherosclerotic heart disease with angina pectoris. The subcategories for these codes are I25.11, Atherosclerotic heart disease of native coronary artery with angina pectoris and I25.7, Atherosclerosis of coronary artery bypass graft(s) and coronary artery of transplanted heart with angina pectoris.

When using one of these combination codes it is not necessary to use an additional code for angina pectoris. A causal relationship can be assumed in a patient with both atherosclerosis and angina pectoris, unless the documentation indicates the angina is due to something other than the atherosclerosis.

If a patient with coronary artery disease is admitted due to an acute myocardial infarction (AMI), the AMI should be sequenced before the coronary artery disease.

See Section I.C.9. Acute myocardial infarction (AMI)

c. Intraoperative and Postprocedural *Cerebrovascular Accident*

Medical record documentation should clearly specify the cause- and-effect relationship between the medical intervention and the cerebrovascular accident in order to assign a code for intraoperative or postprocedural cerebrovascular accident.

Proper code assignment depends on whether it was an infarction or hemorrhage and whether it occurred intraoperatively or postoperatively. If it was a cerebral hemorrhage, code assignment depends on the type of procedure performed.

d. Sequelae of Cerebrovascular Disease

1) Category I69, Sequelae of Cerebrovascular disease

Category I69 is used to indicate conditions classifiable to categories I60-I67 as the causes of late effects (neurologic deficits), themselves classified elsewhere. These "late effects" include neurologic deficits that persist after initial onset of conditions classifiable to categories I60-I67. The neurologic deficits caused by cerebrovascular disease may be present from the onset or may arise at any time after the onset of the condition classifiable to categories I60-I67.

2) Codes from category I69 with codes from I60-I67

Codes from category I69 may be assigned on a health care record with codes from I60-I67, if the patient has a current cerebrovascular **disease** and deficits from an old **cerebrovascular disease**.

3) Code Z86.73

Assign code Z86.73, Personal history of transient ischemic attack (TIA), and cerebral infarction without residual deficits (and not a code from category I69) as an additional code for history of cerebrovascular disease when no neurologic deficits are present.

e. Acute myocardial infarction (AMI)

1) ST elevation myocardial infarction (STEMI) and non ST elevation myocardial infarction (NSTEMI)

The ICD-10-CM codes for acute myocardial infarction (AMI) identify the site, such as anterolateral wall or true posterior wall. Subcategories I21.0-I21.2 and code I21.4 are used for ST elevation myocardial infarction (STEMI). Code I21.4, Non-ST elevation (NSTEMI) myocardial infarction, is used for non ST elevation myocardial infarction (NSTEMI) and nontransmural MIs.

<u>If NSTEMI evolves to STEMI, assign the STEMI code. If STEMI converts to NSTEMI due to thrombolytic therapy, it is still coded as STEMI.</u>

When the patient requires continued care for the myocardial infarction, codes from category I21 may continue to be reported for the duration of 4 weeks (28 days) or less from onset, regardless of the healthcare setting, including when a patient is transferred from the acute care setting to the post-acute care setting if the patient is still within the four weeks time frame. For encounters after the 4 weeks time frame and the patient requires continued care related to the myocardial infarction, the appropriate aftercare code should be assigned, rather than a code from category I21. Otherwise, code I25.2, Old myocardial infarction, may be assigned for old or healed myocardial infarction not requiring further care.

2) Acute myocardial infarction, unspecified

Code I21.3, ST elevation (STEMI) myocardial infarction of unspecified site, is the default for the unspecified term acute myocardial infarction. If only STEMI or transmural MI without the site is documented, query the provider as to the site, or assign code I21.3.

3) AMI documented as nontransmural or subendocardial but site provided
If an AMI is documented as nontransmural or subendocardial, but the site is provided, it is still coded as a subendocardial AMI.

    See Section I.C.21.3 for information on coding status post administration of tPA in a different facility within the last 24 hours.

4) Subsequent acute myocardial infarction
A code from category I22, Subsequent ST elevation (STEMI) and non ST elevation (NSTEMI) myocardial infarction, is to be used when a patient who has suffered an AMI has a new AMI within the 4 week time frame of the initial AMI. A code from category I22 must be used in conjunction with a code from category I21.

    The sequencing of the I22 and I21 codes depends on the circumstances of the encounter. Should a patient who is in the hospital due to an AMI have a subsequent AMI while still in the hospital code I21 would be sequenced first as the reason for admission, with code I22 sequenced as a secondary code. Should a patient have a subsequent AMI after discharge for care of an initial AMI, and the reason for admission is the subsequent AMI, the I22 code should be sequenced first followed by the I21. An I21 code must accompany an I22 code to identify the site of the initial AMI, and to indicate that the patient is still within the 4 week time frame of healing from the initial AMI.

    The guidelines for assigning the correct I22 code are the same as for the initial AMI.

Apply the General Coding Guidelines as found in Chapter 5 and the Procedural Guidelines as found in Chapter 7.

GUIDELINE DIFFERENCES BETWEEN ICD-9-CM AND ICD-10-CM

- There is no Hypertension Table in ICD-10-CM.
- There are no fourth digits to classify hypertension as benign, malignant, or unspecified; all are included in the code for hypertension.
- A causal relationship can be assumed when a patient has both atherosclerosis and angina and an additional code for the angina is not assigned; the combination code is used.

MAJOR DIFFERENCES BETWEEN ICD-9-CM AND ICD-10-CM

- The code for gangrene has been moved from the symptom chapter in ICD-9-CM to Diseases of the Circulatory System in ICD-10-CM.
- The section Late Effects of Cerebrovascular Disease has been expanded to include more specificity and laterality.
- The time limit for assigning the acute MI code is 28 days in ICD-10-CM, whereas in ICD-9-CM, it was 8 weeks.
- A new category has been added for coding a subsequent acute MI, which is an MI that occurs within 28 days of a previous acute MI.
- A new category for complications within 28 days of acute MI has been added.
- Transient ischemic attack has been reclassified to the nervous system chapter.
- Stages of chronic kidney disease are no longer found as fifth digits but are assigned a separate code.
- Subsequent acute MI is new to I10. This is a new MI that occurs in a patient who suffered a previous new MI within the last 4 weeks.

ANATOMY AND PHYSIOLOGY

The circulatory system is composed of the heart and blood vessels (Figure 15-3). Its function is to supply tissue in the body with oxygen and nutrients. This function is accomplished when the arteries carry blood (oxygen) to the cells. The largest artery, the aorta, branches

FIGURE 15-3. The heart and great vessels, posterior view.

off the heart and divides into many smaller arteries. The veins carry deoxygenated blood to the lungs to acquire oxygen and then to the heart, whose job it is to pump oxygenated blood back to the arteries.

The Heart

The function of the heart is to pump oxygen-rich blood to the cells of the body. The heart itself receives oxygenated blood from the coronary arteries; the two major coronary arteries branch off the aorta.

The heart is enclosed laterally by the lungs, posteriorly by the backbone, and anteriorly by the sternum. The wall of the heart is composed of three layers: epicardium, myocardium, and endocardium (Figure 15-4). The epicardium is the outer protective layer, the myocardium is the middle layer and is composed of cardiac muscle, and the endocardium is the inner layer that lines all of the heart chambers and covers the heart valves.

The heart consists of four chambers: right atrium, left atrium, right ventricle, and left ventricle. The atrium and the ventricle on the right side are separated from the left by a septum. The top two chambers, the atria, receive blood via the veins from the body or the lungs. The right ventricle pumps blood to the lungs to pick up oxygen, and the left ventricle pumps blood to the rest of the body. Within the heart are four valves (Figure 15-5), and their job is to direct blood flow. The tricuspid valve is located between the right atrium and the right ventricle. The valve between the left atrium and the left ventricle is the mitral or bicuspid valve. The aortic valve is located in the aorta at the point at which the left ventricle empties into the aorta. The pulmonary valve is located in the pulmonary artery at the point of exit from the right ventricle.

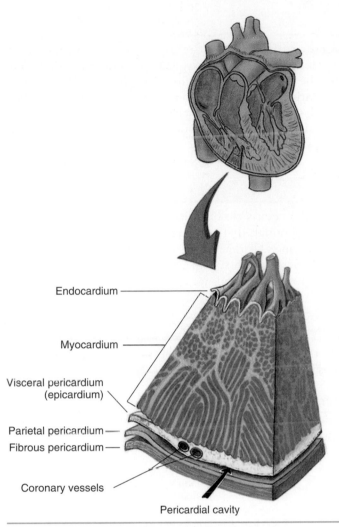

Endocardium

Myocardium

Visceral pericardium
(epicardium)

Parietal pericardium

Fibrous pericardium

Coronary vessels

Pericardial cavity

FIGURE 15-4. Layers of the heart wall.

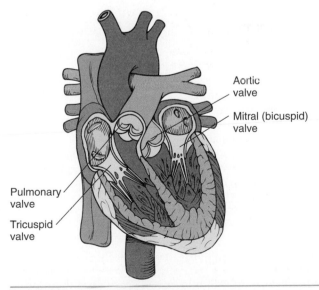

Aortic
valve

Mitral (bicuspid)
valve

Pulmonary
valve

Tricuspid
valve

FIGURE 15-5. Cardiac valves.

Blood Vessels

Blood vessels are the tubes that transport blood from the heart to the cells and back to the heart. Most arteries carry oxygenated blood away from the heart. They continue to get smaller the farther away they are from the heart (arterioles). At this point, arterioles lead to **capillaries**, and exchange is made between blood and body cells; venules and veins return blood to the heart. The circulation of blood that moves throughout the body is referred to as systemic circulation. Blood pressure measured at the arm indicates systemic pressures.

Lymphatic System

The lymphatic system is closely related to the circulatory system. The lymphatic drainage system returns products that have leaked out from the capillaries back to the bloodstream. The lymph system is also made up of lymph nodes, as well as the spleen, thymus, tonsils, and adenoids. The lymph system fights infection by filtering out viruses and bacteria by attacking them with lymphocytes.

DISEASE CONDITIONS

Diseases of the Circulatory System (390-459), Chapter 7 in the ICD-9-CM code book, is divided into the following categories:

CATEGORY	SECTION TITLES
390-392	Acute Rheumatic Fever
393-398	Chronic Rheumatic Heart Disease
401-405	Hypertensive Disease
410-414	Ischemic Heart Disease
415-417	Diseases of Pulmonary Circulation
420-429	Other Forms of Heart Disease
430-438	Cerebrovascular Disease
440-449	Diseases of the Arteries, Arterioles, and Capillaries
451-459	Diseases of the Veins and Lymphatics and Other

Diseases of the Circulatory System (I00-I99), Chapter 9 in the ICD-10-CM code book, is divided into the following categories:

CATEGORY	SECTION TITLES
I00-I02	Acute Rheumatic Fever
I05-I09	Chronic Rheumatic Heart Disease
I10-I15	Hypertensive Diseases
I20-I25	Ischemic Heart Diseases
I26-I28	Pulmonary Heart Disease and Diseases of Pulmonary Circulation
I30-I52	Other Forms of Heart Disease
I60-I69	Cerebrovascular Diseases
I70-I79	Diseases of Arteries, Arterioles, and Capillaries
I80-I89	Diseases of Veins, Lymphatic Vessels, and Lymph Nodes, Not Elsewhere Classified
I95-I99	Other and Unspecified Disorders of the Circulatory System

Acute Rheumatic Fever and Chronic Rheumatic Heart Disease

Acute rheumatic fever is an inflammatory disease usually found in children that may affect the heart, joints, skin, or brain following an infection with streptococcal bacteria such as strep throat or scarlet fever.

EXAMPLE   Patient was admitted with acute rheumatic fever with endocarditis, 391.1 (I01.1).

EXAMPLE   Patient has rheumatic chorea without heart involvement, 392.9 (I02.9).

Chronic rheumatic heart disease is a chronic condition that is usually a late effect of attacks of acute rheumatic fever and most often involves the heart valves. When mitral and aortic valves are both involved, ICD-9-CM assumes a causal relationship to rheumatic heart disease.

Index:
  Insufficiency
    Mitral (valve), 424.0
      With
        Aortic (valve) disease, 396.3.

EXAMPLE   Aortic stenosis, 424.1 (I35.0).

EXAMPLE   Aortic stenosis with mitral stenosis, 396.0 (I08.0).

Mitral stenosis, mitral valve disease unspecified, and mitral valve failure are presumed by ICD-9-CM to be rheumatic in origin.

EXAMPLE   Stenosis, mitral, 394.0 (I05.0).

If one mitral valve condition is presumed rheumatic and more than one mitral valve condition exists, ICD-9-CM assumes that both conditions are rheumatic.

Index:
  Stenosis
    Mitral
      With
        Insufficiency, 394.2.

Unless otherwise specified, diseases of the tricuspid valve are presumed to be rheumatic in nature.

Hypertensive Disease

The codes for hypertension are located in a table (see Figure 15-1) found in the Alphabetic Index of diseases in ICD-9-CM. The three columns within this table identify the course of the disease: malignant, benign, or unspecified. There is no Hypertension Table in ICD-10-CM. The course of the disease in ICD-10-CM (benign, malignant, or unspecified) is not a requirement for assigning a code.

EXAMPLE   Patient has chronic benign hypertension due to renal artery stenosis, 440.1, 405.11 (I70.1, I15.0).

Hypertension is classified by ICD-9-CM as primary (essential) or secondary. Primary hypertension, or high **blood pressure** (BP), is a condition that is defined as abnormally high blood pressure in the arterial system. The American Heart Association defines hypertension as pressures exceeding 140/90. A diagnosis of hypertension can be made only by a physician and should not be assigned on the basis of BP readings alone. Essential hypertension has no known origin, and its symptoms are insidious. ICD-9-CM uses fourth digits that describe the course of the disease. These fourth digits are as follows:

- 0 for malignant
- 1 for benign
- 9 for unspecified

Secondary hypertension is a consequence of other diseases such as kidney diseases, brain tumor, or polycythemia, and coding requires these same fourth digits. When secondary hypertension is documented, the sequencing of the codes is determined by the reason for admission/encounter.

EXAMPLE Patient has hypertension due to Cushing's disease, 255.0, 405.99 (E24.9, I15.2).

Benign, Malignant, and Uncontrolled Hypertension

Malignant hypertension is a very severe form of hypertension and may be a life-threatening condition. The coding of malignant hypertension must be documented by a physician. In cases of malignant hypertension, systolic pressure may be greater than 200, and diastolic may be greater than 120. Malignant hypertension is also known as accelerating or necrotizing hypertension. Patients are at greater risk for malignant hypertension if they experience renal failure.

Coding Clinic (1984:July-Aug:p12)[1] describes malignant hypertension as "rapidly rising blood pressure, usually in excess of 140 mm Hg diastolic with findings of visual impairment and symptoms or signs of progressive cardiac failure." The fact that hypertension is documented as uncontrolled or hypertensive emergency or hypertensive urgency does not make it malignant, and a separate code is not used to describe these conditions. Benign hypertension is rarely documented by physicians; therefore, coders often must assign the unspecified code. Hypertension that is not specifically documented as malignant or benign must be assigned to the unspecified fourth digit. Often, physicians document a history of hypertension when referring to ongoing hypertension that is under control. The current medication list should be reviewed to determine whether the hypertension is currently under treatment.

EXAMPLE Uncontrolled hypertension, 401.9 (I10).

EXAMPLE Hypertension, accelerated, 401.0 (I10).

Medications often used for treating hypertension include Accupril, Aldomet, captopril, Cardizem, diltiazem, Cozaar, losartan, Coreg, dyazide, Hytrin, Inderal, Lopressor, Norvasc, Procardia, Tenormin, atenolol, Vasotec, Toprol, Calan, verapamil, Zestril, and lisinopril.

EXAMPLE Patient has a past history of hypertension, currently taking verapamil, 401.9 (I10).

For a variety of reasons, patients may have elevated blood pressure readings. Per *Coding Clinic* (1990:3Q:p4),[2] unless a patient has an established diagnosis of hypertension, the code 796.2 (R03.0) elevated blood pressure, should be assigned.

Hypertensive Heart, Renal, and Heart and Renal Disease

Per *Coding Clinic* (2003:1Q:p20-21),[3] "ICD-9-CM assumes a cause-and-effect relationship and classifies chronic renal failure with hypertension as hypertensive renal disease." This indicates to the coder that anytime hypertension and chronic renal failure (codes from category 585) (N18) occur in a patient, category 403 (I12) should be assigned. The only time the 403 (I12) category code would not be selected is when the physician documents, "CRF not due to hypertension." On occasion, a patient will have chronic kidney disease (CKD) due to diabetes and also have hypertension; diabetic kidney disease and hypertensive kidney disease would both be assigned in these cases.

Hypertensive heart disease, in contrast to hypertensive renal disease, does not assume a cause-and-effect relationship. A causal relationship must be stated by the physician. For a code from this category to be assigned, the physician must document hypertensive heart disease or must say that heart disease is due to hypertension. This category includes heart failure as a fifth digit. It is important to note that if a patient has hypertensive congestive heart failure, at least two codes—402.x1 (I11.0) and 428.0 (I50.-)—are required; if known, the codes for systolic (428.20-428.23) (I50.2-), diastolic (428.30-428.33) (I50.3-), or a combination systolic and diastolic (428.40-428.43) (I50.4-) should also be assigned.

EXAMPLE	Patient is admitted with both diastolic and systolic congestive heart failure due to long history of hypertension, 402.91, 428.40, 428.0 (I11.0, I50.40).

Hypertensive heart and renal disease requires that the condition be classified to 404.xx (I13.–). It is important to become familiar with the Includes as well as Excludes notes in all of the above categories.

EXAMPLE	Patient is admitted with hypertensive renal disease. The patient also has hypertensive cardiomyopathy, 404.90, 585.9, 425.8 (I13.10, N18.9).

EXERCISE 15-1

Assign codes to the following conditions.

1. Patient is admitted with a diagnosis of hypertensive urgency _____
2. Aortic stenosis with mitral insufficiency _____
3. Malignant hypertension _____
4. Labile hypertension _____
5. Portal hypertension _____
6. Heart failure due to hypertensive heart disease _____
7. Cardiomegaly with hypertension _____
8. Hypertension secondary to coarctation of aorta _____
9. Ocular hypertension _____
10. Essential hypertension _____
11. HCVD (hypertensive cardiovascular disease) with chronic renal failure _____
12. High blood pressure reading _____

Ischemic Heart Disease

Acute Myocardial Infarction

Acute **myocardial infarction** (AMI, or MI) in layman's terms is known as a heart attack. An MI occurs when complete blockage of blood flow occurs in a coronary artery. When this occurs, blood is prevented from reaching the heart muscle (Figure 15-7). Blockage may be caused by fatty deposits (also known as plaque or atherosclerosis) or blood clots. When the blood cannot reach the heart, the heart muscle may become damaged. Signs of a heart attack include chest pain, shortness of breath, nausea, and pain in the arms and chest.

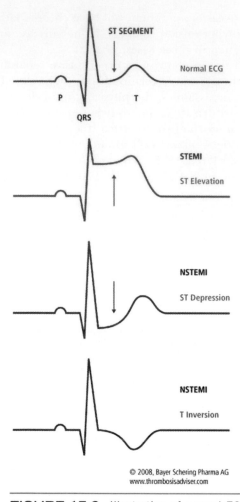

© 2008, Bayer Schering Pharma AG
www.thrombosisadviser.com

FIGURE 15-6. Illustration of normal ECG as well as STEMI and NSTEMI.

To determine whether a patient is having a heart attack, several tests, including various types of blood tests, may be performed. One of these tests is called CPK (creatine phosphokinase, or creatine kinase). CPK is an isoenzyme that occurs in high concentration in the heart and skeletal muscle. The level of CPK-MB (creatine phosphokinase, MB isoenzyme) in the blood rises 3 to 6 hours after an MI and returns to normal 12 to 48 hours after the infarct. Usually, CPK is measured every 8 to 12 hours, and patterns are determined. The normal value for males is 25 to 90; for females, it is 10 to 70. Another type of blood test that is often performed is the measurement of cardiac muscle proteins called troponins. Testing for troponin levels and CPK levels is performed serially. Troponin levels are usually very low, and elevated levels can indicate damage to the heart. Healthcare providers also perform electrocardiograms (EKGs) to determine whether an MI has occurred. The EKG shows ST segment elevations during episodes of chest pain (see Figure 15-6).

Types of MI may be classified as to the area of heart that suffers damage or the extent of damage, as evidenced by an EKG. The most common areas are the following:

- Anterior
- Inferior
- Lateral
- Posterior
- Right ventricular

STEMI (ST elevation MI) occurs when complete obstruction of the coronary artery causes damage involving the full thickness of the heart muscle. This type of MI is also known as an ST elevation MI or a Q wave MI. **NSTEMI** (non–ST elevation) occurs when a coronary artery is partially obstructed and damage does not involve the full thickness of the heart

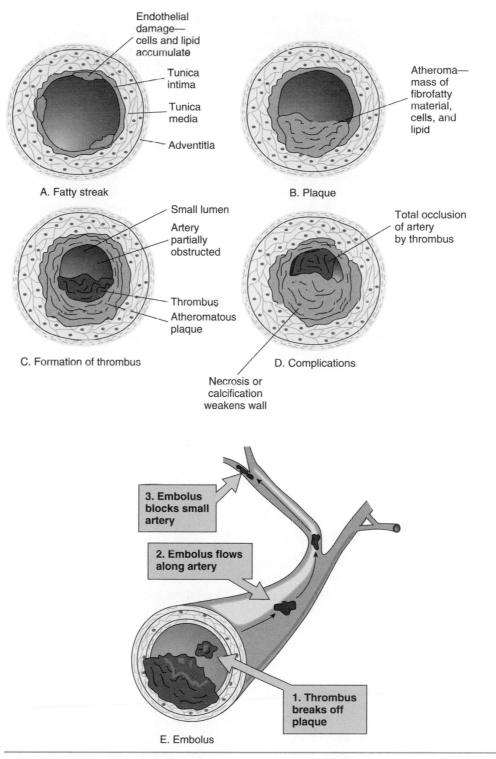

FIGURE 15-7. Development of an atheroma, leading to arterial occlusion.

muscle. This type of MI is often referred to as non–Q wave MI. Old terminology for transmural or nontransmural MI has been replaced by Q or non–Q MI.

Patients suspected of having an MI are usually treated with a combination of medications and/or procedures. Procedures performed to treat the causes of MI include coronary angioplasty (percutaneous transluminal coronary angioplasty [PTCA]), stenting (percutaneous coronary intervention [PCI]), and possibly coronary artery bypass surgery (CABG or CAB). Often, upon presentation of the patient to the Emergency Room (ER), thrombolytic therapy is initiated. Thrombolytics (tissue plasminogen activator [TPA], streptokinase) are used to dissolve blood clots that may be blocking a coronary artery. Thrombolytics must be administered within 6 hours of the onset of chest pain to avoid heart damage. A potential adverse effect of the use of these drugs is severe bleeding; for this reason, they are contraindicated in many patients. All of these procedures are discussed in greater detail in the procedure section of this chapter.

ICD-9-CM provides a fourth digit for the location of the heart attack within the heart and a fifth digit for the episode of care. The record should be reviewed to determine whether the site of the MI is documented. If location of a STEMI or transmural MI is not documented, it may be necessary to query the physician.

Fifth Digits

0 Episode of Care Unspecified This fifth digit would rarely be used in the inpatient setting. The date the infarct occurred is usually documented.

1 Initial Episode of Care This fifth digit is used for a newly diagnosed infarct, regardless of the facility site. In other words, if a patient presents to one facility with an acute MI and then is transferred to another, the fifth digit of one is used in both cases. An MI is coded to this digit if a patient has never been sent home from the hospital after presentation for this diagnosis.

2 Subsequent Episode of Care This fifth digit is used to describe a patient who has had an MI during a previous episode of care but is now being readmitted. This fifth digit is used up to 8 weeks following the original infarct. This digit is used if the patient went home after initial presentation to the hospital for the MI.

Once an MI is greater than 8 weeks old, code 412 (I25.2) is assigned to describe a patient who has had an MI in the past.

EXAMPLE   Patient was admitted with NSTEMI, 410.71 (I21.4).

EXAMPLE   Patient is admitted to hospital A with an acute anterolateral MI. Patient is stabilized and transferred to hospital B for coronary intervention. The principal diagnosis in both cases is, 410.01 (I21.09).

Prior to having an MI, a patient may have had symptoms such as unstable angina (USA), which is often described in today's vernacular as acute coronary syndrome, or ACS. A patient with this condition requires immediate medical treatment, but a patient with chronic angina may be treated with medications on a long-term basis as necessary. Patients with angina may be prescribed sublingual nitroglycerin to relieve pain symptoms. Often, the underlying condition of chest pain, or angina, is coronary artery disease.

Coronary artery disease (CAD), 414.0X may be coded with a fifth digit, which describes what type of coronary artery is involved:

- 414.01 is the native coronary artery. (This is the artery the patient was born with.)
- 414.02 is autologous vein bypass graft. (This is a vein that is taken from the patient, usually the saphenous vein, and is placed during a CABG.)
- 414.03 is a nonautologous biological bypass graft. (This is a vessel taken from another patient that is placed during a CABG.)
- 414.04 is an artery bypass graft. (This artery, most often the internal mammary, is used for a bypass.)

Sometimes a patient will present to the ER with acute chest pain. The attending decides to administer TPA and documents that once TPA was administered, symptoms were relieved and the patient is admitted for observation with a diagnosis of "aborted MI." Per *Coding Clinic* (2001:2Q:p7-8),[4] an aborted MI is coded to 411.1, Intermediate Coronary Syndrome.

When CAD is present in a patient with a previous CABG, but it is not known whether the CAD is of a graft or a native artery, the code 414.00 for unspecified should be used, per

Coding Clinic (1997:3Q:p15).[5] Also assign code V45.81 to show that the patient had coronary artery bypass surgery. When there is no documentation that the patient had a CABG procedure in the past, then the code for CAD should be assigned to native arteries (414.01).

EXERCISE 15-2

Assign codes to the following conditions.

1. Patient had an MI 1 year prior to this admission _____

2. Patient had a nontransmural MI 6 weeks ago and now presents with chest pain _____

3. Patient has CAD and a history of CABG _____

   Recent coronary catheterization shows coronary artery disease of the native arteries _____

4. Patient has CAD and a previous MI and coronary artery bypass _____

5. Patient with an anterolateral MI is transferred to this hospital for further evaluation and treatment _____

Diseases of Pulmonary Circulation

Pulmonary Embolism

A **pulmonary embolism** is a blood clot(s) in the pulmonary artery that causes blockage in the artery. Most often, clots originate in the legs and then travel to the lung. A blood clot that forms and remains in a vein is a **thrombus**. A clot that travels to another part of the body is an **embolus**. Common symptoms of pulmonary embolism include shortness of breath, chest pain, and cough.

A pulmonary embolism may be diagnosed via lung scan or computed tomography (CT) scan. A pulmonary embolism can be life-threatening, and once you have had one, the risk for recurrence is increased.

Pulmonary Hypertension

Pulmonary hypertension (PHT) is high blood pressure in the arteries that supply blood to the lungs. Normal pulmonary systolic pressure is 18 to 25 mm Hg. Two types of pulmonary hypertension—primary and secondary—have been identified. Primary pulmonary hypertension (PPH) is a rare condition of unknown origin that is both progressive and ultimately fatal. In recent years, this condition has been linked with the use of anti-obesity drugs such as Fen/Phen. Secondary pulmonary hypertension is caused by other conditions such as chronic obstructive pulmonary disease (COPD), emphysema, pulmonary embolism, or obstructive sleep apnea (OSA). Patients who have prolonged untreated pulmonary hypertension often develop right ventricular failure. Doppler echocardiography is the most useful test for determining the diagnosis of pulmonary hypertension.

Symptoms of pulmonary hypertension may include dyspnea on exertion (DOE), syncope, fatigue, and chest pain. Treatment for this disease may involve correcting the underlying cause, if possible. Medical treatments may include vasodilators, diuretics, anticoagulants, oxygen, and digoxin. In some cases, lung transplantation may be considered.

EXAMPLE   Patient has pulmonary hypertension due to COPD, 416.8, 496 (I27.2, J44.9).

Other Forms of Heart Disease

Pericarditis

Pericarditis is inflammation of the covering of the heart. It is often a complication of viral infection and systemic disease such as acquired immunodeficiency syndrome (AIDS). Sometimes, pericarditis follows an MI; it may also arise from bacterial infection. The disease presents with symptoms such as chest pain, breathing difficulties, fever, and cough. The heart sound heard through the stethoscope by the physician in cases of pericarditis is called a pericardial rub. Pericarditis is diagnosed through the use of chest x-ray (CXR), echocardiography, and magnetic resonance imaging (MRI). Usually, these patients also have abnormal EKG results.

EXAMPLE | Acute pericardial effusion, 420.90 (I30.9).

EXAMPLE | Uremic pericarditis, 585.9, 420.0 (N18.9, I32).

EXAMPLE | Acute viral pericarditis, 420.91 (I30.1, B97.89).

Endocarditis

Endocarditis is inflammation of the lining of the heart chambers and valves. Most often, bacterial infection is the cause of endocarditis. Patients with intravenous drug use (IVDU), central venous lines, and valve replacements (aortic valve replacement [AVR], mitral valve replacement [MVR]) are at greater risk for developing endocarditis. Patients with endocarditis might present with fever, shortness of breath (SOB), fatigue, night sweats, and muscle aches. In determining this diagnosis, physicians order blood cultures and perform echocardiograms. Treatment always consists of intravenous (IV) antibiotics; therefore, the patient usually is hospitalized. IV antibiotic treatment may take up to 6 weeks.

EXAMPLE | Patient admitted for antibiotics for subacute endocarditis, 421.9 (I33.9).

EXAMPLE | Patient admitted for endocarditis caused by typhoid, 002.0, 421.1 (A01.02).

Valve Disorders

Valve disorders of incompetence, insufficiency, and regurgitation may be classified to the category of 424 (I34.–). A leaking valve is another name for regurgitation, incompetence, or insufficiency. When this occurs, blood flows backward within the valve. If a valve's opening is blocked, or flow of blood is diminished, this is called stenosis. Stenosis, for some valves, is assigned the 424 (I34.–) category. However, tricuspid stenosis is always found under category 397 (I07.–). When diseases of both the mitral valve and the aortic valve are identified, ICD-9-CM assigns them to category 396, whether or not they are specified as rheumatic. Coding of valve disorders requires following the Alphabetic Index closely and paying attention to all instructional notes to assign the appropriate code.

EXAMPLE | Tricuspid stenosis, 397.0 (I07.0).

EXAMPLE | Mitral insufficiency, 424.0 (I34.0).

EXAMPLE | Mitral valve prolapse, 424.0 (I34.1).

Cardiomyopathy

Cardiomyopathy is a disorder of the muscle of the heart chambers that impedes the functioning of the heart. Another term for congestive cardiomyopathy is dilated cardiomyopathy. Cardiomyopathy can be caused by disorders such as CAD, infection, diabetes, or alcohol abuse. Two codes may be required to code cardiomyopathy—one for the underlying condition and one for cardiomyopathy. In subcategories 425.7 and 425.8, the underlying condition would be sequenced first. Cardiomyopathy is diagnosed by echocardiography and is treated with antibiotics if due to an infection, or treatment may be targeted to the underlying cause. Congestive cardiomyopathy may be associated with congestive heart failure. When they occur together, congestive heart failure would be the principal diagnosis because it is often the focus of treatment. The cardiomyopathy would be assigned as an additional code, according to *Coding Clinic* (1990:2Q:p19).[6]

EXAMPLE | Cardiomyopathy due to progressive muscular dystrophy, 359.1, 425.8 (G71.0).

EXAMPLE | Obstructive hypertrophic cardiomyopathy, 425.11 (I42.1).

EXAMPLE | Alcoholic cardiomyopathy, 425.5, 303.90 (I42.6, F10.20).

Conduction Disorders

A **conduction disorder** is a problem that occurs in the electrical impulses that regulate heartbeat. A heartbeat begins when an electrical impulse is sent through the upper chambers of the heart. A human heart usually beats from 60 to 100 times per minute. **Tachycardia** (fast heart rate) means the heartbeat is greater than 100 beats per minute; **bradycardia** (slow heart rate) is a heartbeat of fewer than 60 beats per minute. Sometimes during an electrophysiologic study, ventricular tachycardia is induced. According to *Coding Clinic* (2008:1Q:p14),[7] it is appropriate to assign a code for the sustained or nonsustained ventricular tachycardia.

Heart blocks occur when impulses originating in the upper chambers are unable to pass to the lower chambers at the correct rate. Three types of blocks have been observed:
- First degree: Conduction of beats from upper to lower is slower than normal.
- Second degree: Not all beats pass from upper to lower.
- Third degree: Impulses cannot pass from upper to lower.

EXAMPLE | ECG shows left bundle branch block, anterior fascicular block with posterior fascicular block, 426.3 (I44.7, I44.4, I44.5).

EXAMPLE | The patient has a bifascicular block, 426.53 (I45.2).

Cardiac arrhythmias (Table 15-1) occur when the normal sequence of electrical impulses changes, or the rhythm of the heartbeat is disturbed. (Normal sequence = RA [right atrium] through atrioventricular [AV] node through His bundle to ventricles.)

EXAMPLE | Atrial fibrillation (AF), 427.31 (I48.0).

EXAMPLE | Sick sinus syndrome (SSS), 427.81 (I49.5).

EXAMPLE | Supraventricular tachycardia (SVT), 427.89 (I47.1).

TABLE 15-1 ARRYTHMIAS[8]

Types	Symptoms and Signs	Etiology	Diagnosis	Treatment
Normal sinus rhythm	Rate of 60-100 bpm, regular, P wave uniform	Impulse originates in SA node, conduction normal	Normal	None indicated
Sinus tachycardia	Rate >100 bpm, regular, P wave uniform	Rapid impulse originates in SA node, conduction normal	Rapid rate	Beta blockers, calcium channel blockers
Sinus brachycardia	Rate <60 bpm, regular, P wave uniform	Slow impulse originates in SA node, conduction normal	Slow rate	Atropine
Premature atrial contraction	Rate depends on underlying rhythm, usually normal P wave, morphology different from other P waves	Irritable atrium, single ectopic beat that arises prematurely, conduction through ventricle normal	Irregular heartbeat, diagnosis by ECG	Treatment usually unnecessary; if needed, antiarrhythmic drugs
Atrial tachycardia	Rate of 150-250 bpm, rhythm normal, sudden onset	Irritable atrium, firing at rapid rates, normal conduction	Rapid rate with atrial and ventricular rates identical, diagnosis by ECG	Reflex vagal stimulation, calcium channel–blocking drugs (verapamil), cardioversion
Atrial fibrillation	Atrial rate >350 bpm, ventricular rate <100 bpm (controlled) or ≥100 bpm (rapid ventricular response)	Atrial ectopic foci discharging at too rapid and chaotic a rate for muscles to respond and contract, resulting in quivering of atrium; AV node blocks some impulses, and ventricle responds irregularly	ECG show no P waves, grossly irregular ventricular rate	IV verapamil; if unsuccessful, procainamide; if unsuccessful, cardioversion
First-degree heart block	Rate depends on rate of underlying rhythm, PR interval >0.20 second	Delay at AV node, impulse eventually conducted	ECG shows PR interval >0.20 second	Atropine; if unsuccessful, artificial pacemaker insertion
Second-degree heart block, Wenckebach block	Intermittent block with progressively longer delay in conduction until one beat is blocked; atrial rate normal, ventricular rate slower than normal, rhythm irregular	SA node initiates impulse, conduction through AV node is blocked intermittently	ECG shows normal P waves, some P waves not followed by QRS complex; PR interval progressively longer, followed by block of impulse	Mild forms, no treatment; severe, insertion of artificial pacemaker
Classic second-degree heart block	Ventricular rate slow ($\frac{1}{2}$, $\frac{1}{3}$, or $\frac{1}{4}$ of atrial rate); rhythm, regular; P waves normal, QRS complex dropped every 2nd, 3rd, or 4th beat	SA node initiates impulse, conduction through AV node is blocked	ECG shows P waves present, QRS complex blocked every 2nd, 3rd, or 4th impulse	Artificial pacemaker is inserted

AV, Atrioventricular; *bpm,* beats per minute; *ECG,* electrocardiogram; *IV,* intravenous; *PR,* pulse rate; *PVC,* premature ventricular contraction; *SA,* sinoatrial.

TABLE 15-1 ARRYTHMIAS[8]—cont'd

Types	Symptoms and Signs	Etiology	Diagnosis	Treatment
Third-degree heart block	Atrial rate normal, ventricular rate 20-40 or 40-60 bpm; no relationship between P wave and QRS complex	SA node initiates impulse, which is completely blocked from conduction, causing atria and ventricles to beat independently	ECG shows P waves and QRS complexes with no relationship to each other; rhythms are regular but independent of each other	Insertion of artificial pacemaker is needed
Premature ventricular contraction (single focus)	Single ectopic beat, arising from ventricle, followed by compensatory pause	Ectopic beat originates in irritable ventricle	ECG shows a wide, bizarre QRS complex >0.12 second, usually followed by a compensatory pause	Usually, no treatment if <6 per minute and single focus
Multifocal arrhythmia Coupling, 2 in a row Bigeminy, every other beat Trigeminy, every 3rd beat Quadrigeminy, every 4th beat	Rate dependent on underlying rhythm; rhythm regular or irregular; P wave absent before ectopic beat	Same as single focus	Same as single focus	Same as single focus
Ventricular tachycardia	Rate of 150-250 bpm, rhythm usually regular; focus of pacemaker normally single; patient experiences palpitations, dyspnea, and anxiety followed by chest pain	Four or more consecutive PVCs at a rapid rate due to advanced irritability of myocardium, indicating ventricular command of heart rate	ECG show runs of four or more PVCs; P was buried in QRS complex	Often forerunner of ventricular fibrillation; immediate intervention necessary; IV lidocaine; if unsuccessful, follow by cardioversion; procainamide or bretylium may be used
Ventricular fibrillation (lethal arrhythmia)	Patient loses consciousness immediately after onset; no peripheral pulses palpable, no heart sounds, no blood pressure	Ventricular fibers twitch rather than contract; reason unknown	Pulseless, unconscious patient; ECG shows rapid, repetitive, chaotic waves originating in ventricle	Recognize and terminate rhythm; precordial shock (defibrillation)

AV, Atrioventricular; *bpm,* beats per minute; *ECG,* electrocardiogram; *IV,* intravenous; *PR,* pulse rate; *PVC,* premature ventricular contraction; *SA,* sinoatrial.

Cardiac arrest, the sudden loss of heart function, is assigned code 427.5 (I46.9). Per *Coding Clinic* (1988:2Q:p8),[9] this may be coded as the principal diagnosis in only two instances:

1. When the patient presents to the ER in cardiac arrest and dies before the underlying cause of the arrest has been established
2. When the patient presents to the hospital in cardiac arrest, is resuscitated, admitted as an inpatient, and subsequently dies before the underlying cause of the arrest has been established

Cardiac arrest may be coded as a secondary diagnosis when a patient has a cardiac arrest and is resuscitated on arrival or during the inpatient stay. The arrest is not coded when a physician documents cardiac arrest as the cause of death.

Heart failure is impaired function of the heart's pumping ability. The heart is unable to pump with enough force or to fill with enough blood. This damage to the heart muscle may be caused by a variety of heart conditions such as CAD, MI, cardiomyopathy, hypertension (HTN), valve disease, diabetes mellitus (DM), and CKD. This impaired pumping function in turn results in insufficient blood reaching the kidneys, which causes the body to retain fluid (Figure 15-8). Symptoms of heart failure may include congested lungs, edema, fatigue, and irregular heartbeat.

Two types of heart failure may occur: systolic and diastolic. Systolic heart dysfunction, also known as systolic heart failure, occurs when the heart muscles are not contracting with enough force, and, therefore, not enough blood is being pumped to the body. Diastolic cardiac dysfunction, also known as diastolic heart failure, occurs when the contraction is normal but the ventricle does not allow enough blood to enter the heart. Physicians can measure the percentage of blood that is pumped out of a filled ventricle with each heartbeat (known as ejection fraction) to determine how the heart is functioning. A normal ejection fraction measures 55% to 70%. Ejection fraction can be determined in several ways: echocardiography, MRI, multiple-gated acquisition (MUGA), or computerized tomography (CT) scan. Another test used to determine whether a patient is in heart failure is the brain natriuretic peptide (BNP) test. **BNP** is a hormone that is produced by the heart; a BNP test measures the amount of BNP that is found in the blood. Normally, levels of BNP are low, but in heart failure, these levels become elevated. A normal value of BNP would be 0 to 99 pg/mL. If this level is greater than 100, heart failure is indicated. Sometimes a provider will document the stage of heart failure. This may be described by a classification of the New York Heart Association (NYHA):

- NYHA Class I   Asymptomatic
- NYHA Class II   Symptoms with moderate exertion
- NYHA Class III   Symptoms with minimal exertion
- NYHA Class IV   Symptoms at rest

When coding heart failure, it is appropriate to pick up codes for heart failure as well as codes for systolic, diastolic, or combination systolic/diastolic and codes for the underlying cause, if known. It is also important to look for documentation of acute, chronic, or acute on chronic. It is important to recognize that the terms "exacerbated" and "decompensated" indicate that a chronic condition is now in an acute phase, per *Coding Clinic* (2008:3Q:p12).[10] Patients may be treated for CHF as a chronic condition and may never be hospitalized. However, should the patient have an exacerbation, he or she may be hospitalized per *Coding Clinic* (2002:4Q:p52-55).[11] To assign a code for rheumatic congestive heart failure, the heart failure must be classified as rheumatic by ICD-9-CM, or the physician must document that the heart failure is rheumatic in nature, per *Coding Clinic* (2000:2Q:p16-17; 1995:1Q:p6).[12,13]

EXAMPLE Patient admitted with decompensated diastolic congestive heart failure, 428.33, 428.0 (I50.30).

EXAMPLE Patient admitted with congestive heart failure, acute on chronic combined systolic and diastolic, 428.43, 428.0 (I50.43).

FIGURE 15-8. Chronic passive congestion. Left-sided heart failure leads to pulmonary edema. Right ventricular failure causes peripheral edema that is most prominent in the lower extremities.

In many cases, physicians will refer to heart failure as pulmonary edema or volume overload. Pulmonary edema has other causes, but one of its main causes is heart failure. Also, patients with CHF may have pleural effusions. *Coding Clinic* (1991:3Q:p19)[14] says, "Pleural effusion is commonly seen with CHF with or without pulmonary edema." In cases in which the patient has CHF, pulmonary edema, and pleural effusions, CHF would always be the principal diagnosis. Pleural effusion may be reported as an additional diagnosis if it were specifically evaluated or treated. Pulmonary edema would rarely be coded in addition to CHF. *Coding Clinic* (1991:3Q:p19)[14] also says that if special x-rays are taken to confirm the presence, or if diagnostic or therapeutic **thoracentesis** is performed, then pleural effusion may be additionally coded. Likewise, pulmonary edema is not assigned an additional code.

Assign codes to the following conditions.

1. Pulmonary hypertension with cor pulmonale   _____
2. Acute pericarditis due to tuberculosis   _____
3. Acute bacterial endocarditis   _____
4. Chronic hypertension and pulmonary hypertension   _____
5. Aortic regurgitation   _____
6. Dilated cardiomyopathy   _____
7. Incomplete right bundle branch block (RBBB)   _____
8. Wenckebach heart block   _____
9. Atrial flutter   _____
10. Persistent sinus bradycardia   _____
11. Thyrotoxic cardiomyopathy   _____
12. Hypertensive cardiomyopathy   _____
13. Another name for inflammation of the lining of the heart chambers   _____

Cerebrovascular Disease

A patient who is admitted with a diagnosis of **stroke** (brain infarction or cerebrovascular accident [CVA]) is similar to a patient who is admitted with a diagnosis of heart attack or MI. The blood supply to a part of the brain is blocked by a broken blood vessel, ischemia, or blood clots (Figure 15-9). When the blood supply is cut off, brain cells die. Several types of stroke or brain infarcts may occur (Figure 15-10). Ischemic stroke, which accounts for 80% of all strokes, happens when blockage to the brain, usually by a blood clot, occurs. A clot that develops in another part of the body and then becomes wedged in a brain artery is a free-roaming clot or an embolus (Figure 15-11).

The most common type of stroke is ischemic (thrombotic/embolic). An ischemic stroke occurs when a blood clot or a piece of plaque breaks loose from an artery and lodges in a blood vessel of the brain, which then cuts off the blood supply to that area of the brain. A blood clot that forms and remains in a vein is called a thrombus, whereas a clot that travels to another part of the body is an **embolus**. Sometimes plaque is dislodged and becomes an embolus. The other type of stroke is hemorrhagic.

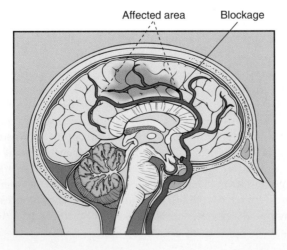

FIGURE 15-9. Cerebrovascular accident (CVA).

Blood flows freely through a normal artery.

Hemorrhagic strokes are caused by cerebral arterial wall rupture.

Embolic (embolitic) strokes are caused by dislodged thrombi (emboli) that occlude cerebral arteries.

Thrombotic strokes are caused by atheromatous plaques that occlude cerebral arteries.

FIGURE 15-10. Types of stroke: ischemic (thrombotic and embolic) and hemorrhagic.

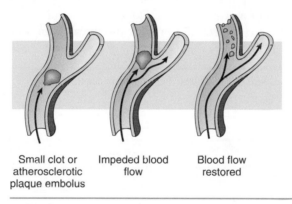

Small clot or atherosclerotic plaque embolus

Impeded blood flow

Blood flow restored

FIGURE 15-11. Embolus causing transient ischemic attack.

EXAMPLE   Embolic cerebral infarction, 434.11 (I63.40).

Ischemic stroke may be caused by narrowing of the arteries, or **stenosis**. Stenosis is often caused by the buildup of plaque in the artery. This may be referred to as small- or large-vessel disease. Often, this is called a lacunar infarction.

EXAMPLE   Ischemic stroke, 434.91 (I63.8).

Hemorrhagic stroke occurs when an artery in the brain bursts and blood seeps into the surrounding tissue, causing the tissue to malfunction. When bleeding from the artery goes into the brain itself, this is called an intracerebral hemorrhage. When bleeding seeps into the meninges or outer membranes, this is called a subarachnoid hemorrhage. Hemorrhagic stroke may be caused by aneurysms, arteriovenous malformations (AVMs), and, possibly, plaque-encrusted walls that rupture. Hypertension can increase the risk of rupture of the artery wall. On occassion an infarction has a hemorrhagic conversion and per *Coding Clinic*

(2010:3Q:p5-6)[15] in these cases, two codes are necessary, one for the infarct and one for the intracerebral hemorhage.

Nontraumatic subarachnoid hemorrhage, 430 (I60.7).

Symptoms of a stroke often appear suddenly. These may occur as weakness or numbness of one side of the body, arm, leg, or face; confusion; difficulty talking or speaking; trouble walking or seeing; dizziness; and headache. A CT scan is often used to determine whether a patient has had a hemorrhagic stroke; MRI is another useful tool in the diagnosis of stroke. The benefit of MRI is that it can rapidly detect small infarcts.

Medication is the most common treatment for stroke patients. Patients with ischemic stroke may be treated with thrombolytic agents such as TPA. Similar to heart attack victims, stroke patients need to be treated with TPA soon after onset of symptoms. Most patients are treated with anticoagulants or with antiplatelet agents.

Sometimes a patient will present to the hospital with symptoms of a stroke, such as difficulty speaking or weakness on one side. TPA may be administered with considerable improvement in the patient's symptoms. According to *Coding Clinic* (2007:1Q:p23-24),[16] if the physician documented aborted CVA, the code 434.91 for CVA would be assigned. Often, a patient is admitted with a stroke with deficits. These deficits are often gone by the time the patient is discharged. Any deficits that a patient exhibits from the stroke, whether present at discharge or not, should be assigned codes. On occassion an infarction has a hemorrhagic conversion and per *Coding Clinic* (2010:3Q:p5-6)[15] in these cases, two codes are necessary, one for the infarct and one for the intracerebral hemorhage.

Subdural hemorrhage, with dysphagia at time of discharge, 432.1, 787.20 (I62.00, I69.291, R13.10).

Patient suffered an embolic stroke. She presented with hemiparesis of the right side and aphasia, both of which were no longer present at discharge. 434.11, 784.3, 342.90 (I63.40, I69.351, I69.320).

Stenosis of the carotid artery with cerebral infarction, 433.11 (I63.239).

Patient has a history of bilateral carotid stenosis. Upon presentation to the hospital, it is determined that the patient has had a CVA due to thrombosis (*Coding Clinic* [1995:2Q:p14]).[17] In this case both the codes for the carotid stenosis without infarct, 433.10 and 433.30, and the code for the CVA, 434.01, would be assigned.

When coding bilateral carotid artery stenosis, it is necessary to assign two codes, one for the site, code 433.1X, as well as one for laterality code, 433.3X (*Coding Clinic* [2006:1Q:p17]).[18]

Transient Ischemic Attack

A **transient ischemic attack** (TIA) is a stroke that lasts for only a few minutes. Patients who present with a TIA usually have the same symptoms that occur with a stroke. Most symptoms of a TIA are gone within an hour, but they may last up to 24 hours.

It is important for the coder to be aware of the Excludes notes in this chapter, excluding codes found in this category that occur during pregnancy or the puerperium and strokes that occur as a result of treatment.

Late Effects of Cerebrovascular Disease

Stroke is one of the leading causes of disability in the United States. Types of disability that may result from stroke consist of paralysis, particularly on one side of the body (hemiplegia), or weakness on one side (hemiparesis). Other disabilities include **cognitive deficits**, **aphasia** (impairment of language comprehension and production), emotional problems, and pain. When an inpatient has had a stroke, has current deficits, and also has late effects from a previous stroke, all codes should be assigned. Late effect codes may be listed as principal diagnoses when the purpose of the admission is to treat the late effect. The code for a history of CVA with no residuals is V12.54 (Z86.73).

EXAMPLE	Patient presents with carotid artery stenosis with infarct and current hemiparesis. Patient has residual aphasia from a previous stroke, 433.11, 342.90, 438.11 (I63.239, I69.359, I69.320).

EXERCISE 15-4

Assign codes to the following conditions.

1. Transient ischemic attack with right-sided weakness, which cleared shortly following admission _____

2. Cerebral hemorrhage _____

3. Patient was admitted with CVA and aphasia; the aphasia cleared before discharge _____

4. Cerebral thrombosis without infarction _____

5. Ruptured berry aneurysm _____

6. Patient with a history of cerebrovascular accident, no residuals _____

7. Quadriplegia resulting from a stroke last year _____

8. Patient is being treated for cognitive deficits following a stroke _____

Diseases of the Arteries, Arterioles, and Capillaries

Atherosclerosis or arteriosclerosis is a stricture or hardening of the artery that is caused by deposits of plaque. These deposits restrict blood flow through the artery; plaques can rupture and travel to other parts of the body or can form blood clots that block a blood vessel. If a blood vessel to the heart is blocked, this causes a heart attack; if a vessel to the brain is blocked, this causes a stroke; and if vessels to the extremities are blocked, this can cause claudication, ulcers, and eventually gangrene. Codes found in subcategory 440.2 are hierarchical. Per *Coding Clinic* (1993:4Q:p27-28),[19] "Thus all patients in this subcategory who have gangrene (regardless of whether ulceration, rest pain, and/or intermittent claudication [is] present) are coded to 440.24." For example, if a patient presents with atherosclerosis of the extremities with ulceration and gangrene, only the code for gangrene, 440.24, is assigned. The ulcer code 707.1X is assigned in addition to the 440.23.

EXAMPLE	Arteriosclerotic renal artery, 440.1 (I70.1).

EXAMPLE	Atherosclerosis of extremity autologous bypass graft, 440.31 (I70.409).

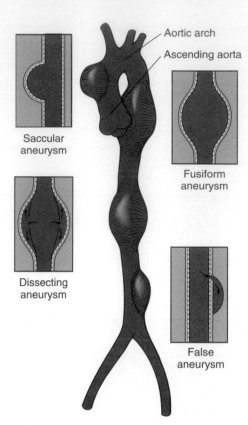

FIGURE 15-12. Types of aortic aneurysm.

An **aneurysm** is a bulging or ballooning out of a vessel. Aneurysms are often caused by atherosclerosis and tend to have no symptoms, unless dissection occurs. Dissection is typically accompanied by severe pain in the area of dissection. Aneurysms tend to form in areas where vessels branch out. Aortic aneurysms (Figure 15-12) can occur anywhere along the aorta, which is the largest artery in the body; it runs from the heart through the chest into the abdominal area and then divides into vessels that supply blood to the legs. The most common aneurysms occur in the abdominal area. Rupture of an aneurysm is a life-threatening event. The risk of rupture increases as the aneurysm becomes larger. Sometimes, an aneurysm becomes **dissecting**, which means a tear begins in the wall of the vessel that causes layers to separate. Physicians use the terms type I, type II, and type III to describe dissecting aneurysms.

Classifications of Dissecting Aneurysms

In the Stanford classification, aneurysms are divided into two types:
- Type A involves the ascending aorta (DeBakey types I and II); requires surgery.
- Type B does not involve the ascending aorta and may be managed medically.

The DeBakey classification divides dissections into three types:
- Type I involves the ascending aorta, aortic arch, and descending aorta.
- Type II is confined to the ascending aorta.
- Type III is confined to the descending aorta distal to the left subclavian artery. Type III dissections are further divided into IIIa and IIIb.
  - Type IIIa refers to dissections that originate distal to the left subclavian artery but extend both proximally and distally, mostly above the diaphragm.
  - Type IIIb refers to dissection that originate distal to the left subclavian artery, extend only distally, and may extend below the diaphragm.

EXAMPLE | Patient presents to hospital with Type I thoracoabdominal aneurysm, 441.03 (I171.03).

Aneurysms are usually not treated until they reach a certain size or begin to enlarge quickly. Treatment for an aneurysm consists of open or endovascular surgery, which is discussed in the Procedure section of this chapter.

| EXAMPLE | Abdominal aortic aneurysm, 441.4 (I71.4). |

| EXAMPLE | Ruptured thoracic aneurysm, 441.1 (I71.1). |

| EXAMPLE | Femoral aneurysm, 442.3 (I72.4). |

An arteriovenous **fistula** is an abnormal passage between an artery and a vein. Blood typically flows from arteries into capillaries and then to veins; however, when blood bypasses the capillaries and goes directly to the vein, an arteriovenous fistula results.

| EXAMPLE | Patient has an arteriovenous fistula, acquired, 447.0 (I77.0). |

Diseases of Veins and Lymphatics and Other Diseases of Circulatory System

Phlebitis, Thrombophlebitis, and Deep Vein Thrombosis

Phlebitis is inflammation of a vein; thrombophlebitis occurs when a clot forms in the vein and then causes phlebitis. **Deep vein thrombosis** (DVT) is a blood clot that forms in a deep vein, usually in the leg or hip (Figures 15-13 and 15-14). *Coding Clinic* (1992:1Q:p15-16)[20] says, "Deep vein thrombosis (DVT) is rarely an acute finding without the associated inflammation leading to thrombophlebitis, and in most cases, DVT is synonymous with thrombophlebitis. If both conditions are present, only the code for 451.xx is assigned."

| EXAMPLE | Patient admitted with an acute femoral DVT of the right leg with inflammation, 451.11 (I82.411). |

Varicose veins are enlarged, twisted veins that usually occur in the legs. Varicose veins can be found in other areas of the body such as the esophagus. Varicose veins often develop complications that require surgical treatment. Stasis dermatitis with varicose veins of the leg is assigned code 454.1 (I83.10).

Stasis dermatitis is a skin condition caused by poor circulation (venous insufficiency) that is characterized by swelling, skin discoloration, weeping, itching, and scaly skin. The legs and particularly the ankles are the areas most often affected. This condition is often seen in the elderly, and risk for developing this condition increases when any of the following conditions is present: obesity, high blood pressure, varicose veins and heart, and/or kidney failure. A common complication of stasis dermatitis is cellulitis.

| EXAMPLE | Stasis dermatitis without varicose veins and ulcer of the calf of the right leg, stage I, 459.81, 707.10 (I87.2, L97.211). |

| EXAMPLE | Patient with alcoholic cirrhosis of the liver with esophageal varices with bleeding, 571.2, 456.20, 303.90 (K70.30, I85.11, F10.20). |

FIGURE 15-13. Common sites of thrombus formation.

NORMAL VEINS

Functional valves aid
in flow of venous blood
back to the heart

VARICOSE VEINS

Failure of valves and
pooling of blood in
superficial veins

— Thrombophlebitis

— Edema

— Pigmented skin

FIGURE 15-14. Normal and varicose veins. Slow flow in the veins makes an individual susceptible to clot formation. Thrombotic occlusion of varicose veins is known as thrombophlebitis. If a thrombus becomes loosened from its place in a vein, it can travel to the lungs (pulmonary embolism) and block a blood vessel there. Then blood pools in the lower part of the leg and fluid leaks from distended small capillaries, causing edema.

EXERCISE 15-5

Assign codes to the following conditions.

1. Atherosclerosis of the extremities with rest pain and   _____
    gangrene
2. Arteriosclerotic cardiovascular disease   _____
3. Arteriosclerosis of a carotid artery   _____
4. Atherosclerosis of a nonautologous bypass graft of the leg   _____
5. Dissection of the thoracic aorta   _____
6. Type II dissection of the aorta   _____
7. Iliac artery aneurysm   _____
8. Acquired arteriovenous aneurysm of the brain   _____
9. Buerger's disease   _____
10. Embolic infarction of the abdominal aorta   _____
11. Thrombosis of the subclavian artery   _____
12. Deep vein thrombosis of the lower extremity   _____
13. Peroneal thrombophlebitic DVT   _____
14. Scrotal varices   _____
15. Varicose veins, asymptomatic   _____

FACTORS INFLUENCING HEALTH STATUS AND CONTACT WITH HEALTH SERVICES (V CODES/Z CODES)

In the past, V/Z codes were considered for use primarily in the outpatient setting. This has changed with the addition of more V/Z codes each year. As was discussed in Chapter 8, it may be difficult to locate V/Z codes in the Index. Coders often say, "I did not know there was a V/Z code for that."

Refer to Chapter 8 for a listing of common main terms used to locate V/Z codes. A review of the Tabular reveals that some V/Z codes pertain to diseases of the circulatory system:

V12.50	Personal history of unspecific coronary disease
V12.51	Personal history of thrombosis and embolism
V12.52	Personal history of thrombophlebitis
V12.53	Personal history of sudden cardiac arrest
V12.54	Personal history of TIA and cerebral infarction without deficits
V12.55	Personal history of pulmonary embolism
V12.59	Personal history of other disease of the circulatory system
V15.1	Surgery of heart and great vessels
V17.1	Family history of stroke
V17.3	Family history of ischemic heart disease
V17.41	Family history of sudden cardiac death
V17.49	Family history of other cardiovascular diseases
V42.1	History of heart transplant
V42.2	History of heart valve transplant
V43.21	Heart replacement by heart-assist device
V43.22	Fully implantable artificial heart
V43.3	Heart valve replaced by artificial valve
V45.00	Postprocedural status of unspecified cardiac device
V45.01	Postprocedural status of cardiac pacemaker
V45.02	Postprocedural status AICD (automatic implantable cardioverter-defibrillator)
V45.09	Postprocedural status of other specified cardiac device
V45.81	Aortocoronary bypass status
V45.82	Percutaneous transluminal coronary angioplasty status
V45.88	Status post administration of tPA (rtPA) in a different facility within the last 24 hours prior to admission to current facility
V47.2	Other cardiorespiratory problems
V49.83	Awaiting organ transplant status
V53.31	Fitting and adjustment of cardiac pacemaker
V53.32	Fitting and adjustment of AICD (automatic implantable cardioverter-defibrillator)
V53.39	Fitting and adjustment of other cardiac device
V58.73	Aftercare following surgery of the circulatory system, not elsewhere classified (NEC)
V58.61	Long-term (current) drug use—anticoagulant
V58.63	Long-term (current) drug use—antiplatelet/antithrombotic
V58.66	Long-term (current) drug use—aspirin
V71.7	Observation for suspected cardiovascular disease not found
V72.81	Preoperative cardiovascular examination
V81.0	Screening for ischemic heart disease
V81.1	Screening for hypertension
V81.2	Screening for other and unspecified cardiovascular conditions

EXAMPLE | Patient admitted with chest pain. Has a history of PTCA, 786.50, V45.82 (R07.9, Z98.61).

EXAMPLE Patient admitted for DVT right lower extremity. On Coumadin for previous stroke, 453.40, V58.61, V12.54 (I82.401, Z79.01, Z86.73).

EXAMPLE Patient admitted to Hospital A with a CVA and tPA was administered. The patient was stabilized and transferred to Hospital B for treatment of CVA.
   Hospital A: 434.91, 99.20 (I63.50; not enough information to code 99.20 in ICD-10-CM PCS).
   Hospital B: 434.91, V45.88 (I63.50, Z92.82).

EXERCISE 15-6

Assign codes to the following conditions.

1. Patient is admitted to the hospital with chest pain; the only risk factor he has is a family history of CAD _____

2. Patient is admitted with pulmonary edema, history of CHF, and history of a heart valve replaced by a prosthesis _____

3. Patient is admitted to the hospital with an acute MI and history of a five-vessel CABG _____

4. Patient is admitted to the hospital with ACS and has a history of angioplasty _____

5. Patient is admitted to the hospital with syncope and has previously had a pacemaker inserted _____

6. Patient is awaiting a heart transplant and is on a heart-assist device _____

COMMON TREATMENTS

CONDITION	MEDICATION/TREATMENT
Angina	Nitroglycerin, beta blockers, and calcium channel blockers
	Coreg, Lopressor, Norvasc, Verapamil, Procardia
Atrial fibrillation	Blood thinners (Coumadin, Plavix, Ticlid)
	Rate control: calcium channel blockers: Cardizem, verapamil
	Beta blockers: atenolol, Lopressor, Inderal, Digoxin, Lanoxin, Amiodarone
Congestive heart failure	Diuretics: Lasix, Bumex, Zaroxolyn, Furosemide
	Beta blockers: Dyazide, Lanoxin, HCTZ
Hypertension	Diuretics, Aldactone
	Beta blockers: atenolol, Vasotec, Cozaar, Calan, Cardizem, Aldomet
Stroke/CVA (nonhemorrhagic)	Blood thinners (Coumadin, Plavix, Ticlid) and clot-busting agents such as tPA and streptokinase

PROCEDURES

Some of the procedures that may be related to diseases of the circulatory system may be located in the following chapters of the Procedure Tabular:
   0. Procedures and Interventions, Not Elsewhere Classified (00)
   7. Operations on the Cardiovascular System (35-39)

Left ventricle

Aorta

Catheter inserted in femoral artery

FIGURE 15-15. Left-sided cardiac catheterization. The catheter is passed retrograde (backward) from the femoral artery into the aorta and then into the left ventricle. For right-sided cardiac catheterization, the cardiologist inserts a catheter through the femoral vein and advances it to the right atrium and right ventricle and into the pulmonary artery.

Procedures related to the cardiovascular system in ICD-10-PCS may be found in the following tables:

Heart and Great Vessels	021-02Y
Upper Arteries	031-03W
Lower Arteries	041-04W
Upper Veins	051-05W
Lower Veins	061-06W

Diagnostic Cardiac Catheterization

Diagnostic cardiac catheterization (Figure 15-15) is a procedure that may be performed on a patient with chest pain, angina, or an acute MI to determine if coronary artery disease is present. This procedure allows the physician to view the heart chambers, valves, and arteries. A hollow needle or catheter is inserted into the vein for a right heart catheterization and into an artery in the arm or groin for a left heart catheterization. Usually, this catheter is inserted into the groin in the femoral artery and winds its way up into the coronary artery. Pictures of the arteries are then taken. These pictures are called coronary arteriograms or angiograms. When a cardiac catheterization is coded, the procedure codes listed in Table 15-2 may be assigned. The most common set of codes for a cardiac catheterization includes the codes 37.22, Left cardiac catheterization, 88.53, Left ventriculography, and 88.56, Coronary angiography. In ICD-10-PCS, cardiac caths are found in the measurement and monitoring section with the root operation of measurement.

Once the cardiologist has determined the extent of the patient's problem, he or she decides on medical therapy, refers the patient for bypass, or performs a therapeutic procedure right then and there while the catheter is in place. The cardiologist may go on to perform the procedures as described below.

Angioplasty

Angioplasty is a procedure that is usually done with a balloon (Figure 15-16). The device inflates, and the plaque is compressed against the wall of the artery. This procedure is often abbreviated as PTCA (percutaneous transluminal coronary angioplasty). The root operation for an angioplasty procedure in ICD-10-PCS is dilation.

TABLE 15-2 COMMON PROCEDURE CODES FOR CARDIAC CATHETERIZATION

Test	Procedure	Comment
Left heart cath	37.22 (4A023N7)	Most commonly done alone when used to diagnose coronary artery disease (CAD)
Right heart cath	37.21 (4A023N6)	Most commonly used for assessment of ventricular function, especially for patients who also have congestive heart failure (CHF)
Combined right and left	37.23 (4A023N8)	
Right angiogram	88.52 (B204YZZ)	All of these angiograms are also called ventriculograms
Left angiogram	88.53 (B205YZZ)	
Combined right and left angiogram	88.54 (B206YZZ)	
Coronary arteriography	88.55 (B200YZZ)	Also known as Sones technique; uses single cath
Coronary arteriography	88.56 (B200YZZ)	Also known as Judkins technique; uses two caths
Coronary arteriography	88.57 (B200YZZ)	Other and unspecified coronary arteriography

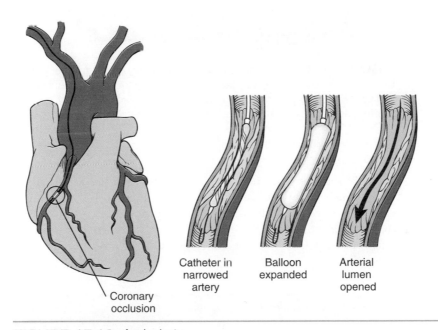

Coronary occlusion

Catheter in narrowed artery

Balloon expanded

Arterial lumen opened

FIGURE 15-16. Angioplasty.

EXAMPLE Patient with CAD presents for PTCA of left anterior descending and left circumflex, 414.01, 00.66, 00.41 (I25.10, 02713ZZ).

One of the most common complications of angioplasty is restenosis, which occurs in about one third of cases. To try to avoid restenosis, physicians may use a stent. Sometimes, they also treat a restenosed patient with intravascular radiation therapy. Most often, an angioplasty is performed prior to insertion of a stent.

Atherectomy is the removal of plaque from a vessel. This may be done with the use of a catheter with a shaver or rotablator on the end. A laser is also used to perform atherectomy. An atherectomy is assigned the same code as a PTCA.

Stent insertion into the coronary artery is a procedure that may be performed after completion of an angioplasty (Figure 15-17). The stent helps to keep the artery open. Inserted stents may be drug-eluting (DES) or non–drug-eluting.

Three types of drug-eluting stents are currently in use in the United States. These include a paclitaxel eluting stent, a sirolimus-eluting stent, and an everolimus stent. These

FIGURE 15-17. Placement of an intracoronary stent. **A,** The stent is positioned at the site of the lesion. **B,** The balloon is inflated, thereby expanding the stent. **C,** The balloon is then deflated and removed, and the implanted stent is left in place. Coronary stents are stainless steel scaffolding devices that help hold open arteries such as the coronary, renal, and carotid arteries.

drug-eluting stents are not to be confused with a stent that may be coated with antiplatelet drug, which would be assigned 36.06. The coding of stenting usually requires four procedures codes: a code for the angioplasty/atherectomy, a code for the number of stents inserted, a code for the number of vessels treated, and a code for the type of stent inserted. In ICD-10-PCS the root operation for insertion of a stent into a coronary artery is dilation.

EXAMPLE The patient had a percutaneous coronary intervention (PCI), which included inserting a drug-eluting stent into the LAD for coronary atherosclerosis, 414.01, 00.66, 36.07, 00.45, 00.40 (I25.10, 027034Z).

Coronary Artery Bypass Graft

Coronary artery bypass graft (CABG or CAB) is surgery that is performed to bypass blood around the clogged arteries to the heart (Figure 15-18). The procedure is performed by taking a healthy blood vessel from another part of the body, usually the internal mammary artery or the saphenous vein. Surgeons should document in their operative notes the number of arteries bypassed and the types of blood vessels used. The root operation for a CABG in ICD-10-PCS is bypass.

When reading a bypass operative report, it is helpful to know the coronary arteries that may be bypassed. Two main coronary arteries are located on the left (LCA) and on the right (RCA). The LCA divides into two arteries: the LAD and the circumflex. The RCA divides into the posterior descending artery (PDA) and the marginal branch. Smaller branches consist of the acute marginal, the obtuse marginal (OM), and the diagonals (Figure 15-19).

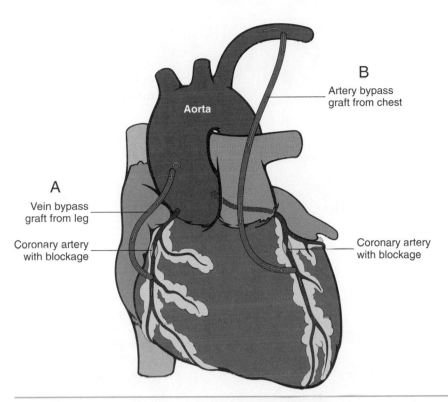

FIGURE 15-18. Coronary artery bypass graft (CABG) surgery with anastomosis of vein and arterial grafts. **A,** Section of a vein is removed from the leg and is anastomosed (upside-down because of its directional valves) to a coronary artery to bypass the area of arteriosclerotic blockage. **B,** An internal mammary artery is grafted to a coronary artery to bypass a blockage.

EXAMPLE

For example, it might be documented as follows:
   Coronary bypass times three. Saphenous vein graft from the left leg to the LAD and to the obtuse marginal and left internal mammary to the right posterior descending. Codes assigned would be as follows:
   36.12 for bypass of the two coronary arteries using the saphenous veins and
   36.15 for the internal mammary bypass
   (021109W, 02100Z9, 06BQ4ZZ)

Per *Coding Clinic* (1997:3Q:p14),[21] the axis used in assignment of the code for aorto-coronary grafts is the number of coronary arteries that were involved in a graft from the aorta to the coronary artery. When coding CABGs, coders should be aware that code 39.61, cardiopulmonary bypass, should be assigned if it is performed. The note under category 36.1 also advises the coding of 00.16 (pressurized treatment of venous bypass graft with pharmaceutical substance) if it is performed.

It is not appropriate to assign additional codes for other procedures that are auxiliary to heart surgery such as hypothermia, cardioplegia, intraoperative cardiac pacing, and chest tube insertion. These procedures are considered integral to the bypass surgery procedure and do not require separate codes. This information is taken from *Coding Clinic* (1995:1Q:p5-6).[22]

Electrophysiologic Studies/Procedures

Electrophysiologic studies (EPS) are used to analyze the electrical conduction system of the heart. In ICD-10-PCS, the root operation for eletrophysiologic studies is found in the medical- and surgical-related sections under measurement and monitoring. Patients with symptoms such as light-headedness, palpitations, or syncope may have EP tests done to

FIGURE 15-19. Anterior view of coronary arterial system.

determine the cause of these symptoms. Other patients with known heart rhythm disturbances may have EP studies so that the severity of the heart disturbance can be determined. During these studies, catheters are inserted into a vein in the leg and are threaded to the heart. They measure electrical signals and conduction of these signals and look for abnormal heart rhythms. The **electrophysiologist** (physician trained in electrical disorders of the heart) may administer electrical stimuli to check the heart's response.

Ablation is correction of abnormal heart rhythm by destroying abnormal heart tissue through radiofrequency or other methods such as laser, microwave, or freezing. Radiofrequency ablation (RFA) can be performed with the use of an EP catheter. The root operation for ablation in ICD-10-PCS is destruction.

EXAMPLE   Patient is admitted through the ER with atrial fibrillation and a history of COPD. She is taken to the EPS lab for EPS testing, mapping, and radiofrequency ablation, 427.31, 496, 37.34, 37.27, 37.26 (I48.0, J44.9, 02583ZZ, 02K83ZZ, 4A023FZ).

Pacemaker/Defibrillators (AICD)

A pacemaker is a device that is used to correct abnormally slow heartbeats, complete heart blocks (CHB) and other abnormalities of heart conduction. The root operation for pacemaker generator insertion is insertion of device into subcutaneous tissue of the chest. The root operation for insertion of leads (electrodes) is insertion of intraluminal device into the atrium. Patients who present with syncope and studies determined that they have a heart

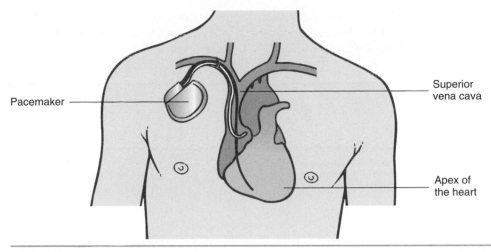

FIGURE 15-20. Cardiac leads in the atrium and in the ventricle enable a dual-chamber pacemaker to sense and pace in both heart chambers.

block often require a pacemaker. A pacemaker has two functions: sensing and pacing. Pacing is the sending of electrical signals to the heart from the pacemaker via the lead. If the rhythm of the heart is too slow, the pacemaker paces the heart to a faster rhythm. Sensing involves monitoring the heart's electrical activity; when the heart is functioning normally, no pacing is required.

The pacemaker system consists of the pulse generator (device, battery) and the leads (Figure 15-20). Leads are placed into the heart chambers and are then attached to the generator. These can be temporary or permanent. A temporary pacemaker is used for emergencies or intraoperatively. Code assignment for a temporary pacemaker does not require codes for the leads or codes for removal.

A permanent pacemaker is usually implanted through an incision near the collarbone. Wires are inserted into a vein and are advanced into the heart; they are then connected to a generator, which is implanted under the skin. Coding of initial insertion of permanent pacemakers requires two codes: one for the insertion of the generator/device and one for insertion of the leads or electrodes. Leads can be placed inside the heart or outside the heart (epicardially). Pacemaker pockets for epicardial leads are usually placed in the abdominal wall; this is typically done for children who are still growing.

Insertion/replacement/revision requires that the coder must know the type of device that is being inserted. Codes for initial insertion and replacement require knowledge as to whether this is a single-chamber or a dual-chamber device and whether the device is rate-responsive. A rate-responsive device has a sensor that detects changes in movement of the body and reacts accordingly.

EXAMPLE Initial insertion of single-chamber device into the right atrium using a single lead, 37.81 and 37.73 (0JH60P0, 02H63MA; approach and location must be specified for accurate coding in ICD-10-PCS).

EXAMPLE Initial insertion of dual-chamber pacemaker into right atrium and right ventricle using two leads, 37.83, and 37.72 (0JH60P2, 02H63MA, 02HK3MA).

Separate codes are used for replacement of devices and leads and removal of devices and leads. When a replacement is performed, the removal code is included in the replacement code. The code V53.31 (Z45.018), Fitting and adjustment of cardiac pacemaker, is assigned as the principal diagnosis when a patient is admitted for removal, replacement, or reprogramming. Often, surgeons document that a patient is being admitted for end of life of the battery or pacemaker. Root operations in ICD-10-PCS may be insertion or removal depending on what is being performed.

EXAMPLE | Removal of a pacemaker and leads, V53.31, 37.77, 37.89 (Z45.010, Z45.018, 02PA3MZ, 0JPT0PZ).

EXAMPLE | Replacement of a single-chamber pacemaker with a dual-chamber device with retention of the atrial lead and open removal of the single chamber device, with transvenous right ventricular lead insertion, 37.87, 37.71 (0JH60P2, 02HK3MA).

An automatic implantable cardioverter-defibrillator (AICD) is a device that is used for treating patients with tachyarrhythmias. Similar to a pacemaker, it has a pulse generator and electrodes that both sense and defibrillate. The root operation in ICD-10-PCS for the insertion of both leads and the generator is insertion. Defibrillators give shocks that attempt to convert the heart rhythm. Implantation of this system is usually done via thoracotomy or sternotomy. The code for this procedure is 37.94, which is assigned for insertion or replacement of the total system. On occasion, this may be done as a two-stage procedure, in which the leads may be implanted on one day and the generator on the next day. The staged procedure would then use codes 37.95 and 37.96. Additional codes are used for replacement of both leads and generators.

EXAMPLE | Patient is admitted with ventricular tachycardia and has an AICD placed with leads in the right atrium and right ventricle, 427.1, 37.94 (I47.2, 0JH60P4, 02H63ME, 02HK3ME).

Biventricular pacing is also known as cardiac resynchronization therapy (CRT). Biventricular pacemakers come as a stand-alone device or with a built-in implantable cardioverter (ICV). They are used primarily to treat heart failure. Similar to a pacemaker, a generator and leads are included. The biventricular pacemaker uses a third lead. This third lead, which is attached to the wall of the left ventricle in the vein of the coronary sinus, causes both ventricles to contract at the same time or in sync. In contrast to regular pacemakers, biventricular pacemakers do not increase heart rate. Some biventricular pacers include internal cardiac defibrillators (ICDs) for patients with fast irregular rhythms. These systems have biventricular pacing, anti-tachycardia pacing, and internal defibrillators. There are codes for implantation and replacement of both systems, with the ICD and without.

EXAMPLE | Implantation of a cardiac resynchronization treatment pacemaker (CRT-P) without mention of defibrillation, total system CRT-P, or biventricular pacing without ICD with insertion of left ventricular lead, 00.50 (0JH63P3, 02HL3MA).

EXAMPLE | Implantation of cardiac resynchronization treatment defibrillator (CRT-D), total system CRT-D, or biventricular pacing and ICD total system, 00.51 (0JH63P5, 02H63ME, 02HL3ME, 02H43ME).

Often, surgeons will upgrade to a biventricular pacing system. A patient who currently has an AICD and is upgraded to a biventricular pacer with a defibrillator would be assigned code 00.51. For further information on this subject, refer to *Coding Clinic* (2002:4Q:p100).[23]

Aneurysm Repair

Aneurysms can be repaired either by resection using an open transperitoneal approach, with either an anastomosis or graft repair or endovascular repair where an endograft is introduced through the femoral artery via a catheter, which avoids the major abdominal incision. The root operations in ICD-10-PCS for an abdominal aortic aneurysm repair depend on the type of procedure performed. If the aneurysm is repaired openly by replacement with a graft, the root operation is replacement. If the aneurysm is repaired openly by an anastomosis, the root operation is excision. Lastly if the repair is performed endovascularly, the root operation is restriction.

EXAMPLE Patient presents for repair of an abdominal aortic aneurysm. The repair is performed endovascularly, 441.4, 39.71 (I71.4, 04V03DZ).

Central Lines/Catheters

Central venous lines are used for several purposes. They may be used to administer chemotherapy, total parenteral nutrition (TPN), antibiotics, and for dialysis. Hickman, Groshong, triple lumen, and double lumen are all types of central lines. Usually, central venous catheters are inserted into the subclavian or jugular vein and are then advanced into the vena cava. The root operation for insertion of a central line is insertion. A central line has a catheter that is NOT totally implanted under the skin. A peripherally inserted central catheter (PICC) (Figure 15-21) is assigned the same code as a central line. It is inserted in a slightly different manner. Separate procedure codes are used for venous catheterization for renal dialysis, arterial lines, and vascular access devices. Sometimes a provider will document a diagnosis of poor IV access when a line is being inserted. Per *Coding Clinic,* "There is no diagnosis code for poor IV access. The diagnosis for the underlying condition being treated should be coded" (2008:2Q:p14).[24]

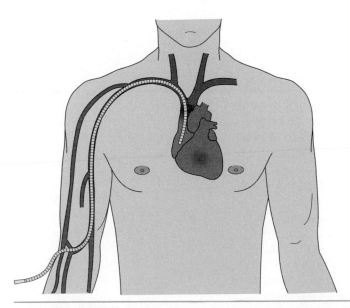

FIGURE 15-21. A peripherally inserted central catheter is threaded through the vein until the end is near the heart.

EXAMPLE

Patient is admitted to the hospital for bacterial endocarditis. A central line is inserted into the right subclavian for administration of antibiotics to treat the endocarditis, 421.0, 38.93 (I33.0, 05H533Z).

EXERCISE 15-7

Assign codes to the following conditions.

1. Patient is admitted for a diagnostic left cardiac catheterization with a diagnosis of chest pain _____

2. Patient is admitted with a diagnosis of CAD for a PTCA with CYPHER stent insertion into the LAD _____

3. Patient is admitted 3 days status post angioplasty with restenosis of a stent; a non–drug-eluting stent is inserted into the RCA _____

4. Patient with CAD is admitted, and a bypass of four coronary arteries is performed; bypass grafts were performed with use of the left internal mammary to the LAD, and saphenous vein grafts were used to bypass PDA, circumflex, and obtuse marginal _____

5. Patient is admitted with ventricular fibrillation, and RF ablation is performed _____

6. Patient is admitted with bradycardia, and a complete dual-chamber pacemaker system is inserted _____

7. Patient is admitted for a pacemaker battery change for the end of life of the battery _____

8. Patient with CHF is admitted for total biventricular pacing with internal cardiac defibrillation _____

9. Patient is admitted with cerebral aneurysm, and a clipping is performed _____

10. Patient with a tachyarrhythmia has a total AICD placed _____

DOCUMENTATION/REIMBURSEMENT/MS-DRGS

Often, documentation difficulties are due to lack of documentation. Sometimes pathology and other test results are not available at the time of discharge or when the physician is dictating the discharge summary or is reporting the final diagnoses.

Frequently missed complications/comorbidities from this chapter include:

- Prinzmetal angina
- Cardiac arrest
- Cardiomyopathy
- Cor pulmonale
- Hypertensive heart and kidney disease
- Ventricular fibrillation
- Atrial flutter
- Myocardial infarction
- Coronary ischemia, acute
- Phlebitis
- Paroxysmal supraventicular tachycardia
- Cardiogenic shock

MS-DRG With and Without MCC/CC

EXAMPLE Patient was admitted with subendocardial MI; patient also was treated for acidosis, 410.71, 276.2 (I21.4, E87.2).

DIAGNOSES	CODES	MS-DRG	RW
Acute subendocardial MI	410.71 (I21.4)	282	0.8064
Acute subendocardial MI with acidosis	410.71 (I21.4) 276.2 (E87.2)	281	1.192

Coronary Artery Disease/Unstable Angina/Chest Pain

It is important to note that on several occasions *Coding Clinic* has addressed the issue of CAD and angina. Per *Coding Clinic* (1997:2Q:p13),[25] if angina and CAD have been previously linked, it is appropriate to sequence CAD as the principal diagnosis. Likewise, if a patient has had a previous CABG and then presents with USA (unstable angina), the principal diagnosis would again be CAD (*Coding Clinic* [2001:3Q:p15][26]). If a patient presents with USA and a cardiac catheterization is performed that determines that the patient has CAD that is causing the angina, then the principal diagnosis would once again be CAD. In other words, the underlying cause or CAD would always be the principal diagnosis if it has been determined in the current visit or in previous visits to be the cause of angina. These above stated rules do NOT apply to chest pain. Also of note, *Coding Clinic* (1993:1Q:p25)[27] advises that when a patient presents with chest pain due to cocaine intoxication, the poisoning code is the principal diagnosis.

EXAMPLE

DIAGNOSES	CODES	MS-DRG	RW
Chest pain with or without complication/comorbidity	786.59 (R07.89)	313	0.5499
Unstable angina	411.1 (I120.0)	311	0.5070
Unstable angina With left heart cath	411.1 (I120.0) 37.22 (4A023N7)	287	1.0879
CAD without complication/comorbidity	414.01 (I25.10)	303	0.5830
CAD with left heart cath	414.01 (I25.10) 37.22 (4A023N7)	287	1.0879

EXAMPLE Patient presents to the hospital complaining of chest pain. The patient is admitted to the coronary care unit (CCU), and cardiology performs a cardiac cath. The left heart cath determines that the patient does not have coronary artery disease. The principal diagnosis in this case is noncardiac chest pain, 786.59, with 37.22, 88.53, 88.56 (R07.89, 4A023N7, B211YZZ, B215YZZ).

EXAMPLE Patient presents to the hospital with chest pain. The emergency physician determines that the patient has unstable angina. The patient is admitted to the CCU, and cardiology performs a left heart cath. The cath determines that the patient has severe coronary artery disease. The principal diagnosis in this case is 414.01 for CAD; a secondary diagnosis is 411.1 for unstable angina, 37.22, 88.53, 88.56 for left cardiac catheterization (I25.110, 4A023N7, B211YZZ, B215YZZ).

Pacemakers/ICDs/Cardioverter/Defibrillators

Insertion of pacemakers, as mentioned earlier in the chapter, will require two codes more often than not. One code will be assigned for insertion of the generator and the other for insertion of the leads. As illustrated below, if the leads are not coded, the payment would be significantly lower.

EXAMPLE

DIAGNOSES/PROCEDURES	CODES	MS-DRG	RW
Sick sinus syndrome (SSS) with insertion of dual chamber pacemaker (coded only the device, not the leads)	427.81 (I49.5) 37.83 (0JH63P2)	310	0.5709
SSS with insertion of dual chamber pacemaker (both leads and device) generator inserted chest subcutaneous via percutaneous approach with leads in right atrium and right ventricle	427.81 (I49.5) 37.83, 37.72 (0JH63P2, 02H63MA, 02HK3MA, 02HX3MZ)	244	2.0398

EXAMPLE

DIAGNOSES/PROCEDURES	CODES	MS-DRG	RW
SSS with insertion of total biventricular pacemaker CRT-P generator inserted into chest subcutaneous via percutaneous approach with a lead in the right atrium and right ventricle	427.81 (I49.5) 00.50 (0JH63P3, 02HK3MA, 02H63MA)	244	2.0398
SSS with insertion of total biventricular defibrillator CRT-D generator inserted into chest subcutaneous via percutaneous approach with 3 leads: one in right atrium, one in left ventricle, and one in coronary sinus vein	427.81 (I49.5) 00.51 (0JH63P5, 02H63ME, 02H43ME, 02HL3ME)	227	5.1936

CHAPTER REVIEW EXERCISE

Assign codes for all diagnoses and procedures including all applicable V/Z codes and external cause codes.

1. Patient has atrial fibrillation with rapid ventricular response _____

2. Patient had a previous CVA and now has left hemiparesis _____

3. Patient has orthostatic hypotension _____

4. Patient has mitral and tricuspid insufficiency _____

5. Patient has congestive heart failure, rheumatic _____

6. Patient has both acute and chronic renal failure and a history of hypertension; patient is currently taking verapamil and is on dialysis _____

7. Patient has congestive heart failure with pleural effusion and hypertension _____

8. Patient has chest pain and elevated troponins _____

9. Patient presents with a non–Q wave myocardial infarction (NQMI), is taken to the cath lab for a left heart cath, and has a drug-eluting stent inserted in RCA for coronary artery disease _____

10. Patient with a previous CABG presents to the hospital with USA _____

11. Patient with ACS presents to the hospital; patient is taken to the cath lab and following a left cardiac cath and diagnosis of CAD, the patient was immediately taken to surgery, where a 2-vessel CABG is performed _____

12. Patient has a left anterior fascicular block _____

13. Patient is admitted through the ER with chest pain that is determined to be coronary artery disease following a left heart cath. Following the cath procedure, the patient dies of cardiac arrest _____

14. Patient has congestive systolic and diastolic heart failure _____

15. Patient presents to the hospital with pulmonary edema and a history of hypertensive congestive heart failure for which the patient currently takes Lasix and verapamil _____

16. Patient is admitted for a stroke with left-side weakness and dysphagia. Upon discharge the weakness has resolved _____

17. Patient has a history of stroke and is currently admitted with atrial fibrillation and dysphagia due to the old stroke _____

18. Patient has arteriosclerosis of the extremities and is admitted with an ulcer and gangrene of the foot _____

19. Patient is admitted to the hospital with deep vein thrombosis and a pulmonary embolism _____

20. History of heart valve replaced with porcine valve _____

21. Patient had a left heart catheterization, a left ventriculography, and a single-catheter coronary arteriography to determine the cause of chest pain _____

22. Patient had an angioplasty with atherectomy of the right coronary artery for CAD _____

23. Patient with CAD had a coronary bypass times two using one saphenous vein and one internal mammary; the cardiac bypass pump was used _____

24. Patient had a complete pacemaker inserted for syncope, which was attributed to bradycardia _____

25. Patient had congestive heart failure and was treated with CRT _____

26. Patient had an abdominal aortic aneurysm (AAA) and was treated with endovascular repair _____

27. Patient was admitted with endocarditis and had a Hickman catheter inserted for antibiotic administration _____

Write the correct answer in the space provided.

28. Which MS-DRG is better reimbursed—the one for CAD or for USA? _____

CHAPTER GLOSSARY

Ablation: correction of abnormal heart rhythm by burning of abnormal heart tissue through radiofrequency or other methods such as laser, microwave, or freezing.

Aneurysm: bulging or ballooning out of a vessel.

Angioplasty: a procedure performed to treat coronary artery disease. An inflated balloon compresses plaque against artery walls.

Aphasia: impairment of speech expression and/or word understanding.

Atherosclerosis: type of arteriosclerosis wherein fatty substances such as plaque block or clog the arteries.

Blood pressure: the force that blood puts on the arterial walls when the heart beats.

BNP: (brain natriuretic peptide) a hormone that is produced by the heart; a BNP test measures the amount of BNP that is found in the heart.

Bradycardia: slow heart rate, generally fewer than 60 beats per minute.

Capillaries: smallest blood vessel through which material passes to and from the bloodstream.

Cardiac arrest: sudden loss of heart function.

Cardiomyopathy: a disorder of the muscles of the heart chambers that impedes heart function.

Cognitive deficit: disorder in thinking, learning, awareness, or judgment.

Conduction disorder: abnormalities of cardiac impulses.

Coronary artery bypass graft: surgery performed to bypass an occluded coronary artery.

Deep vein thrombosis: a blood clot that forms in a deep vein.

Dissection: a tear in wall of a vessel.

Electrophysiologist: physician trained in electrical disorders of the heart.

Embolus: clot that travels to another part of the body.

Endocarditis: inflammation of the lining of the heart chambers and valves.

Fistula: an abnormal passage between an artery and a vein.

Heart failure: impaired function of the heart's pumping ability.

Malignant hypertension: rapidly rising blood pressure, usually in excess of 140 mm Hg diastolic with findings of visual impairment and symptoms or signs of progressive cardiac failure.

Myocardial infarction: heart attack.

NSTEMI: non–ST elevation myocardial infarction.

Pericarditis: inflammation of the covering of the heart.

Phlebitis: inflammation of a vein.

Pulmonary embolism: a blood clot(s) in the pulmonary artery that causes blockage in the artery.

Pulmonary hypertension: high blood pressure in the arteries that supply blood to the lungs.

Stasis dermatitis: skin condition due to poor circulation (venous insufficiency) that is characterized by swelling, skin discoloration, weeping, itching, and scaly skin.

STEMI: ST elevation myocardial infarction.

Stenosis: abnormal narrowing.

Stroke: cerebrovascular accident or brain infarction.

Tachycardia: fast heart rate, generally greater than 100 beats per minute.

Thoracentesis: puncture of the chest wall to remove fluid (pleural effusion) from the space between the lining of the outside of the lungs (pleura) and the wall of the chest.

Thrombus: a blood clot that forms and remains in a vein.

Transient ischemic attack: a stroke that lasts for only a few minutes.

Varicose veins: enlarged, twisted veins that usually occur in the legs.

REFERENCES

1. American Hospital Association. *Coding Clinic for ICD-9-CM* 1984:July-Aug:p12. Benign and malignant hypertension—Guidelines.
2. American Hospital Association. *Coding Clinic for ICD-9-CM* 1990:3Q:p4. Blood pressure, elevated.
3. American Hospital Association. *Coding Clinic for ICD-9-CM* 2003:1Q:p20-21. Renal failure due to diabetic nephropathy in patient with hypertension.
4. American Hospital Association. *Coding Clinic for ICD-9-CM* 2001:2Q:p7-8. Aborted myocardial infarction.
5. American Hospital Association. *Coding Clinic for ICD-9-CM* 1997:3Q:p15. Clarification—Coronary artery disease of unspecified type of vessel.
6. American Hospital Association. *Coding Clinic for ICD-9-CM* 1990:2Q:p19. Congestive cardiomyopathy and CHF.
7. American Hospital Association. *Coding Clinic for ICD-9-CM* 2008:1Q:p14. Sustained and nonsustained ventricular tachycardia.
8. From Frazier ME, Drzymkowski JW. Essentials of Human Diseases and Conditions, 3rd ed. St. Louis, Saunders, 2004, Table 10-1, pp 457-459.
9. American Hospital Association. *Coding Clinic for ICD-9-CM* 1988:2Q:p8. Cardiac arrest.
10. American Hospital Association. *Coding Clinic for ICD-9-CM* 2008:3Q:p12. Chronic diastolic congestive heart failure.
11. American Hospital Association. *Coding Clinic for ICD-9-CM* 2002:4Q:p52-55. CHF due to diastolic dysfunction due to hypertension.
12. American Hospital Association. *Coding Clinic for ICD-9-CM* 2000:2Q:p16-17. Heart failure.
13. American Hospital Association. *Coding Clinic for ICD-9-CM* 1995:1Q:p6. Rheumatic congestive heart failure.

14. American Hospital Association. *Coding Clinic for ICD-9-CM* 1991:3Q:p19. Pleural effusion w/ congestive heart failure.

15. American Hospital Association. *Coding Clinic for ICD-9-CM* 2010:3Q:p5-6. Hemorrhagic conversion of cerebral infarction.

16. American Hospital Association. *Coding Clinic for ICD-9-CM* 2007:1Q:p23-24. Aborted cerebrovascular accident (CVA).

17. American Hospital Association. *Coding Clinic for ICD-9-CM* 1995:2Q:p14. Clarification—Explanation of fifth digits for categories 433 and 434.

18. American Hospital Association. *Coding Clinic for ICD-9-CM* 2006:1Q:p17. Clarification—Bilateral carotid artery stenosis.

19. American Hospital Association. *Coding Clinic for ICD-9-CM* 1993:4Q:p27-28. Athcrosclerotic peripheral vascular disease—Guidelines.

20. American Hospital Association. *Coding Clinic for ICD-9-CM* 1992:1Q:p15-16. Clarification—Thrombosis with thrombophlebitis.

21. American Hospital Association. *Coding Clinic for ICD-9-CM* 1997:3Q:p14. Clarification—Coronary artery bypass.

22. American Hospital Association. *Coding Clinic for ICD-9-CM* 1995:1Q:p5-6. Auxiliary procedures to heart surgery—Guidelines.

23. American Hospital Association. *Coding Clinic for ICD-9-CM* 2002:4Q:p100. Implantation of biventricular defibrillator.

24. American Hospital Association. *Coding Clinic for ICD-9-CM* 2008:2Q:p14. Poor IV access.

25. American Hospital Association. *Coding Clinic for ICD-9-CM* 1997:2Q:p13. Clarification—Unstable angina and coronary artery disease.

26. American Hospital Association. *Coding Clinic for ICD-9-CM* 2001:3Q:p15. Unstable angina status post CABG.

27. American Hospital Association. *Coding Clinic for ICD-9-CM* 1993:1Q:p25. Cocaine intoxication with chest pain.

16

Diseases of the Respiratory System

(ICD-9-CM Chapter 8, Codes 460-519, and ICD-10-CM Chapter 10, Codes J00-J99)

CHAPTER OUTLINE

ICD-9-CM Official Guidelines for Coding and Reporting
ICD-10-CM Official Guidelines for Coding and Reporting
Guideline Differences Between ICD-9-CM and ICD-10-CM
Major Differences Between ICD-9-CM and ICD-10-CM Guidelines
Anatomy and Physiology
Disease Conditions
    Acute Respiratory Infections and Other Diseases of the Upper Respiratory Tract
    Pneumonia and Influenza
    Chronic Obstructive Pulmonary Disease and Allied Conditions
    Pneumoconioses and Other Lung Diseases Due to External Agents
    Other Diseases of the Respiratory System
Factors Influencing Health Status and Contact with Health Services (V Codes/Z Codes)
Common Treatments
Procedures
    Mechanical Ventilation
    Noninvasive Ventilation
    Bronchoscopy
    Thoracentesis
    Thoracostomy
    Tracheostomy
    Pulmonary Resection
Documentation/Reimbursement/MS-DRGs
    Pneumonia and Causative Organism
    Two Diagnoses That Equally Meet the Definition for Principal Diagnosis
    MS-DRG With and Without MCC/CC
    Respiratory Failure Versus Another Acute Condition
Chapter Review Exercise
Chapter Glossary
References

LEARNING OBJECTIVES

1. Apply and assign the correct ICD-9-CM and ICD-10-CM codes in accordance with Official Guidelines for Coding and Reporting.
2. Identify major differences between ICD-9-CM and ICD-10-CM related to the respiratory system
3. Identify pertinent anatomy and physiology of the respiratory system
4. Identify diseases of the respiratory system

5. Assign the correct V/Z codes and procedure codes related to the respiratory system
6. Identify common treatments, medications, laboratory values, and diagnostic tests
7. Explain the importance of documentation in relation to MS-DRGs for reimbursement

ABBREVIATIONS/ ACRONYMS

ABG arterial blood gas

AIDS acquired immunodeficiency syndrome

AMI acute myocardial infarction

BAL bronchoalveolar lavage

BIPAP bilevel positive airway pressure

CAP community-acquired pneumonia

CC complication/comorbidity

CHF congestive heart failure

COPD chronic obstructive pulmonary disease

CPAP continuous positive airway pressure

CVA cerebrovascular accident

E. coli *Escherichia coli*

ER Emergency Room

GERD gastroesophageal reflux disease

H. flu *Haemophilus influenzae*

HIV human immunodeficiency virus

ICD-9-CM *International Classification of Diseases, 9th Revision, Clinical Modification*

ICD-10-CM *International Classification of Diseases, 10th Revision, Clinical Modification*

ICD-10-PCS *International Classification of Diseases, 10th Revision, Procedure Coding System*

IPPV intermittent positive pressure ventilation

IV intravenous

LLL left lower lobe

MS-DRG Medicare Severity diagnosis-related group

NEC not elsewhere classifiable

NOS not otherwise specified

NPPV noninvasive positive pressure ventilation

O₂ oxygen

OIG Office of the Inspector General

OR Operating Room

Paco₂ partial pressure of carbon dioxide in arterial blood

Pao₂ partial pressure of oxygen in arterial blood

PCP *Pneumocystis carinii* pneumonia

RAD reactive airway disease

RSV respiratory syncytial virus

RUL right upper lobe

RW relative weight

STAPH aureus *Staphylococcus aureus*

TRALI transfusion-related acute lung injury

VATS video-assisted thoracic surgery

ICD-9-CM

Official Guidelines for Coding and Reporting

Please refer to the companion Evolve website for the most current guidelines.

8. Chapter 8: Diseases of Respiratory System (460-519)
   See I.C.17.f. for ventilator-associated pneumonia.
   a. Chronic Obstructive Pulmonary Disease [COPD] and Asthma
      1) Conditions that comprise COPD and Asthma
         The conditions that comprise COPD are obstructive chronic bronchitis, subcategory 491.2, and emphysema, category 492. All asthma codes are under category 493, Asthma. Code 496, Chronic airway obstruction, not elsewhere classified, is a nonspecific code that should only be used when the documentation in a medical record does not specify the type of COPD being treated.
      2) Acute exacerbation of chronic obstructive bronchitis and asthma
         The codes for chronic obstructive bronchitis and asthma distinguish between uncomplicated cases and those in acute exacerbation. An acute exacerbation is a worsening or a decompensation of a chronic condition. An acute exacerbation is not equivalent to an infection superimposed on a chronic condition, though an exacerbation may be triggered by an infection.
      3) Overlapping nature of the conditions that comprise COPD and asthma
         Due to the overlapping nature of the conditions that make up COPD and asthma, there are many variations in the way these conditions are documented. Code selection must be based on the terms as documented. When selecting the correct code for the documented type of COPD and asthma, it is essential to first review the index, and then verify the code in the tabular list. There are many instructional notes under the different COPD subcategories and codes. It is important that all such notes be reviewed to assure correct code assignment.

4) Acute exacerbation of asthma and status asthmaticus

An acute exacerbation of asthma is an increased severity of the asthma symptoms, such as wheezing and shortness of breath. Status asthmaticus refers to a patient's failure to respond to therapy administered during an asthmatic episode and is a life threatening complication that requires emergency care. If status asthmaticus is documented by the provider with any type of COPD or with acute bronchitis, the status asthmaticus should be sequenced first. It supersedes any type of COPD including that with acute exacerbation or acute bronchitis. It is inappropriate to assign an asthma code with 5th digit 2, with acute exacerbation, together with an asthma code with 5th digit 1, with status asthmatics. Only the 5th digit 1 should be assigned. (See Figure 16-1.)

b. Chronic Obstructive Pulmonary Disease [COPD] and Bronchitis

1) Acute bronchitis with COPD

Acute bronchitis, code 466.0, is due to an infectious organism. When acute bronchitis is documented with COPD, code 491.22, Obstructive chronic bronchitis with acute bronchitis, should be assigned. It is not necessary to also assign code 466.0. If a medical record documents acute bronchitis with COPD with acute exacerbation, only code 491.22 should be assigned. The acute bronchitis included in code 491.22 supersedes the acute exacerbation. If a medical record documents COPD with acute exacerbation without mention of acute bronchitis, only code 491.21 should be assigned.

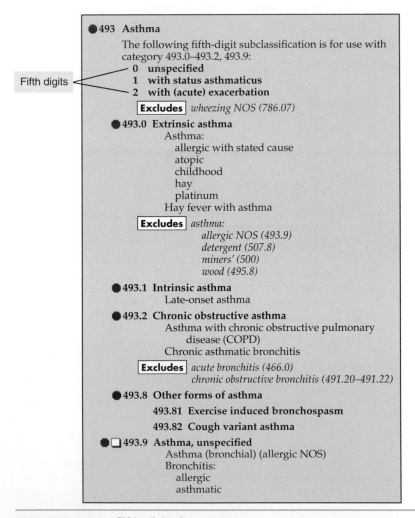

FIGURE 16-1. Fifth digits for asthma.

c. Acute Respiratory Failure

1) Acute respiratory failure as principal diagnosis

Code 518.81, Acute respiratory failure, may be assigned as a principal diagnosis when it is the condition established after study to be chiefly responsible for occasioning the admission to the hospital, and the selection is supported by the Alphabetic Index and Tabular List. However, chapter-specific coding guidelines (such as obstetrics, poisoning, HIV, newborn) that provide sequencing direction take precedence.

EXAMPLE

The patient presented to the ER in acute respiratory failure and was intubated and admitted to ICU. Following admission, the patient was started on antibiotics for pneumonia. The patient was on mechanical ventilation for 24 hours. 518.81, 486, 96.71, 96.04 (J96.00, J18.9, 5A1945Z, 0BH17EZ).

(Per guidelines, if respiratory failure and another acute condition are equally responsible for occasioning the admission, the guidelines regarding two or more diagnoses that equally meet the definition for principal diagnoses may be applied.)

2) Acute respiratory failure as secondary diagnosis

Respiratory failure may be listed as a secondary diagnosis if it occurs after admission, or if it is present on admission, but does not meet the definition of principal diagnosis.

EXAMPLE

The patient was admitted from the clinic for IV antibiotics for pneumonia. A couple of hours after admission, the patient's condition deteriorated and acute respiratory failure developed, 486, 518.81 (J18.9, J96.00).

3) Sequencing of acute respiratory failure and another acute condition

When a patient is admitted with respiratory failure and another acute condition, (e.g., myocardial infarction, cerebrovascular accident, aspiration pneumonia), the principal diagnosis will not be the same in every situation. This applies whether the other acute condition is a respiratory or nonrespiratory condition. Selection of the principal diagnosis will be dependent on the circumstances of admission. If both the respiratory failure and the other acute condition are equally responsible for occasioning the admission to the hospital, and there are no chapter-specific sequencing rules, the guideline regarding two or more diagnoses that equally meet the definition for principal diagnosis (*Section II, C.*) may be applied in these situations.

If the documentation is not clear as to whether acute respiratory failure and another condition are equally responsible for occasioning the admission, query the provider for clarification.

EXAMPLE

Patient was admitted to the hospital in acute respiratory failure due to congestive heart failure. The patient was intubated and placed on mechanical ventilation for 2 days. The patient responded well to IV diuretics, 518.81, 428.0, 96.71, 96.04 (J96.00, I50.9, 5A1945Z, 0BH17EZ).

d. Influenza due to certain identified viruses

Code only confirmed cases of avian influenza (codes 488.**01-488.02, 488.09**, Influenza due to identified avian influenza virus) or novel H1N1 influenza virus (H1N1 or swine flu, code 488.**11-488.12, 488.19**). This is an exception to the hospital inpatient guideline Section II, H. (Uncertain Diagnosis).

In this context, "confirmation" does not require documentation of positive laboratory testing specific for avian or novel H1N1 influenza. However, coding should be based on the provider's diagnostic statement that the patient has avian or novel H1N1 (H1N1 or swine flu) influenza.

If the provider records "suspected or possible or probable avian or novel H1N1 influenza (H1N1 or swine flu)," the appropriate influenza code from category 487 should be assigned. A code from category 488, Influenza due to certain identified influenza viruses, should not be assigned.

EXAMPLE

Patient was admitted with a confirmed case of avian influenza, 488.02 (J09.02).

EXAMPLE

Patient was admitted with possible H1N1 influenza, 487.1 (J11.1).

Apply the General Coding Guidelines as found in Chapter 5 and the Procedural Guidelines as found in Chapter 6.

ICD-10-CM

Official Guidelines for Coding and Reporting

Please refer to the companion Evolve website for the most current guidelines.

10. Chapter 10: Diseases of Respiratory System (J00-J99)

a. Chronic Obstructive Pulmonary Disease [COPD] and Asthma

1) Acute exacerbation of chronic obstructive bronchitis and asthma

The codes in categories J44 and J45 distinguish between uncomplicated cases and those in acute exacerbation. An acute exacerbation is a worsening or a decompensation of a chronic condition. An acute exacerbation is not equivalent to an infection superimposed on a chronic condition, though an exacerbation may be triggered by an infection.

b. Acute Respiratory Failure

1) Acute respiratory failure as principal diagnosis

A code from subcategory J96.0, Acute respiratory failure, or **subcategory** J96.2, Acute and chronic respiratory failure, may be assigned as a principal diagnosis when it is the condition established after study to be chiefly responsible for occasioning the admission to the hospital, and the selection is supported by the Alphabetic Index and Tabular List. However, chapter-specific coding guidelines (such as obstetrics, poisoning, HIV, newborn) that provide sequencing direction take precedence.

2) Acute respiratory failure as secondary diagnosis

Respiratory failure may be listed as a secondary diagnosis if it occurs after admission, or if it is present on admission, but does not meet the definition of principal diagnosis.

3) Sequencing of acute respiratory failure and another acute condition

When a patient is admitted with respiratory failure and another acute condition, (e.g., myocardial infarction, cerebrovascular accident, aspiration pneumonia), the principal diagnosis will not be the same in every situation. This applies whether the other acute condition is a respiratory or nonrespiratory condition. Selection of the principal diagnosis will be dependent on the circumstances of admission. If both the respiratory failure and the other acute condition are equally responsible for occasioning the admission to the hospital, and there are no chapter-specific sequencing rules, the guideline regarding two or more diagnoses that equally meet the definition for principal diagnosis *(Section II, C.)* may be applied in these situations.

If the documentation is not clear as to whether acute respiratory failure and another condition are equally responsible for occasioning the admission, query the provider for clarification.

c. Influenza due to *certain identified influenza* influenza *viruses*

Code only confirmed cases of avian influenza (code J09.0-, Influenza due to identified avian influenza virus) or novel H1N1 or swine flu, code J09.1-. This is an exception to the hospital inpatient guideline Section II, H. (Uncertain Diagnosis).

In this context, "confirmation" does not require documentation of positive laboratory testing specific for avian or novel H1N1 (H1N1 or swine flu) influenza. However, coding should be based on the provider's diagnostic statement that the patient has avian influenza.

If the provider records "suspected or possible or probable avian influenza," the appropriate influenza code from category J11, Influenza due to **unspecified** influenza virus, should be assigned. A code from category J09, Influenza due to certain identified influenza viruses, should not be assigned.

d. *Ventilator associated Pneumonia*

  1) **Documentation of Ventilator associated Pneumonia**
  As with all procedural or postprocedural complications, code assignment is based on the provider's documentation of the relationship between the condition and the procedure.

  Code J95.851, Ventilator associated pneumonia, should be assigned only when the provider has documented ventilator associated pneumonia (VAP). An additional code to identify the organism (e.g., Pseudomonas aeruginosa, code B96.5) should also be assigned. Do not assign an additional code from categories J12-J18 to identify the type of pneumonia.

  Code J95.851 should not be assigned for cases where the patient has pneumonia and is on a mechanical ventilator but the provider has not specifically stated that the pneumonia is ventilator-associated pneumonia. If the documentation is unclear as to whether the patient has a pneumonia that is a complication attributable to the mechanical ventilator, query the provider.

  2) **Ventilator associated Pneumonia Develops after Admission**
  A patient may be admitted with one type of pneumonia (e.g., code J13, Pneumonia due to Streptococcus pneumonia) and subsequently develop VAP. In this instance, the principal diagnosis would be the appropriate code from categories J12-J18 for the pneumonia diagnosed at the time of admission. Code J95.851, Ventilator associated pneumonia, would be assigned as an additional diagnosis when the provider has also documented the presence of ventilator associated pneumonia.

Apply the General Coding Guidelines as found in Chapter 5 and the Procedural Guidelines as found in Chapter 7.

GUIDELINE DIFFERENCES BETWEEN ICD-9-CM AND ICD-10-CM GUIDELINES

There are fewer guidelines in ICD-10-CM related to the coding of COPD.

MAJOR DIFFERENCES BETWEEN ICD-9-CM AND ICD-10-CM GUIDELINES

- ICD-10-CM uses codes that identify acute recurrent sinusitis to the individual sinuses.
- In ICD-9-CM, asthma is coded by specific type (e.g., extrinsic, intrinsic, chronic obstructive, or unspecified) and by whether the condition is exacerbated or status asthmaticus is present. ICD-10-CM divides asthma into the following subcategories:
  - Mild intermittent asthma
  - Mild persistent asthma
  - Moderate persistent asthma
  - Severe persistent asthma
  - Other and unspecified asthma
- Under code category J44, Other chronic obstructive pulmonary disease, there is an instructional notation to code also the type of asthma if applicable (J45.-). In ICD-9-CM, asthma associated with COPD is only one combination code. In ICD-10-CM, both conditions are assigned codes if the specific type of asthma is documented.
- In ICD-10-CM, an instructional note at the beginning of the chapter states that if a respiratory condition occurs in more than one site, and it is not specifically indexed,

it should be classified to the lower anatomic site, such as tracheobronchitis would be classified to bronchitis.

■ Procedural complications affecting the respiratory system are included in Chapter 10, Diseases of the Respiratory System, of ICD-10-CM. Some of the complications include:
  • Tracheostomy complication
  • Acute pulmonary insufficiency following thoracic surgery
  • Acute pulmonary insufficiency following nonthoracic surgery
  • Postprocedural pneumothorax
  • Postprocedural respiratory failure
  • Intraoperative hemorrhage, hematoma, or accidental laceration
  • Transfusion-related acute lung injury (TRALI)
  • Mechanical complication of respiratory (ventilator)

ANATOMY AND PHYSIOLOGY

The primary function of the **respiratory system** (Figure 16-2) is to supply the body with oxygen (O_2). Respiration occurs through the nose and mouth, bringing oxygen through the larynx and trachea and into the lungs, where oxygen is delivered and carbon dioxide is exhaled. Dome-shaped muscles at the bottom of the lungs, or the **diaphragm**, assist in the process of breathing and in the exchange of oxygen/carbon dioxide. The lungs are the major organ of the respiratory system. The right lung is made up of three lobes; the left lung is smaller and contains two lobes. The **bronchi** are the two air tubes that branch off the trachea and deliver air to both lungs. The **trachea**, or windpipe, is responsible for filtering the air that we breathe.

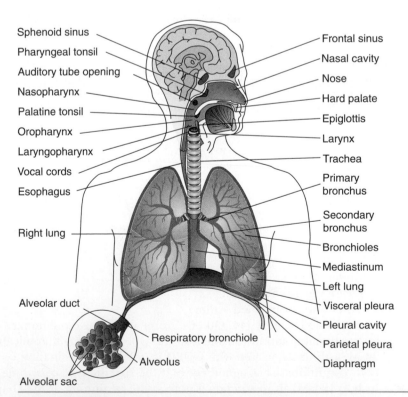

FIGURE 16-2. Anatomy of the respiratory system.

DISEASE CONDITIONS

Diseases of the Respiratory System (460-519), Chapter 8 in the ICD-9-CM code book, is divided into the following categories:

CATEGORY	SECTION TITLES
460-466	Acute Respiratory Infections
470-478	Other Diseases of the Upper Respiratory Tract
480-488	Pneumonia and Influenza
490-496	Chronic Obstructive Pulmonary Disease and Allied Conditions
500-508	Pneumoconioses and Other Lung Disease Due to External Agents
510-519	Other Disease of Respiratory System

Diseases of the Respiratory System, Chapter 10 in the ICD-10-CM code book, are divided into the following categories:

CATEGORY	SECTION TITLES
J00-J06	Acute Upper Respiratory Infections
J09-J18	Influenza and Pneumonia
J20-J22	Other Acute Lower Respiratory Infections
J30-J39	Other Diseases of Upper Respiratory Tract
J40-J47	Chronic Lower Respiratory Diseases
J60-J70	Lung Diseases Due to External Agents
J80-J84	Other Respiratory Diseases Principally Affecting the Interstitium
J85-J86	Suppurative and Necrotic Conditions of the Lower Respiratory Tract
J90-J94	Other Diseases of the Pleura
J95	Intraoperative and Postprocedural Complications and Disorders of Respiratory System, Not Elsewhere Classified
J96-J99	Other Diseases of the Respiratory System

At the very beginning of Chapter 8 is an instruction to use an additional code to identify the infectious organism (Figure 16-3). In the Respiratory chapter, some codes are provided that do include the organisms. When the organism is included, it is not necessary to assign an additional code.

EXAMPLE Pneumonia due to respiratory syncytial virus, 480.1 (J12.1).

This is a combination code that includes the disease process, pneumonia, and the causative organism, respiratory syncytial virus (RSV). No additional code is necessary to identify the organism.

EXAMPLE Acute laryngitis due to *Haemophilus influenzae*, 464.00, 041.5 (J04.0, B96.3).

In this case, laryngitis is due to *Haemophilus influenzae* bacteria *(H flu)*. The code for acute laryngitis, 464.0 (J04.0) makes no mention of the causative bacteria; therefore, code 041.5 (B96.3) is assigned as an additional code to identify the bacteria.

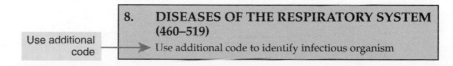

FIGURE 16-3. Instruction to use additional code to identify infectious organism.

Acute Respiratory Infections and Other Diseases of the Upper Respiratory Tract

Infection is invasion of the body by organisms that have the potential to cause disease. This section deals with infections of the upper respiratory tract and the bronchus. It must be noted that diseases in this section are identified as acute infections. It is possible that an acute infection may be superimposed upon a chronic infection or inflammation. Following general guidelines, "If the same condition is described as both acute (subacute) and chronic, and separate subentries exist in the Alphabetic Index at the same indentation level, code both and sequence the acute (subacute) code first" (Figure 16-4).

EXAMPLE   Acute and chronic bronchitis, 466.0, 491.9 (J20.9, J42).

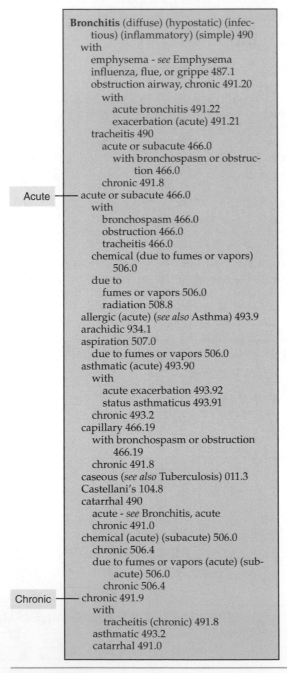

```
Bronchitis (diffuse) (hypostatic) (infec-
    tious) (inflammatory) (simple) 490
  with
      emphysema - see Emphysema
      influenza, flue, or grippe 487.1
      obstruction airway, chronic 491.20
          with
              acute bronchitis 491.22
              exacerbation (acute) 491.21
      tracheitis 490
          acute or subacute 466.0
              with bronchospasm or obstruc-
                  tion 466.0
          chronic 491.8
  acute or subacute 466.0
      with
          bronchospasm 466.0
          obstruction 466.0
          tracheitis 466.0
      chemical (due to fumes or vapors)
          506.0
      due to
          fumes or vapors 506.0
          radiation 508.8
  allergic (acute) (see also Asthma) 493.9
  arachidic 934.1
  aspiration 507.0
      due to fumes or vapors 506.0
  asthmatic (acute) 493.90
      with
          acute exacerbation 493.92
          status asthmaticus 493.91
      chronic 493.2
  capillary 466.19
      with bronchospasm or obstruction
          466.19
      chronic 491.8
  caseous (see also Tuberculosis) 011.3
  Castellani's 104.8
  catarrhal 490
      acute - see Bronchitis, acute
      chronic 491.0
  chemical (acute) (subacute) 506.0
      chronic 506.4
      due to fumes or vapors (acute) (sub-
          acute) 506.0
          chronic 506.4
  chronic 491.9
      with
          tracheitis (chronic) 491.8
      asthmatic 493.2
      catarrhal 491.0
```

Acute — acute or subacute 466.0

Chronic — chronic 491.9

FIGURE 16-4. Alphabetic Index for acute and chronic bronchitis.

Acute **sinusitis** occurs when the linings of one or more sinuses become infected, usually because of viruses or bacteria. Sinuses may swell, causing an obstruction and interfering with the normal drainage of mucus. This may occur as the result of a cold. Sinusitis can cause considerable discomfort and may lead to more serious infection.

EXAMPLE Acute maxillary sinusitis, 461.0 (J01.00).

EXAMPLE Chronic maxillary sinusitis, 473.0 (J32.0).

Acute **bronchitis** is a lower respiratory tract or bronchial tree infection that may be characterized by cough, sputum production, and wheezing. Most cases of acute bronchitis are caused by viruses such as RSV, influenza, and parainfluenza. Bacterial infection with *Mycoplasma pneumoniae*, *Chlamydia pneumoniae*, and *Bordetella pertussis* (whooping cough), particularly in young adults, can lead to acute bronchitis. Bronchitis may progress to pneumonia or may aggravate respiratory symptoms in those who have chronic respiratory conditions.

EXAMPLE Subacute bronchitis with bronchospasm, 466.0 (J20.9).

EXERCISE 16-1

Assign codes to the following conditions.

1. Headache due to acute pansinusitis _____
2. Laryngotracheitis _____
3. Acute streptococcal pharyngitis _____
4. Acute bronchiolitis due to RSV _____
5. Upper respiratory infection _____
6. Acute and chronic maxillary sinusitis _____
7. Deviated nasal septum _____
8. Paralysis, vocal cords, bilateral _____
9. Allergic rhinitis _____
10. Spasm larynx _____

Pneumonia and Influenza

Pneumonia is an infection of the lungs that can be caused by a variety of organisms, including viruses, bacteria, and parasites. Pneumonia frequently follows an upper respiratory infection, and symptoms depend on age and cause of the pneumonia. More than 50 different types of pneumonia have been identified. High-risk individuals include the elderly, the very young, and those with underlying health problems such as chronic obstructive pulmonary disease (COPD), diabetes mellitus, congestive heart failure, asthma, and sickle cell anemia. Those with impaired immune systems as the result of human immunodeficiency virus (HIV)/acquired immunodeficiency syndrome (AIDS), cancer therapy, steroid therapy, or anti-rejection medications are also at risk for developing pneumonia.

Some common symptoms of pneumonia include the following:

- Fever/chills
- Cough
- Chest pain

TABLE 16-1 **COMMON CAUSES OF PNEUMONIA**[2]	
Causative Agents	**Percentage of All Diagnosed Cases**
Bacteria	50
Streptococcus pneumoniae	10
Haemophilus influenzae	5
Staphylococcus aureus	5
Mycobacterium tuberculosis	10
Viruses	
Influenza virus	–
Fungi*	
Aspergillus fumigatus	–
Candida albicans	–
Pneumocystis jiroveci	–
Bacterium-like organisms	
Mycoplasma pneumoniae	10

*Opportunistic infection: rare except in immunosuppressed, debilitated, or terminally ill patients.

- Shortness of breath
- Rapid breathing and heart rate

Community-acquired pneumonia (CAP) is a broad term that is used to refer to pneumonias that are contracted outside of the hospital or nursing home setting. The most common cause of CAP is *Streptococcus pneumoniae*. **Nosocomial pneumonia** refers to a pneumonia that is acquired while the patient is hospitalized. Hospital patients are most susceptible to Gram-negative bacteria and staphylococcal pneumonia. **Nursing home-acquired pneumonia** refers to a pneumonia that is acquired in a nursing home or extended care facility. More than one organism may be responsible for pneumonia. In this case, pneumonia codes would be assigned to identify both types of pneumonia. If this was the reason for the hospital stay, either could be sequenced as the principal diagnosis. See Table 16-1 for other pathogens responsible for pneumonia. Complications of pneumonia include the formation of abscesses, respiratory failure, bacteremia, pleural effusion, empyema, and pneumothorax.

According to *Coding Clinic* (1998:2Q:p3),[1] different types of diagnostic tests may be used as part of a "diagnostic workup" to find the "causative organism" that is responsible for the patient's illness. This could include various cultures, x-rays, other minimally invasive tests, such as bronchoscopy, or a lung biopsy, if necessary. A sputum culture from a healthy person would generally have no growth. A mixture of microorganisms, normally found in or on a patient's body, may be identified in a culture. This does not necessarily mean that this organism is responsible for a particular infection. A physician may document that a particular organism is a **contaminant.** This means that the physician does not believe that this organism is responsible for causing the infection. No code would be assigned for an organism that was described as a contaminant. *Coding Clinic* (1998:2Q:p3)[1] goes on to say that it "is inappropriate for coders to assume a causal organism on the basis of laboratory or radiology" findings alone. All code assignments should be based on the physician's documentation. If the documentation is vague or not available, query the physician to confirm whether the culture findings identify the causative organism or identify a contaminant."

Sometimes, pneumonia may be described as to the lobe that it is located in; for example, right upper lobe (RUL) pneumonia or left lower lobe (LLL) pneumonia. Both of these diagnostic statements are coded to 486, pneumonia, unspecified. The location of the pneumonia should not be misinterpreted to mean **lobar pneumonia**, which is a synonym for pneumococcal pneumonia or pneumonia due to *Streptococcus pneumoniae* pneumonia.

Often, **empiric** treatment (initiation of treatment prior to making a definite diagnosis) with antibiotic will be administered before the organism has been identified or the type of pneumonia determined. For example, patients with HIV may be treated empirically with antibiotics that treat both *Pneumocystis carinii* pneumonia (PCP) and CAP. Once PCP has been ruled out, the treatment and the type of antibiotic used may be modified. Because *Pneumocystis carinii* pneumonia was ruled out, it cannot be coded, even though the condition was treated as such until test results were complete.

EXAMPLE	Pneumonia due to Gram-negative bacteria, 482.83 (J15.6).

EXAMPLE	Bronchopneumonia, 485 (J18.0).

Influenza is a contagious viral infection of the respiratory tract that causes coughing, difficulty breathing, headache, muscle aches, and weakness. Possible complications include pneumonia, encephalitis, bronchitis, and sinus and ear infections. Three types of influenza virus have been identified: Types A, B, and C. Types A and B cause flu epidemics each winter and are the types that may be prevented with a flu shot. Type A is the most common and the most serious. Influenza Type C is a very mild respiratory illness that is not thought to be responsible for epidemics. Code 487.0 (J10.1) has an instructional note to assign an additional code to identify the type of pneumonia.

H1N1 influenza is an influenza virus that is a subtype of influenza A. Because it is a new virus, people may not have any immunity to it. H1N1 influenza poses a greater risk to certain groups of people such as:

- Pregnant women
- Persons who are 6 months to 24 years of age
- Persons who are 25 to 64 years who have health conditions that put them at risk for medical complications due to influenza

Bacterial pneumonia is the most common complication of influenza.

EXAMPLE	Influenza with *Klebsiella* pneumonia, 487.0, 482.0 (J11.08, J15.0)

EXAMPLE	Influenza, Type A, 487.1 (J10.1).

EXERCISE 16-2

Assign codes to the following conditions.

1. Legionnaires' disease _____
2. Pneumonia due to aspergillosis _____
3. Influenza with *Staph aureus* pneumonia _____
4. Viral pneumonia _____
5. *Mycoplasma* pneumonia _____
6. Avian influenza _____
7. Pneumonia due to *E. coli* _____
8. Cough and fever due to pneumonitis _____
9. Community-acquired pneumonia; empiric treatment was started for *Pneumocystis carinii* pneumonia. PCP was ruled out. Patient has AIDS. _____
10. Headache and weakness due to influenza A _____

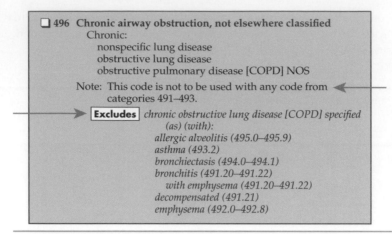

FIGURE 16-5. Note and Excludes note for category 496.

Chronic Obstructive Pulmonary Disease and Allied Conditions

COPD, or **chronic obstructive pulmonary disease,** is a general term that is used to describe a lung disease in which the airways become obstructed, making it difficult for air to get into and out of the lungs. Although cigarette smoking is the most common culprit, other irritants such as pollution, chemicals, or dust can also play a role. Various diseases can be classified as COPD; these include asthmatic bronchitis, chronic bronchitis, and emphysema. All three affect the bronchial tree and result in wheezing, coughing, and shortness of breath. It may be clinically difficult to distinguish among these disorders.

A specific note under category 496, Chronic airway obstruction, not elsewhere classified, instructs as follows: "This code is not to be used with any code from categories 491-493." An Excludes note also assists with proper code assignment (Figure 16-5).

Chronic bronchitis is characterized by a mucus-producing cough most days of the month, 3 months out of a year, for 2 successive years, with no other underlying disease that explains the cough. Smoking cigarettes is the most common cause of chronic bronchitis. Chronic bronchitis often remains untreated because it is thought to be just a "smoker's cough."

Emphysema is a chronic lung disease of gradual onset that can be attributed to chronic infection and inflammation or irritation from cigarette smoke (Figure 16-6).

EXAMPLE Patient was admitted with exacerbation of chronic obstructive bronchitis, 491.21 (J44.1).

Asthma is a disease that affects the airways that carry air into and out of the lungs. Asthma can be controlled to minimize serious symptoms or attacks. Physicians use the terms "asthma" and "reactive airway disease" (RAD) interchangeably.

Asthma is category 493 and the following fifth-digit classifications must be assigned with codes 493.0-493.2, and 493.9:

0   unspecified
1   with status asthmaticus
2   with acute exacerbation

Per *Coding Clinic* (1988:3Q:p9-10),[3] "status asthmaticus can be described with the following terms:

- Intractable asthmatic attack
- Refractory asthma
- Severe, prolonged asthmatic attack
- Airway obstruction (mucous plug) not relieved by bronchodilators
- Severe, intractable wheezing"

FIGURE 16-6. A, Emphysema. **B,** Bullous emphysema with large subpleural bullae. **C,** Emphysematous lung with tumor.

The presence of status asthmaticus should be queried if it is not documented by the physician.

If respiratory failure occurs, it should also be coded, and sequencing would depend on whether respiratory failure was present on admission and meets the criteria for principal diagnosis.

Asthmatic bronchitis refers to an underlying asthmatic problem in patients in whom asthma has become so persistent that clinically significant chronic airflow obstruction is present despite antiasthmatic therapy. Symptoms of chronic bronchitis are generally also present.

EXAMPLE

Patient was admitted in respiratory failure caused by an intractable asthmatic attack, 518.81, 493.91 (J96.90, J45.902).

(Per guidelines, if both the respiratory failure and another acute condition are equally responsible for occasioning the admission, the guidelines regarding two or more diagnoses that equally meet the definition for principal diagnosis may be applied.)

EXAMPLE

Patient was admitted with acute exacerbation of asthmatic bronchitis. The patient went into acute respiratory failure 6 hours after admission, 493.92, 518.81 (J45.901, J96.00).

Category 495 (J67.–), Extrinsic allergic alveolitis, includes conditions that are due to inhalation of organic materials such as grain dust, cotton dust, or animal dander.

EXAMPLE   Patient was diagnosed with farmers' lung, 495.0 (J67.0).

EXERCISE 16-3

Assign codes to the following conditions.

1. Exercise-induced asthma   _____
2. Bronchiectasis   _____
3. Asthma exacerbation with pneumonia   _____
4. Emphysema with chronic bronchitis   _____
5. Ventilation pneumonitis   _____
6. Acute bronchitis with COPD   _____
7. Decompensated COPD   _____
8. Asthma with exacerbation of COPD   _____
9. End-stage COPD with emphysema   _____
10. Mushroom worker's lung   _____

Pneumoconioses and Other Lung Diseases Due to External Agents

Pneumoconioses are lung diseases that are caused by chronic inhalation of inorganic (mineral) dust and are often due to occupational exposure. Examples include **siderosis**, which results from inhalation of iron oxide; **baritosis**, caused by inhalation of barium; **stannosis**, resulting from inhalation of tin particles; **black lung** or **coal workers' pneumoconiosis** (Figure 16-7), caused by inhalation of coal dust; and **asbestosis**, which is caused by inhalation of asbestos.

EXAMPLE   Patient has silicosis, caused by working as a sandblaster for many years, 502 (J62.8).

Aspiration pneumonia is an inflammation of the lungs and bronchial tubes that is due to the aspiration of foreign material (e.g., food, saliva, vomit) into the lung. Disorders that

FIGURE 16-7.   Coal workers' lung shows deposits of carbon particles *(black areas).*

affect normal swallowing include disorders of the esophagus, decreased or absent gag reflex, old age, dental problems, use of sedative drugs, anesthesia, coma, and excessive alcohol consumption. These disorders may cause aspiration.

Per *Coding Clinic* (1991:3Q:p16-17),[4] if both aspiration pneumonia and bacterial pneumonia are present, it is acceptable to assign codes for both.

EXAMPLE   Aspiration pneumonia with superimposed pneumonia due to *Staphylococcus aureus*, 507.0, 482.41 (J69.0, J15.21).
If both were present on admission, either could be sequenced as the principal diagnosis.

Several respiratory conditions can be induced by chemical fumes and vapors. These range from acute conditions such as bronchitis and pneumonitis to chronic respiratory conditions such as emphysema and pulmonary fibrosis. The appropriate E code should also be assigned to identify the cause.

EXAMPLE   Acute pulmonary edema due to smoke inhalation from grass fire, 506.1, E892 (T59.811A, J68.1, X01.1xxA).

EXERCISE 16-4

Assign codes to the following conditions.

1. Aspiration pneumonia; patient has dysphagia due to old CVA   _____
2. Fibrosis due to radiation treatments   _____
3. Black lung disease   _____
4. Pleural effusion due to asbestosis   _____

Other Diseases of the Respiratory System

Pleural Effusion

Pleural effusion is accumulation of fluid in the pleural space caused by trauma or disease. If blood is present in the accumulating fluid, the condition is called **hemothorax**; if pus is present, it is called **empyema**; if chyle (milky fluid consisting of lymph and fat) is present, it is called **chylothorax**. The most common causes of pleural effusion include the following:

- Cardiac: congestive heart failure
- Liver: liver failure
- Kidney: nephrotic syndrome, peritoneal dialysis, uremia
- Lung: infection, pulmonary embolism, pulmonary infarction, cancer (primary lung and metastatic), asbestosis
- Vascular: collagen vascular disease (systemic lupus erythematosus, rheumatoid arthritis)
- Trauma: hemothorax, chylothorax, rupture of the esophagus
- Miscellaneous: pancreatitis, post abdominal or coronary artery bypass graft surgery, and drug reactions

According to *Coding Clinic* (1991:3Q:p19-20),[5] pleural effusion is not usually reported if it appears in conjunction with congestive heart failure because the condition is not separately treated. When the only documentation is a diagnostic x-ray, the coder should not report the condition. However, in certain cases, "special x-rays such as decubitus views are required to confirm the presence of pleural effusion or diagnostic thoracentesis may be performed to identify its etiology. In other cases, it may be necessary to address the effusion by therapeutic thoracentesis or chest tube drainage. In any of these situations, it is acceptable to report pleural effusion as an additional diagnosis since the condition was specifically evaluated or treated, but reporting is not required."

EXAMPLE
EXAMPLE   Hemothorax due to pulmonary embolism, 415.19, 511.89 (I26.99, J94.2).

Pneumothorax

When air enters the pleural space, this is called **pneumothorax**. A pneumothorax may be classified as spontaneous (not caused by trauma), traumatic, or iatrogenic. **Spontaneous pneumothorax** may occur in individuals who have no history of lung disease and often is the result of a ruptured subpleural bleb. **Iatrogenic** pneumothorax is the result of a complication of a diagnostic or therapeutic intervention or procedure. Traumatic pneumothorax occurs as the result of an injury and is assigned an injury code.

EXAMPLE   Spontaneous pneumothorax, no specific cause found, 512.81 (J93.1).

Pulmonary Edema

Pulmonary edema is a condition whereby fluid accumulates in the lungs. In most cases, heart problems are the cause. According to *Coding Clinic* (1988:3Q:p3),[6] the following codes for heart failure include pulmonary edema that is cardiac in origin.

EXAMPLE   Patient admitted with exacerbation of left ventricular heart failure with pulmonary edema confirmed by chest x-ray, 428.1 (I50.1).

Acute Pulmonary Edema of Noncardiac Origin

According to *Coding Clinic* (1988:3Q:p3-4),[7] pulmonary edema is not always related to a cardiac condition. The "noncardiogenic" type of acute pulmonary edema may also be caused by lung disease or related to patient trauma, and it occurs in a variety of conditions. Some of these conditions include the following:

■ Postoperative pulmonary edema that is not caused by left ventricular failure or CHF, both of which are cardiac in nature.

■ Postoperative pulmonary edema specifically caused by fluid overload is reported with 518.4 (J81.0) and 276.69 (E87.7) (Fluid overload).

■ Acute pulmonary edema caused by bacterial pneumonia, or viral pneumonia, is reported with 518.4 (J81.0) unless caused by left ventricular failure or congestive heart failure because the latter conditions are cardiac in nature.

■ Acute pulmonary edema is reported with an additional code when in conjunction with endotoxic shock, uremia, or septicemia.

Respiratory Failure

Respiratory failure is a general term that describes ineffective gas exchange across the lungs by the respiratory system. An arterial blood gas (ABG) measurement may be used to detect the presence of respiratory failure. A partial pressure of oxygen in arterial blood (Pao_2) of less than 60 torr and a partial pressure of carbon dioxide in arterial blood ($Paco_2$) greater than 50 torr indicate respiratory failure.

Some of the most common causes of respiratory failure include the following:

• Obstruction of the airways (chronic bronchitis, emphysema, cystic fibrosis, etc.)

• Weak breathing due to drugs and alcohol, extreme obesity, or sleep apnea

• Muscle weakness from muscular dystrophy, polio, stroke, spinal cord injury, or Lou Gehrig's disease

• Abnormality of lung tissue such as pneumonia, fluid in lungs, lung cancer, pulmonary fibrosis, sarcoidosis, and radiation

• Abnormal chest wall from scoliosis or severe injury to chest wall

Respiratory failure is classified on the basis of acuity. Acute respiratory failure is the result of a sudden, catastrophic event. Chronic respiratory failure is the result of a gradual worsening of respiratory function. Acute on chronic respiratory failure occurs when a patient has chronic respiratory failure that has decompensated or deteriorated.

EXAMPLE Patient presents to the Emergency Room (ER) in acute respiratory failure and is admitted. Following admission, the patient was started on antibiotics for pneumonia, 518.81, 486 (J96.00, J18.9).
(Per guidelines, if both the respiratory failure and another acute condition are equally responsible for occasioning the admission, the guidelines regarding two or more diagnoses that equally meet the definition for principal diagnosis may be applied in these situations.)

EXAMPLE Patient is admitted from the clinic for intravenous (IV) antibiotics for pneumonia. A couple of hours after admission, the patient deteriorated and developed acute respiratory failure, 486, 518.81 (J18.9, J96.00).

EXAMPLE Patient is admitted to the hospital in acute respiratory failure and is found to have suffered a myocardial infarction, 410.91, 518.81, or 518.81, 410.91 (I21.3, J96.00 or J96.00, I21.3).
(Per guidelines, if both the respiratory failure and another acute condition are equally responsible for occasioning the admission, the guidelines regarding two or more diagnoses that equally meet the definition for principal diagnosis may be applied in these situations.)

Lung Involvement in Conditions Classified Elsewhere

Code 516.1 and code category 517 identify conditions that affect the lung that are caused by other diseases. These codes are identified by *italics*, with instructions to "code first underlying disease." Examples of these codes are shown in Figures 16-8 and 16-9.

EXAMPLE Systemic lupus erythematosus that has affected the patient's lungs, 710.0, 517.8 (M32.13).

● 516.1 *Idiopathic pulmonary hemosiderosis*
        Essential brown induration of lung
        → *Code first underlying disease (275.01 - 275.09)*

FIGURE 16-8. Manifestation code for hemosiderosis.

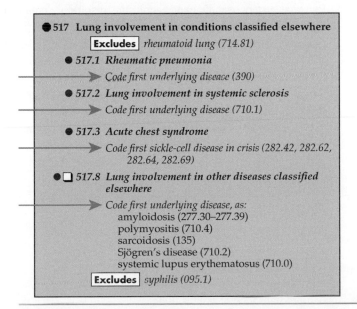

●517 **Lung involvement in conditions classified elsewhere**
      Excludes *rheumatoid lung (714.81)*
  ● 517.1 *Rheumatic pneumonia*
        → *Code first underlying disease (390)*
  ● 517.2 *Lung involvement in systemic sclerosis*
        → *Code first underlying disease (710.1)*

  ● 517.3 *Acute chest syndrome*
        → *Code first sickle-cell disease in crisis (282.42, 282.62, 282.64, 282.69)*
  ●☐ 517.8 *Lung involvement in other diseases classified elsewhere*
        → *Code first underlying disease, as:*
            amyloidosis (277.30–277.39)
            polymyositis (710.4)
            sarcoidosis (135)
            Sjögren's disease (710.2)
            systemic lupus erythematosus (710.0)
      Excludes *syphilis (095.1)*

FIGURE 16-9. Manifestation lung involvement codes for conditions classified elsewhere.

EXERCISE 16-5

Assign codes to the following conditions.

1. Empyema   _____

2. Sickle cell disease with vaso-occlusive crisis with acute   _____
   chest syndrome

3. Tracheal stenosis due to tracheostomy   _____

4. Acute respiratory failure due to pneumonia; patient was   _____
   intubated and was placed on mechanical ventilation for 48
   hours; the respiratory failure developed after admission

5. Asthma with allergic rhinitis   _____

6. Acute respiratory failure due to Lou Gehrig's disease   _____

7. Acute respiratory distress following surgery   _____

8. Acute on chronic respiratory failure in patient with severe   _____
   emphysema; patient is oxygen-dependent

9. Acute pulmonary edema following surgery   _____

10. Respiratory failure due to exacerbation of COPD   _____

FACTORS INFLUENCING HEALTH STATUS AND CONTACT WITH HEALTH SERVICES (V CODES/Z CODES)

In the past, V/Z codes have been considered for use primarily in the outpatient setting. This has changed with the addition of more V/Z codes each year. As was discussed in Chapter 8, it is difficult to locate V/Z codes in the Index. Coders will often say, "I did not know there was a V/Z code for that." Refer to Chapter 8 for a listing of common main terms to locate V/Z codes.

V/Z codes that may be used with diseases of the respiratory system include the following:

V10.11	Personal history of malignant neoplasm—bronchus and lung
V10.12	Personal history of malignant neoplasm—trachea
V10.20	Personal history of malignant neoplasm—respiratory organ, unspecified
V10.21	Personal history of malignant neoplasm—larynx
V10.22	Personal history of malignant neoplasm—nasal cavities, middle ear, and accessory sinuses
V10.29	Personal history of malignant neoplasm—other
V12.60	Personal history—unspecified disease of respiratory system
V12.61	Personal history—pneumonia (recurrent)
V12.69	Personal history—other diseases of the respiratory system
V15.82	History of tobacco use
V15.84	History of exposure to asbestos
V16.1	Family history of malignant neoplasm—trachea, bronchus, and lung
V16.2	Family history of malignant neoplasm—other respiratory and intrathoracic organs
V17.5	Family history of asthma
V17.6	Family history of other chronic respiratory conditions
V42.6	Organ or tissue replaced by transplant—lung
V43.81	Organ or tissue replaced by other means—larynx
V44.0	Artificial opening status—tracheostomy
V45.76	Acquired absence of organ—lung
V46.0	Other dependence on machines—aspirator

V46.11	Other dependence on machines—respirator, status
V46.12	Encounter for respiratory dependence during power failure
V46.13	Encounter for weaning from respirator (ventilator)
V46.14	Mechanical complication of respirator (ventilator)
V46.2	Other dependence on machines—supplemental oxygen
V47.2	Other cardiorespiratory problems
V55.0	Attention to artificial openings—tracheostomy
V57.0	Care involving use of rehabilitation procedures—breathing exercises
V58.44	Aftercare following organ transplant (lung)
V58.74	Aftercare following surgery of the respiratory system, not elsewhere classified (NEC)
V64.42	Thoracoscopic surgical procedure converted to open procedure
V72.5	Radiologic examination, not elsewhere classified
V72.82	Preoperative respiratory examination
V76.0	Special screening for malignant neoplasms—respiratory organs
V81.3	Special screening for chronic bronchitis and emphysema
V81.4	Special screening for other and unspecified respiratory conditions

EXAMPLE   Exposure to asbestos, V15.84, (Z77.090).

EXERCISE 16-6

Assign codes to the following conditions.

1. Status post lung transplant   _____

2. Preoperative examination to assess COPD status prior to   _____
   elective surgery for cholelithiasis

3. Patient has a tracheostomy and is dependent on a respirator   _____

4. Personal history of lung cancer with previous surgery to   _____
   remove lung; no recurrence

5. Family history of asthma   _____

COMMON TREATMENTS

Smoking cessation may be beneficial in the prevention of exacerbations and progression of many respiratory conditions. Annual vaccinations against influenza and a once-only vaccination against bacterial pneumococcal pneumonia may help prevent the pulmonary complications of infection.

CONDITION	MEDICATION/TREATMENT
Sinusitis	Decongestant to help sinuses drain; antibiotics
Bronchitis	If viral—rest, fluids, cough medicine
	If bacterial—an antibiotic may be prescribed
Asthmatic bronchitis	Bronchodilators, steroids, and antibiotics for acute infection
Chronic bronchitis	Bronchodilators, steroids, and antibiotics for acute infection
Emphysema	Bronchodilators, steroids, oxygen therapy, and antibiotics for acute infection
Asthma	Corticosteroids, albuterol (Proventil, Ventolin), theophylline (TheoDur, Slo-Bid, Uniphyl), Serevent, Xopenex, Azmocort, Advair, Singulair, and Symbicort
COPD	Prednisone, albuterol (Proventil, Ventolin), Combivent, Serevent, Alupent, and Atrovent

CONDITION	MEDICATION/TREATMENT
Pneumonia	Sputum culture and antibiotics, if suspected to be bacterial
Influenza	Influenza vaccination, nasal swab, amantadine, zanamivir, and treatment of symptoms
Respiratory failure	Oxygen, mechanical ventilation, treatment of underlying cause
Pleural effusion	Treatment of underlying cause
Pulmonary edema	Treatment of underlying cause

PROCEDURES

Some of the procedures that may be related to diseases of the respiratory system may be located in the following chapters of the Procedure Tabular:

5. Operations on the Respiratory System (30-34)

Procedures related to the respiratory system in ICD-10-PCS can be located in the following tables:

0B1-0BY	Respiratory System
0C0-0CX	Mouth and Throat
5A0-5A2	Extracorporeal Assistance and Performance

Mechanical Ventilation

Mechanical ventilation is the use of a machine to induce alternating inflation and deflation of the lungs for the purpose of regulating the exchange rate of gases in the blood. The root operation for mechanical ventilation is performance. The most common type of ventilator (or respirator) delivers inspiratory gases directly into the person's airway. Mechanical ventilation codes are time-based as follows:

- Continuous mechanical ventilation of unspecified duration
- Continuous mechanical ventilation for less than 96 consecutive hours
- Continuous mechanical ventilation for 96 consecutive hours or longer

Instructions are provided for coding of any associated endotracheal tube insertions or tracheostomy. Specific instructions also explain the calculation of mechanical ventilator hours. To calculate the number of hours (duration) of continuous mechanical ventilation during a hospitalization, begin the count from the start of the (endotracheal) intubation. The duration ends with (endotracheal) extubation. If a patient is intubated prior to admission, begin counting the duration from time of admission. If a patient is transferred (discharged) while intubated, the duration would end at the time of transfer (discharge).

For patients who have been (endotracheal) intubated and subsequently undergo a tracheostomy, duration begins with the (endotracheal) intubation and ends when the mechanical ventilation is turned off (after the weaning period).

In a patient with a tracheostomy, to calculate the number of hours of continuous mechanical ventilation during hospitalization, begin counting the duration when mechanical ventilation is started. Duration ends when the mechanical ventilator is turned off (after the weaning period). If a patient has received a tracheostomy prior to admission and is on mechanical ventilation at the time of admission, begin counting the duration from the time of admission. If a patient is transferred (discharged) while still on mechanical ventilation via tracheostomy, duration would end at the time of transfer (discharge).

For certain procedures or for particular patients, mechanical ventilation may be used during surgery and in the immediate postoperative period. Per *Coding Clinic* (1992:2Q:p14),[8] mechanical ventilation during surgery does not require a code assignment unless the ventilation is required for "an extended period (several days)" during the post surgical period. *Coding Clinic* (2004:3Q:p11)[9] states "the term 'several' is defined as more than two. Therefore, unless the physician has clearly documented an unexpected extended period of mechanical ventilation (several days), do not assign a code for the mechanical ventilation."

If ventilation is required for a longer period than normal, a medical reason for continuing ventilation should be documented. If this is not well-documented, the coder may have to query the physician. To calculate the hours, begin counting from the time of intubation.

If a patient has been extubated and is no longer on mechanical ventilation but his or her condition deteriorates, requiring reintubation and mechanical ventilation, this would begin a new ventilation period, and a second code based on hours of ventilation would be assigned, per *Coding Clinic* (1991:4Q:p16-21).[10]

EXAMPLE

> Patient was intubated and placed on mechanical ventilation for respiratory failure due to myasthenia gravis. Patient was ventilated for 3 days, 518.81, 358.00, 96.71, 96.04 (J96.90, G70.00, 5A1945Z, 0BH17EZ).

Noninvasive Ventilation

Noninvasive ventilation is a form of ventilation without an invasive artificial airway (endotracheal tube or tracheostomy). The root operation for noninvasive ventilation is assistance. The use of noninvasive ventilation preserves the speech, swallowing, and cough functions of the patient. Noninvasive ventilation is divided into two categories:

- Negative-pressure ventilation
- Noninvasive positive-pressure ventilation (NPPV)

Negative-pressure ventilators provide ventilatory support by reducing the pressure surrounding the chest wall during inspiration and reversing the pressure during expiration. Machines such as iron lungs and body ventilators are used.

Noninvasive positive-pressure ventilation is being used more often in the hospital setting. NPPV is delivered by a nasal or face mask and may be administered with the following devices:

- Intermittent positive-pressure ventilation (IPPV)
- Bilevel positive airway pressure (BIPAP)
- Continuous positive airway pressure (CPAP)

NPPV is more comfortable for the patient and complications that are associated with invasive ventilation such as pneumothorax, airway injury, and ventilator-associated pneumonia can be minimized.

It is important to note that when BIPAP, CPAP, or PPV is administered via endotracheal tube or tracheostomy, it becomes invasive ventilation and would be assigned a code from the 96.7X category.

Bronchoscopy

Bronchoscopy is a diagnostic endoscopic procedure in which a tube with a tiny camera on the end is inserted through the nose or mouth into the lungs (Figure 16-10). The root operation for a diagnostic bronchoscopy is inspection. Different procedure codes are available for a bronchoscopy done through a tracheostomy. This procedure provides a view of the airways of the lung and allows doctors to collect lung secretions or tissue specimens (biopsy). Bronchoalveolar lavage (BAL) is done via bronchoscope. Fluid is squirted into a small part of the lung and is recollected for cytologic examination, microscopy, and culture. The root operation for BAL is irrigation. Bronchoalveolar lavage is very useful for diagnosing infections such as PCP in a patient with HIV.

EXAMPLE

> Bronchoalveolar lavage (left lung) confirmed the diagnosis of PCP in a patient with HIV, 042, 136.3, 33.24 (B20, B59, 3E1F88X).

EXAMPLE

> Transbronchial biopsy of the right lung, which confirmed carcinoma of the lung, 162.9, 33.27 (C34.91, 0BBK87X).

FIGURE 16-10. A, Fiberoptic bronchoscopy—a bronchoscope is passed through the nose, throat, larynx, and trachea into the bronchus. **B,** A bronchoscope with a brush catheter, ready for biopsy of bronchial tissue.

FIGURE 16-11. Thoracentesis. The needle is inserted close to the base of the effusion so that gravity will help with drainage.

Thoracentesis

Thoracentesis is puncture of the chest wall to remove fluid (pleural effusion) from the space between the lining of the outside of the lungs (pleura) and the wall of the chest (pleural cavity) (Figure 16-11). The root operation for thoracentesis is drainage. Physicians may perform a diagnostic thoracentesis or a therapeutic thoracentesis. The fluid collected is sent to the laboratory for analysis. This may also relieve any shortness of breath caused by compression on the lung by the fluid.

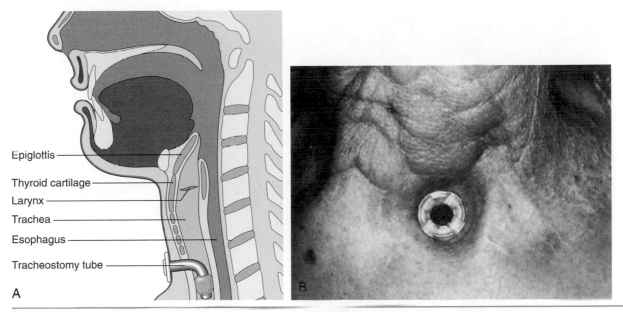

Epiglottis
Thyroid cartilage
Larynx
Trachea
Esophagus
Tracheostomy tube
A
B

FIGURE 16-12. A, Tracheostomy with tube in place. **B,** Healed tracheostomy incision.

EXAMPLE	Patient with pneumonia and large right pleural effusion requiring thoracentesis right pleural cavity, 486, 511.9, 34.91 (J18.9, J90, 0W993ZZ).

Thoracostomy

Tube thoracostomy is the term used for insertion of chest tube(s) to drain blood, fluid, or air and to allow full expansion of the lungs. The root operation for tube thoracostomy is drainage. A tube is placed between the ribs and into the space between the inner lining and the outer lining of the lung (pleural space); fluid is allowed to drain. A suction machine may be used to facilitate drainage. Reasons why chest tubes may be used include pneumothorax, hemothorax, abscess, empyema, and cancer; they also may be used after surgery.

EXAMPLE	Insertion of chest tube on the right side for continuous drainage of empyema, 510.9, 34.04 (J86.9, 0W9930Z).

Tracheostomy

Tracheostomy is a procedure in which an artificial opening is made in the front of the windpipe (trachea) through the skin of the neck (Figure 16-12). The root operation for tracheostomy is bypass. A tube is inserted, through which breathing may continue until the normal airway can be restored. A tracheostomy may be performed during an emergency at the patient's bedside. In some cases, a tracheostomy is planned and is performed in the Operating Room (OR). If it is not documented as a permanent tracheostomy, the code for temporary or unspecified tracheostomy should be assigned. If any question arises about the type of tracheostomy, a physician query may be necessary.

EXAMPLE	Temporary open tracheostomy was performed in the OR because of the patient's recurrent aspiration pneumonitis, 507.0, 31.1 (J69.0, 0B110F4).

FIGURE 16-13. Pulmonary resections. **A,** Wedge resection. **B,** Segmental resection. **C,** Lobectomy. **D,** Pneumonectomy.

Pulmonary Resection

The type of pulmonary resection undertaken may depend on the condition that is being diagnosed and/or treated. Wedge resection (Figure 16-13, *A*) is the removal of a small, localized area of diseased tissue near the surface of the lung. Segmental resection (Figure 16-13, *B*) involves the removal of a bronchiole and its alveoli in one or more lung segments. Removal of an entire lobe of the lung is a lobectomy (Figure 16-13, *C*), and the removal of an entire lung is known as pneumonectomy (Figure 16-13, *D*). The root operation for resection of any part of the lung will depend on the portion of the lung that is resected. Resection is the root operation when all of a body part is cut out or off without replacement. "All of a body part" includes any anatomical subdivision that has its own body part value. Although a lobectomy is not the removal of the entire lung, it is the removal of a body part that has its own value; therefore, it is a resection. For partial resections the root operation is excision.

A surgical technique known as video-assisted thoracic surgery (VATS) has allowed surgeons to perform thoracic surgery in a minimally invasive manner. Depending on the type of procedure performed, a hospital stay may last only 1 to 3 days, intensive care may not be needed, and recovery may be quicker. Patients may return to their normal activities much sooner than when an "open" procedure is performed.

EXERCISE 16-7

Assign codes for all diagnosis and procedures.

1. Thoracoscopy with removal of lung cancer (left lower lobe) _____

2. Pleurodesis with administration of talc for recurrent spontaneous pneumothorax on the right _____

3. Diagnostic thoracentesis for large right-sided pleural effusion _____

4. Bronchoalveolar lavage of right lung to assess type of pneumonia _____

5. Temporary percutaneous tracheostomy in patient with laryngeal cancer who will be having surgery in a couple of weeks _____

6. Endotracheal intubation with mechanical ventilation for 3 days because of acute respiratory failure due to exacerbation of congestive heart failure _____

7. Lobectomy for squamous cell carcinoma, right lung, upper lobe _____

8. Transbronchial biopsy of the left lung and bronchus; histologic exam confirms pulmonary tuberculosis _____

DOCUMENTATION/REIMBURSEMENT/MS-DRGs

Often, coding difficulties are due to lack of documentation. Sometimes pathology and other test results are not available at the time of discharge or when the physician is dictating the discharge summary or is reporting the final diagnoses.

Assigning the correct code to identify the COPD can be difficult because of conflicting documentation. Physicians frequently use the general term COPD rather than more specific terminology.

Documentation of pneumonia and the causative organism or sputum culture results may not be directly linked, making it necessary to query the physician. Physicians often document exacerbation of COPD but fail to document any condition that may be responsible for the exacerbation such as pneumonia.

It may be difficult to calculate mechanical ventilation time with the use of physician documentation, and it may be necessary to use respiratory therapy notes to determine the exact length of time. It is also possible that a patient could have more than one continuous episode of ventilation.

Procedures that can be performed at bedside such as tracheostomy, thoracentesis, and insertion of a chest tube may not be well-documented by the physician or may be documented only within a progress note and therefore are easy to miss.

An abnormal laboratory test may not necessarily be clinically significant. If abnormal laboratory tests are noted and treatment is given, it would be appropriate to query the physician regarding the abnormal laboratory test(s). An abnormal laboratory test must be clinically significant to be coded, per *Coding Clinic* (1990:2Q:p15-16).[11]

Frequently missed complications/comorbidities from the respiratory chapter include the following:

- Atelectasis
- Bronchiectasis with acute exacerbation
- Bronchitis, chronic, with exacerbation
- COPD exacerbation
- Effusion, pleural
- Failure, respiratory
- Pneumonia
- Pneumothorax

Pneumonia and Causative Organism

EXAMPLE Patient has a long history of chronic obstructive pulmonary disease and was admitted for the treatment of pneumonia. Sputum cultures grew *Klebsiella*. The physician should be queried to determine whether the pneumonia is due to *Klebsiella*. The patient's COPD was treated due to flare up.

DIAGNOSES	CODES	MS-DRG	RW
Pneumonia in patient with COPD	486, 491.21 (J18.9, J44.1)	194	1.0152
Klebsiella pneumonia with COPD	482.0, 491.21 (J15.0, J44.1)	178	1.4887

The causative organism of pneumonia can make a significant difference in the MS-DRG assignment. Also, the presence of a complication/comorbidity such as an exacerbation of COPD can make a difference in reimbursement, depending on the principal diagnosis and the MS-DRG assigned.

Two Diagnoses That Equally Meet the Definition for Principal Diagnosis

EXAMPLE Patient was admitted with aspiration pneumonia and *pneumococcal* pneumonia. Patient had severe gastroesophageal reflux disease (GERD). The patient was admitted with both types of pneumonia, and both diagnoses fit the definition of principal diagnosis.

DIAGNOSES	CODES	MS-DRG	RW
Aspiration pneumonia with *pneumococcal* pneumonia	507.0, 481, 530.81 (J69.0, J13, K21.9)	179	0.9861
Pneumococcal pneumonia with aspiration pneumonia	481, 507.0, 530.81 (J13, J69.0, K21.9)	195	0.7096

Note that the aspiration pneumonia groups to an MS-DRG with a higher weight. If both pneumonias meet the definition of a principal diagnosis, it is perfectly acceptable to sequence aspiration pneumonia as the principal. If a patient was admitted with *pneumococcal* pneumonia, and a couple of days after admission aspirated and developed aspiration pneumonia, *pneumococcal* pneumonia is the principal diagnosis and aspiration pneumonia is a secondary diagnosis.

MS-DRG With and Without MCC/CC

In other MS-DRGs, either of the pneumonia diagnoses would qualify as complications/comorbidities, but with pneumonia as the principal and pneumonia as a secondary diagnosis, these case scenarios are grouped into MS-DRGs without complications/comorbidities. Further optimization could be accomplished by reviewing the chart for additional diagnoses, as in the following example:

EXAMPLE Patient was admitted with aspiration pneumonia and *pneumococcal* pneumonia. Patient has severe GERD. The patient was admitted with both types of pneumonia, and both diagnoses fit the definition of principal diagnosis. It is noted on the history and physical that the patient has a chronic kidney disease, stage IV.

DIAGNOSES	CODES	MS-DRG	RW
Aspiration pneumonia with *pneumococcal* pneumonia CKD, stage IV	507.0, 481, 530.81, 585.4 (J69.0, J13, K21.9, N18.4)	178	1.4887
Pneumococcal pneumonia with aspiration pneumonia, CKD, stage IV	481, 507.0, 530.81, 585.4 (J13, J69.0, K21.9, N18.4)	194	1.0152

Both MS-DRGs are optimized by the addition of 585.4 (N18.4) stage IV CKD, which is a complication/comorbidity in these cases. The difference in relative weight when aspiration pneumonia is sequenced as the principal diagnosis should also be noted.

Respiratory Failure Versus Another Acute Condition

EXAMPLE

Patient was admitted with acute respiratory failure due to pneumonia.
(Per guidelines, if both the respiratory failure and another acute condition are equally responsible for occasioning the admission, the guidelines regarding two or more diagnoses that equally meet the definition for principal diagnosis may be applied in these situations.)

DIAGNOSES	CODES	MS-DRG	RW
Respiratory failure due to pneumonia	518.81, 486 (J96.00, J18.9)	189	1.2809
Pneumonia with respiratory failure	486, 518.81 (J18.9, J96.00)	193	1.4796

In this case, either the respiratory failure or the pneumonia could be selected as the principal diagnosis; the reimbursement is higher if the respiratory failure is the principal diagnosis. In MS-DRG 193, the respiratory failure is an MCC.

CHAPTER REVIEW EXERCISE

Assign codes for all diagnoses and procedures.

1. Cough due to *Streptococcus pneumoniae* pneumonia _____

2. Patient with severe emphysema who is dependent on oxygen; quit smoking 5 years ago. NPPV (48 hours) was initiated for the patient's chronic respiratory failure _____

3. Patient is high-risk for lung disease due to on-the-job exposure to asbestos; patient has a 20–pack-year history of smoking; currently active _____

4. Croup _____

5. Left tonsillar abscess; abscess was drained _____

6. Patient with whooping cough has pneumonia _____

7. *Haemophilus influenzae* pneumonia in a patient who is being treated for influenza _____

8. Edema larynx _____

9. Status asthmaticus _____

10. Bronchospasm with acute exacerbation of COPD _____

11. Acute on chronic respiratory failure due to sarcoidosis involving the lungs; mechanical ventilation for 3 days; patient was intubated at transferring facility and was transferred for evaluation of sarcoidosis _____

12. Retractive airway disease _____

13. Inhalation anthrax with pneumonia _____

14. Bronchiolitis obliterans organizing pneumonia _____

15. Acute and chronic sinusitis _____

16. Chronic tonsillitis and adenitis; tonsillectomy with adenoidectomy performed _____

17. Nasal cavity polyps with endoscopic polypectomy _____

18. Solitary pulmonary nodule   _____

19. Empyema with insertion of left chest tube; empyema was due to   _____
    Staphylococcus aureus

20. Double lung transplant for diffuse idiopathic pulmonary fibrosis;   _____
    cardiopulmonary bypass was performed in this transplant from a
    cadaver

21. Congestive heart failure with left pleural effusion that was treated   _____
    with thoracentesis at bedside

22. Granuloma lung   _____

23. Iatrogenic pneumothorax   _____

24. Acute bronchitis with chronic obstructive bronchitis   _____

25. Pulmonary edema   _____

Write the correct answer(s) in the space(s) provided.

26. Define contamination of a culture.

    _____

27. Define empiric treatment.

    _____

28. Define iatrogenic.

    _____

29. List two problems/conditions that could cause a patient to aspirate.

    _____

    _____

30. List two terms that describe status asthmaticus.

    _____

    _____

CHAPTER GLOSSARY   **Asbestosis:** lung disease due to inhalation of asbestos.

Aspiration pneumonia: inflammation of the lungs and bronchial tubes due to aspiration of foreign
material into the lung.

Asthma: chronic disease that affects the airways that carry air into and out of the lungs.

Asthmatic bronchitis: underlying asthmatic problem in patients in whom asthma has become so
persistent that clinically significant chronic airflow obstruction is present despite antiasthmatic
therapy.

Baritosis: lung disease due to inhalation of barium.

Black lung: lung disease due to inhalation of coal dust.

Bronchi: the two air tubes that branch off the trachea and deliver air to both lungs.

Bronchitis: lower respiratory tract or bronchial tree infection characterized by cough, sputum
production, and wheezing.

Bronchoscopy: diagnostic endoscopic procedure in which a tube with a tiny camera on the end is
inserted through the nose or mouth into the lungs.

Chronic bronchitis: condition defined by a mucus-producing cough most days of the month,
3 months out of a year for 2 successive years with no other underlying disease to explain the
cough.

Chronic obstructive pulmonary disease: general term used to describe a lung disease in which the
airways become obstructed, making it difficult for air to get into and out of the lungs.

Chylothorax: milky fluid consisting of lymph and fat (chyle) that accumulates in the pleural space.

Coal workers' pneumoconiosis: lung disease due to inhalation of coal dust.

Community-acquired pneumonia: broad term used to define pneumonias that are contracted outside of the hospital or nursing home setting.

Contaminant: a cultured organism that a physician does not believe is responsible for causing a particular infection.

Diaphragm: dome-shaped muscles at the bottom of the lungs that assist in the process of breathing and in the exchange of oxygen/carbon dioxide.

Emphysema: chronic lung disease of gradual onset that can be attributed to chronic infection and inflammation or irritation from cigarette smoke.

Empiric: initiation of treatment prior to making a definite diagnosis.

Empyema: pus that accumulates in the pleural space.

Hemothorax: blood that accumulates in the pleural space.

Iatrogenic: caused by medical treatment.

Infection: invasion of the body by organisms that have the potential to cause disease.

Influenza: contagious viral infection of the respiratory tract that causes coughing, difficulty breathing, headache, muscle aches, and weakness.

Lobar pneumonia: synonym for pneumococcal pneumonia or pneumonia due to *Streptococcus pneumoniae.*

Mechanical ventilation: use of a machine to induce alternating inflation and deflation of the lungs and to regulate the exchange rate of gases in the blood.

Noninvasive ventilation: ventilation without an invasion artificial airway (i.e., endotracheal tube or tracheostomy).

Nosocomial pneumonia: pneumonia that is acquired while the patient is residing in a hospital-type setting.

Nursing home-acquired pneumonia: pneumonia that is acquired in a nursing home or extended care facility.

Pleural effusion: fluid that accumulates in the pleural space because of trauma or disease.

Pneumoconioses: lung diseases due to chronic inhalation of inorganic (mineral) dust that are often due to occupational exposure.

Pneumonia: infection of the lungs that may be caused by a variety of organisms, including viruses, bacteria, and parasites.

Pneumothorax: air in space around the lung.

Pulmonary edema: condition in which fluid accumulates in the lungs.

Respiratory failure: general term that describes ineffective gas exchange across the lungs by the respiratory system.

Respiratory system: system that supplies the body with oxygen (O_2).

Siderosis: lung disease due to inhalation of iron oxide.

Sinusitis: a condition in which the linings of one or more sinuses become infected, usually because of viruses or bacteria.

Spontaneous pneumothorax: pneumothorax that is not caused by trauma.

Stannosis: lung disease due to inhalation of tin particles.

Thoracentesis: puncture of the chest wall to remove fluid (pleural effusion) from the space between the lining of the outside of the lungs (pleura) and the wall of the chest.

Trachea (windpipe): body part that is responsible for filtering the air that we breathe.

Tracheostomy: procedure in which an artificial opening is made in the front of the windpipe (trachea) through the skin of the neck.

Tube thoracostomy: insertion of chest tube(s) to drain blood, fluid, or air and allow full expansion of the lungs.

REFERENCES

1. American Hospital Association. *Coding Clinic for ICD-9-CM* 1998:2Q:p3. Pneumonia: infection or inflammation of the lung.
2. Damjanov I. Pathology for the Health Professions, 3rd ed. St Louis, Saunders, 2006, Table 8-1, p 177.
3. American Hospital Association. *Coding Clinic for ICD-9-CM* 1988:3Q:p9-10. Status asthmaticus.
4. American Hospital Association. *Coding Clinic for ICD-9-CM* 1991:3Q:p16-17. Aspiration pneumonia with growth of *Staphylococcus aureus.*
5. American Hospital Association. *Coding Clinic for ICD-9-CM* 1991:3Q:p19-20. Pleural effusion with congestive heart failure.
6. American Hospital Association. *Coding Clinic for ICD-9-CM* 1988:3Q:p3. Acute pulmonary edema of cardiac origin.
7. American Hospital Association. *Coding Clinic for ICD-9-CM* 1988:3Q:p3-4. Pulmonary edema.
8. American Hospital Association. *Coding Clinic for ICD-9-CM* 1992:2Q:p14. Mechanical ventilation during surgery and mechanical ventilation for extended period following surgery.
9. American Hospital Association. *Coding Clinic for ICD-9-CM* 2004:3Q:p11. Clarification—Postoperative mechanical ventilation.
10. American Hospital Association. *Coding Clinic for ICD-9-CM* 1991:4Q:p16-21. Mechanical ventilation—Guidelines.
11. American Hospital Association. *Coding Clinic for ICD-9-CM* 1990:2Q:p15-16. Abnormal findings—Reporting guidelines.

17

Diseases of the Digestive System

(ICD-9-CM Chapter 9, Codes 520-579, and ICD-10-CM Chapter 11, Codes K00-K94)

LEARNING OBJECTIVES

1. Apply and assign the correct ICD-9-CM and ICD-10-CM codes in accordance with Official Guidelines for Coding and Reporting
2. Identify major differences between ICD-9-CM and ICD-10-CM related to diseases of the digeslive system
3. Identify pertinent anatomy and physiology of the digestive system
4. Identify diseases of the digestive system
5. Assign the correct V/Z codes and procedure codes related to the digestive system
6. Identify common treatments, medications, laboratory values, and diagnostic tests
7. Explain the importance of documentation in relation to MS-DRGs for reimbursement

ABBREVIATIONS/ ACRONYMS

AVM arteriovenous malformation

EGD esophagogastroduodenoscopy

ERCP endoscopic retrograde cholangiopancreatography

ESWL extracorporeal shock wave lithotripsy

GERD gastroesophageal reflux disease

GI gastrointestinal

ICD-9-CM *International Classification of Diseases,*

9th Revision, Clinical Modification

ICD-10-CM *International Classification of Diseases, 10th Revision, Clinical Modification*

ICD-10-PCS *International Classification of Diseases, 10th Revision, Procedure Coding System*

IV intravenous

LGIB lower gastrointestinal bleed

MS-DRG Medicare Severity diagnosis-related group

NSAID nonsteroidal antiinflammatory drug

PEG percutaneous endoscopic gastrostomy

PUD peptic ulcer disease

TIPS transjugular intrahepatic portosystemic shunt

UGIB upper gastrointestinal bleed

ICD-9-CM OFFICIAL GUIDELINES FOR CODING AND REPORTING

There are currently no official guidelines for Diseases of the Digestive System. Apply the General Coding Guidelines as found in Chapter 5.

ICD-10-CM OFFICIAL GUIDELINES FOR CODING AND REPORTING

There are currently no official guidelines for diseases of the digestive system. Apply the General Coding Guidelines as found in Chapter 5 of this text.

GUIDELINE DIFFERENCES BETWEEN ICD-9-CM AND ICD-10-CM

As there are no guidelines relating to the digestive system in either ICD-9-CM or ICD-10-CM, there are no differences.

MAJOR DIFFERENCES BETWEEN ICD-9-CM AND ICD-10-CM

- ICD-10-CM has expanded Crohn's disease to fourth, fifth, and sixth characters. These characters specify site, whether there was a complication present, and what the specific complication was.
- ICD-9-CM classified GI ulcers by the presence or absence of an obstruction. ICD-10-CM eliminates the reference to obstruction.
- ICD-10-CM expands on the hernia categories with characters for laterality and recurrence.
- ICD-10-CM expands the section on cholelithiasis to incorporate cholangitis.

ANATOMY AND PHYSIOLOGY

The digestive system (Figure 17-1) consists of the mouth, pharynx, esophagus, stomach, small intestine and large intestine (the **alimentary canal**), and accessory organs, which include the salivary glands, liver, gallbladder, and pancreas. The purpose of the digestive system is to process food so that it may be absorbed by cells.

The mouth is where digestion begins. The tongue, which is composed of muscle, the teeth, and saliva, facilitates **mastication** and assists in moving food to the pharynx, where swallowing occurs and food moves to the esophagus. **Peristalsis**, or the squeezing movement of food toward the stomach, occurs in the esophagus. Once the food arrives in the stomach, it is churned with gastric juices and begins the movement toward the small intestine.

The pancreas, the liver, and the gallbladder all aid in the digestive process. The purpose of the pancreas is to excrete juices that aid in the digestive process. The pancreatic duct connects with the duodenum in the same area in which the bile duct from the liver and the gallbladder intersect the duodenum. The liver secretes bile to aid in the digestive process, and the gallbladder stores bile and releases it as needed. The gallbladder is attached to the liver by the cystic duct, which joins the hepatic duct. Together, they form the common bile duct, which enters into the duodenum.

The function of the liver, in addition to aiding the digestive process, is to remove poisons from the blood, produce immune agents to control infection, and remove germs and bacteria from the blood. The liver serves as a filter for the body; a person cannot live without a functioning liver.

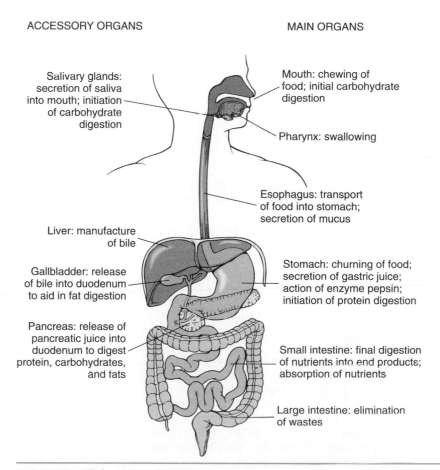

ACCESSORY ORGANS

Salivary glands: secretion of saliva into mouth; initiation of carbohydrate digestion

Liver: manufacture of bile

Gallbladder: release of bile into duodenum to aid in fat digestion

Pancreas: release of pancreatic juice into duodenum to digest protein, carbohydrates, and fats

MAIN ORGANS

Mouth: chewing of food; initial carbohydrate digestion

Pharynx: swallowing

Esophagus: transport of food into stomach; secretion of mucus

Stomach: churning of food; secretion of gastric juice; action of enzyme pepsin; initiation of protein digestion

Small intestine: final digestion of nutrients into end products; absorption of nutrients

Large intestine: elimination of wastes

FIGURE 17-1. Main and accessory organs of the digestive system.

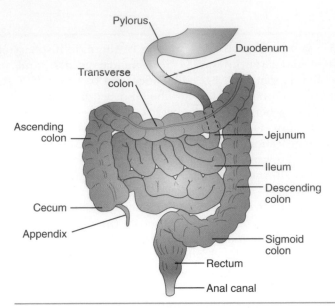

FIGURE 17-2. Small and large intestines.

The small intestine contains three areas: the duodenum, the jejunum, and the ileum. The small intestine completes the digestion begun in the stomach, absorbs products of digestion, and transports residue to the large intestine. The small intestine is suspended and is attached to the abdomen by a fold of peritoneum known as the mesentery. The small intestine joins the large intestine at the ileocecal valve.

The large intestine (Figure 17-2) is composed of the cecum, colon, rectum, and anal canal. The appendix is an appendage off the cecum. The purpose of the large intestine is to absorb electrolytes and store feces until the time of elimination.

DISEASE CONDITIONS

Diseases of the Digestive System (520-579), Chapter 9 in the ICD-9-CM code book, is divided into the following categories:

CATEGORY	SECTION TITLES
520-529	Diseases of the Oral Cavity, Salivary Glands, and Jaws
530-538	Diseases of the Esophagus, Stomach, and Duodenum
540-543	Appendicitis
550-553	Hernia of Abdominal Cavity
555-558	Noninfectious Enteritis and Colitis
560-569	Other Diseases of Intestines and Peritoneum
570-579	Other Diseases of Digestive System

Diseases of the Digestive System (K00-K94), Chapter 11 in the ICD-10-CM code book, are divided into the following categories:

CATEGORY	SECTION TITLES
K00-K14	Diseases of Oral Cavity and Salivary Glands
K20-K31	Diseases of the Esophagus, Stomach, and Duodenum
K35-K38	Diseases of Appendix
K40-K46	Hernia
K50-K52	Noninfective Enteritis and Colitis
K55-K63	Other Diseases of Intestines
K65-K68	Diseases of Peritoneum and Retroperitoneum
K70-K77	Diseases of Liver
K80-K87	Disorders of Gallbladder, Biliary Tract, and Pancreas
K90-K94	Other Diseases of the Digestive System

Diseases of the Oral Cavity, Salivary Glands, and Jaws

Many of the conditions in these categories concern the teeth and their structures, which are often treated in the outpatient setting. Some of these conditions, however, may be treated when a patient is admitted for another condition. In the exam section of the record, a healthcare provider might document whether the patient has dentures due to **edentulism**, which is the complete loss of teeth. The loss of teeth might affect the patient's ability to eat and therefore their nutritional state.

EXAMPLE

> Patient is admitted to the hospital with severe malnutrition and dehydration. During the exam it is identified that the patient has Class I complete edentulism, 261, 276.51, 525.41, 525.10 (E43, E86.0, K08.101).

Sialolithiasis is caused by stones in the salivary glands. Patients usually present with swollen, painful glands around the neck. When the stones are obstructing the gland, an infection, which is known as sialoadenitis, can result. Surgery may be required to remove the stone.

EXAMPLE

> Patient with known sialolithiasis is admitted through the ER with very painful glands in the neck and fever. After CT scan to determine the location of the stones and administration of antibiotics, the patient is taken to the OR for open removal, 527.5, 26.0 (K11.5, 0CCJ0ZZ).

Mucositis is an inflammation/ulceration of the digestive tract commonly occurring in the oral cavity. It can be found in up to 40% of patients being treated with chemotherapy. The condition can range from mild to severe. In the severest cases the patient may be unable to eat due to the pain caused by ulcerations in the mouth. It can be treated with viscous lidocaine.

EXAMPLE

> Patient admitted for chemotherapy for pancreatic cancer and develops ulcerative mucositis due to gemcitabine, V58.11, 157.9, 528.01, E933.1, 99.25 (Z51.11, C25.9, T45.1x5A, K12.31, 3E04305).

EXERCISE 17-1

Assign codes to the following conditions.

1. Canker sore _____
2. Ulcerative stomatitis _____
3. Hypertrophy of the salivary gland _____
4. Impacted teeth _____

Diseases of the Esophagus, Stomach, and Duodenum

Esophageal Conditions

Esophageal varices (Figure 17-3), one of the most common causes of esophageal hemorrhage, are excluded from the code for gastrointestinal hemorrhage. The codes for esophageal hemorrhage due to esophageal varices are found in the Circulatory System chapter.

EXAMPLE

> Patient has esophageal varices due to cirrhosis of the liver, 571.5, 456.21 (K74.60, I85.10).

Varices
(dilated veins)

FIGURE 17-3. Esophageal varices.

Mallory-Weiss is the name for bleeding laceration of the esophagogastric junction that usually occurs after severe vomiting. If the bleeding is severe, an EGD may be performed to control bleeding. One of the most common conditions is esophageal reflux, which is also known as gastroesophageal reflux disease (GERD). It is treated with proton pump inhibitors such as Prilosec or, in more severe cases, by Nissen fundoplication surgery.

Barrett's esophagus is a precancerous condition that usually occurs in people with chronic GERD. The normal cells lining the esophagus change type. Symptoms may include heartburn, indigestion, difficulty swallowing solid foods, and nocturnal regurgitation.

EXAMPLE | Patient with chronic GERD who is having difficulty swallowing is found to have Barrett's esophagus, 530.85, 530.81, 787.20 (K22.70, K21.9, R13.10).

Arteriovenous malformations (AVM) may occur in the gastrointestinal tract. The terms AVM and **angiodysplasia** often are used interchangeably, although an angiodysplasia is a type of AVM characterized by dilated or fragile blood vessels. AVMs may be congenital or acquired. A congenital AVM is a defect that arises during fetal development. An acquired AVM is one that develops as the result of a variety of factors during one's lifetime. Unless specified as congenital, a gastrointestinal AVM should be coded as acquired, according to *Coding Clinic* (1996:3Q:p9-10; 1986:Nov-Dec:p11).[1,2] For indexing of gastrointestinal AVMs, see Figure 17-4.

EXAMPLE | Patient presents to hospital with a GI bleed. During the workup for the cause of the bleed, it is determined that the patient has an AVM of the colon, 569.85 (K55.21).

EXERCISE 17-2

Assign codes to the following conditions.

1. Esophageal ulcer due to ingestion of aspirin _____

2. Inflammation of the esophagus due to reflux _____

3. Mallory-Weiss tear _____

4. GERD _____

Malformation (congenital) - *see also*
Anomaly
bone 756.9
bursa 756.9
Chiari
type I 348.4
type II (*see also* Spina bifida)
741.0 ☑
type III 742.0
type IV 742.2
circulatory system NEC 747.9
specified type NEC 747.89
cochlea 744.05
digestive system NEC 751.9
lower 751.5
specified type NEC 751.8
upper 750.9

Anomaly, anomalous — *continued*
alimentary tract — *continued*
specified type NEC 751.8
upper (any part, except tongue) 750.9
tongue 750.10
adrenal (gland) 759.1
alveolar 524.70
ridge (process) 525.8
specified NEC 524.79
ankle (joint) 755.69
anus, anal (canal) 751.5
aorta, aortic 747.20
arch 747.21
coarctation (postductal) (preductal)
747.10
cusp or valve NEC 746.9
septum 745.0
specified type NEC 747.29
aorticopulmonary septum 745.0
apertures, diaphragm 756.6
appendix 751.5
aqueduct of Sylvius 742.3
with spina bifida (*see also* Spina
bifida) 741.0 ☑
arm 755.50
reduction (*see also* Deformity, reduction, upper limb) 755.20
arteriovenous (congenital) (peripheral)
NEC 747.60
brain 747.81
cerebral 747.81
coronary 746.85
gastrointestinal 747.61
acquired - *see* Angiodysplasia
lower limb 747.64
renal 747.62
specified site NEC 747.69
spinal 747.82
upper limb 747.63

Angioblastoma (M9161/1) - *see* Neoplasm, connective tissue, uncertain
behavior
Angiocholecystitis (*see also* Cholecystitis,
acute) 575.0
Angiocholitis (*see also* Cholecystitis,
acute) 576.1
Angiodysgensis spinalis 336.1
Angiodysplasia (intestinalis) (intestine)
569.84
with hemorrhage 569.85
duodenum 537.82
with hemorrhage 537.83
stomach 537.82 ◄
with hemorrhage 537.83

FIGURE 17-4. Indexing of gastrointestinal arteriovenous malformation (AVM).

Gastrointestinal Hemorrhage

Gastrointestinal (GI) hemorrhage is a common reason for a patient to seek medical attention. The healthcare provider must determine whether the bleed is lower or upper GI in origin, so appropriate treatment can be provided. To make this determination, the provider must evaluate how the patient presents.

- In lower GI bleeds (LGIB), the patient may present with the following:
Hematochezia—bright red blood in stool
- In upper GI bleeds (UGIB), the patient may present with the following:
Hematemesis—vomiting of blood

If a patient presents with **melena** (dark blood in stool) or **occult blood** in the stool (this can be found only by laboratory inspection), it is unknown without further workup whether this is an upper or a lower GI bleed. Often, when a patient presents with acute anemia without a causative condition, the healthcare provider may suspect a GI bleed.

EXAMPLE | Blood in feces, occult, lab finding, 792.1 (R19.5).

GI hemorrhage has many causes; the most common causes consist of gastric or intestinal ulcers, hemorrhoids, diverticulitis, and angiodysplasia of the intestine.

EXAMPLE | Patient admitted with GI bleed caused by angiodysplasia of the stomach, 537.83 (K31.811).

FIGURE 17-5. If an ulcer is drug- or chemical-induced, assign an E code for the responsible drug or chemical.

EXAMPLE	Patient is being treated for diverticulitis of the sigmoid colon with hemorrhage, 562.13 (K57.33).

Per *Coding Clinic* (2005:3Q:p17-18),[3] if a patient presents with a GI bleed and then undergoes diagnostic testing such as esophagogastroduodenoscopy (EGD) to determine the site of the bleed, unless the physician specifies a causal relationship between the findings on this test and the bleed, the code 578.9 (K92.2) should be assigned. Codes for any other findings such as gastritis should be coded as without hemorrhage.

Ulcers of the Stomach and Small Intestine

An ulcer of the stomach or the intestine is an open sore in the lining of the stomach or intestine. An ulcer occurs when the lining is damaged. Damage to the lining may occur when production of stomach acid is increased, or it may be caused by a bacterium known as *Helicobacter pylori*, or *H. pylori*. When locating the code for a bacterium, the main term "Infection" should be referenced in the Alphabetic Index. Ulcers may be drug-induced. The Tabular List contains instructions for the use of additional E codes to identify the responsible drug (Figure 17-5).

Symptoms of gastric ulcer may include pain when eating, vomiting, and tarry bowel movements. Ulcers can be diagnosed by means of an upper GI x-ray, blood tests that look for *H. pylori*, stool samples, or endoscopy. Treatment for ulcers may include antacids, drugs such as proton pump inhibitors or histamine receptor blockers, which stop the stomach from making acids, or antibiotics, and finally, in the worst case scenario, gastrectomy. Some conditions that may accompany ulcers are chronic or acute blood loss anemia and gastric outlet syndrome. A gastric ulcer is a stomach ulcer. A peptic ulcer can occur in the esophagus, stomach, duodenum, jejunum, and/or ileum. If no site is specified, 533.xx (K27.-) is assigned for peptic ulcer.

EXAMPLE	Patient has a peptic ulcer of the esophagus, secondary to aspirin use, 530.20, E935.3 (T39.015A, K22.10).

EXAMPLE	Patient is admitted for a bleeding gastric ulcer with obstruction and perforation, 531.61 (K25.6).

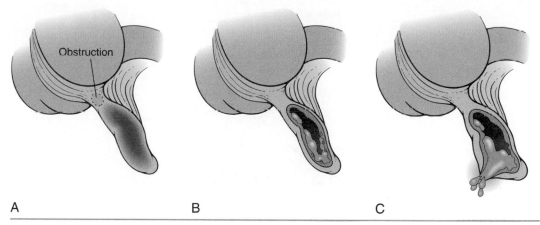

A   B   C

FIGURE 17-6. Stages of appendicitis. **A,** Obstruction that causes inflammation. **B,** Pus and bacteria invade the wall of the appendix. **C,** Pus perforates the wall of the appendix, leading to peritonitis.

EXERCISE 17-3

Assign codes to the following conditions.

1. Angiodysplasia with hemorrhage of the duodenum and chronic blood loss anemia   _____

2. Acute penetrating peptic ulcer of the duodenum   _____

3. GI bleed due to peptic ulcer   _____

4. Bleeding esophageal varices   _____

5. Blood in stool   _____

Appendicitis

Appendicitis is inflammation of the appendix that is usually caused by obstruction, which, in turn, results in infection (Figure 17-6). A patient who presents with appendicitis may have some or all of the following signs and symptoms: abdominal pain (right lower quadrant, also known as **McBurney's point**), vomiting, **anorexia** (loss of appetite), fever, constipation, and elevated white blood cell count.

If the appendix ruptures, peritonitis develops. Patients with appendicitis are usually treated with antibiotics and surgery (appendectomy). It is important to review the pathology report for documentation of abscess or perforation of appendix.

On occasion, all signs and symptoms lead the surgeon to believe that a patient has appendicitis, but the pathology report does not confirm this diagnosis. When the pathology report indicates a normal appendix, *Coding Clinic* (1990:2Q:p26)[4] instructs the coder to use the symptom the patient presented with as the principal diagnosis.

EXAMPLE   Patient admitted with acute appendicitis with peritoneal abscess, 540.1 (K35.3).

EXAMPLE   Patient has a ruptured appendicitis, 540.0 (K35.2).

A   HIATAL (DIAPHRAGMATIC) HERNIA   INGUINAL HERNIAS   B

FIGURE 17-7. A, Hiatal hernia. **B,** Inguinal hernia. Direct inguinal hernia passes through the abdominal wall. Indirect hernia passes through the inguinal canal.

Hernia of Abdominal Cavity

A **hernia** (Figure 17-7) is a protrusion of an organ or tissue through an abnormal opening in the body. Hernias can be present at birth or may develop over time. Most commonly, a hernia is a protrusion of the intestine through a weakness in the abdominal cavity. Hernias are classified by type or site.

Some types of hernias
- Inguinal—common in men; intestines protrude into the inguinal canal
- Femoral—more common in women; intestine protrudes through the femoral canal at the top of the thigh
- Umbilical—most common in children; abdominal wall is weakened at the point of the umbilical cord
- Ventral—this is when scar tissue in the abdominal wall weakens following surgery or trauma. If the cause of the ventral hernia is surgery, it may also be called an incisional hernia
- Diaphragmatic—abnormal opening in the diaphragm that allows parts of organs from the abdominal cavity (e.g., intestines, stomach) to move into the chest cavity. Also known as a hiatal hernia

Once the site of the hernia is known, then it must be determined whether it is obstructed or gangrenous. An obstructed abdominal hernia is one in which the bowel is trapped and obstructed but viable (still working); when it becomes nonviable, it can become gangrenous (deficient blood supply to trapped bowel, making it **necrotic**). Some codes require documentation as to whether the hernia is unilateral or bilateral, and whether it is recurrent. Hernia repairs require more information and are discussed in the procedure section of this chapter.

EXAMPLE Patient was seen in consultation for an inguinal hernia, unilateral, recurrent, with obstruction, 550.11 (K40.31).

Noninfectious Enteritis and Colitis

Crohn's Disease

Crohn's disease is characterized by inflammation of the GI tract, especially the small and large intestine. It is an inflammatory bowel disease that appears to run in families. It is typically diagnosed first at the age of 20 to 30. Often there is difficulty determining Crohn's versus ulcerative colitis. Crohn's may also be known as ileitis or enteritis. People presenting with Crohn's may exhibit symptoms of abdominal pain and diarrhea. Depending on the severity and location of the disease, patients may be treated with drugs to control inflammation, steroids, immunosuppressive agents, biologic response modifiers, antibiotics, and medications to control diarrhea, along with fluid replacement. Almost 75% of the patients with Crohn's require surgery at some point in their lives to remove the diseased intestine, and they often require an ostomy.

Ulcerative Colitis

Ulcerative colitis, like Crohn's disease, is an inflammatory bowel disease. Ulcerative colitis is a disease that produces ulcers in the lining of the rectum and colon, whereas Crohn's disease causes inflammation deep within the intestinal wall and can occur in other parts of the digestive system, including the small intestine, mouth, esophagus, and stomach.

Coding Clinic (2008:2Q:p15)[5] has also advised that when GI bleeding is due to acute ischemic colitis, only the code 557.0 (K55.0), for the acute vascular insufficiency of intestine, is assigned. The Includes note makes it inappropriate to assign an additional code for GI bleed.

EXAMPLE | Patient is admitted to the hospital with abdominal pain and dehydration. After testing is completed, a diagnosis of ulcerative enterocolitis is confirmed, 556.0, 276.51 (K51.80, E86.0).

Gastroenteritis is an inflammation of the stomach and intestines. Two of the main causes of this condition are viruses and bacteria. Viral gastroenteritis usually runs its course in 1 to 2 days, whereas bacterial gastroenteritis can last for up to a week or more. The most common causes of viral gastroenteritis, which often spreads via poor handwashing habits in schools and daycare centers, are adenoviruses, rotaviruses, and norovirus. The noroviruses are the leading cause of acute gastroenteritis. The most common bacterial causes are *E. coli*, salmonella, campylobacter, and shigella. Gastroenteritis due to particular viruses or bacteria may be indexed under "Gastroenteritis" with a subterm for the bacterium/virus. If the bacterium/virus is not listed, the Index has an instruction to *see also* enteritis. Codes for gastroenteritis caused by viruses or bacteria may be located in the infectious and parasitic diseases chapter. Gastroenteritis may also be caused by chemical toxins such as those found in medications or foods. These types of gastroenteritis are not infectious.

The symptoms of gastroenteritis can include vomiting, diarrhea, low grade fever, and abdominal pain. Treatment in a hospital usually consists of IV fluids for rehydration, and if the patient is suffering from bacterial gastroenteritis, antibiotics may be used. If vomiting is severe, antiemetics and antidiarrheal agents may also be used.

EXAMPLE | Patient is admitted to hospital with severe vomiting and diarrhea. After testing is performed, it is determined that she is suffering from a bout of gastroenteritis, 558.9 (K52.9).

Other Diseases of Intestines and Peritoneum

Intestinal Obstruction

This condition occurs when the content of the intestines cannot move forward. The intestines can be completely blocked or partially blocked. Obstruction may be mechanical or functional. Mechanical obstruction can be caused by a variety of conditions, such as neoplasm, **impaction**, stricture, adhesion, **intussusception**, **volvulus**, and herniation (Figure 17-8). When the obstruction is functional, it is called an **ileus**.

EXAMPLE | Patient with intestinal obstruction due to fecal impaction, 560.32 (K56.41).

EXAMPLE | Patient with obstruction due to ileus, 560.1 (K56.69).

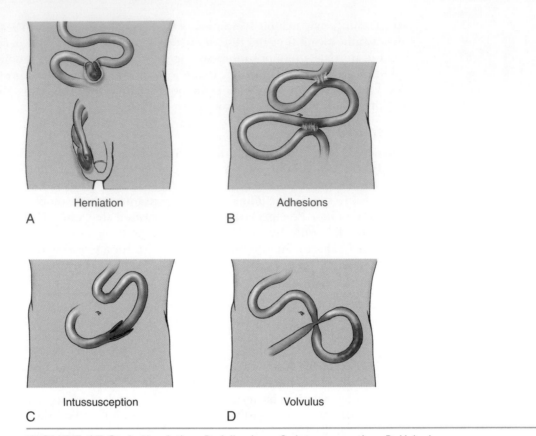

A Herniation

B Adhesions

C Intussusception

D Volvulus

FIGURE 17-8. **A,** Herniation. **B,** Adhesions. **C,** Intussusception. **D,** Volvulus.

EXAMPLE Patient has intussusception of the intestine, 560.0 (K56.1).

Diverticulitis and Diverticulosis

Diverticula (Figure 17-9), also known as tics, are small pouches in the lining of the mucous membranes of an organ. When a patient has diverticula, the condition is referred to as diverticulosis. If these pouches become inflamed or infected, the condition becomes diverticulitis. It is not necessary in ICD-9-CM to code both conditions; if a patient has diverticulitis, it is assumed that he or she also has diverticulosis. If the condition is described as diverticulosis without site, it is assumed by ICD-9-CM to be a condition of the colon.

EXAMPLE Patient has diverticulosis of the duodenum with diverticulitis and hemorrhage, 562.03 (K57.13).

EXERCISE 17-4

Assign codes to the following conditions.

1. Patient with acute abdominal pain is taken to the Operating _____
   Room (OR) for appendectomy with suspected appendicitis.
   Pathology report reveals normal appendix

2. Incisional hernia _____

3. Gangrenous ventral hernia _____

4. Congenital diaphragmatic hernia _____

5. Obstructed unilateral femoral hernia _____

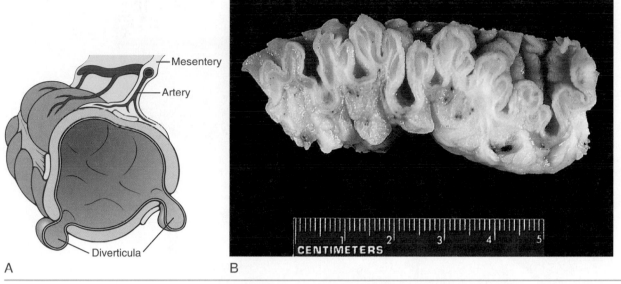

FIGURE 17-9. A, Diverticula. **B,** Diverticulosis.

6.	Meckel's diverticulitis	_____
7.	Hemorrhagic diverticulitis	_____
8.	Diverticulosis	_____
9.	Volvulus causing intestinal obstruction	_____
10.	Adhesions causing intestinal obstruction	_____
11.	Regional enteritis of the colon	_____
12.	Gastroenteritis due to *E. coli*	_____
13.	Allergic gastroenteritis due to milk allergy	_____
14.	Gastroenteritis due to radiation	_____
15.	Pseudopolyposis of the colon	_____

Other Diseases of Digestive System

Cholelithiasis and Cholecystitis

Cholelithiasis is an abnormal condition of stones in the gallbladder (gallstones). The condition is generally asymptomatic until gallstones block the cystic duct or the common bile duct, which does not allow the gallbladder to drain stored bile; the patient then develops acute cholecystitis (Figure 17-10). If the cystic duct is blocked, a patient generally has right upper quadrant crampy abdominal pain. This pain is often made worse by ingestion of fatty or greasy foods. When the common bile duct is blocked, a patient may develop cholangitis; when the stone is blocking the lower end of the common bile duct, secretion from the pancreas may be blocked, and pancreatitis may occur. **Choledocholithiasis** is the term used for a stone lodged in the bile duct. Endoscopic retrograde cholangiopancreatography (ERCP) may be used to detect the presence of gallstones.

EXAMPLE Patient has acute cholecystitis with cholelithiasis and choledocholithiasis, 574.60 (K80.62).

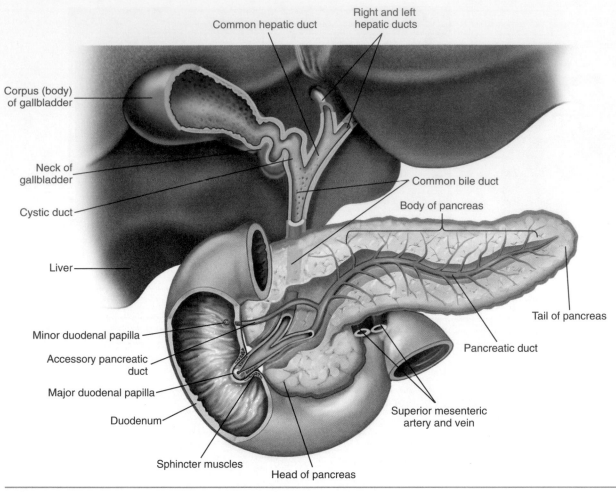

FIGURE 17-10. Ducts that carry bile from the liver and gallbladder. Obstruction of either the common hepatic duct or the common bile duct by a stone or spasm prevents bile from being ejected into the duodenum. From Patton KT. *Anatomy and Physiology, 7th ed.* St. Louis, Mosby, 2010.

Cirrhosis of the Liver

Cirrhosis of the liver is degeneration of liver tissue that causes blockage of blood through the organ and inhibits the function of this organ. Cirrhosis may be caused by a variety of factors; alcoholism and hepatitis are the most common.

EXAMPLE | Alcoholic cirrhosis of liver. Patient is a recovering alcoholic and no longer drinking, 571.2, 303.93 (K70.30, F10.21).

Hepatitis

Hepatitis, which is an inflammation of the liver, can last for a short time, or it may be chronic and last a lifetime. Most commonly, hepatitis is caused by a virus. When it is caused by a virus, hepatitis is coded from the infectious disease chapter of ICD-9-CM. However, other less common types of hepatitis are coded to the chapter on Digestive Diseases. Because the liver metabolizes both alcohol and drugs, a patient may develop alcoholic hepatitis or drug-induced hepatitis. When coding drug-induced hepatitis, it is important to also assign the E code for the responsible drug.

EXAMPLE | Patient has chronic hepatitis C, 070.54 (B18.2).

EXAMPLE	Patient has chronic hepatitis, 571.40 (K73.9).

EXERCISE 17-5

Assign codes to the following conditions.

1. Alcoholic hepatitis   _____
2. Drug-induced hepatitis by ibuprofen   _____
3. Hepatitis due to cytomegalovirus   _____
4. Fatty liver   _____
5. Portal hypertension   _____
6. Patient admitted to hospital with chronic cholecystitis for a   _____
   laparoscopic cholecystectomy; during the surgery, the surgeon
   decides to convert to open
7. Patient is admitted with gallstone pancreatitis; this is treated   _____
   and the patient is sent home

FACTORS INFLUENCING HEALTH STATUS AND CONTACT WITH HEALTH SERVICES (V CODES/Z CODES)

In the past, V/Z codes have been considered for use primarily in the outpatient setting. This has changed with the addition of more V/Z codes each year. As was discussed in Chapter 8, it is difficult to locate V/Z codes in the Index. Coders will often say, "I did not know there was a V/Z code for that." Refer to Chapter 8 for a listing of common main terms used to locate V/Z codes.

V/Z codes that may be used with digestive system conditions include the following:

V12.70	Personal history of unspecified digestive disorder
V12.71	Personal history of peptic ulcer disease
V12.72	Personal history of colonic polyps
V18.59	Family history of digestive disorders
V42.83	History of pancreas replaced by transplant
V42.84	History of intestines replaced by transplant
V44.1	Gastrostomy status
V44.2	Ileostomy status
V44.3	Colostomy status
V45.3	Intestinal bypass or anastomosis status
V45.72	Acquired absence of intestine
V45.75	Acquired absence of the stomach
V45.86	Bariatric sugery status
V53.50	Fitting and adjustment of intestinal appliance and device
V53.51	Fitting and adjustment of gastric lap band
V53.59	Fitting and adjustment of other gastrointestinal appliance and device
V55.1	Attention to gastrostomy
V55.2	Attention to ileostomy
V55.3	Attention to colostomy
V55.4	Attention to other artificial openings of the digestive tract
V59.6	Liver donor

EXAMPLE	Patient is admitted to donate a liver. An open right lobe liver lobectomy is performed, V59.6, 50.3 (Z52.6, 0FT10ZZ).

EXERCISE 17-6

Assign codes to the following conditions.

1. Patient is admitted for takedown of a colostomy _____

2. Patient had gastric bypass 1 year ago _____

3. Physician notes that the patient has a history of having the pancreas replaced by a transplant _____

4. Patient has a remote history of PUD _____

COMMON TREATMENTS

Many digestive disorders are treated with surgery.

CONDITION	MEDICATION
GERD	Propulsid, Reglan, Prilosec, Prevacid, Zantac, Tagamet
Crohn's disease	Azulfidine, Remicade, corticosteroids, Rowasa
Diverticulitis	Metronidazole, Ciprofloxacin
Gastric ulcer	Pepcid, Axid, Prilosec, Nexium
Gastroenteritis	Antiemetics such as Promethazine (Phenergan), prochlorperazine (Compazine), ondansetron (Zofran)
	Antidiarrheals, such as diphenoxylate atropine (Lomotil, Lofene, Lonox) or loperamide hydrochloride (Imodium)
	IV fluids
Pancreatitis	Antibiotics such as gentamicin, clindamycin

PROCEDURES

Some procedures that may be related to diseases of the digestive system may be located in the following chapter of the Procedure Tabular:

Chapter 9   Operations on the Digestive System (42-54)

Procedures related to the digestive system in ICD-10-PCS may be found in the following tables:

Mouth and Throat	0C0-0CX
Gastrointestinal System	0D1-0DY
Hepatobiliary System and Pancreas	0F1-0FY

Procedures of the Stomach

Nissen **fundoplication** (Figure 17-11) is a surgical treatment for GERD. The root operation in ICD-10-PCS for a Nissen fundoplication is restriction of the esophagogastric junction. This procedure takes the fundus (the upper portion) of the stomach and wraps it around

FIGURE 17-11. Nissen fundoplication.

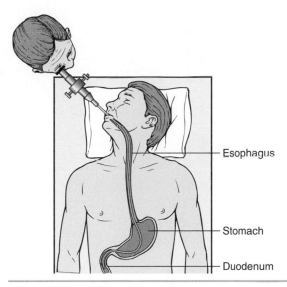

FIGURE 17-12. Esophagogastroduodenoscopy (EGD).

the lower portion of the esophagus to prevent the reflux of stomach contents back into the esophagus.

Percutaneous endoscopic gastrostomy (PEG) is the placement of a tube through the abdominal wall into the stomach with the use of a scope. The root operation for a PEG in ICD-10-PCS is insertion of a feeding device into the stomach. PEGs are used as feeding tubes for patients who are having difficulty eating (e.g., malnourished patients, patients who aspirate food). Per *Coding Clinic* (1993:5th issue:p16),[6] if a patient is admitted for insertion of a PEG tube because of carcinoma of the soft palate, and he or she now has dysphagia and dehydration, the principal diagnosis would be 145.3 (C05.1), carcinoma, and additional codes 787.20 (R13.10) (for dysphagia) and 276.51 (E86.0) (for dehydration) would be assigned.

If a patient presents to the hospital with a chief complaint of a PEG tube falling out, the principal diagnosis would be V55.1 (Z43.1), or attention to gastrostomy, because no complications resulted from the gastrostomy itself. This is described in detail in *Coding Clinic* (1997:3Q:p8).[7]

Procedures of the Intestine

Esophagogastroduodenoscopy (EGD) (Figure 17-12) is a diagnostic procedure that is used to identify disease conditions in the esophagus, stomach, and duodenum. The root operation for an EGD in ICD-10-PCS is inspection. Many times additional procedures are performed, such as biopsy, lesion removal, ablation, hemorrhage control, and dilations.

EXAMPLE   Patient with bleeding gastric ulcer taken to the OR for EGD to control bleeding in the stomach. Bleeding is controlled by electrocautery, 531.40, 44.43 (K25.4, 0D568ZZ).

Colostomy (Figure 17-13) is a procedure that uses the colon to create an artificial opening (**stoma**) to the exterior of the abdomen. The root operation for a colostomy in ICD-10-PCS is bypass. This artificial opening serves as a substitute anus through which the intestines excrete waste until the colon heals or other corrective surgery is performed. The location of the stoma depends on which part of the colon is involved in the surgery. Most colostomies are temporary. A sigmoid colostomy is the most commonly performed type.

Per *Coding Clinic* (1997:3Q:p9-10),[8] when a patient is admitted for a colostomy closure (takedown), the principal diagnosis should be V55.3 (Z43.3). Most often, when closing a

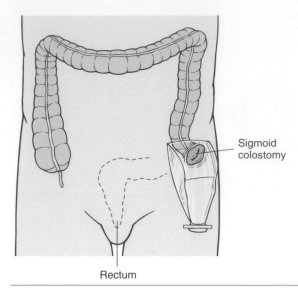

Sigmoid colostomy

Rectum

FIGURE 17-13. Colostomy. The opening of the colon is brought to the surface of the skin to divert feces into an external pouch worn by the patient.

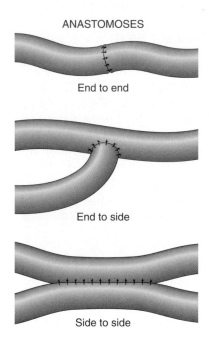

ANASTOMOSES

End to end

End to side

Side to side

FIGURE 17-14. Types of anastomoses.

colostomy, the surgeon must perform minor trimming of the colon to complete the anastomosis, but sometimes it is necessary to actually excise portions of the colon; in that case, it would be appropriate to code the intestinal resection as an additional code.

An **ileostomy** is very similar to a colostomy, except that the end of the small intestine is brought out through the abdominal wall.

Bowel resection can be performed for many reasons such as neoplasms, severe diverticulitis, bowel perforation, and bowel obstruction. Surgeons remove a portion of the bowel and then connect the bowel back together (anastomosis). In bowel resection in which an end-to-end anastomosis is performed, an additional code for the anastomosis is not assigned. This includes small intestine anastomosed to large intestine. Figure 17-14 illustrates various types of anastomoses.

EXAMPLE | Patient with malignant neoplasm of the descending colon is admitted for an open left hemicolectomy, and temporary colostomy, 153.2, 45.75, 46.11 (C18.6, 0DTG0ZZ, 0DIM0Z4).

    Appendectomy is removal of the appendix. The root operation for an appendectomy in ICD-10-PCS is resection. Codes are available for appendectomy done by incision and those done by laparoscopy. Often, when a surgeon is performing an abdominal operation, an incidental appendectomy may be performed. An **incidental appendectomy** is one that is performed at the time of another procedure with no known disease process in the appendix.

EXAMPLE | Patient with acute appendicitis is admitted for a laparoscopic appendectomy, 540.9, 47.01 (K35.80, 0DTJ4ZZ).

Procedures of the Gallbladder and Biliary System

Cholecystectomy, or removal of the gallbladder, can be performed by incision or by laparoscope (Figure 17-15). The root operation for a cholecystectomy in ICD-10-PCS is resection. Cholecystotomy may also be performed to remove stones from the gallbladder. This can be performed by open incision as well as by scope.

EXAMPLE | Patient with acute cholecystitis with cholelithiasis has a laparoscopic cholecystectomy, 574.00, 51.23 (K80.00, 0FT44ZZ).

    Common bile duct stones can be removed in three different ways (i.e., by incision, endoscopy, or percutaneously). Occasionally a cholecystectomy is performed along with removal of common duct stones. Codes should be assigned for both the cholecystectomy and the common bile duct stone removal. Fragmentation of stones of the gallbladder by extracorporeal shock wave lithotripsy, or ESWL, is the breaking apart of stones by shock waves.

FIGURE 17-15. Trocar placement for laparoscopic cholecystectomy.

EXAMPLE | Patient with common bile duct stones presents for stone removal by ERCP, 574.50, 51.88 (K80.50, 0FC98ZZ).

An endoscopic retrograde cholangiopancreatography (ERCP) is often done for diagnosis, but it may be done for stent insertion, or may be done in combination with a sphincterotomy or for removal of stones. In all of these cases, both the ERCP and the additional codes are assigned. The root operation in ICD-10-PCS for a diagnostic ERCP is located under Section B, imaging. If the ERCP is done for stent insertion, the root operation is dilation. If the ERCP is done for stone removal, the root operation is extirpation.

EXAMPLE | Patient with abdominal pain that is suspected to be due to a pancreatic malignancy presents for a diagnostic ERCP with low osmolar contrast. The ERCP reveals no malignancy, 789.00, 51.10 (R10.9, BF111ZZ).

Lysis of Adhesions

Lysis of adhesions is a procedure that is performed to destroy adhesions. The root operation in ICD-10-PCS for lysis of adhesions is release. **Adhesions**, which are very often found in the peritoneal area, are fibrous bands of tissue that adhere abdominal organs to one another or to the abdominal wall. Adhesions are often synonymous with scar tissue and can develop after surgery, often causing abdominal pain. To code adhesion removal, look in the Index under Lysis, adhesions. Attention should be paid to the instructional note in the Alphabetic Index under lysis of adhesions to omit this code if the surgeon uses terminology such as blunt, digital, manual, mechanical, and without instrumentation. *Coding Clinic* (1990:4Q:p18-19)[9] discusses when it is appropriate to include this code in combination with other procedure codes.

EXAMPLE | Patient with chronic cholecystitis admitted for laparoscopic cholecystectomy. The surgeon performed manual lysis of adhesions of the gallbladder, prior to laparoscopic cholecystectomy, 575.11, 51.23 (K81.1, 0FT44ZZ). No code for lysis of adhesions required.

EXAMPLE | Patient with abdominal pain is admitted. The surgeon performed laparoscopic lysis of adhesions of the peritoneum, 568.0, 54.51 (K66.0, 0DNW4ZZ).

Hernia Repair

Herniorrhaphy is repair of a hernia. The root operation in ICD-10-PCS for hernia repair is repair. When the hernia is repaired with mesh, the root operation becomes supplement. Coding hernia repairs requires attention to location, laterality, whether direct or indirect, and whether performed with a prosthesis or a graft. In a direct hernia, the protrusion occurs through the abdominal wall; an indirect hernia results when the protrusion occurs through the inguinal ring into the inguinal canal.

EXAMPLE | Patient had a bilateral inguinal hernia repair direct and indirect with prosthesis, 550.92, 53.16 (K40.20, 0YUA0JZ).

Whipple Procedure

Whipple procedure is also known as a pancreaticoduodenectomy. This procedure generally involves removal of the gallbladder, common bile duct, part of the duodenum, and the head of the pancreas. The root operation in ICD-10-PCS for a whipple procedure includes both resection and bypass. This procedure may be performed for chronic pancreatitis, pancreatic pseudocysts, or pancreatic malignancies.

EXAMPLE

> Patient with pancreatic cancer in the head of the pancreas presents for Whipple procedure, the head of the pancreas, a portion of the bile duct, the gallbladder, and part of the duodenum were removed during this procedure, 157.0, 52.7 (C25.0, OFT40ZZ, OFBG0ZZ, OFB90ZZ, OD160ZA, ODB90ZZ, OF198Z3, OF1G0ZC).

Transjugular Intrahepatic Portosystemic Shunt (TIPS)

TIPS (transjugular intrahepatic portosystemic shunt): This procedure is often performed by interventional radiologists for patients with severe complications of liver disease. The root operation in ICD-10-PCS for a TIPS procedure is bypass. The interventionalist percutaneously makes a tunnel through the liver with a needle and connects the portal vein to one of the hepatic veins. A stent is inserted into this tunnel to keep the tract open. This procedure does not improve the functioning of the liver but helps in treatment of the complications.

EXAMPLE

> A patient with portal hypertension is admitted for a TIPS procedure, 572.3, 39.1 (K76.6, O6183DY).

EXERCISE 17-7

Assign codes to the following conditions.

1. Insertion percutaneous endoscopic gastrostomy for dysphagia   _____

2. Incidental appendectomy during cholecystectomy for gallstones   _____

3. Repair of ventral hernia   _____

4. ERCP with endoscopic sphincterotomy and stone removal from pancreatic duct   _____

5. Patient with GERD admitted for Nissen fundoplication   _____

DOCUMENTATION/REIMBURSEMENT/MS-DRGS

Often, coding difficulties are due to lack of documentation. Sometimes pathology and other test results are not available at the time of discharge or when the physician is dictating the discharge summary or is reporting the final diagnoses.

Frequently missed complications/comorbidities from this chapter include the following:

- Cholangitis
- Hematemesis
- GI hemorrhage
- Ileus
- Melena
- Pancreatitis
- Peritonitis

Types of Appendicitis

It is important to check pathology reports when appendectomies are performed and to review the record for documentation of appendiceal rupture, abscess, or generalized peritonitis. Different MS-DRGs are assigned for appendicitis with a complicated principal diagnosis.

EXAMPLE

DIAGNOSES/PROCEDURES	CODES	MS-DRG	RW
Acute appendicitis with	540.9 (K35.9)	343	0.9568
Appendectomy, laparoscopic	47.01 (0DTJ8ZZ)		
Ruptured appendicitis with	540.0 (K35.0)	340	1.2393
Appendectomy, laparoscopic	47.01 (0DTJ8ZZ)		

Two or More Interrelated Conditions, Each Potentially Meeting the Definition of Principal Diagnosis

EXAMPLE

DIAGNOSES	CODES	MS-DRG	RW
Dehydration	276.51 (E86.0)	641	0.6916
Gastroenteritis	558.9 (K52.9)		
Gastroenteritis	558.9 (K52.9)	392	0.7173
Dehydration	276.51 (E86.0)		

Coding Clinic (1984:July-Aug:p19-20; 1988:2Q:p10)[10,11] reminds the coder that the reason the patient is admitted for treatment should be the principal diagnosis. If the patient had dehydration caused by gastroenteritis and was admitted for IV fluids, then the principal diagnosis would be the dehydration. However, if the patient had gastroenteritis and dehydration and the patient was admitted for treatment of both of these diagnoses, then either diagnosis could be sequenced as the principal.

Lysis of Adhesions

It is always important to review the operative report for lysis of adhesions. Per *Coding Clinic* (1990:4Q:p18)[8] if multiple adhesions prevent the surgeon from gaining access to the organ that is being removed, thereby requiring lysis before the operation can be completed, both diagnosis of adhesions and the lysis procedure should be coded.

EXAMPLE

DIAGNOSES/PROCEDURES	CODES	MS-DRG	RW
Acute appendicitis	540.9 (K35.9)	343	0.9568
Adhesions	568.0 (K66.0)		
Appendectomy	47.01 (0DTJ8ZZ)		
Acute appendicitis	540.9 (K35.9)	337	1.4789
Adhesions	568.0 (K66.0)		
Appendectomy	47.01 (0DTJ8ZZ)		
Lysis of adhesions	54.51 (0DNW4ZZ)		

Coding Clinic (1990:4Q:p18)[9] goes on to say that frequently, however, adhesions may exist without being organized and without causing any symptoms in the patient or increasing the difficulty of performing the operative procedure. When such minor adhesions exist and are easily lysed as part of the principal procedure, coding a diagnosis of adhesions and the procedure would be inappropriate.

Blood Loss Anemia With GI Bleeds

In cases of GI bleed, it would be prudent to check laboratory values with regard to falling hematocrit or hemoglobin, as well as orders for transfusions. Many GI bleeds have as a common comorbidity acute or chronic blood loss anemia. This is often not well documented by physicians, and a query may be required.

EXAMPLE

DIAGNOSES	CODES	MS-DRG	RW
GI bleed	578.9 (K92.2)	379	0.7146
GI bleed with acute blood loss anemia	578.9 (K92.2)	378	1.0274
	285.1 (D62)		

Types of Cholecystectomies and Additional Procedures Performed

Cholecystectomies have a separate set of MS-DRGs for those done with common bile duct exploration. Common bile duct exploration is a procedure that allows the clinician to see whether a stone is blocking the flow of bile from the liver and gallbladder to the intestine. Close attention must be paid to the method by which the cholecystectomy is performed as there is a separate MS-DRG for cholecystectomies performed by laparoscopy.

EXAMPLE

DIAGNOSES/PROCEDURES	CODES	MS-DRG	RW
Calculus of bile duct with acute cholecystitis and cholecystectomy	574.30 (K80.62) 51.22 (0FT40ZZ)	416	1.3080

EXAMPLE

DIAGNOSES/PROCEDURES	CODES	MS-DRG	RW
Calculus of bile duct with acute cholecystitis and cholecystectomy with exploration of the common bile duct	574.30 (K80.62) 51.22 (0FT40ZZ) 51.51 (0FJ90ZZ)	413	1.7180

EXAMPLE

DIAGNOSES/PROCEDURES	CODES	MS-DRG	RW
Calculus of bile duct with acute cholecystitis and laparoscopic cholecystectomy	574.30 (K80.62) 51.24 (0FB44ZZ)	419	1.1698

CHAPTER REVIEW EXERCISE

Where applicable, assign codes for diagnoses, procedures, V/Z codes, and external causes codes.

1. What makes up the alimentary canal?

   _____

2. What are the three areas of the small intestines?
   1. _____
   2. _____
   3. _____

3. What three organs assist the digestive process?
   1. _____
   2. _____
   3. _____

4. A patient is admitted to the hospital with severe GERD and is treated by Nissen fundoplication.   _____

5. A patient presents to the Emergency Room (ER) with hematochezia and hematemesis. The patient is admitted, and it is determined that acute blood loss anemia is caused by diverticulosis.   _____

6. A patient has a bleeding gastric ulcer caused by *Helicobacter pylori*.   _____

7. A patient is admitted to the hospital with what the surgeon believes to be acute appendicitis. The surgeon takes the patient to the Operating Room (OR) and removes the appendix; the pathology report reveals a ruptured appendix.   _____

8. A patient is admitted to the hospital with an incisional hernia. The patient is taken to the OR, and herniorrhaphy is performed with a graft. _____

9. A patient is admitted to the hospital with a bilateral indirect inguinal hernia that is repaired with a graft. _____

10. A patient with diverticulitis and diverticulosis is taken to the OR for an endoscopic diverticulectomy of the large intestine. _____

11. A patient with cholecystitis presents to the ER. ERCP reveals cholelithiasis. The surgeon performs a laparoscopic partial cholecystectomy. _____

12. A patient with severe Crohn's disease is taken to the OR for a Hartmann procedure on the left with an end-to-end anastomosis and a temporary colostomy. _____

13. A patient with cholelithaisis has an ESWL. _____

14. A patient with severe chronic pancreatitis is admitted to the hospital, where a surgeon performs a Whipple procedure. _____

15. A patient with ascites due to alcoholic cirrhosis is admitted to the hospital for a TIPS procedure. _____

16. A patient with a bleeding duodenal ulcer is admitted to the hospital, where the gastroenterologist provides endoscopic control of the hemorrhage. _____

17. A patient with severe malnutrition is admitted to the hospital for endoscopic placement of a gastrostomy tube. _____

18. Acute hemorrhagic gastric ulcer caused by NSAID _____

19. Gallstone of common bile duct, status post cholecystectomy, 1 year PTA _____

20. GI bleed due to acute vascular insufficiency _____

CHAPTER GLOSSARY

Adhesion: scar tissue that forms an abnormal connection between body parts.

Alimentary canal: comprises the mouth, pharynx, esophagus, stomach, small intestine, and large intestine.

Angiodysplasia: type of AVM characterized by dilated or fragile blood vessels.

Anorexia: loss of appetite.

Appendectomy: removal of the appendix.

Appendicitis: inflammation of the appendix.

Arteriovenous malformation: defect that arises during fetal development.

Barrett's esophagus: precancerous condition that usually occurs in people with chronic GERD.

Bowel resection: removal of a portion of the bowel.

Choledocholithiasis: stone lodged in the bile duct.

Cholelithiasis: an abnormal condition of stones in the gallbladder.

Cirrhosis: liver disease wherein scar tissue replaces healthy tissue and blocks blood flow.

Colostomy: a procedure that uses the colon to create an artificial opening.

Crohn's disease: inflammation of the GI tract, especially the small and large intestine.

Diverticula: small pouches in the lining of the mucous membranes of an organ.

Edentulism: the complete loss of teeth.

Fundoplication: surgery in which the fundus of the stomach is wrapped around the esophagus.

Gastroenteritis: inflammation of the stomach and intestines.

Hematemesis: vomiting of blood.

Hematochezia: bright red blood in stool.

Hepatitis: an inflammation of the liver.

Hernia: protrusion of an organ or tissue through an abnormal opening in the body.

Herniorrhaphy: repair of a hernia.

Ileostomy: end of small intestine brought out through the abdominal wall.

Ileus: absence of normal movement within the intestine.

Impaction: condition that occurs when stool in the rectum becomes so hard that it cannot be passed normally.

Incidental appendectomy: appendectomy performed at the time of another procedure with no known disease process in the appendix.

Intussusception: bowel becomes obstructed when a portion of the intestine telescopes into another portion.

Lysis: destruction of adhesions.

Mallory-Weiss: bleeding laceration of the esophagogastric junction.

Mastication: chewing of food.

McBurney's point: area of the abdomen that, when touched, causes pain that may be indicative of appendicitis.

Melena: dark blood in stool

Mucositis: an inflammation/ulceration of the digestive tract commonly occurring in the oral cavity.

Necrotic: dead tissue that lacks a blood supply.

Occult blood: blood only found by laboratory inspection.

Percutaneous endoscopic gastrostomy: a tube put through the abdominal wall into the stomach with the use of a scope.

Peristalsis: rhythmic muscle contractions that move food down the digestive tract.

Sialolithiasis: stones in the salivary glands.

Stoma: an artificial opening.

TIPS (transjugular intrahepatic portosystemic shunt): a procedure in which the portal vein is connected to one of the hepatic veins and a stent is inserted.

Ulcerative colitis: an inflammatory bowel disease.

Volvulus: an abnormal twisting of the intestine that may impair blood flow to the intestine.

Whipple procedure: a procedure that generally involves removal of the gallbladder, common bile duct, part of the duodenum, and the head of the pancreas.

REFERENCES

1. American Hospital Association. *Coding Clinic for ICD-9-CM* 1996:3Q:p9-10. Gastric arteriovenous malformation.
2. American Hospital Association. *Coding Clinic for ICD-9-CM* 1986:Nov-Dec:p11. Arteriovenous (A-V) malformation of colon.
3. American Hospital Association. *Coding Clinic for ICD-9-CM* 2005:3Q:p17-18. GI bleeding with multiple possible causes.
4. American Hospital Association. *Coding Clinic for ICD-9-CM* 1990:2Q:p26. Appendicitis, unqualified.
5. American Hospital Association. *Coding Clinic for ICD-9-CM* 2008:2Q:p15. Acute ischemic colitis with hemorrhage.
6. American Hospital Association. *Coding Clinic for ICD-9-CM* 1993:5th issue:p16. Dysphagia and dehydration due to CA with PEG feeding tube placement.
7. American Hospital Association. *Coding Clinic for ICD-9-CM* 1997:3Q:p8. Dislodged gastrostomy tube.
8. American Hospital Association. *Coding Clinic for ICD-9-CM* 1997:3Q:p9-10. Admission for colostomy closure.
9. American Hospital Association. *Coding Clinic for ICD-9-CM* 1990:4Q:p18-19. Lysis of adhesions—Guidelines.
10. American Hospital Association. *Coding Clinic for ICD-9-CM* 1984:July-Aug:p19-20. Dehydration due to gastroenteritis—Sequencing.
11. American Hospital Association. *Coding Clinic for ICD-9-CM* 1988:2Q:p10. Gastroenteritis with diarrhea and dehydration.

18

Diseases of the Skin and Subcutaneous Tissue

(ICD-9-CM Chapter 12, Codes 680-709, and ICD-10-CM Chapter 12, Codes L00-L99)

LEARNING OBJECTIVES

1. Apply and assign the correct ICD-9-CM and ICD-10-CM codes in accordance with Official Guidelines for Coding and Reporting
2. Identify major differences between ICD-9-CM and ICD-10-CM related to the skin and subcutaneous tissue
3. Identify pertinent anatomy and physiology of the skin and subcutaneous tissue
4. Identify diseases of the skin and subcutaneous tissue
5. Assign the correct V/Z codes and procedure codes related to the skin and subcutaneous tissue
6. Identify common treatments, medications, laboratory values, and diagnostic tests
7. Explain the importance of documentation in relation to MS-DRGs for reimbursement

ABBREVIATIONS/ ACRONYMS

CEA cultured epidermal autograft

FTSG full-thickness skin graft

ICD-9-CM *International Classification of Diseases, 9th Revision, Clinical Modification*

ICD-10-CM *International Classification of Diseases, 10th Revision, Clinical Modification*

ICD-10-PCS *International Classification of Diseases, 10th Revision, Procedure Coding System*

I&D incision and drainage

MS-DRG Medicare Severity diagnosis-related group

STSG split-thickness skin graft

ICD-9-CM

Official Guidelines for Coding and Reporting

Please refer to the companion Evolve website for the most current guidelines.

Chapter 12: Diseases Skin and Subcutaneous Tissue (680-709)

a. Pressure ulcer stage codes

1) Pressure ulcer stages

Two codes are needed to completely describe a pressure ulcer: A code from subcategory 707.0, Pressure ulcer, to identify the site of the pressure ulcer and a code from subcategory 707.2, Pressure ulcer stages.

The codes in subcategory 707.2, Pressure ulcer stages, are to be used as an additional diagnosis with a code(s) from subcategory 707.0, Pressure ulcer. Codes from 707.2, Pressure ulcer stages, may not be assigned as a principal or first-listed diagnosis. The pressure ulcer stage codes should only be used with pressure ulcers and not with other types of ulcers (e.g., stasis ulcer).

The ICD-9-CM classifies pressure ulcer stages based on severity, which is designated by stages I-IV and unstageable.

EXAMPLE

The patient was admitted to the hospital from the nursing home. Upon examination the physician noted a stage II pressure ulcer on the sacrum, 707.03, 707.22 (L89.152).

2) Unstageable pressure ulcers

Assignment of code 707.25, Pressure ulcer, unstageable, should be based on the clinical documentation. Code 707.25 is used for pressure ulcers whose stage cannot be clinically determined (e.g., the ulcer is covered by eschar or has been treated with a skin or muscle graft) and pressure ulcers that are documented as deep tissue injury but not documented as due to trauma. This code should not be confused with code 707.20, Pressure ulcer, stage unspecified. Code 707.20 should be assigned when there is no documentation regarding the stage of the pressure ulcer.

EXAMPLE

Patient is in the hospital for pneumonia. It is noted in the physical exam that the patient was recently treated for a pressure ulcer of the heel by skin graft. The graft looks to be progressing as planned, 486, 707.07, 707.25 (J18.9, L89.609).

3) Documented pressure ulcer stage

Assignment of the pressure ulcer stage code should be guided by clinical documentation of the stage or documentation of the terms found in the index. For clinical terms describing the stage that are not found in the index, the provider should be queried.

4) Bilateral pressure ulcers with same stage

When a patient has bilateral pressure ulcers (e.g., both buttocks) and both pressure ulcers are documented as being the same stage, only the code for the site and one code for the stage should be reported.

5) Bilateral pressure ulcers with different stages

When a patient has bilateral pressure ulcers at the same site (e.g., both buttocks) and each pressure ulcer is documented as being at a different stage, assign one code for the site and the appropriate codes for the pressure ulcer stage.

> **6) Multiple pressure ulcers of different sites and stages**
> When a patient has multiple pressure ulcers at different sites (e.g., buttock, heel, shoulder) and each pressure ulcer is documented as being at different stages (e.g., stage 3 and stage 4), assign the appropriate codes for each different site and a code for each different pressure ulcer stage.

EXAMPLE

Patient has stage IV pressure ulcers on both heels, 707.07, 707.24 (L89.624, L89.614).

EXAMPLE

Patient has pressure ulcers on both buttocks. The buttock on the right has a stage II ulcer while the left buttock has a stage III ulcer, 707.05, 707.22, 707.23 (L89.323, L89.312).

EXAMPLE

Patient is transferred from the nursing home with a fever and infected decubitus ulcers. There is an ulcer of the left hip stage III and ulcers of both elbows. The right elbow has a stage I ulcer and the left elbow has a stage II ulcer, 707.04, 707.01, 707.23, 707.21, 707.22 (L89.223, L89.011, L89.022).

> **7) Patients admitted with pressure ulcers documented as healed**
> No code is assigned if the documentation states that the pressure ulcer is completely healed.
>
> **8) Patients admitted with pressure ulcers documented as healing**
> Pressure ulcers described as healing should be assigned the appropriate pressure ulcer stage code based on the documentation in the medical record. If the documentation does not provide information about the stage of the healing pressure ulcer, assign code 707.20, Pressure ulcer stage, unspecified.
>   If the documentation is unclear as to whether the patient has a current (new) pressure ulcer or if the patient is being treated for a healing pressure ulcer, query the provider.

EXAMPLE

On the discharge summary, the provider documents the following discharge diagnoses: Exacerbation of COPD, hypertension, hyperlipidemia, and a healed sacral decubitus, 491.21, 401.9, 272.4 (J44.1, I10, E78.5).

EXAMPLE

On the discharge summary, the provider documents the following discharge diagnoses: Exacerbation of COPD, hypertension, hyperlipidemia, and a healing sacral decubitus, 491.21, 401.9, 272.4, 707.03, 707.20 (J44.1, I10, E78.5, L89.159).

> **9) Patient admitted with pressure ulcer evolving into another stage during the admission**
> If a patient is admitted with a pressure ulcer at one stage and it progresses to a higher stage, assign the code for highest stage reported for that site.

EXAMPLE

Patient is admitted to the hospital from the nursing home for aspiration pneumonia. The admitting provider documents that the patient has a stage II sacral ulcer. At the time of transfer back to the nursing home, the provider documents the ulcer as stage III, 507.0, 707.03, 707.23 (J69.0, L89.153).

Apply the General Coding Guidelines as found in Chapter 5 and the Procedural Guidelines as found in Chapter 6.

ICD-10-CM

Official Guidelines for Coding and Reporting

Please refer to the companion Evolve website for the most current guidelines.

12. Chapter 12: Diseases of Skin and Subcutaneous Tissue (L00-L99)

  a. Pressure ulcer stage codes

    1) Pressure ulcer stages

      Codes from category L89, Pressure ulcer, are combination codes that indentify the site of the pressure ulcer as well as the stage of the ulcer.

      The ICD-10-CM classifies pressure ulcer stages based on severity, which is designated by stages 1-4, unspecified stage and unstageable.

      Assign as many codes from category L89 as needed to identify all the pressure ulcers the patient has, if applicable.

    2) Unstageable pressure ulcers

      Assignment of the code for unstageable pressure ulcer (L89.–0) should be based on the clinical documentation. These codes are used for pressure ulcers whose stage cannot be clinically determined (e.g., the ulcer is covered by eschar or has been treated with a skin or muscle graft) and pressure ulcers that are documented as deep tissue injury but not documented as due to trauma. This code should not be confused with the codes for unspecified stage (L89.–9). When there is no documentation regarding the stage of the pressure ulcer, assign the appropriate code for unspecified stage (L89.–9).

    3) Documented pressure ulcer stage

      Assignment of the pressure ulcer stage code should be guided by clinical documentation of the stage or documentation of the terms found in the **Alphabetic Index**. For clinical terms describing the stage that are not found in the **Alphabetic Index**, and there is no documentation of the stage, the provider should be queried.

    4) Patients admitted with pressure ulcers documented as healed

      No code is assigned if the documentation states that the pressure ulcer is completely healed.

    5) Patients admitted with pressure ulcers documented as healing

      Pressure ulcers described as healing should be assigned the appropriate pressure ulcer stage code based on the documentation in the medical record. If the documentation does not provide information about the stage of the healing pressure ulcer, assign the appropriate code for unspecified stage.

      If the documentation is unclear as to whether the patient has a current (new) pressure ulcer or if the patient is being treated for a healing pressure ulcer, query the provider.

    6) Patient admitted with pressure ulcer evolving into another stage during the admission

      If a patient is admitted with a pressure ulcer at one stage and it progresses to a higher stage, assign the code for the highest stage reported for that site.

Apply the General Coding Guidelines as found in Chapter 5 and the Procedural Guidelines as found in Chapter 7.

GUIDELINE CHANGES BETWEEN ICD-9-CM AND ICD-10-CM

The only major guideline difference between ICD-9-CM and ICD-10-CM is in ICD-10-CM only one code covers both site of ulcer and stage of ulcer. Also in ICD-10-CM there are more specific codes for bilateral ulcers of the same site; therefore, the guidelines from ICD-9-CM addressing this issue are no longer applicable.

MAJOR DIFFERENCES BETWEEN ICD-9-CM AND ICD-10-CM

- In ICD-9-CM, the coding of decubitus ulcers required two codes, whereas ICD-10-CM uses a combination code.
- ICD-10-CM introduces a new term, "androgenic alopecia."
- In ICD-10-CM, the terms "dermatitis" and "eczema" are used interchangeably.

- Instructions in ICD-10-CM for allergic contact dermatitis state to code first the responsible drug or substance with codes T36-T65.
- Intraoperative and procedural complications of the skin and subcutaneous tissue include:
  - Intraoperative hemorrhage of skin
  - Accidental puncture or laceration of the skin
  - Postprocedural hemorrhage or hematoma of the skin

ANATOMY AND PHYSIOLOGY

The skin and its accessory organs constitute the **integumentary** system (Figure 18-1), whose functions include protection, temperature regulation, sensory reception, and vitamin D synthesis.

The skin is composed of three layers: epidermis, dermis, and subcutaneous layers. The outer layer of the skin, or the **epidermis,** serves as a protective barrier and prevents the entrance of disease-causing organisms. The **dermis**, or middle layer, is composed of fibrous connective tissues that make it strong and elastic. This middle layer contains blood vessels, nerve fibers, sebaceous glands, and some hair follicles. The **subcutaneous** layer contains fat, sweat glands, and additional hair follicles.

The integumentary system also has accessory organs; these include hair, glands, and nails. Three types of glands are located in the skin: sweat glands, sebaceous glands, and mammary glands. The sweat glands assist in temperature regulation, and the sebaceous glands secrete an oily substance, **sebum,** which lubricates the hair and skin.

FIGURE 18-1. The skin. **A,** Three layers of the skin. **B,** Epidermis.

DISEASE CONDITIONS

Diseases of the Skin and Subcutaneous Tissue (680-709), Chapter 12 in the ICD-9-CM code book, is divided into the following categories:

CATEGORY	SECTION TITLES
680-686	Infections of Skin and Subcutaneous Tissue
690-698	Other Inflammatory Conditions of Skin and Subcutaneous Tissue
700-709	Other Diseases of Skin and Subcutaneous Tissue

Diseases of the Skin and Subcutaneous Tissue (L00-L99), Chapter 12 in the ICD-10-CM code book, are divided into the following categories:

CATEGORY	SECTION TITLES
L00-L08	Infections of the skin and subcutaneous tissue
L10-L14	Bullous disorders
L20-L30	Dermatitis and eczema
L40-L45	Papulosquamous disorders
L50-L54	Urticaria and erythema
L55-L59	Radiation-related disorders of the skin and subcutaneous tissue
L60-L75	Disorders of skin appendages
L76	Intraoperative and postprocedural complications of skin and subcutaneous tissue
L80-L99	Other disorders of the skin and subcutaneous tissue

Infections of the Skin and Subcutaneous Tissue

Carbuncle and Furuncle

Another name for a **furuncle** is a boil, and a cluster of boils is known as a **carbuncle** (Figure 18-2). The organism that is responsible for a boil is *Staphylococcus*. This organism enters the body through a hair follicle. An additional code is required to identify the organism responsible.

FIGURE 18-2. A, Furuncle. **B,** Carbuncle.

Cellulitis/Abscess of the Skin

Cellulitis is an acute inflammation of tissue that is characterized by swelling, redness, and tenderness that are most often caused by a bacterial infection. An **abscess** is a localized collection of pus that causes swelling. Cellulitis is generally treated with antibiotics; an abscess may be treated with antibiotics and also may require incision and drainage.

As is noted in these code categories, acute lymphangitis is included and is **NOT** coded separately in a patient with cellulitis or abscess. An additional code is used to identify the organism causing the cellulitis, when documented.

Cellulitis associated with a superficial injury, burn, or frostbite requires the use of two codes: one code for the injury/burn/frostbite and one code for the cellulitis. Per *Coding Clinic* (1991:2Q:p5-7),[1] the sequence of these codes is dependent on the focus of treatment. For superficial injuries with cellulitis, it is likely that treatment will be focused on the cellulitis.

EXAMPLE

> Patient with cat scratch of the right hand with localized cellulitis admitted for treatment of cellulitis, 682.4, 914.9, E906.8 (L03.113, S60.511A, W55.03xA).

Cellulitis associated with a traumatic open wound requires the use of two codes: one code for the open wound, complicated, and one code for the cellulitis. The sequence of these codes is dependent on the focus of treatment. If the focus of treatment is the open wound, the code for the wound is sequenced first, followed by the code for cellulitis. If, on the other hand, the focus of the treatment is the cellulitis and the wound is trivial, or if the wound was treated on a separate occasion, the cellulitis would be sequenced first.

EXAMPLE

> Patient stepped on a piece of glass and injured his foot 2 days ago. He is now being admitted to the hospital for treatment of cellulitis in the left leg, 682.6, 892.1, E920.8 (L03.116, S91.312A, W25.xxxA).

Gangrenous cellulitis is assigned only the code for gangrene—NOT a code for cellulitis. Cellulitis associated with a skin ulcer requires the use of two codes: one for the ulcer and one for the cellulitis. The sequence of codes is dependent on the focus of treatment.

EXAMPLE

> Patient has a chronic right leg ulcer with cellulitis. She is admitted to the hospital for treatment of the leg ulcer, 707.10, 682.6 (L97.919, L03.115).

Cellulitis occurring in areas other than the skin is coded to the chapter that is most appropriate. The coder will find direction in the Alphabetic Index.

EXAMPLE

> Patient has cellulitis of the lip, 528.5 (K13.0).

EXERCISE 18-1

Assign codes to the following conditions.

1. Cellulitis of the face _____
2. Cellulitis with lymphangitis of the breast. *Staphylococcus aureus* infection _____
3. Cellulitis of the foot due to patient stepping on a nail with open wound of the foot _____
4. Gangrenous cellulitis of toe _____
5. Neck abscess _____
6. Cellulitis, rectum _____

Other Inflammatory Conditions of Skin and Subcutaneous Tissue

Dermatitis

Dermatitis is an inflammation of the skin that is also referred to as **eczema**. Dermatitis, which is characterized by redness, itching, scaling, and crusting skin, is caused by contact with a substance (**exogenous**) or ingestion of a substance (**endogenous**).

Contact dermatitis in ICD-9-CM contains a variety of fourth-digit codes that are used to identify the substance the patient came into contact with that caused the dermatitis. This category also includes dermatitis due to the effects of solar radiation. When coding dermatitis due to drugs or medicines, the coder must first determine whether the drug was taken as correctly prescribed, causing an adverse reaction, or if the drug was not taken as prescribed, making this a poisoning. An adverse reaction is coded with the dermatitis code first, followed by a therapeutic E code that describes the type of drug that caused the dermatitis.

EXAMPLE   Patient with dermatitis caused by drinking tomato juice, 693.1 (L27.2).

Stasis dermatitis is an inflammation of the lower legs that is often associated with venous incompetence. It is important to follow the Index carefully. Often, patients have ulcers associated with stasis dermatitis. Per *Coding Clinic* (1991:2Q:p20),[2] these are coded to 454.0, which represents varicose veins with ulcer.

EXAMPLE   Patient is being treated for stasis ulcer of the leg without varicose veins, 459.81, 707.10 (I87.2). In ICD-10-CM stasis ulcer is indexed to this code with no instructions to assign an additional code for the ulcer.

EXAMPLE   Patient has a stasis ulcer of the right calf with varicose veins, 454.0 (I83.012, L97.219).

EXAMPLE   Patient has varicose veins of the left leg with inflammation, 454.1 (I83.12).

Intertriginous dermatitis, a type of rash that is found in body folds, is a common condition in the overweight patient, possibly because of skin chafing and the inability of sweat to evaporate. This condition is not found under the Dermatitis heading in the Index but may be located under **Intertrigo**.

Psoriasis is an inflammation of the skin caused by a fault in the immune system. There are several types of psoriasis, the most common of which is plaque psoriasis. The skin on the elbows, knees, lower back, and scalp are the most common areas plaques are found. Psoriasis usually itches, and the skin may crack and bleed. This is a life-long condition for which there is no cure. Some people develop psoriatic arthritis, which is a systemic rheumatic disease.

"**Hives**" and "**urticaria**" are synonymous terms that refer to vascular reactions of the skin that present as wheals, welts, or reddened patches (Figure 18-3) and are associated with **pruritus** (itching). Hives usually occur as an allergic reaction to food, bug bites, or drugs.

EXAMPLE   Patient is treated for hives due to peanuts, 708.0 (L50.0).

EXAMPLE   Patient presented with hives. No cause can be determined, 708.9 (L50.9).

FIGURE 18-3. Urticaria.

FIGURE 18-4. Ulcers.

EXERCISE 18-2

Assign codes to the following conditions.

1. Contact dermatitis due to mascara _____
2. Contact dermatitis due to tanning bed _____
3. Hives due to penicillin _____
4. Contact dermatitis due to milk _____
5. Dermatitis, intertriginous _____

Other Diseases of Skin and Subcutaneous Tissue

Skin **ulcers** are open sores of the skin (Figure 18-4). Ulcers may have a variety of causes such as diabetes, skin cancers, venous insufficiency, arteriosclerosis, and pressure sores (**decubitus ulcer**). In ICD-9-CM, there are basically two types of ulcers located in the skin: decubitus ulcers and all others. When coding ulcers, note should be taken of the instructions found under the heading 707.1. This note instructs coders that if applicable the code for the underlying condition should be coded first. Per *Coding Clinic* (1991:2Q:p5-7),[1]

FIGURE 18-5. Decubitus ulcer.

Cellulitis is coded in addition to the ulcer. The sequencing of the cellulitis and ulcer is dependent on the focus of treatment. When coding gangrene with an ulcer, the ulcer is sequenced first.

Pressure Ulcer

A pressure ulcer is more commonly known as a bed sore or decubitus ulcer (Figure 18-5). These ulcers occur over bony areas (e.g., heel, hip, sacrum, ankle, and elbow) of patients who are immobile. Conditions found under this heading are chronic in nature, although the ulcer may be described as infected.

When coding a pressure ulcer in ICD-9-CM, two codes are required: a code from subcategory 707.0X that identifies the site of the ulcer and a code from 707.2X that identifies the stage of the ulcer. These codes identifying the stage are NEVER to be used as the principal or first-listed diagnosis. The stage codes are only used with pressure ulcers and never used with other types of ulcers. For classification purposes these ulcers are identified by stages 1–4 and unstageable.

- Stage 1: Red skin with warmth—persistent focal erythema
- Stage 2: Skin swollen with abrasion, blister, and partial thickness skin loss
- Stage 3: Full-thickness skin loss with subcutaneous necrosis
- Stage 4: Necrosis of soft tissues through to underlying muscle/tendon/bone
- Unstageable: Ulcers that have either been previously treated or covered with an eschar and the clinician is unable to determine the stage or they are documented as deep tissue injury not due to trauma

Selecting the stage of the pressure ulcer is determined by clinical documentation or terms listed in the Index. Stage of ulcer can be documented by clinicians who are not the patient's provider. The stage of ulcer may be assigned from nursing documentation but not the ulcer itself. If a term describing an ulcer is not listed in the Index and there is no documentation of stage, the provider should be queried.

EXAMPLE Patient has a decubitus ulcer on the left buttock with skin loss to bone, 707.05, 707.24 (L89.324).

When coding bilateral pressure ulcers of the same site, only one code is assigned if both ulcers are the same stage. However, if the ulcer on one side is a different stage from the ulcer on the other side, then codes for each site and for each different stage should be assigned.

EXAMPLE Patient is admitted with a pressure ulcer on each buttock. The pressure ulcer on the right buttock is documented as a stage 2 and the pressure ulcer on the left buttock is documented as a stage 4, 707.05, 707.24, 707.22 (L89.324, L89.312).

If a patient has a healed pressure ulcer documented, no code is assigned. However, if the pressure ulcer is documented as healing, then the ulcer and the stage of the ulcer are assigned codes. Should the documentation be unclear as to whether the patient has a healing or healed pressure ulcer, the physician should be queried.

EXAMPLE

> Patient is admitted with pneumonia. During the physical exam, the physician identifies a decubitus ulcer of the right heel that appears to be healing. The physician cannot give the ulcer a stage as it is covered by a skin graft, 486, 707.07, 707.25 (J18.9, L89.610).

If a patient has a pressure ulcer on admit that is documented as stage 2 and then during the admission this ulcer progresses to a stage 3, only the most severe stage of the ulcer is assigned.

EXAMPLE

> Patient is admitted to the hospital with, among other conditions, a stage 1 decubitus ulcer of the left ankle. During this admission, this ankle ulcer progresses to a stage 3, 707.06, 707.23 (L89.523).

EXAMPLE

> Patient has a sacral stage 4 decubitus ulcer with gangrene, 707.03, 785.4, 707.24 (I96, L89.154).

Ulcer of the Lower Limb, Except Decubitus

Ulcers of the lower limb have a fifth digit that describes the area of the limb in which they are located. These ulcers may be caused by other disease conditions. When an ulcer is described as having a causal relationship with another disease condition, the other disease condition is coded first.

EXAMPLE

> A patient has an ulcer of the right heel caused by diabetes, 250.80, 707.14 (E11.621, L97.419).

Stasis Ulcer

A **stasis ulcer** is associated with varicose veins. These ulcers are not coded as skin ulcers but as ulcers associated with varicose veins. If physician documentation states that the stasis ulcer is caused by a condition other than varicose veins, the Index directs the coder to the code 459.81 and to use an additional code for the ulcer (707.10-707.9).

EXAMPLE

> The patient has stasis dermatitis of the right leg due to varicose veins, 454.1 (I83.11).

EXERCISE 18-3

Assign codes to the following conditions.

1. Decubitus ulcer of the heel, stage 2 _____
2. Stasis ulcer without varicose vein calf _____
3. Diabetic ulcer of the toe _____
4. Arteriosclerotic ulcer of the leg with gangrene _____
5. Ischemic ulcer of the calf _____
6. Ulcer of the buttocks _____

FACTORS INFLUENCING HEALTH STATUS AND CONTACT WITH HEALTH SERVICES (V CODES/Z CODES)

In the past, V/Z codes have been considered for use primarily in the outpatient setting. This has changed with the addition of more V/Z codes each year. As was discussed in Chapter 8, it is difficult to locate V/Z codes in the Index. Coders will often say, "I did not know there was a V/Z code for that." Refer to Chapter 8 for a listing of common main terms used to locate V/Z codes.

V/Z codes that may be used with diseases of the skin and subcutaneous tissue include the following:

V13.3	Diseases of the skin and subcutaneous tissue
V19.4	Family history of skin conditions
V42.3	Skin replaced by transplant
V43.83	Skin replaced by other means
V58.31	Attention to surgical dressings and sutures
V58.77	Aftercare following surgery of the skin and subcutaneous tissue, NEC
V67.51	Following completed treatment with high-risk medications, NEC
V82.0	Special screening for skin conditions

EXAMPLE Patient presents to dermatologist's office for a rash on the cheeks and nose. Patient has a family history of skin disorders, 782.1, V19.4 (R21, Z84.0).

EXERCISE 18-4

Assign codes to the following conditions.

1. Patient with a history of eczema _____
2. Patient with a family history of dermatitis _____

COMMON TREATMENTS

CONDITION	MEDICATION
Acne	Tetracycline (Achromycin), isotretinoin (Accutane)
Boils	Bacitracin, Neosporin
Cellulitis	Antibiotics such as nafcillin, oxacillin, cefazolin, vancomycin, linezolid
Psoriasis	Topical corticosteroids

PROCEDURES

Some procedures that may be related to diseases of the skin and subcutaneous tissue may be located in the following chapter of the Procedure Tabular:

Chapter 15   Operations of the Integumentary System (85-86)

Procedures related to the Diseases of the Skin and Subcutaneous Tissue section in ICD-10-PCS may be located in the following tables:

Skin and Breast	0H0-0HY
Subcutaneous Tissue and Fascia	0J0-0JX

Incision and Drainage

Incision and drainage (I&D) is a common form of treatment for abscesses of the skin. The physician cuts into the lining of the abscess, which allows the pus to drain. Usually, the physician cleans the cavity with warm saline. If the abscess is deep, the physician may insert a drainage tube. It is important to be aware that I&D can also be used to describe incision and debridement. In cases in which the documentation is questionable, a physician query may be necessary.

EXERCISE 18-5

Assign codes to the following conditions.

1. Incision and drainage of neck abscess   _____
2. I&D of boil on arm   _____
3. Incision and drainage of pilonidal sinus   _____

Debridement

Excisional Debridement

Excisional debridement, as defined by *Coding Clinic* (1988:4Q:p5),[3] is "the surgical removal or cutting away of devitalized tissue, necrosis, or slough." The root operation for debridement in ICD-10-PCS is excision if it is excisional and extraction if it is nonexcisional. Excisional debridements may be performed in a variety of settings (Operating Room, Emergency Room, or bedside) and by a variety of healthcare providers (physicians, nurse practitioners, physician assistants, and physical therapists). For a debridement to qualify as excisional, documentation provided by the healthcare provider performing this service must indicate that the procedure was excisional, per *Coding Clinic* (2008:1Q:p3-4).[4]

According to *Coding Clinic* (1999:1Q:p8-9),[5] when an extensive debridement goes beyond the skin and subcutaneous tissue into the muscle, tendon, and/or bone, it is appropriate to "assign only a code for the deepest layer of debridement when multiple layers of the same site are débrided." If a patient had a debridement of skin, subcutaneous tissue, muscle, and bone, the bone is the deepest layer and debridement of the bone is the only procedure code assigned.

EXAMPLE   Patient with a stage 4 decubitus ulcer of the sacrum is taken to the OR for debridement. The debridement is performed through the skin, muscle, and bone, 707.03, 707.24, 77.69 (L89.154, 0QB10ZZ).

Nonexcisional Debridement

Any debridement that does not meet the criteria described earlier for excisional debridement would be coded as nonexcisional. A nonexcisional debridement may be performed by brushing, irrigating, scrubbing, or washing to remove devitalized tissue. Once again, this procedure may be performed in a variety of settings by a variety of healthcare providers.

It is important to remember that if debridement of the skin is performed in preparation for further surgery, the debridement should not be coded separately. For example, prior to reduction of an open fracture, a debridement may be performed.

EXAMPLE   Pulse lavage debridement is performed by wound care nurse on a patient with a stage 3 decubitus ulcer of the right ankle, 707.06, 707.23, 86.28 (L89.513, 0HDKXZZ).

Assign codes to the following conditions.

1. Excisional debridement of decubitus ulcer of the left heel _____

2. Skin tissue of the lower left leg ulcer removed by scrubbing _____

3. Debridement of a fungus of the nail bed of the right index finger _____

Skin Grafts

Skin grafts are composed of pieces of skin that are removed from one body area (donor) and are used to cover a defect in another body area (recipient). Several types of skin graft classifications are included in ICD-9-CM. In ICD-10-PCS skin grafts are coded to the root operation replacement.

Free Skin Grafts

Free skin grafts in ICD-CM include the removal of skin from one body area and transplantation to another body area. These may be split-thickness (STSGs) or full-thickness skin grafts (FTSGs) (Figure 18-6). It is important to note the differences between autografts, allografts (**homografts**), and xenografts (heterografts).

- **Autograft**—graft from one area of the body to another in the same individual
- **Allograft**—graft from one person to another
- **Xenograft**—also known as a **heterograft**; graft to an individual from another species such as a pig

A fourth category of graft source is the dermal regenerative graft, which is also known as a cultured epidermal autograft (CEA). These types of grafts are available in several varieties; they may be referred to as artificial skin.

EXAMPLE | Patient presents for full-thickness skin graft to the left thigh from the abdomen to repair a skin contracture from third-degree burn of the left thigh. Patient spilled boiling water on himself several months ago, 709.2, 906.7, E929.8, 86.63 (L905, T24.312S, 0HB7XZZ, X12XXXS).

Pedicle Grafts or Flaps

Pedicle grafts or **flaps** differ from STSG and FTSG in that part of the graft or flaps remains attached to the donor site. A pedicle graft is a full-thickness skin and subcutaneous tissue flap/graft that is attached by tissue (Figure 18-7), through which it receives its blood supply. The ICD-10-PCS root operation for a pedicle graft and for skin transfer flaps is transfer.

Assign codes to the following conditions.

1. STSG from patient's thigh to cover scar contracture due to burn from fire on right arm _____

2. FTSG to left hand from buttock due to scar from necrotizing fasciitis _____

3. Advancement flap to nose following surgery to remove skin cancer from nose _____

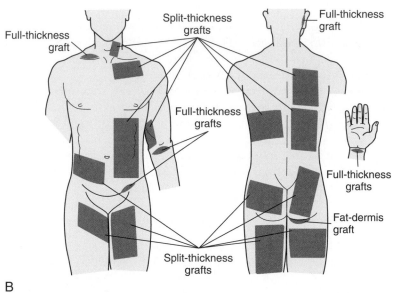

B

FIGURE 18-6. Split-thickness and full-thickness skin grafts.

FIGURE 18-7. Pedicle graft.

DOCUMENTATION/REIMBURSEMENT/MS-DRGs

Often, coding difficulties are due to lack of documentation. Sometimes pathology and other test results are not available at the time of discharge or when the physician is dictating the discharge summary or is reporting the final diagnoses.

It is very important for coding to make sure that healthcare providers fully describe the type of debridement that was performed. If sharp instruments were used to cut away devitalized tissue, this must be documented. This can make a significant difference in MS-DRG assignment and reimbursement.

When physicians state that an I&D was performed, it is imperative to identify whether the physician means incision and drainage or incision and debridement. These terms may be used interchangeably. In most cases, the term "I&D" stands for incision and drainage; however, if it seems unlikely that the condition would require this procedure, a query to the physician is warranted.

Frequently missed complications/comorbidities from this chapter include:

- Abscess
- Cellulitis
- Pressure ulcers

Incision and Drainage Versus Debridement

EXAMPLE

DIAGNOSES/PROCEDURES	CODES	MS-DRG	RW
Stage 2 decubitus ulcer of right heel	707.07, 707.22 (L89.612)	594	0.7591
Incision and drainage	86.04 (0H9MXZZ)		
Stage 4 decubitus ulcer of right heel	707.07, 707.24 (L89.614)	575	1.0899
Excisional debridement	86.22 (0HBMXZ)		

MS-DRG With and Without MCC/CC

The appropriate assignment of codes to identify the stage of a pressure ulcer may affect MS-DRG assignment.

EXAMPLE

DIAGNOSES/PROCEDURES	CODES	MS-DRG	RW
Patient with pneumonia and stage 2 decubitus ulcer heel of the right heel	486, 707.07, 707.20 (J18.9, L89.612)	195	0.7096
Patient with pneumonia and stage 4 decubitus ulcer heel of the right heel	486, 707.07, 707.24 (J18.9, L89.614)	193	1.4796

CHAPTER REVIEW EXERCISE

Answer the following and assign codes to the following conditions.

1. Abscess of the leg with cellulitis _____
2. Pressure ulcer of the foot with cellulitis, stage 3 _____
3. Eczema _____
4. Dermatitis caused by Cipro _____
5. Dermatitis due to poison sumac _____
6. Stasis dermatitis with ulcer _____
7. Diabetic PVD with foot ulcer _____
8. Incision and drainage of abscess of the leg _____
9. Excision of a pilonidal cyst _____
10. Excisional debridement of decubitus ulcer of the buttock (stage 4) by the attending physician _____

Write the correct answer(s) in the space(s) provided.

11. What is the difference between a pedicle graft and a split-thickness skin graft?

_____

12. Name one documentation challenge about which coders must be aware in diseases of the skin and subcutaneous tissue.

_____

13. What are the three accessory organs of the skin?

_____

_____

_____

14. Where in ICD-9-CM and ICD-10-CM would a coder find the skin condition herpes zoster?

_____

15. What is another name for a decubitus ulcer?

_____

16. Name and describe three types of skin grafts.

_____

_____

_____

CHAPTER GLOSSARY

Abscess: a localized collection of pus that causes swelling.

Allograft: graft of tissue between individuals of the same species.

Autograft: graft of tissue from another site on the same individual.

Carbuncle: cluster of boils.

Cellulitis: inflammation of the tissue with possible abscess.

Decubitus ulcer: skin ulcer also known as a bed sore.

Dermatitis: inflammation of the skin.

Dermis: layer of skin below the epidermis.

Eczema: type of dermatitis characterized by itching.

Endogenous: type of dermatitis caused by something taken internally, such as medication.

Epidermis: outermost layer of skin.

Excisional Debridement: removal by surgical cutting of devitalized tissue, necrosis, or slough.

Exogenous: type of dermatitis caused by contact with a substance.

Furuncle: a boil.

Heterograft: graft of skin from another species, such as a graft from a pig to a human.

Hives: skin condition also known as urticaria, wherein the skin reacts with welts; characterized by itching.

Homograft: graft from one individual to another of the same species; also known as an allograft.

Integumentary: another name for skin.

Intertrigo: dermatitis in areas where friction may occur.

Pedicle graft or flap: involves identifying a flap that remains attached to its original blood supply and tunneling it under the skin to a particular area such as the breast.

Pruritus: itching.

Psoriasis: inflammation of skin caused by a fault in the immune system.

Sebum: substance secreted from the sebaceous gland.

Stasis ulcer: ulcer associated with varicose veins.

Subcutaneous: inner layer of the skin that contains fat and sweat glands.

Ulcer: open sore of skin.

Urticaria: another name for hives.

Xenograft: graft to an individual from another species; also known as a heterograft.

REFERENCES

1. American Hospital Association. *Coding Clinic for ICD-9-CM* 1991:2Q:p5-7. Cellulitis of skin.
2. American Hospital Association. *Coding Clinic for ICD-9-CM* 1991:2Q:p20. Stasis dermatitis in chronic venous insufficiency w/o varicose veins.
3. American Hospital Association. *Coding Clinic for ICD-9-CM* 1988:4Q:p5. Debridement of wound, excisional vs nonexcisional—Guidelines.
4. American Hospital Association. *Coding Clinic for ICD-9-CM* 2008.1Q:p3-4. Excisional debridement.
5. American Hospital Association. *Coding Clinic for ICD-9-CM* 1999:1Q:p8-9. Extensive wound debridement.

19

Diseases of the Musculoskeletal System and Connective Tissue

(ICD-9-CM Chapter 13, Codes 710-739, and ICD-10-CM Chapter 13, Codes M00-M99)

CHAPTER OUTLINE

ICD-9-CM Official Guidelines for Coding and Reporting
ICD-10-CM Official Guidelines for Coding and Reporting
Guideline Differences Between ICD-9-CM and ICD-10-CM
Major Differences Between ICD-9-CM and ICD-10-CM
Anatomy and Physiology
Disease Conditions
    Arthropathies and Related Disorders
    Dorsopathies
    Rheumatism, Excluding the Back
    Osteopathies, Chondropathies, and Acquired Musculoskeletal Deformities
Factors Influencing Health Status and Contact with Health Services (V Codes/Z Codes)
Common Treatments
Procedures
    Arthroscopic Surgery
    Joint Replacement
    Vertebroplasty/Kyphoplasty
    Spinal Decompression/Fusion
Documentation/Reimbursement/MS-DRGs
    Pathologic Fracture Versus Traumatic Fracture
    Correct Procedure Code
Chapter Review Exercise
Chapter Glossary
References

LEARNING OBJECTIVES

1. Apply and assign the correct ICD-9-CM and ICD-10-CM codes in accordance with Official Guidelines for Coding and Reporting
2. Identify major differences between ICD-9-CM and ICD-10-CM related to the musculoskletal system and connective tissue
3. Identify pertinent anatomy and physiology of the musculoskeletal system and connective tissue

4. Identify diseases of the musculoskeletal system and connective tissue

5. Assign the correct V codes and procedure codes related to the musculoskeletal system and connective tissue

6. Identify common treatments, medications, laboratory values, and diagnostic tests

7. Explain the importance of documentation as it relates to MS-DRGs for reimbursement

ABBREVIATIONS/ ACRONYMS

AKA above-knee amputation

DEXA dual-energy x-ray absorptiometry (bone density)

DIC disseminated intravascular coagulation

DJD degenerative joint disease

ICD-9-CM *International Classification of Diseases, 9th Revision, Clinical Modification*

ICD-10-CM *International Classification of Diseases, 10th Revision, Clinical Modification*

ICD-10-PCS *International Classification of Diseases, 10th Revision, Procedure Coding System*

IV intravenous

JRA juvenile rheumatoid arthritis

MAO monoamine oxidase

MRI magnetic resonance imaging

MS-DRG Medicare Severity diagnosis-related group

NSAIDs nonsteroidal anti-inflammatory drugs

OA osteoarthritis

PMR polymyalgia rheumatica

PV percutaneous vertebroplasty

RA rheumatoid arthritis

SLE systemic lupus erythematosus

ICD-9-CM

Official Guidelines for Coding and Reporting

Please refer to the companion Evolve website for the most current guidelines.

13. Chapter 13: Diseases of Musculoskeletal and Connective Tissue (710-739)

   a. Coding of Pathologic Fractures

   1) Acute Fractures vs. Aftercare

   Pathologic fractures are reported using subcategory 733.1, when the fracture is newly diagnosed. Subcategory 733.1 may be used while the patient is receiving active treatment for the fracture. Examples of active treatment are: surgical treatment, emergency department encounter, evaluation and treatment by a new physician.

EXAMPLE The patient underwent a percutaneous vertebroplasty (synthetic substitute) for pathologic fracture of the L1 vertebra due to delayed healing. Patient has osteoporosis of vertebrae, 733.13, 733.00, 81.65 (M80.88xG, 0QU03JZ).

Fractures are coded using the aftercare codes (subcategories V54.0, V54.2, V54.8 or V54.9) for encounters after the patient has completed active treatment of the fracture and is receiving routine care for the fracture during the healing or recovery phase. Examples of fracture aftercare are: cast change or removal, removal of external or internal fixation device, medication adjustment, and follow-up visits following fracture treatment.

EXAMPLE The patient was seen for follow-up after vertebroplasty for pathologic fracture of the L1 vertebra. Patient has osteoporosis of vertebrae, V54.27, 733.00 (M80.88xD).

Care for complications of surgical treatment for fracture repairs during the healing or recovery phase should be coded with the appropriate complication codes.
Care of complications of fractures, such as malunion and nonunion, should be reported with the appropriate codes.
See Section I. C. 17.b for information on the coding of traumatic fractures.

Apply the General Coding Guidelines as found in Chapter 5 and the Procedural Guidelines as found in Chapter 6.

ICD-10-CM

Official Guidelines for Coding and Reporting

Please refer to the companion Evolve website for the most current guidelines.

13. Chapter 13: Diseases of the Musculoskeletal System and Connective Tissue (M00-M99)

a. Site and laterality

Most of the codes within Chapter 13 have site and laterality designations. The site represents the bone, joint or the muscle involved. For some conditions where more than one bone, joint or muscle is usually involved, such as osteoarthritis, there is a "multiple sites" code available. For categories where no multiple site code is provided and more than one bone, joint or muscle is involved, multiple codes should be used to indicate the different sites involved.

1) Bone versus joint

For certain conditions, the bone may be affected at the upper or lower end, (e.g., avascular necrosis of bone, M87, Osteoporosis, M80, M81). Though the portion of the bone affected may be at the joint, the site designation will be the bone, not the joint.

b. Acute traumatic versus chronic or recurrent musculoskeletal conditions

Many musculoskeletal conditions are a result of previous injury or trauma to a site, or are recurrent conditions. Bone, joint or muscle conditions that are the result of a healed injury are usually found in chapter 13. Recurrent bone, joint or muscle conditions are also usually found in chapter 13. Any current, acute injury should be coded to the appropriate injury code from chapter 19. Chronic or recurrent conditions should generally be coded with a code from chapter 13. If it is difficult to determine from the documentation in the record which code is best to describe a condition, query the provider.

c. Coding of Pathologic Fractures

7th character A is for use as long as the patient is receiving active treatment for the fracture. Examples of active treatment are: surgical treatment, emergency department encounter, evaluation and treatment by a new physician. 7th character, D is to be used for encounters after the patient has completed active treatment. The other 7th characters, listed under each subcategory in the Tabular List, are to be used for subsequent encounters for treatment of problems associated with the healing, such as malunions, nonunions, and sequelae.

Care for complications of surgical treatment for fracture repairs during the healing or recovery phase should be coded with the appropriate complication codes.

See Section I.C.19. Coding of traumatic fractures.

d. Osteoporosis

Osteoporosis is a systemic condition, meaning that all bones of the musculoskeletal system are affected. Therefore, site is not a component of the codes under category M81, Osteoporosis without current pathological fracture. The site codes under category M80, Osteoporosis with current pathological fracture, identify the site of the fracture, not the osteoporosis.

1) Osteoporosis without pathological fracture

Category M81, Osteoporosis without current pathological fracture, is for use for patients with osteoporosis who do not currently have a pathologic fracture due to the osteoporosis, even if they have had a fracture in the past. For patients with a history of osteoporosis fractures, status code **Z87.310**, Personal history of **(healed)** osteoporosis fracture, should follow the code from M81.

2) Osteoporosis with current pathological fracture

Category M80, Osteoporosis with current pathological fracture, is for patients who have a current pathologic fracture at the time of an encounter. The codes under M80 identify the site of the fracture. A code from category M80, not a traumatic fracture code, should be used for any patient with known osteoporosis who suffers a fracture, even if the patient had a minor fall or trauma, if that fall or trauma would not usually break a normal, healthy bone.

Apply the General Coding Guidelines as found in Chapter 5 and the Procedural Guidelines as found in Chapter 7.

GUIDELINE DIFFERENCES BETWEEN ICD-9-CM AND ICD-10-CM

Because there are significant differences in the coding of musculoskeletal and connective tissue diseases in ICD-10-CM, there are guidelines that address these differences.

ICD-10-CM codes identify laterality with different code assignments for right versus left. The guidelines address the issue of acute traumatic injury versus a chronic/recurrent musculoskeletal condition. Any current acute injury is assigned a code from Chapter 19 in ICD-10-CM, Injury, Poisoning, and Certain Other Consequences of External Causes. Chronic/recurrent conditions are generally assigned codes from Chapter 13 in ICD-10-CM, Diseases of the Musculoskeletal System and Connective Tissue.

The seventh-character extension is a new concept in ICD-10-CM. These character extensions are used in this chapter to code pathologic fractures.

ICD-10-CM uses a combination code for osteoporosis with pathologic fracture, and guidelines address the coding of osteoporosis with or without pathologic fracture. In ICD-9-CM, these two conditions were coded separately.

MAJOR DIFFERENCES BETWEEN ICD-9-CM AND ICD-10-CM

Some of the differences have already been identified in the guidelines section. Other differences include:

- ICD-10-CM identifies three different causes for pathologic fractures:
  - Neoplastic disease
  - Osteoporosis
  - Other specified disease
- The code assigned is a combination code that identifies the pathologic fracture and the cause of the fracture.
- In ICD-10-CM, bacterial organisms are included in some of the infectious arthropathy codes. A code from the infectious disease chapter may still need to be assigned to completely identify the organism.
- Codes for gout have been moved to the Musculoskeletal System chapter in ICD-10-CM from the Endocrine, Nutritional and Metabolic Disease chapter in ICD-9-CM.
- Some codes in Chapter 13 of ICD-10-CM require the seventh-character extension that describes the type of encounter, the stage of the fracture's healing process, and any residual effects or sequelae from the fracture. These extensions are as follows:
  A Initial encounter for fracture
  D Subsequent encounter for fracture with routine healing
  G Subsequent encounter for fracture with delayed healing
  K Subsequent encounter for fracture with nonunion
  P Subsequent encounter for fracture with malunion
  S Sequela
- Procedural complications affecting the musculoskeletal system are included in Chapter 13 of ICD-10-CM. Some of the complications include:
  - Pseudoarthrosis after a fusion or arthrodesis
  - Postlaminectomy syndrome
  - Fractures following insertion of orthopedic implants, prosthesis, or bone plates
  - Intraoperative hemorrhage, hematoma, or accidental laceration

ANATOMY AND PHYSIOLOGY

The musculoskeletal system is made up of muscles, bones, ligaments, tendons, cartilage, and the joints they form. The purposes of the musculoskeletal system are to provide a framework and to protect the internal organs. Bones also are important for hematopoiesis and for storing calcium and phosphate. **Hematopoiesis** is the development of blood cells that occurs in the bone marrow and lymphatic tissue of normal adults.

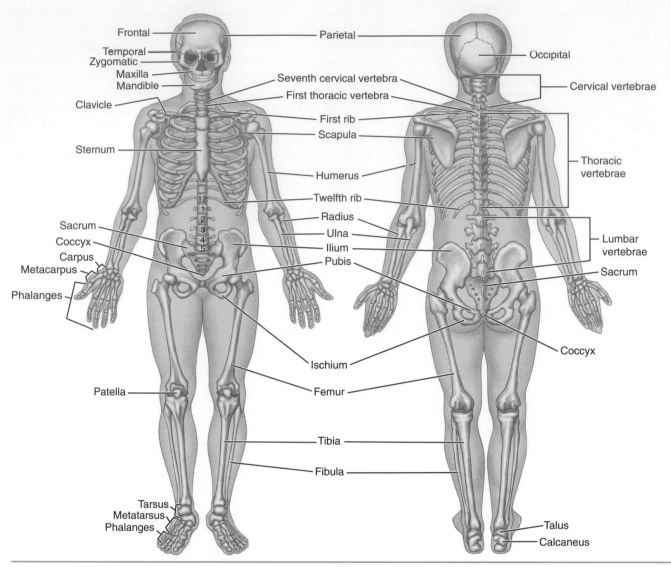

FIGURE 19-1. Anterior and posterior views of the human skeleton.

A good grasp of anatomy is essential in coding conditions of the musculoskeletal system. It is important to know that the femur is the long bone in the thigh area, and that the radius and the ulna are two bones in the forearm. Pictures are best for illustrating the locations of the skeletal structures (Figure 19-1) and muscles (Figure 19-2). It is particularly important to understand the terms used in the musculoskeletal chapter to describe the location of structures relative to the body as a whole or to other body structures (Figure 19-3). **Anterior** or **ventral** describes the front of the body or an organ. **Posterior** or **dorsal** relates to the back of the body or an organ. The terms medial and lateral describe the position of the body or an organ relative to the median sagittal plane that divides the body in half. **Medial** refers to a structure that is closer to the median plane than is another structure in the body. The eyes are medial to the ears. **Lateral** refers to a structure that is to the side of the body. The ears are lateral to the eyes. The terms **superior** (above) and **inferior** (below) describe the position of the body or an organ relative to the vertical axis of the body. The shoulders are superior to the hips, and the ankles are inferior to the knees. Other terms that may be used are **cranial**, which means toward the head, and **caudal**, which means toward the tail. **Proximal** (closer to the point of reference) and **distal** (farther from the point of reference) are often used to describe a location in the limbs. The shoulder is

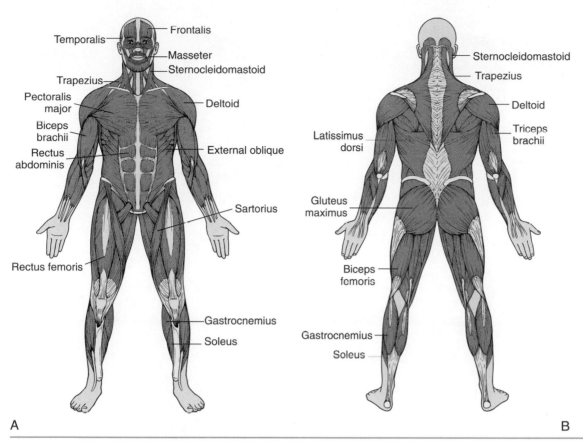

FIGURE 19-2. Normal muscular system. **A**, Anterior view. **B**, Posterior view.

proximal to the elbow, and the wrist is distal to the elbow. **Supine** refers to lying on the back, face up. **Prone** is lying on the stomach, face down.

The **joints** are the means of joining two bones together; they assist with body movement. **Ligaments** are dense fibrous bands of connective tissue that provide stability for the joint. Ligaments can be injured by overstretching or tearing (sprain). **Tendons** are the connective tissue that attaches muscle to bone. Tendons are susceptible to strain injuries. The **fascia** is the tissue just below the skin that covers and separates the underlying layers of muscle.

DISEASE CONDITIONS

Diseases of the Musculoskeletal System and Connective Tissue (710-739), Chapter 13 in your ICD-9-CM code book, is divided into the following categories:

CATEGORY	SECTION TITLES
710-719	Arthropathies and Related Disorders
720-724	Dorsopathies
725-729	Rheumatism, Excluding the Back
730-739	Osteopathies, Chondropathies, and Acquired Musculoskeletal Deformities

Diseases of the Musculoskeletal System and Connective Tissue (M00-M99), Chapter 13 in the ICD-10-CM code book, are divided into the following categories:

CATEGORY	SECTION TITLES
M00-M02	Infectious Arthropathies
M05-M14	Inflammatory Polyarthropathies
M15-M19	Osteoarthritis

FIGURE 19-3. Directions and planes of the body.

CATEGORY	SECTION TITLES
M20-M25	Other Joint Disorders
M26-M27	Dentofacial Anomalies, Including Malocclusion, and Other Disorders of the Jaw
M30-M36	Systemic Connective Tissue Disorders
M40-M43	Deforming Dorsopathies
M45-M49	Disorders of Muscles
M65-M67	Disorders of Synovium and Tendon
M70-M79	Other Soft-Tissue Disorders
M80-M85	Disorders of Bone and Bone Density
M86-M90	Other Osteopathies
M91-M94	Chondropathies
M95	Other Disorders of the Musculoskeletal System and Connective Tissue
M96	Intraoperative and Postprocedural Complications and Disorders of Musculoskeletal System, Not Elsewhere Classified
M99	Biomechanical Lesions, Not Elsewhere Classified

One of the most important parts of this chapter in ICD-9-CM is the breakdown of the fifth-digit subclassifications that are used with categories 711-712, 715-716, 718-719, and 730; this information appears at the very beginning of the chapter (Figure 19-4) and is provided to assist in making the proper fifth-digit assignment. One may not remember whether the wrist fits into the subclassification of 3 for forearm, or 4 for hand. The appropriate fifth-digit subclassification for wrist joint is 3, forearm.

EXERCISE 19-1

Using Figure 19-4, assign the appropriate fifth digits to the following conditions.

1.	Pyogenic arthritis of the right elbow	711.0_____
2.	Traumatic arthropathy left foot	716.1_____
3.	Osteoarthritis both wrists	715.3_____
4.	Recurrent dislocation right thumb	718.3_____
5.	Acute osteomyelitis sacrum	730.0_____

13. **DISEASES OF THE MUSCULOSKELETAL SYSTEM AND CONNECTIVE TISSUE (710–739)**

The following fifth-digit subclassification is for use with categories 711–712, 715–716, 718–719, and 730:

☐ **0 site unspecified**
   1 shoulder region
      Acromioclavicular joint(s)
      Clavicle
      Glenohumeral joint(s)
      Scapula
      Sternoclavicular joint(s)
   2 upper arm
      Elbow joint
      Humerus
   3 forearm
      Radius
      Ulna
      Wrist joint
   4 hand
      Carpus
      Metacarpus
      Phalanges [fingers]
   5 pelvic region and thigh
      Buttock
      Femur
      Hip (joint)
   6 lower leg
      Fibula
      Knee joint
      Patella
      Tibia
   7 ankle and foot
      Ankle joint
      Digits [toes]
      Metatarsus
      Phalanges, foot
      Tarsus
      Other joints in foot
☐ **8 other specified sites**
      Head
      Neck
      Ribs
      Skull
      Trunk
      Vertebral column
☐ **9 multiple sites**

FIGURE 19-4. Fifth-digit subclassifications for use with categories 711-712, 715-716, 718-719, and 790, as shown in the Tabular List.

Arthropathies and Related Disorders

Collagen Diseases

The main component of connective tissue is collagen. Collagen diseases result from immune system malfunctions in which the immune system identifies the body's connective tissue as foreign and attacks it. A patient's heart, lungs, and kidneys may also suffer damage. No cure is known for these diseases. The most common conditions include systemic lupus erythematosus, scleroderma, and rheumatoid arthritis.

Systemic lupus erythematosus (SLE) is a chronic, inflammatory autoimmune disease that can damage connective tissue anywhere in the body. It causes inflammation of the skin, joints, nervous system, kidneys, lungs, and other organs. A butterfly rash that spreads from one cheek across the nose to the other cheek is a common symptom (Figure 19-5). Fever, fatigue, weight loss, and joint deformity may also be present.

Scleroderma is a chronic, progressive disease that is characterized by hardening of the skin and scarring of internal organs. No cure is known for scleroderma; treatment is supportive and varies according to the organs that are affected. CREST syndrome is a form of scleroderma that includes the following:

Calcinosis—calcification of the skin

Raynaud's phenomenon—a disorder that is characterized by vasospastic attacks in which blood vessels to the fingers, toes, and sometimes the ears and nose constrict, causing discoloration and pain

Esophageal dysfunction—such as reflux or difficulty in swallowing

Sclerodactyly—hardening of the skin of the fingers or toes

Telangiectasia—dilatation of tiny blood vessels, particularly of the skin

Rheumatoid arthritis (RA) is a chronic, inflammatory, systemic disease that affects the joints, often causing deformity (Figure 19-6). RA is one of the most severe and disabling forms of arthritis. Damage may extend beyond the joints, affecting the heart and blood vessels and producing damage within the layers of skin.

FIGURE 19-5. Butterfly rash that may accompany systemic lupus erythematosus.

FIGURE 19-6. Joint deformity from rheumatoid arthritis.

Juvenile rheumatoid arthritis (JRA) affects children, usually between the ages of 2 and 5 years. Various forms of JRA may affect only a few joints, may affect many joints, or may be systemic in nature (also known as Still's disease).

EXAMPLE | Patient is being treated for CREST syndrome, 710.1 (M34.1).

EXAMPLE | Fourteen year old child is being treated for Still's disease, 714.30 (M08.20).

Arthropathy is a disease that affects the joints. In categories 711, 712, and 713, many of the codes describe arthropathies or arthritis as a manifestation of other diseases or conditions; these appear in italics with instructions to code first underlying disease (Figure 19-7).

EXAMPLE | Patient has arthritis due to hypothyroidism, 244.9, 713.0 (E03.9, M14.80).

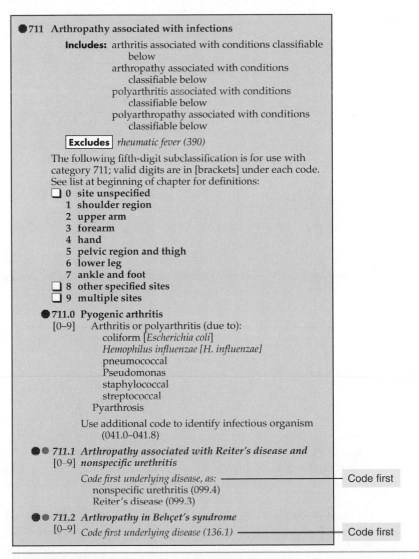

FIGURE 19-7. Most codes in categories 711, 712, and 713 are given in italics and include instructions to code first the underlying disease.

FIGURE 19-8. Pathologic changes of osteoarthritis.

Osteoarthritis

Osteoarthritis is a type of arthritis that develops as the result of wear and tear on the joints. It occurs because of breakdown and loss of cartilage within the joints (Figure 19-8). Osteoarthritis (OA) or degenerative joint disease (DJD), the most common form of arthritis, is more common in the elderly. Weight-bearing joints such as the knees and hips are often affected. The most common symptoms include sore and stiff joints, particularly in the morning or with changes of weather. Edema and deformity may also be present. Treatment depends on the severity of the condition and the success of conservative medical treatments (i.e., anti-inflammatory medications, exercise, steroid injections). In severe cases, surgery may be required to replace affected joints.

Primary osteoarthritis is an idiopathic condition that occurs in previously intact joints and has no apparent initiating factor. Primary osteoarthritis is related to the aging process and typically occurs in older individuals. **Secondary osteoarthritis** refers to degenerative disease of the joints that results from a predisposing condition such as trauma or disease. Secondary osteoarthritis may occur in relatively young individuals and usually affects the joints of one area. Under category 715, a note indicates that "localized, in the subcategories below, includes bilateral involvement of the same site"; for example, in a patient with OA of both knees, the condition would be considered localized because it is present in both lower extremities at the same site.

Coding Clinic (1995:2Q:p5)[1] states that "when the degenerative joint disease affects only one site but is not identified as primary or secondary it is coded to 715.3X, Osteoarthrosis, localized, not specified whether primary or secondary. If it involves more than one site, but is not specified as generalized, assign code 715.8X, Osteoarthrosis involving, or with mention of more than one site but not specified as generalized."

EXAMPLE	Patient has osteoarthritis of both hips, 715.35 (M16.0).

EXAMPLE	Patient is being treated for osteoarthritis hands and wrists, 715.89 (M15.9).

EXERCISE 19-2

Assign codes to the following conditions.

1. Pain both knees due to DJD   _____
2. Juvenile RA   _____
3. Arthritis due to Lyme disease   _____
4. Loose body in left knee joint   _____
5. Sicca syndrome   _____
6. SLE with nephrotic syndrome   _____
7. Arthritis due to sarcoidosis   _____

Dorsopathies

Dorsopathies are conditions or diseases that affect the back or spine. Code assignment may depend on the location or region that is affected. The spinal column contains 33 vertebrae, as indicated in Figure 19-9. Seven cervical vertebrae are found in the neck. Twelve thoracic, or dorsal, vertebrae are found in the region of the chest, or thorax; these provide attachment for 12 pairs of ribs. Five lumbar vertebrae are located in the lower back. Five fused sacral vertebrae form the sacrum, a solid bone that fits like a wedge between the bones of the hip and the coccyx. The coccyx consists of three or four vertebrae fused together at the bottom of the sacrum. Between each vertebra is a thick, fibrous disc of cartilage known as an intervertebral disc. Intervertebral discs may become displaced, herniated, ruptured, and/or prolapsed with resultant pain.

Spondylosis (spinal osteoarthritis) is a degenerative disorder that may cause loss of normal spinal structure and function. Although aging is the primary cause, the location and rate of degeneration are individualized. The degenerative process of spondylosis may affect the cervical, thoracic, and/or lumbar regions of the spine, including the intervertebral discs and facet joints. **Facet joints** are small, stabilizing joints located between and behind adjacent vertebrae.

Spondylolisthesis occurs when one vertebra slips on another (Figure 19-10). Symptoms usually appear when the spinal nerves are pinched by the vertebrae. Symptoms such as back, buttock, and leg pain are often aggravated by activity and relieved with rest. The amount of slippage is identified by grades.

Spinal stenosis is a narrowing of the central spinal canal, or areas of the spine where the nerve roots exit (neuroforamina). This narrowing is often caused by arthritis and therefore is most often found in persons from older age groups. Spinal stenosis may be caused by other factors such as injury, infection, tumor, or congenital abnormality. Stenosis does not necessarily cause symptoms; if symptoms do appear, they usually indicate the presence of **radiculopathy** (nerve root compression) or **myelopathy** (spinal cord compression).

EXAMPLE	The patient's magnetic resonance imaging (MRI) showed stenosis of cervical vertebrae, 723.0 (M48.02).

EXAMPLE	Patient's CT shows spondylosis of lumbosacral region with myelopathy, 721.42 (M47.17).

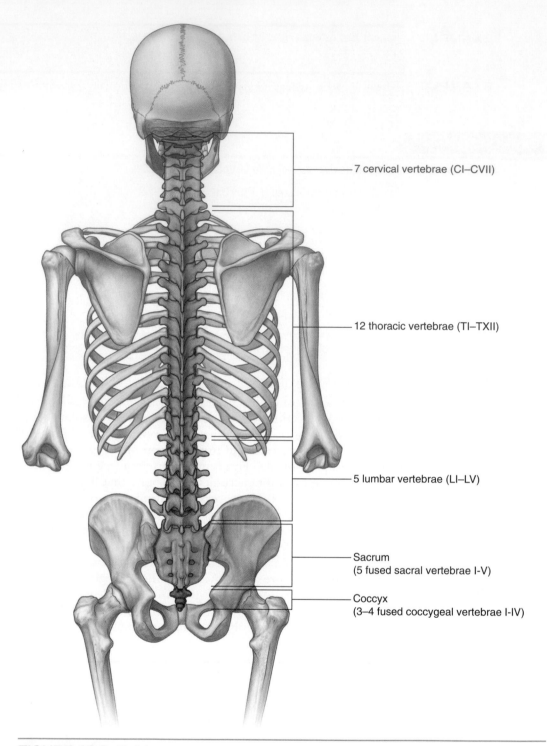

7 cervical vertebrae (CI–CVII)

12 thoracic vertebrae (TI–TXII)

5 lumbar vertebrae (LI–LV)

Sacrum
(5 fused sacral vertebrae I-V)

Coccyx
(3–4 fused coccygeal vertebrae I-IV)

FIGURE 19-9. Vertebrae.

Postlaminectomy Syndrome

"Postlaminectomy syndrome" is a term that is used to describe the condition of patients who have undergone spine surgery and have some degree of recurrent spinal and/or leg pain. Treatment varies according to the cause. *Coding Clinic* (1997:2Q:p15)[2] states that "**postlaminectomy syndrome** is a buildup of scar tissue after a laminectomy has been performed. The patient is in constant pain and the physician documents that this is due to the scar tissue that has formed."

FIGURE 19-10. Spondylolysis with resulting grade 2 spondylolisthesis.

EXERCISE 19-3

Assign codes to the following conditions.

1. Cervical spondylosis without myelopathy   _____
2. Degenerative disc disease lumbar spine   _____
3. Right-sided sciatica due to sitting on wallet   _____
4. Chronic low back pain   _____
5. Torticollis   _____
6. Pain in neck   _____
7. OA thoracic spine   _____
8. Stenosis lumbosacral vertebra   _____
9. Lumbago due to disc herniation at L4-L5   _____
10. Back pain due to postlaminectomy syndrome   _____

Rheumatism, Excluding the Back

Polymyalgia Rheumatica

Polymyalgia rheumatica, or PMR, is a syndrome that is characterized by severe aching and stiffness in the neck, shoulder girdle, and pelvic girdle. It is classified as a rheumatic disease, although its origin remains undetermined. It has been closely linked to temporal arteritis.

Fibromyalgia

Fibromyalgia, one of the most common diseases affecting the muscles, is characterized by widespread muscle pain associated with chronic fatigue. Other common symptoms of this condition include "brain fog," irritable bowel syndrome, sleep disorders, chronic headaches, anxiety, and depression. Fibromyalgia is a chronic condition that may be aggravated by weather conditions, infection, allergies, hormones, stress, and overexertion. Most available treatments focus on improving sleep and controlling pain.

Bursitis

Bursitis is inflammation of a bursa, which is a tiny, fluid-filled sac found between muscles, tendons, and bones designed to reduce friction and facilitate movement. Symptoms of bursitis include pain and tenderness when the affected body part is moved, limited range of motion, and edema or swelling. Areas most affected are the shoulders, elbows, hips, and knees. Bursitis may be caused by trauma, overuse of the joint, infection, or diseases such as gout and RA.

EXAMPLE Patient is being seen for bursitis left olecranon process, 726.33 (M70.22).

EXAMPLE Patient is being treated for subpatellar bursitis, 726.69 (M70.50).

Rhabdomyolysis

Rhabdomyolysis is the breakdown of muscle fibers that results in the release of muscle fiber contents into the circulation. Some of these contents are toxic to the kidney, frequently resulting in kidney damage. Some inherited disorders such as carnitine palmityltransferase, phosphofructokinase deficiency, and phosphoglycerate kinase deficiency can lead to muscle injury with exercise and rhabdomyolysis. Some of the most common causes include the following:

- Muscle exertion (physical, related to convulsions or to heat injury)
- Trauma-crush syndromes and pseudo-crush syndrome
- Muscle ischemia related to arterial occlusion or insufficiency
- Burns
- Repetitive muscle injury (bongo drumming, torture)
- Status epilepticus
- Drug overdose
- Extended periods of muscle pressure

EXAMPLE Traumatic rhabdomyolysis due to intractable status epilepticus
Patient was diagnosed with epilepsy 2 years ago, 345.3, 728.88 (G40.911, T79.6xxA).

Necrotizing Fasciitis

Necrotizing fasciitis or "flesh-eating disease," is a rare but serious condition in which an infection occurs in the tissues below the skin (Figure 19-11). The tissues may quickly die because of poor blood supply, possibly leading to the death of the patient. Necrotizing fasciitis is usually caused by group A streptococcus (the same bacterium that causes strep throat) and is often preceded by an injury to the skin.

FIGURE 19-11. Necrotizing fasciitis.

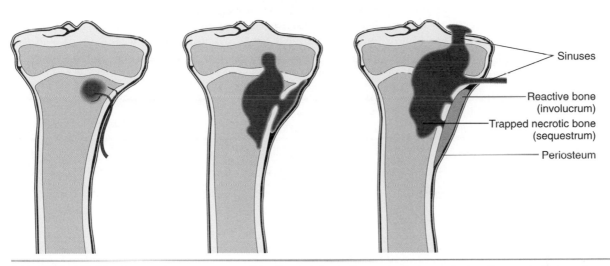

Sinuses

Reactive bone (involucrum)

Trapped necrotic bone (sequestrum)

Periosteum

FIGURE 19-12. Progression of osteomyelitis. Bacterial growth results in bone destruction and abscess formation.

EXERCISE 19-4

Assign codes to the following conditions.

1. Necrotizing fasciitis due to group A strep with gangrene right leg _____

2. Acute renal failure due to rhabdomyolysis _____

3. Pain due to bursitis left shoulder _____

4. Insomnia due to fibromyalgia _____

5. De Quervain's disease _____

Osteopathies, Chondropathies, and Acquired Musculoskeletal Deformities

Osteomyelitis

Osteomyelitis is an infection of the bone that often starts in another part of the body and spreads to the bone via the blood (Figure 19-12). In children, the long bones are usually affected. In adults, the vertebrae and the pelvis are the most commonly affected areas. *Staphylococcus aureus* bacteria are usually the cause of acute osteomyelitis. This organism may enter the bloodstream through a wound or a contaminated intravenous needle. Chronic osteomyelitis results when bone tissue dies as a result of the lost blood supply. Risk factors include recent trauma, diabetes, hemodialysis, and intravenous (IV) drug abuse. People who have had a splenectomy are also at higher risk for osteomyelitis. Prolonged IV antibiotic therapy may be required.

EXAMPLE Subacute osteomyelitis sacrum with decubitus sacral ulcer, stage III.
Staphylococcus aureus is the causative organism, 730.08, 707.03, 707.23, 041.11 (M46.27, L89.153, B95.6).

EXAMPLE Chronic osteomyelitis left tibia, 730.16 (M86.662).

Osteoporosis

Osteoporosis is a metabolic bone disorder that results in decreased bone mass and density. Osteoporosis, which is most common in older persons, particularly postmenopausal women, may also occur as the result of other diseases such as hyperparathyroidism or Cushing's syndrome; use of steroids may contribute to bone loss. Individuals with osteoporosis are susceptible for pathologic fractures. These fractures most often occur in the vertebrae of the spine, wrists, and hips (Figure 19-13).

EXAMPLE Patient is being treated for postmenopausal osteoporosis, 733.01 (M81.0).

EXAMPLE Patient has osteoporosis due to disuse, 733.03 (M81.8).

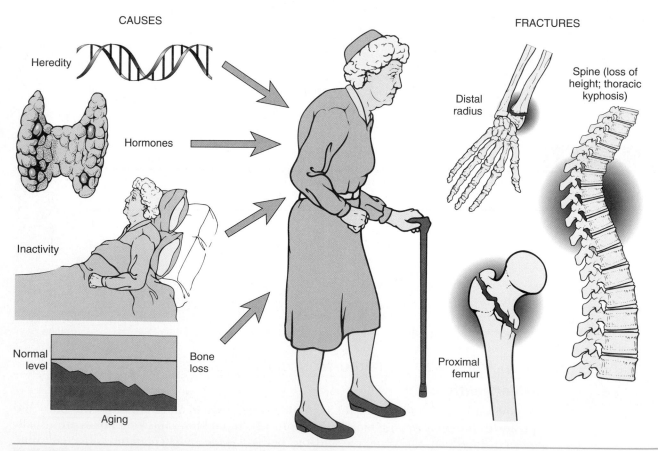

FIGURE 19-13. Causes and results of osteoporosis.

Pathologic Fractures and Fracture Aftercare

A **pathologic fracture** is a break in a bone that occurs because of underlying disorders that weaken the bone, including malignancy, benign bone tumors, metabolic disorders, infection, and osteoporosis. A pathologic fracture may result from normal stress placed on an abnormal bone. Fractures may occur spontaneously in individuals with diseased bones as the result of minor exertion or trauma. Because the bone is already diseased, the healing process of the fracture can be complicated by delayed healing, nonunion, pseudarthrosis, necrosis, and infection. A fracture cannot be coded as both a traumatic fracture and a pathologic fracture; it is one or the other. Only a physician can determine whether the severity of trauma corresponds with the injury. Compression fractures of the spine are often pathologic, but a thorough review of the record and/or a physician query may be necessary to determine the appropriate fracture code.

Active treatment for a pathologic fracture includes surgery, an Emergency Room encounter, and/or evaluation and treatment by a new physician. According to the guidelines, when a patient is receiving active treatment, the acute fracture code is assigned. If a pathologic fracture is documented as being chronic and is being treated in some way, it is acceptable to code it as an active pathologic fracture according to *Coding Clinic* (2008:3Q:p4).[3]

Following the period of active treatment of a pathologic fracture, other encounters may be necessary. These encounters are assigned aftercare V codes. Aftercare may include a cast change or removal, removal of a fixation device, medication adjustments, and other follow-up visits.

EXAMPLE | Elderly woman with osteoporosis sustains a spontaneous fracture of the lumbar spine after removing a heavy turkey roaster from the oven, 733.13, 733.00 (M80.88xA).

EXAMPLE | Patient had a cast change for pathologic right radial fracture, V54.22, 97.11 (M84.433D, 2W0CX2Z).

EXAMPLE | Pathologic fracture distal left femur due to osteosarcoma femur, 733.15, 170.7 (M84.552A, C40.22).

Spinal Deformities

Sometimes, the normal curvatures of the spine are altered. **Lordosis** is an exaggerated inward curvature of the spine that may be caused by increased abdominal girth due to obesity, pregnancy, or abdominal tumor (Figure 19-14, *A*). Improved posture, exercise, and weight loss can often alleviate symptoms. **Kyphosis** is an excessive posterior curvature of the thoracic spine that may not be detected until a hump in the upper back is noticeable (Figure 19-14, *B*). In older people, particularly women, osteoporosis is often the cause. If it occurs in children or adolescents, the exact cause may have to be determined, so that the best treatment approach can be selected. **Scoliosis** is a lateral or sideways curvature of the spine (Figure 19-15). School screening programs may detect spinal abnormalities. Varying degrees of abnormality may be observed, and often, conservative medical management is attempted. In severe cases, the performance of procedures that fuse the vertebrae and the application of internal fixation devices such as rods, wires, plates, and/or screws may be necessary to correct the problem.

EXAMPLE | The patient is being treated conservatively for kyphoscoliosis, 737.30 (M41.9).

EXAMPLE | Postlaminectomy lordosis, 737.21 (M96.4).

EXAMPLE | Patient has back, buttock, and leg pain due to acquired lumbar spondylolisthesis, 738.4 (M43.16)

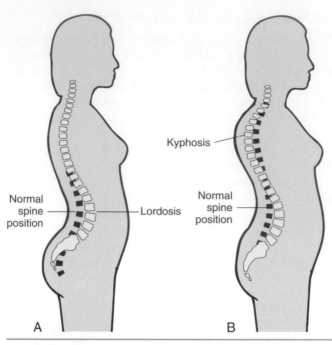

FIGURE 19-14. A, Lordosis. **B,** Kyphosis.

FIGURE 19-15. Scoliosis. **A,** Note scapular asymmetry in the upright position. **B,** Bending forward reveals a mild rib hump deformity.

EXERCISE 19-5

Assign codes to the following conditions.

1. Kyphosis due to osteoporosis _____

2. Osteomyelitis with periostitis, right tibia. Cultures did not grow any organisms. _____

3. Osteochondritis dissecans _____

4. Pathologic fracture, left wrist, due to osteoporosis _____

5. Stress fracture, right lower leg _____

6. Talipes planus, right (acquired) _____

7. Chest pain due to costochondritis _____

8. Pectus excavatum, acquired _____

9. Cast change for pathologic fracture, right radius _____

10. Nontraumatic slipped upper left femoral epiphysis _____

FACTORS INFLUENCING HEALTH STATUS AND CONTACT WITH HEALTH SERVICES (V CODES/Z CODES)

In the past, V/Z codes have been considered primarily for use in the outpatient setting. This has changed with the addition of more V/Z codes each year. As was discussed in Chapter 8, it may be difficult to locate V/Z codes in the Index. Coders often say, "I did not know there was a V/Z code for that." Refer to Chapter 8 for a listing of common main terms used to locate V/Z codes.

It is important for the coder to be familiar with different types and uses of V/Z codes.

V13.4	Personal history of arthritis
V13.51	Personal history of pathologic fracture
V13.52	Personal history of stress fracture
V13.59	Personal history of other musculoskeletal disorders
V17.7	Family history of arthritis
V17.81	Family history of osteoporosis
V17.89	Family history of other musculoskeletal disease
V43.60	Organ or tissue replaced by other means—unspecified joint
V43.61	Organ or tissue replaced by other means—shoulder
V43.62	Organ or tissue replaced by other means—elbow
V43.63	Organ or tissue replaced by other means—wrist
V43.64	Organ or tissue replaced by other means—hip
V43.65	Organ or tissue replaced by other means—knee
V43.66	Organ or tissue replaced by other means—ankle
V43.69	Organ or tissue replaced by other means—other
V43.7	Organ or tissue replaced by other means—limb
V45.4	Arthrodesis status
V49.0	Deficiencies of limbs
V49.1	Mechanical problems with limbs
V49.2	Motor problems with limbs
V49.3	Sensory problems with limbs
V49.4	Disfigurements of limbs
V49.5	Other problems of limbs
V49.60	Upper limb amputation status—unspecified level
V49.61	Upper limb amputation status—thumb

V49.62	Upper limb amputation status—other fingers
V49.63	Upper limb amputation status—hand
V49.64	Upper limb amputation status—wrist
V49.65	Upper limb amputation status—below elbow
V49.66	Upper limb amputation status—above elbow
V49.67	Upper limb amputation status—shoulder
V49.70	Lower limb amputation status—unspecified level
V49.71	Lower limb amputation status—great toe
V49.72	Lower limb amputation status—other toe(s)
V49.73	Lower limb amputation status—foot
V49.74	Lower limb amputation status—ankle
V49.75	Lower limb amputation status—below knee
V49.76	Lower limb amputation status—above knee
V49.77	Lower limb amputation status—hip
V52.0	Fitting and adjustment of prosthetic device/implant—artificial arm
V52.1	Fitting and adjustment of prosthetic device/implant—artificial leg
V52.8	Fitting and adjustment of prosthetic device/implant—other specified prosthetic device
V53.7	Fitting and adjustment of orthopedic devices
V54.01	Encounter for removal of internal fixation device
V54.02	Encounter for lengthening/adjustment of growth rod
V54.09	Other aftercare involving internal fixation device
V54.20	Aftercare for healing pathologic fracture of arm, unspecified
V54.21	Aftercare for healing pathologic fracture of upper arm
V54.22	Aftercare for healing pathologic fracture of lower arm
V54.23	Aftercare for healing pathologic fracture of hip
V54.24	Aftercare for healing pathologic fracture of leg, unspecified
V54.25	Aftercare for healing pathologic fracture of upper leg
V54.26	Aftercare for healing pathologic fracture of lower leg
V54.27	Aftercare for healing pathologic fracture of vertebra
V54.29	Aftercare for healing pathologic fracture of other bone
V54.81	Aftercare following joint replacement
V54.82	Aftercare following explantation of joint prosthesis
V54.89	Other orthopedic aftercare
V54.9	Unspecified orthopedic aftercare
V57.1	Other physical therapy
V57.21	Encounter for occupational therapy
V57.81	Orthotic training
V57.89	Other specified rehabilitation procedure
V58.68	Long term (current) use of bisphosphonates
V58.78	Aftercare following surgery of the musculoskeletal system, not elsewhere classified (NEC)
V64.43	Arthroscopic surgical procedure converted to open procedure
V67.4	Follow-up examination—following treatment of healed fracture
V82.1	Special screening—rheumatoid arthritis
V82.2	Special screening—other rheumatic disorder
V82.3	Special screening—congenital dislocation of hip
V82.81	Special screening—osteoporosis
V88.21	Acquired absence of hip joint
V88.22	Acquired absence of knee joint
V88.29	Acquired absence of other joint

EXAMPLE	Patient is status post knee replacement 1 year ago, V43.65 (Z96.659).

EXAMPLE	Patient with a family history of rheumatoid arthritis is being screened for rheumatoid arthritis, V82.1, V17.7 (Z13.828, Z82.61).

EXAMPLE	Patient is receiving aftercare for healing pathologic fracture of left humerus V54.21 (M84.422D).

EXERCISE 19-6

Assign codes to the following conditions.

1. Status post right knee replacement   _____
2. Dual-energy x-ray absorptiometry (DEXA) scan screening for osteoporosis   _____
3. Aftercare for healing pathologic fracture of cervical spine   _____
4. Amputation status of right foot   _____
5. Encounter to remove screw from left tibia   _____
6. Aftercare for pathologic fracture of right femur   _____

COMMON TREATMENTS

Many conditions or diseases of the musculoskeletal system cause pain and inflammation. Anti-inflammatory agents reduce inflammation in joints and muscles, antiarthritics are used to treat arthritic symptoms, and muscle relaxants may be helpful for acute low back pain and muscle spasms. Physical therapy and chiropractic treatment may be beneficial for many conditions. Medical treatment is usually tried before surgical intervention is considered.

CONDITION	MEDICATION/TREATMENT
Rheumatoid arthritis	Celecoxib (Celebrex), gold compounds such as Ridaura and Myochrysine
Osteoarthritis	Analgesics
	Nonsteroidal anti-inflammatory drugs (NSAIDs) for pain and inflammation (aspirin, ibuprofen [Motrin, Advil], nabumetone [Relafen], naproxen [Aleve, Naprosyn], diclofenac [Voltaren], indomethacin [Indocin], etodolac [Lodine], oxaprozin [Daypro], celecoxib [Celebrex])
Fibromyalgia	Analgesics for pain, muscle relaxants, antidepressants, and sleep aids
Bursitis	Rest, immobilization, ice, NSAIDs
Rhabdomyolysis	Provide treatment of the cause; watch for and treat manifestations such as hypovolemia, hyperkalemia, metabolic acidosis, acute renal failure, or disseminated intravascular coagulation (DIC)
Necrotizing fasciitis	Aggressive antibiotic therapy with surgical debridement
Osteomyelitis	Antibiotics depending on causative organism
Osteoporosis	Alendronate (Fosamax), Boniva (ibandronate), calcitonin, calcium with vitamin D

PROCEDURES

Some procedures that may be related to diseases of the musculoskeletal system and connective tissue may be located in the following chapter of the Procedure Tabular:

Chapter 14 Operations on the Musculoskeletal System (76-84)

Procedures related to the musculoskeletal system and connective tissue in ICD-10-PCS can be located in the following tables:

OK2-OKX	Muscles
OL2-OLX	Tendons
OM2-OMX	Bursae and Ligaments
ON2-ONW	Head and Facial Bones
OP2-OPW	Upper Bones
OQ2-OQW	Lower Bones
OR2-ORW	Upper Joints
OS2-OS2	Lower Joints

Arthroscopic Surgery

Arthroscopic surgery is a minimally invasive surgery that involves the use of highly specialized instruments to perform surgery through very small incisions (½ inch) on joints. Advantages of arthroscopic surgery include small incisions, minimal scar tissue, and less pain after surgery with quicker recovery. Arthroscopic procedures can be performed on any of the joints and joint structures. If an arthroscopic approach is used to perform a definitive procedure (e.g., biopsies, meniscectomies, ligament repairs), the approach is not coded. Occasionally, an arthroscopic procedure is performed for diagnostic purposes, and no additional therapeutic procedures are performed (Figure 19-16). The root operation for a diagnostic arthroscopic examination is inspection.

EXAMPLE Arthroscopic examination of the left knee for chronic pain. All joint structures appear to be intact, 719.46, 80.26 (M25.562, 0SJD4ZZ).

EXAMPLE Arthroscopic meniscectomy for torn right medial meniscus (old injury), 717.3, 80.6 (M23.231, 0SBC4ZZ).

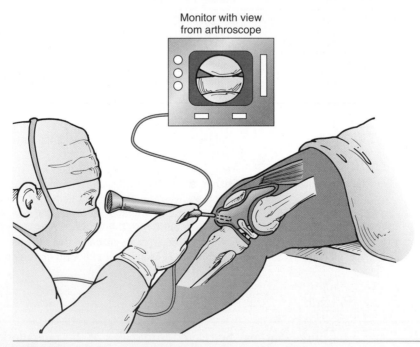

Monitor with view from arthroscope

FIGURE 19-16. Arthroscopic examination of a joint.

Joint Replacement

Joint replacement consists of removal of an arthritic or damaged joint and replacement with an artificial joint, which is also known as a prosthesis. Materials used in total joint replacement are designed to enable the joint to move similarly to a normal joint. The root operation for a total joint replacement is replacement. The prosthesis is generally composed of two parts; a metal piece fits closely into a matching sturdy plastic piece (Figure 19-17). Several metals, including stainless steel, alloys of cobalt and chrome, and titanium, are used. The plastic material is durable and wear resistant (polyethylene). A plastic bone cement may be used to anchor the prosthesis into the bone. Hip and knee replacements are the most common joint replacements, but other joints, including the ankle, foot, shoulder, elbow, and fingers, can be replaced. When the same procedure is performed on bilateral joints, the procedure code should be assigned twice. In cases in which the disease process does not affect the entire joint, partial joint replacement may be performed. Other options besides total joint replacement procedures are available. A resurfacing procedure may be an option. A surface replacement procedure leaves more of the patient's bone in place with resurfacing of the affected area of the joint.

Codes 00.70 to 00.73 are assigned for revisions of hip joint replacements and identify the specific components that are being revised.

- 00.70 Total hip revision (both acetabular and femoral components)
- 00.71 Revision acetabular component
- 00.72 Revision femoral component
- 00.73 Revision acetabular liner and/or femoral head only

If only a component of a joint was previously replaced, the procedure is still considered a revision even if the part of the component is being replaced for the first time.

FIGURE 19-17. Total knee replacement for osteoarthritis.

EXAMPLE Patient who had a previous right hip hemiarthroplasty was admitted because of loosening of the femoral prosthesis. The femoral component was replaced, 996.41, V43.64, E878.1, 00.72 (T84.030A, Z96.641, Y83.1, 0SRR0JZ, 0SP90JZ).

Procedures for knee replacement revisions are identified according to the component (00.80-00.84) revised similar to the hip revisions. The root operations for a revision of a joint replacement are removal and replacement of the prosthetic device.

Codes 00.74-00.77 identify different types of bearing surface materials used in hip prosthetic implants such as metal-on-polyethylene, metal-on-metal, and ceramic-on-ceramic and ceramic-on-polyethylene. If the specific type of bearing surface is known, an additional code should be assigned. These codes can be used with hip replacement or revision procedures.

As with replacement procedures, resurfacing can involve partial or total joint resurfacing. The root operation for a resurfacing procedure is supplement.

Common complications of joint replacement include infection, blood clot, nerve injury, loosening, dislocation, wear and tear, and breakage of the prosthesis. It may be necessary to remove the prosthesis and insert a new prosthesis. According to *Coding Clinic* (1997:3Q:p13),[4] "any time the joint is replaced or revised after the initial replacement this would be considered a revision."

EXAMPLE Primary osteoarthritis both knees. Patient is hospitalized for right partial knee replacement (femoral surface) with synthetic substitute, 715.16, 81.54 (M17.0, 0SRT0JZ).

Vertebroplasty/Kyphoplasty

Percutaneous vertebroplasty (PV) is a technique that is used to treat pain caused by compression fractures of the vertebrae. The root operation for a vertebroplasty is supplement. Under x-ray guidance, an acrylic cement is injected through a needle into a collapsed or weakened vertebra. This stabilizes the fracture, allowing the patient to resume normal activity and decrease the use of analgesics. PV does not reverse osteoporosis or prevent future compression fractures. This procedure is usually performed by interventional radiologists. According to *Coding Clinic* (2002:2Q:p14-15),[5] the code 81.65 for vertebroplasty includes stabilization of the fracture, so it is not necessary to assign an additional code for the stabilization.

Kyphoplasty, similar to PV, is used to treat fractures of the spine; however, in kyphoplasty, a special balloon device is inserted into the compacted vertebrae in an attempt to restore vertebrae to a more normal state by improving the alignment of the spine. The root operations for a kyphoplasty are reposition and supplement. After the balloon has been removed, the cavity is filled with a cement-like material to stabilize the fracture. Kyphoplasty is usually performed under fluoroscopic guidance through a small incision in the back.

EXAMPLE Compression fractures T11-T12 due to osteoporosis. Percutaneous vertebroplasty (synthetic substitute) was performed in radiology, 733.13, 733.00, 81.65 (M80.88xA, 0PU43JZ).

Spinal Decompression/Fusion

Spinal decompression is a surgical procedure that frees space for nerves in the spinal canal. A number of different surgical methods, including laminectomy, laminotomy, laminoplasty, foraminotomy, and anterior discectomy, can be performed to accomplish a decompression. Although in many cases, decompression involves removal of tissue that is constricting or compressing nerve structures, in some cases the spine becomes unstable, and spinal fusion is performed at the time of the decompression. At times the spine becomes unstable and painful following a decompression; at this point, a fusion may be required.

Spinal fusion is the creation of a solid bone bridge between two or more adjacent vertebrae to create stability between levels of the spine. The root operation for spinal fusion is fusion. Fusion is a gradual process (6-9 months or longer) in which bone is grown across desired areas to form a solid fusion. Bone grafts, spinal instrumentation, casts, and/or braces are used to facilitate and promote the fusion process. If a fusion fails to heal or fuse properly, this is called a nonunion or pseudarthrosis; repeat or revision surgery may be required. A bone graft may be obtained from a variety of sources. Bone may be harvested from the patient's (autologous) spine or from the iliac crest. Bone graft material can also be obtained from a bone bank (harvested from cadavers [allograft]). Synthetic bone materials made from demineralized bone matrix (DBM) and calcium phosphates or hydroxyapatites (some derived from sea coral) may also be used. The use of metal devices, also called implants or instrumentation (e.g., screws, rods, plates, cables, wires), can facilitate correction of a deformed spine and may increase the probability of attaining solid spinal fusion. Spinal instrumentation can be placed in the front or in the back portion of the spine. Devices are usually made of metal, commonly stainless steel or titanium. Spinal instrumentation is gradually covered by scar tissue and sometimes by new growth of bone. Even when the spine has healed solidly, the instrumentation is rarely removed.

A 360-degree spinal fusion is defined in *Coding Clinic* (2003:2Q:p20)[6] as "a spinal fusion of both the anterior and posterior portions of the spine during the same operative session. Historically, this procedure was performed using both an anterior approach and a posterior approach by making incisions both in the front and back. Advances in medical technology and surgical techniques now allow the fusion of the anterior and posterior vertebra during the same operative session using a single incision—usually via the lateral transverse approach." Sometimes a spinal fusion is performed as a "staged procedure" with a posterior fusion performed one day, and an anterior fusion is performed a few days later.

During any spinal fusion procedure, the documentation should be reviewed to ascertain whether this is a new fusion or a refusion. To correctly assign the spinal fusion code, it must be determined whether the approach was anterior or posterior, or whether some other approach was used. In addition to the appropriate code to identify spinal fusion, an additional code (81.62-81.64) must be assigned for the total number of vertebrae fused (Figure 19-18).

Also, if an interbody spinal fusion device has been inserted or if recombinant bone morphogenetic protein (BMP) has been used, an additional code is assigned.

EXAMPLE The patient was admitted for surgical intervention for cervical disc herniation with myelopathy. Partial discectomy at C3 and spinal fusion of C3-C4 and C4-C5 were performed via the anterior approach (anterior column) using internal instrumentation, 722.71, 81.02, 81.62, 80.51 (M50.02, 0RG2040, 0RB30ZZ).

EXERCISE 19-7

Assign codes for all diagnoses and procedures.

1. Open bone biopsy left upper femur, which confirmed acute and chronic osteomyelitis _____

2. Excision Baker's cyst, right _____

3. Partial hip replacement (femoral head) for OA right hip _____

4. Removal of fixation device lumbar spine _____

5. Arthroscopy right knee. Mild osteoarthritis _____

6. Hammer toe repair with fusion of left third toe distal interphalangeal joint with internal fixation device _____

7. Necrotizing fasciitis with excisional debridement of subcutaneous tissue and fascia, right forearm _____

8. Pathologic fracture T12 due to postmenopausal osteoporosis. Percutaneous kyphoplasty with synthetic substitute was performed _____

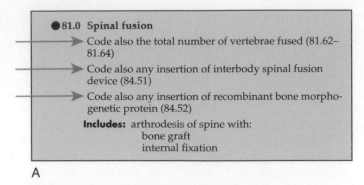

A

B

FIGURE 19-18. Entries for spinal fusion (**A**) and other spine procedures (**B**) require the assignment of additional codes to indicate the number of vertebrae fused.

DOCUMENTATION/REIMBURSEMENT/MS-DRGs

Often, coding difficulties are due to lack of documentation. Sometimes pathology, radiology, and other test results are not available at the time of discharge or when the physician is dictating the discharge summary or is reporting the final diagnoses.

Frequently missed complications/comorbidities from this chapter include:

- Avascular necrosis
- Pathologic fractures
- Malunion/nonunion of fracture

Pathologic Fracture Versus Traumatic Fracture

EXAMPLE

Patient was admitted from the Emergency Room with a fractured right hip. The patient has osteoporosis and had fallen on the morning of admission.

DIAGNOSES	CODES	MS-DRG	RW
Pathologic fracture hip due to osteoporosis	733.14, 733.00 (M80.051A)	544	0.7775
Traumatic fracture hip in patient with osteoporosis	820.8, 733.00, E888.9 (S72.001A, M81.0, W19.xxxA)	536	0.7191

A physician query may be necessary to make sure that the appropriate MS-DRG is assigned for optimal reimbursement.

Correct Procedure Code

	Patient was admitted for resurfacing of left femoral head with resurfacing device due to osteoarthritis, 715.35, 00.86.			
EXAMPLE	**DIAGNOSES**	**CODES**	**MS-DRG**	**RW**
	Osteoarthritis hip	715.35 (M16.12)	470	2.1039
	Resurfacing femoral	00.86 (0SUS0BZ)		
	Osteoarthritis hip	715.35 (M16.12)	468	2.5728
	Revision hip replacement, femoral component	00.72 (0QP70JZ, 0QR70JZ)		

In this example, an error was made when resurfacing of the femoral head was coded as a revision. This error would have resulted in an overpayment to the facility.

CHAPTER REVIEW EXERCISE

Assign codes for all diagnoses and procedures.

1. Osteitis deformans _____
2. Wry neck _____
3. Hallux valgus, left big toe _____
4. Frozen right shoulder _____
5. Plantar fasciitis _____
6. Recurrent dislocation right thumb _____
7. Osteoporosis due to long-term use of steroids _____
8. Instability left ankle _____
9. Ganglion tendon sheath of the right wrist with removal _____
10. Tennis elbow, right _____
11. Polymyalgia rheumatica _____
12. Myositis _____
13. Pain in both wrists _____
14. Avascular necrosis (left femur) due to sickle cell (hemoglobin SS) disease _____
15. Osteogenesis imperfecta _____
16. Right above the knee amputation (AKA) _____
17. Housemaid's knee (right) _____
18. Scleroderma with lung involvement _____
19. Arthropathy due to Crohn's disease _____
20. Felty's syndrome _____
21. Pyogenic arthritis left knee due to *Staphylococcus aureus* _____
22. Osteoarthritis right shoulder treated with intra-articular steroid injection _____
23. Paget's disease, left thigh _____
24. Chondromalacia right patella _____

Write the correct answer(s) in the blank(s) provided.

25. What is the appropriate fifth-digit subclassification for knee joint?

_____

26. Which MS-DRG has higher reimbursement: pathologic fracture or traumatic fracture?

_____

Why? _____

27. Another name for osteoarthritis.

_____

28. List 4 symptoms of SLE.
1. _____
2. _____
3. _____
4. _____

29. Which individuals are at risk for osteoporosis?

_____

30. List 3 examples of aftercare for a pathologic fracture.
1. _____
2. _____
3. _____

CHAPTER GLOSSARY

Anterior: front of the body or an organ.

Arthropathy: disease that affects the joints.

Arthroscopic: minimally invasive surgery that involves the use of highly specialized instruments to perform surgery through very small incisions on joints.

Bursitis: inflammation of a bursa, which is a tiny, fluid-filled sac that is found between muscles, tendons, and bones that reduces friction and facilitates movement.

Caudal: toward the tail.

Cranial: toward the head.

Distal: farther from the median plane; term is often used to describe a location in the limbs.

Dorsal: back of the body or an organ.

Dorsopathies: conditions or diseases that affect the back or spine.

Facet joints: small, stabilizing joints located between and behind adjacent vertebrae.

Fascia: tissue just below the skin that covers and separates the underlying layers of muscle.

Fibromyalgia: one of the most common diseases affecting the muscles; it is characterized by widespread muscle pain associated with chronic fatigue.

Hematopoiesis: development of blood cells that occurs in the bone marrow and lymphatic tissue of normal adults.

Inferior: position of the body or an organ relative to the vertical axis of the body.

Joints: means of joining two bones together.

Juvenile rheumatoid arthritis: type of arthritis that affects children, usually between the ages of 2 and 5 years.

Kyphoplasty: procedure performed to treat and stabilize fractures of the spine.

Kyphosis: excessive posterior curvature of the thoracic spine that may not be detected until a hump in the upper back is noticeable.

Lateral: position of a structure that is to the side of the body.

Ligaments: dense, fibrous bands of connective tissue that provide stability for the joint.

Lordosis: exaggerated inward curvature of the spine that may be caused by increased abdominal girth due to obesity, pregnancy, or abdominal tumor.

Medial: position of a structure closer to the median plane than is another structure in the body.

Myelopathy: compression of the spinal cord.

Necrotizing fasciitis (or "flesh-eating disease"): a rare but serious condition in which an infection occurs in the tissues below the skin.

Osteoarthritis: type of arthritis that develops as the result of wear and tear on the joints.

Osteomyelitis: infection of the bone that often starts in another part of the body and spreads to the bone via the blood.

Osteoporosis: metabolic bone disorder that results in decreased bone mass and density.

Pathologic fracture: break in a bone that occurs because of underlying disorders that weaken the bone, including malignancy, benign bone tumor, metabolic disorder, infection, and osteoporosis.

Percutaneous vertebroplasty: technique in which x-ray guidance is used to inject an acrylic cement through a needle into a collapsed or weakened vertebra; procedure is performed to treat pain caused by compression fractures of the vertebrae.

Polymyalgia rheumatica: syndrome classified as a rheumatic disease that is characterized by severe aching and stiffness in the neck, shoulder girdle, and pelvic girdle.

Posterior: back of the body or an organ.

Postlaminectomy syndrome: term used to describe patients who have undergone spine surgery and have some degree of recurrent spinal and/or leg pain due to the build up of scar tissue.

Primary osteoarthritis: idiopathic degenerative condition that occurs in previously intact joints, with no apparent initiating factor.

Prone: lying on the stomach, face down.

Proximal: closer to the median plane.

Radiculopathy: compression of a nerve root.

Rhabdomyolysis: breakdown of muscle fibers resulting in the release of muscle fiber contents into the circulation.

Rheumatoid arthritis: chronic, inflammatory systemic disease that affects the joints, often causing deformity.

Scleroderma: chronic, progressive disease characterized by hardening of the skin and scarring of internal organs.

Scoliosis: deviation of the vertical line of the spine.

Secondary osteoarthritis: degenerative disease of the joints that results from some predisposing condition such as trauma or disease.

Spinal decompression: surgical procedure that frees space for the nerves in the spinal canal.

Spinal fusion: the creation of a solid bone bridge between two or more adjacent vertebrae to enhance stability between levels of the spine.

Spinal stenosis: narrowing of the central spinal canal or the areas of the spine where the nerve roots exit (neuroforamina).

Spondylolisthesis: condition in which one vertebra slips on another.

Spondylosis (or spinal osteoarthritis): degenerative disorder that may cause loss of normal spinal structure and function.

Superior: position of the body or an organ relative to the vertical axis of the body.

Supine: lying on the back, face up.

Systemic lupus erythematosus: chronic, inflammatory autoimmune disease that can damage connective tissue anywhere in the body.

Tendons: connective tissue that attaches muscle to bone.

Ventral: front of the body or an organ.

REFERENCES

1. American Hospital Association. *Coding Clinic for ICD-9-CM* 1995:2Q:p5. Degenerative joint disease, bilateral.
2. American Hospital Association. *Coding Clinic for ICD-9-CM* 1997:2Q:p15. Clarification—Postlaminectomy syndrome.
3. American Hospital Association. *Coding Clinic for ICD-9-CM* 2008:3Q:p4. Chronic vertebral compression fracture.
4. American Hospital Association. *Coding Clinic for ICD-9-CM* 1997:3Q:p13. Hip prosthesis removal with total hip replacement.
5. American Hospital Association. *Coding Clinic for ICD-9-CM* 2002:2Q:p14-15. Vertebroplasty and stabilization of vertebral fracture.
6. American Hospital Association. *Coding Clinic for ICD-9-CM* 2003:2Q:p20. 360-Degree spinal fusion—Clarification.

20

Diseases of the Genitourinary System

(ICD-9-CM Chapter 10, Codes 580-629, and ICD-10-CM Chapter 14, Codes N00-N99)

CHAPTER OUTLINE

ICD-9-CM Official Guidelines for Coding and Reporting
ICD-10-CM Official Guidelines for Coding and Reporting
Guideline Differences Between ICD-9-CM and ICD-10-CM
Major Differences Between ICD-9-CM and ICD-10-CM

Anatomy and Physiology
    Urinary Tract
    Male Genital Tract
    Female Genital Tract
    Breast

Disease Conditions
    Nephritis, Nephrotic Syndrome, and Nephrosis
    Other Diseases of the Urinary System
    Diseases of the Male Genital Organs
    Disorders of Breast
    Inflammatory Disease of Female Pelvic Organs
    Other Disorders of Female Genital Tract

Factors Influencing Health Status and Contact with Health Services (V Codes/Z Codes)

Common Treatments

Procedures
    Dialysis
    Kidney Transplantation
    Prostate Procedures
    Breast Biopsies and Reconstruction
    Removal of Stones

Documentation/Reimbursement/MS-DRGs
    Urosepsis Versus Sepsis
    MS-DRG With and Without MCC/CC

Chapter Review Exercise
Chapter Glossary
References

LEARNING OBJECTIVES

1. Apply and assign the correct ICD-9-CM and ICD-10-CM codes in accordance with Official Guidelines for Coding and Reporting
2. Identify major differences between ICD-9-CM and ICD-10-CM related to the genitourinary system
3. Identify pertinent anatomy and physiology of diseases of the genitourinary system

4. Identify diseases of the genitourinary system
5. Assign the correct V/Z codes and procedure codes related to the genitourinary system
6. Identify common treatments, medications, laboratory values, and diagnostic tests
7. Explain the importance of documentation in relation to MS-DRGs for reimbursement

**ABBREVIATIONS/
ACRONYMS**

ARF acute renal failure

ARI acute renal insufficiency

AV arteriovenous

BUN blood urea nitrogen

CAPD continuous ambulatory peritoneal dialysis

CC chief complaint

CCPD continuous cycling peritoneal dialysis

CIN cervical intraepithelial neoplasia

CKD chronic kidney disease

CRF chronic renal failure

CRI chronic renal insufficiency

D&C dilatation and curettage

DIEP deep inferior epigastric perforator

ESRD end-stage renal disease

ESWL extracorporeal shock wave lithotripsy

FSG focal segmental glomerulosclerosis

GAP gluteal artery perforator

GFR glomerular filtration rate

GN glomerulonephritis

HSIL high-grade squamous intraepithelial lesion

ICD-9-CM *International Classification of Diseases, 9th Revision, Clinical Modification*

ICD-10-CM *International Classification of Diseases, 10th Revision, Clinical Modification*

ICD-10-PCS *International Classification of Diseases, 10th Revision, Procedure Coding System*

Ig immunoglobulin

LAVH laparoscopically assisted vaginal hysterectomy

LDMF latissimus dorsi musculocutaneous flap

LSIL low-grade squamous intraepithelial lesion

LUTS lower urinary tract symptoms

MRSA methicillin-resistant *Staphylococcus aureus*

MS-DRG Medicare Severity diagnosis-related group

NEC not elsewhere classifiable

NKF National Kidney Foundation

NOS not otherwise specified

OIG Office of the Inspector General

PID pelvic inflammatory disease

PSA prostate-specific antigen

RPGN rapidly progressive glomerulonephritis

SIEA superficial inferior epigastric artery

SIL squamous intraepithelial lesion

TRAM transverse rectus abdominis musculocutaneous

TULIP transurethral ultrasound-guided laser-induced prostatectomy

TUMT transurethral microwave thermotherapy

TUNA transurethral needle ablation of prostate

TURP transurethral resection of the prostate

UHDDS Uniform Hospital Discharge Data Set

UTI urinary tract infection

VIN vulvular intraepithelial neoplasia

VLAP visual laser ablation of the prostate

ICD-9-CM

Official Guidelines for Coding and Reporting

Please refer to the companion Evolve website for the most current guidelines.

10. Chapter 10: Diseases of Genitourinary System (580-629)

a. Chronic kidney disease

1) Stages of chronic kidney disease (CKD)

The ICD-9-CM classifies CKD based on severity. The severity of CKD is designated by stages I-V. Stage II, code 585.2, equates to mild CKD; stage III, code 585.3, equates to moderate CKD; and stage IV, code 585.4, equates to severe CKD. Code 585.6, End stage renal disease (ESRD), is assigned when the provider has documented end-stage-renal disease (ESRD).

If both a stage of CKD and ESRD are documented, assign code 585.6 only.

2) Chronic kidney disease and kidney transplant status

Patients who have undergone kidney transplant may still have some form of CKD, because the kidney transplant may not fully restore kidney function. Therefore, the presence of CKD alone does not constitute a transplant complication. Assign the appropriate 585 code for the patient's stage of CKD and code V42.0. If a transplant complication such as failure or rejection is documented, see section I.C.17.f.2.b for information on coding complications of a kidney transplant. If the documentation is unclear as to whether the patient has a complication of the transplant, query the provider.

3) Chronic kidney disease with other conditions
Patients with CKD may also suffer from other serious conditions, most commonly diabetes mellitus and hypertension. The sequencing of the CKD code in relationship to codes for other contributing conditions is based on the conventions in the Tabular List.

See I.C.3.a.4 for sequencing instructions for diabetes.
See I.C.4.a.1 for anemia in CKD.
See I.C.7.a.3 for hypertensive chronic kidney disease.
See I.C.17.f.1.b, Kidney transplant complications, for instructions on coding of documented rejection or failure.

EXAMPLE   Patient was admitted to the hospital for fluid overload due to noncompliance with attending renal dialysis sessions. Patient has stage V CKD. Hemodialysis was performed, 276.69, 585.6, V45.12, 39.95 (E87.7, N18.6, Z91.15, 5A1D00Z).

Apply the General Coding Guidelines as found in Chapter 5 and the Procedural Guidelines as found in Chapter 6.

ICD-10-CM

Official Guidelines for Coding and Reporting

Please refer to the companion Evolve website for the most current guidelines.

14. Chapter 14: Diseases of Genitourinary System (N00-N99)
a. Chronic kidney disease
1) Stages of chronic kidney disease (CKD)
The ICD-10-CM classifies CKD based on severity. The severity of CKD is designated by stages **1-5**. Stage **2**, code N18.2, equates to mild CKD; stage **3**, code N18.3, equates to moderate CKD; and stage **4**, code N18.4, equates to severe CKD. Code N18.6, End stage renal disease (ESRD), is assigned when the provider has documented end-stage-renal disease (ESRD).
If both a stage of CKD and ESRD are documented, assign code N18.6 only.
2) Chronic kidney disease and kidney transplant status
Patients who have undergone kidney transplant may still have some form of chronic kidney disease (CKD) because the kidney transplant may not fully restore kidney function. Therefore, the presence of CKD alone does not constitute a transplant complication. Assign the appropriate N18 code for the patient's stage of CKD and code Z94.0, Kidney transplant status. If a transplant complication such as failure or rejection or other transplant complication is documented, see section I.C.19.g for information on coding complications of a kidney transplant. If the documentation is unclear as to whether the patient has a complication of the transplant, query the provider.
3) Chronic kidney disease with other conditions
Patients with CKD may also suffer from other serious conditions, most commonly diabetes mellitus and hypertension. The sequencing of the CKD code in relationship to codes for other contributing conditions is based on the conventions in the Tabular List.
See I.C.9. Hypertensive chronic kidney disease.
See I.C.19. Chronic kidney disease and kidney transplant complications.

Apply the General Coding Guidelines as found in Chapter 5 and the Procedural Guidelines as found in Chapter 7.

GUIDELINE DIFFERENCES BETWEEN ICD-9-CM AND ICD-10-CM

There are no differences in the guidelines.

MAJOR DIFFERENCES BETWEEN ICD-9-CM AND ICD-10-CM

- In ICD-10-CM the various stages of dysplasia of the vagina are identified.
- In ICD-10-CM laterality is used to identify conditions under the N60 category, benign mammary dysplasia.
- Procedural complications affecting the genitourinary system are included in Chapter 14 of ICD-10-CM. Some of the complications include:
  - Postprocedural renal failure
  - Postprocedural urethral stricture
  - Prolapse of the vaginal vault after hysterectomy
  - Complications of urinary tract stoma
  - Intraoperative hemorrhage, hematoma, or accidental laceration

ANATOMY AND PHYSIOLOGY

Urinary Tract

The kidneys, ureters, urinary bladder, and urethra form the urinary tract (Figure 20-1). Its main function involves producing, storing, and excreting urine. The kidneys and ureters make up the upper urinary tract, and the bladder and urethra constitute the lower urinary tract. The kidneys are two bean-shaped organs that are located on either side of the spine or retroperitoneally. The kidneys form a complex filtration system that cleanses the blood of waste products that become urine. Each kidney has a ureter that allows the urine to travel to the bladder for storage. The bladder is expandable, and openings into the ureters close so that urine cannot flow backward or reflux into the kidneys. The urine is excreted out of the body through a tube called the urethra. It is easy to confuse the terminology for urethra and ureter. Less than half of a single kidney is needed to do all the work that can be accomplished by two kidneys. The main difference between the male and female urinary tracts is the length of the urethra. The male urethra is 20 cm long; the female urethra measures only 3 cm.

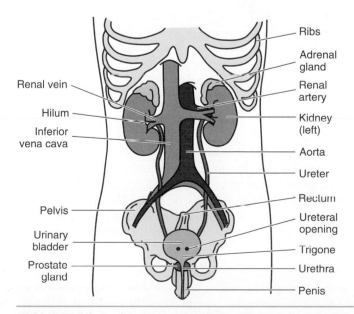

FIGURE 20-1. Gross anatomy of the urinary system (male).

FIGURE 20-2. Normal male reproductive system.

Male Genital Tract

The main parts of the male genital or reproductive tract are the testes, epididymis, vas deferens, seminal vesicles, prostate, and penis (Figure 20-2). Its primary function is the production of sperm. The main diseases related to the male genital tract are infertility, infection, and tumor.

Female Genital Tract

The main parts of the female genital or reproductive tract are the vulva, vagina, uterus, fallopian tubes, and ovaries (Figure 20-3). Reproduction is its primary function. The main diseases and conditions of the female genital tract are related to infection, tumor, hormonal disorders, and pregnancy.

Breast

Male and female breasts are similar in that they are formed embryologically from the same tissues. It is possible for males to have breast disorders also. The female breast (Figure 20-4) will start to develop during puberty due to the hormone estrogen. Female breasts are considered an accessory organ of reproduction and are composed of fat and fibrous tissue with mammary glands for the production of milk (**lactation**).

DISEASE CONDITIONS

Diseases of the genitourinary system (580-629) are located in Chapter 10 of the ICD-9-CM code book and are divided into the following categories:

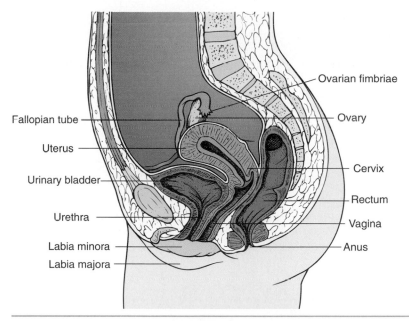

FIGURE 20-3. Normal female reproductive system.

FIGURE 20-4. Views of the breast. **A,** Sagittal. **B,** Frontal. Notice the numerous lymph nodes.

CATEGORY	SECTION TITLES
580-589	Nephritis, Nephrotic Syndrome, and Nephrosis
590-599	Other Diseases of the Urinary System
600-608	Disease of the Male Genital Organs
610-611	Disorders of Breast
614-616	Inflammatory Disease of Female Pelvic Organs
617-629	Other Disorders of Female Genital Tract

It is important to note that disorders of the breast are classified as Diseases of the Genitourinary System in ICD-9-CM and ICD-10-CM.

Diseases of the Genitourinary System (N00 to N99), Chapter 11 in the ICD-10-CM code book, are divided into the following categories:

CATEGORY	SECTION TITLES
N00-N08	Glomerular Diseases
N10-N16	Renal Tubulo-Interstitial Diseases
N17-N19	Acute Renal Failure and Chronic Kidney Disease
N20-N23	Urolithiasis
N25-N29	Other Disorders of the Kidney and Ureter
N30-N39	Other Diseases of the Urinary System
N40-N51	Diseases of Male Genital Organs
N60-N65	Disorders of the Breast
N70-N77	Inflammatory Diseases of Female Pelvic Organs
N80-N98	Noninflammatory Disorders of the Female Genital Tract
N99	Intraoperative and Postprocedural Complications and Disorders of Genitourinary System, Not Elsewhere Classified

Nephritis, Nephrotic Syndrome, and Nephrosis

Glomerulonephritis

Glomerulonephritis (GN) (Figure 20-5) is inflammation of the glomeruli of the kidneys. (See Figure 20-6 for illustration of the anatomy of the kidney.) Glomerulonephritis can be a temporary, reversible condition, or it may be a chronic progressive condition that results in chronic renal failure and end-stage renal disease. GN may cause hypertension and may not be discovered until the hypertension becomes difficult to control. Specific disorders that are associated with glomerulonephritis include the following:

- Focal segmental glomerulosclerosis (FSG)
- Goodpasture's syndrome
- Immunoglobulin (Ig)A nephropathy (Berger's disease)
- IgM mesangial proliferative glomerulonephritis
- Lupus nephritis
- Membranoproliferative glomerulonephritis I
- Membranoproliferative glomerulonephritis II
- Poststreptococcal glomerulonephritis
- Rapidly progressive (crescentic) glomerulonephritis
- Rapidly progressive glomerulonephritis (RPGN)

FIGURE 20-5. End-stage glomerulopathy–chronic glomerulonephritis.

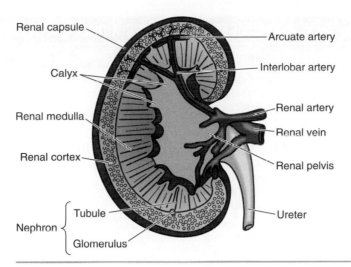

FIGURE 20-6. Anatomy of the kidney.

EXAMPLE   Minimal change glomerulonephritis, 581.3 (N05.0).

EXAMPLE   RPGN, 583.4 (N01.9).

Nephrotic Syndrome/Nephrosis

Nephrotic syndrome is a condition that is marked by **proteinuria** (protein in the urine), low levels of protein in the blood, hypercholesterolemia, and swelling of the eyes, feet, and hands. Damage to the kidneys' glomeruli can result in nephrotic syndrome. Treatment focuses on identifying the underlying cause and reducing cholesterol, blood pressure, and protein in urine through diet and medications.

EXAMPLE   Lupus nephritis, 710.0, 583.81 (M32.14).

Acute Renal Failure

Acute renal failure (ARF) is sudden and severe impairment in renal function characterized by oliguria, increased serum urea, and acidosis. With treatment, ARF is usually reversible. ARF often occurs in hospitalized patients with serious systemic illness such as infection, low blood pressure, shock, and as an adverse effect of the use of certain antibiotics and drugs. Obstruction of the urinary tract and dehydration may also cause ARF. It is possible for a patient with chronic renal failure or chronic kidney disease to also develop ARF. In this case, codes are assigned for both the acute and chronic renal failure.

   If a patient is admitted for multiple reasons including ARF, the guidelines for principal diagnosis selection need to be applied. Often times, the acute renal failure is a result of another condition and should be coded as a secondary diagnosis.

EXAMPLE   Patient is admitted with an exacerbation of congestive heart failure. The patient is also in acute renal failure. This physician documents that the ARF is due to the patient's fluid overload, 428.0, 584.9 (I50.9, N17.9).

   When a patient is admitted to the hospital with acute renal failure and dehydration, according to *Coding Clinic* (2002:3Q:p21-22),[1] ARF is the principal diagnosis, and the dehydration is a secondary diagnosis. Patients with both conditions are generally treated with

TABLE 20-1 FIVE STAGES OF CHRONIC KIDNEY DISEASE

Stage	Description	Glomerular Filtration Rate (GFR)
At increased risk	Risk factors for kidney disease (e.g., diabetes, high blood pressure, family history, older age, ethnic group)	Higher than 90
1	Kidney damage (protein in the urine) and normal GFR	Higher than 90
2	Kidney damage and mild decrease in GFR	60-89
3	Moderate decrease in GFR	30-59
4	Severe decrease in GFR	15-29
5	Kidney failure (dialysis or kidney transplant needed)	Less than 15

Data from the national kidney foundation.

IV fluids, and ARF is more serious than dehydration. A patient who is dehydrated and has no impairment in renal function may be given IV fluids and sent home instead of being admitted to the hospital.

EXAMPLE Acute renal failure due to dehydration, 584.9, 276.51 (N17.9, E86.0).

Chronic Renal Failure (CRF)/Chronic Kidney Disease (CKD)

According to *Coding Clinic* (2005:4Q:p77-79),[2] "Changes were made to the ICD-9-CM classification to recognize more current terminology related to chronic kidney disease (CKD) rather than imprecise terms like chronic renal failure [CRF] and chronic renal insufficiency (CRI). The descriptor for code 585, Chronic renal failure, has been changed to chronic kidney disease. Code 585 has been expanded to recognize current staging of chronic kidney disease developed by the National Kidney Foundation (NKF)" (Table 20-1).

Using these NKF guidelines, levels of kidney damage and kidney function must be determined to accurately assign the code for CKD. A patient's glomerular filtration rate (GFR) indicates the level of kidney function and indicates the stage of the disease, which may slowly progress over many years. Early detection through laboratory tests and proper treatment can limit the effects of CKD, if the disease is discovered in the early stages.

If CKD is left untreated, a patient will develop end-stage renal disease (ESRD). This condition is characterized by the near or complete failure of kidney function, which leaves the patient unable to process waste material. Dialysis or transplantation may be needed to treat the condition.

CRF or CKD can develop from ARF if renal function is not restored through dialysis or treatment. This may take several weeks or months. Documentation in the health record that might indicate the presence of renal failure could include the following:
1. Markedly elevated values of serum creatinine or blood urea nitrogen (BUN), or diminished creatinine clearance
2. Other clinical and laboratory manifestations of renal impairment are as follows:
   - Anemia
   - Hyperphosphatemia
   - Hypocalcemia
   - Hyperkalemia
   - Renal osteodystrophy
   - Uremic symptoms: nausea, vomiting, itching, hemorrhagic conditions, hypertension, edema, dyspnea, lethargy, coma, etc.

EXAMPLE Hyperkalemia due to chronic kidney disease (CKD), 276.7, 585.9 (E87.5, N18.9).

Hypertension and Chronic Kidney Disease/Renal Failure

ICD-9-CM presumes a cause-and-effect relationship with hypertension and chronic renal failure or chronic kidney disease. This is addressed in the coding guidelines. Code 585 (N18.–) has instructions to code first hypertensive chronic kidney disease, if applicable. The physician would have to specifically document that CKD or renal failure is NOT due to hypertension to negate the cause-and-effect relationship. Hypertension and hypertensive manifestations are discussed more extensively in Chapter 15, Diseases of the Circulatory System.

EXAMPLE	Patient has chronic kidney disease, stage III, and benign hypertension, 403.10, 585.3 (I12.9, N18.3).

EXAMPLE	Patient has chronic renal insufficiency and hypertension, 403.90, 585.9 (I12.9, N18.9).

Diabetic Nephropathy

Diabetes mellitus can have effects on many organs, including the kidneys. If diabetes is not well controlled, it may cause renal complications such as glomerulosclerosis, pyelonephritis, and papillary necrosis. Diabetic patients with renal manifestations may be prone to infections that can cause further damage to the kidneys.

Unlike the relationship between renal failure/chronic kidney disease and hypertension, diabetes and renal disease must be linked in a manner that denotes a direct relationship. For example, diabetic nephropathy or intercapillary glomerulosclerosis due to diabetes shows a cause-and-effect relationship with diabetes. It is possible for a patient to have nephropathy and diabetes, and no documentation indicates that nephropathy is due to diabetes. In Chapter 12 of this book, diabetes mellitus and manifestations of the disease are discussed in greater depth.

EXAMPLE	Patient is admitted for treatment of uncontrolled diabetes mellitus, type II. Patient is on hemodialysis for end-stage renal disease, 250.02, 585.6, V45.11 (E11.65, N18.6, Z99.2).

EXAMPLE	Patient had intercapillary glomerulosclerosis due to diabetes mellitus type I, 250.41, 581.81 (E10.21).

EXERCISE 20-1

Assign codes to the following conditions.

1. Acute on chronic renal failure _____
2. Nephrotic syndrome _____
3. Nephritis due to tuberculosis _____
4. Focal segmental glomerulosclerosis _____
5. Essential hypertension; stage IV CKD _____

Other Diseases of the Urinary System

Hematuria

Hematuria is the presence of blood in the urine. Hematuria may be grossly visible, or it may be detected only through microscopic analysis. The causes of hematuria are varied, and some are more serious than others. The extent of diagnostic investigation required to determine a cause depends on the amount of hematuria, its duration, and risk factors the patient may have that indicate a more serious disease. Causes include inflammation due to drugs or medications, stones, infections, cancers or malignancies, trauma, and blockages or obstructions of flow. A patient with renal stones often has hematuria. Hematuria would not be assigned as an additional code because it is considered integral to the renal stones according to *Coding Clinic* (1995:3Q:p8).[3] This corresponds with the general coding guideline that signs and symptoms that are integral to the disease process should not be assigned as additional codes.

EXAMPLE   Hematuria due to nephrolithiasis, 592.0 (N20.0).

Urinary Tract Infections

"**Urinary tract infection**" (UTI) is a general term that is used to describe infection of any area of the urinary tract. **Cystitis** is a lower tract infection that affects the bladder (Figure 20-7), and **urethritis** affects the urethra. An upper tract infection that involves the kidneys is called **pyelonephritis** (Figure 20-8).

According to *Coding Clinic* (1999:2Q:p15-16),[4] "physicians commonly use the term 'urinary tract infection' when referring to cystitis, urethritis, or pyelonephritis. UTIs are

FIGURE 20-7. Acute cystitis. The mucosa of the bladder is red and swollen.

FIGURE 20-8. Small, shrunken, irregularly scarred kidney of a patient with chronic pyelonephritis. The other kidney is of normal size but has scarring on the upper pole.

assigned codes based on the site of infection, if known, although it is not always possible to distinguish between the three conditions on clinical grounds alone." Based on this reference, only 595.9, cystitis, should be assigned when the physician indicates the bladder as the infection site. Additional sites may be coded if the infection has spread. However, if the documentation includes both UTI and cystitis as diagnoses, only 595.9 (N30.90) should be used. If the site of the UTI is not documented or identified, code 599.0 (N39.0), urinary tract infection, NOS, should be assigned; this code can ONLY be used if the site is not identified and not in combination with any other codes where the site is identified.

EXAMPLE

Urinary tract infection due to acute pyelonephritis, 590.10 (N10).
The code 599.0 (N39.0) is not assigned because the site of infection has been identified as the kidneys. No bacteria have been identified, so no organism code is assigned.

Most UTIs are due to bacteria. Urinalysis (Table 20-2) and culture and sensitivity tests may be performed to identify the causative organism and to determine which drugs are more effective in treating the infection. Less common are infections caused by viruses, fungi, or parasites. Infections that are due to sexually transmitted disease such as chlamydia or candidiasis are discussed in the infectious and parasitic disease chapter. An instructional

TABLE 20-2 ROUTINE URINALYSIS*[6]

	Normal	Abnormal	Pathology
Characteristics			
Color and clarity	Pale to darker yellow, and clear	Very pale	Excessive water
		Cloudy, milky white blood cells	Pus, urinary tract infection
		Hematuria, red blood cells, reddish to reddish brown	Bleeding in infection, calculi, or cancer
Odor	Aromatic	Fishy	Cystitis
		Fruity	Diabetes mellitus
		Foul	Urinary tract infection
Chemical nature	pH is generally slightly acidic, 6.5	Alkaline	Infections cause ammonia to form
Specific gravity	1.003-1.030—reflects quantity of waste, minerals, and solids in urine	Higher—causes precipitation of solutes	Kidney stones, diabetes mellitus, diabetes insipidus
		Lower—polyuria	
Constituent Compounds			
Protein	None, or small	Albuminuria	Nephritis, renal failure, amount infection
Glucose	None	Glycosuria	Faulty carbohydrate metabolism, as in diabetes mellitus
Ketone bodies	None	Ketonuria	Diabetic acidosis
Bile and bilirubin	None	Bilirubinuria	Hepatic or gallbladder disease
Casts	None—or small number of hyaline casts	Urinary casts composed of red or white blood cells, fat, or pus	Nephritis, renal disease, inflammation, metal poisoning
Nitrogenous wastes	Ammonia, creatinine, urea, and uric acid	Azoturia, creatinine, and urea clearance tests disproportionate to normal BUN/creatinine ratio	Hepatic disease, renal disease
Crystals	None to trace	Acidic urine, alkaline urine, hypercalcemia, metabolism error	Not significant unless the crystals are large (stones); certain types are interpreted by physician
Fat droplets	None	Lipoiduria	Nephrosis

BUN, Blood urea nitrogen.
*Routine urinalysis is the physical, chemical, and microscopic examination of urine for abnormal elements; this may help the clinician to estimate renal function and may provide clues of systemic disease. This table includes some important characteristics and elements that are screened for in basic urinalysis. Other normal constituents of urine that are studied routinely for diagnosis include calcium, potassium, sodium, phosphorus, creatinine, and volume in a 24-hour period.

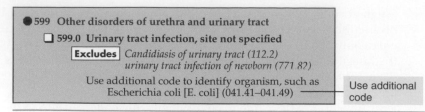

FIGURE 20-9. Instruction is given to use an additional code to identify the organism.

note is provided about the use of an additional code to identify the organism as well as the code for the urinary tract infection (Figure 20-9). The following are the most common organisms responsible for UTIs:

- *Escherichia coli* (*E. coli*)
- *Proteus* (*mirabilis*) (*morganii*)
- Methicillin-susceptible *Staphylococcus aureus*
- Methicillin-resistant *Staphylococcus aureus*
- *Staphylococcus saprophyticus*
- Group B *Streptococcus*
- *Klebsiella pneumoniae*

If a causative organism is documented by the physician, this should be coded in addition to the infection. It would not be appropriate to code an organism on the basis of a urine culture or sensitivity report only. Sometimes the documentation will indicate that the urine grew gram negative bacteria, awaiting sensitivity report. The next progress note will indicate that the urine culture is positive for *Escherichia coli* (*E. coli*). The *E. coli* is the gram negative bacteria that was identified and the only code necessary to show the causative organism is 041.49 (B96.2) for the *E. coli*. It would be incorrect to also assign 041.85 (A49.9), other gram negative organisms.

EXAMPLE | Urinary tract infection due to *E. coli,* 599.0, 041.49 (N39.0, B96.2).

EXAMPLE | Acute cystitis due to Friedlander's bacillus, 595.0, 041.3 (N30.00, B96.1).

Some patients are plagued by recurrent (chronic) UTIs. For this reason, they are sometimes treated with a daily dose of antibiotic to prevent an infection or for prophylactic measures. According to *Coding Clinic* (1996:2Q:p7),[5] "the patient doesn't have any symptoms of UTI, so it would be inappropriate to assign a code for the condition." This should be coded as V58.62 (Z79.2), long-term (current) use of antibiotic, and V13.02 (Z87.41) to identify the personal history of urinary tract infection.

The term "urosepsis" can cause confusion. Some physicians use the term "urosepsis" to mean an infection of the urinary tract without systemic infection. Other physicians may document urosepsis and mean that the patient has a UTI that has progressed to sepsis. Thus, a physician query may be required to establish the appropriate code(s). According to the Alphabetic Index in ICD-9-CM, the term "urosepsis" defaults to 599.0, so unless other information is available, the urinary tract infection code should be assigned. In the Alphabetic Index of ICD-10-CM, the term "urosepsis" does not have a code listed but instructs to code to the condition. A physician query may be necessary to determine what that condition is.

EXAMPLE | Urosepsis due to *Proteus mirabilis,* 599.0, 041.6 (ICD-10-CM Alphabetic Index entry for urosepsis instructs to code to condition. According to the guidelines, the physician should be queried).

EXAMPLE | Sepsis due to *Staphylococcus aureus* with urinary tract infection as the source, 038.11, 995.91, 599.0 (A41.0, N39.0).

FIGURE 20-10. Irregularly shaped struvite stone in the renal pelvis.

Calculus

Calculi or stones (Figure 20-10) may develop anywhere in the urinary tract and can vary in size. "**Urolithiasis**" describes a stone in the urinary tract. The terms "**nephrolithiasis**" and "**ureterolithiasis**" provide greater specificity with regard to location of the stone. Patients with stones are often asymptomatic unless they result in infection or start to move and obstruct the flow of urine. Obstructions due to stones are very painful and may result in admission to the hospital for pain control, identification, and treatment of the stone. Procedures such as extracorporeal shock wave lithotripsy (ESWL) and laser lithotripsy can be used to break up larger stones. "**Renal colic**" describes the intense pain associated with the body's efforts to try to force the stone through the ureters. According to *Coding Clinic* (1991:1Q:p11),[7] renal colic is not coded separately from a renal or ureteral calculus. Pain or renal colic is integral to the presence of urinary tract calculus.

On the other hand, hydronephrosis (due to urinary obstruction) should be assigned as an additional code. **Hydronephrosis** is abnormal dilatation of the renal pelvis that is caused by pressure from urine that cannot flow past an obstruction in the urinary tract (Figure 20-11). **Hydroureter** is the accumulation of urine in the ureters. These conditions may be documented in x-ray reports, ultrasound, or other diagnostic tests, but they must be documented by a physician before code assignment. Obstruction can result from a stone, tumor, infection, prostatic hypertrophy, or congenital abnormalities.

EXAMPLE	Hydroureter due to ureterolithiasis, 592.1, 593.5 (N13.4, N20.1).

EXAMPLE	Hematuria due to renal stone, 592.0 (N20.0).

EXERCISE 20-2

Assign codes to the following conditions.

1. Acute and chronic pyelonephritis due to *Pseudomonas* _____
2. Neurogenic bladder _____
3. Flank pain due to ureteral stone _____
4. Stricture of the urethra _____
5. Hydronephrosis due to kinking of ureter _____

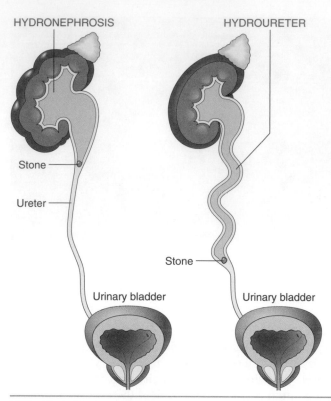

HYDRONEPHROSIS   HYDROURETER

Stone

Ureter

Stone

Urinary bladder   Urinary bladder

FIGURE 20-11. Hydronephrosis caused by a stone (obstruction) in the proximal part of the ureter and hydroureter with hydronephrosis caused by a stone in the distal part of the ureter.

Diseases of the Male Genital Organs

Prostate

The most common diseases of the male genitourinary tract are those that affect the prostate. The prostate gland can become inflamed or enlarged, causing urinary problems. The prostate surrounds the urethra, through which urine flows. The flow of urine can be obstructed by the prostate. **Benign prostatic hyperplasia** and **benign prostatic hypertrophy** are conditions that result in enlargement of the prostate gland; these conditions usually occur in men who are older than 50 years of age (Figure 20-12). Symptoms may include frequency, nocturia, difficulty starting urination, a weak stream of urine, and inability to completely empty the bladder. Some subclassifications within the 600 code category contain special instructions for coding lower urinary tract symptoms (LUTS) (Figure 20-13). This corresponds with the general coding guideline that signs and symptoms that are integral to the disease process should not be assigned as additional codes, *unless otherwise instructed by the classification.*

    Prostatitis or inflammation of the prostate may be acute and/or chronic in nature and may be due to bacteria or to inflammation that is not caused by a bacterial infection. Bacterial infections can be easily treated with antibiotics. Nonbacterial prostatitis involves treatment of urinary symptoms, which may be ongoing. There is an instructional note to use an additional code to identify the organism, if known (Figure 20-14). Use the Index and the Tabular to verify the accuracy of organism codes as referenced in the Tabular instructional note. If the code 041.1 is assigned as shown in Figure 20-14 for staphylococcal infection, an invalid code would have been assigned. A fifth digit is required to identify the type of staphylococcal infection.

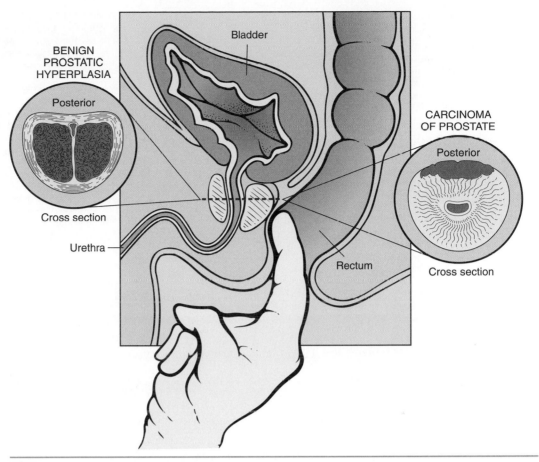

FIGURE 20-12. Digital prostate or rectal examination to identify prostatic abnormalities.

041.1	*Staphylococcus* (invalid code because a fifth digit is available, see below)
041.10	*Staphylococcus,* unspecified
041.11	Methicillin-susceptible *Staphylococcus aureus*
041.12	Methicillin-resistant *Staphylococcus aureus*
041.19	Other *Staphylococcus*

EXAMPLE   Chronic prostatitis due to staphylococcus 601.1, 041.10 (N41.10, B95.8).

Prostate-specific antigen (PSA) is a protein produced by the prostate gland. A blood test to measure PSA is a means of screening for prostate cancer. The risk of cancer is based on the following:
- PSA levels under 4 ng/mL: "normal"
- 4 to 10 ng/mL: 20 to 30% risk
- 10 to 20 ng/mL: 50 to 75% risk
- Above 20 ng/mL: 90%.

Elevated levels do not always indicate cancer, but may be elevated due to other prostate problems such as BPH or prostatitis.

EXAMPLE   Patient was seen in the clinic for an elevated PSA. It was determined that the patient's severe benign prostatic hypertrophy was the cause, 600.00 (N40.0).

EXAMPLE   Patient was referred to a urologist for elevated PSA, 790.93 (R97.2).

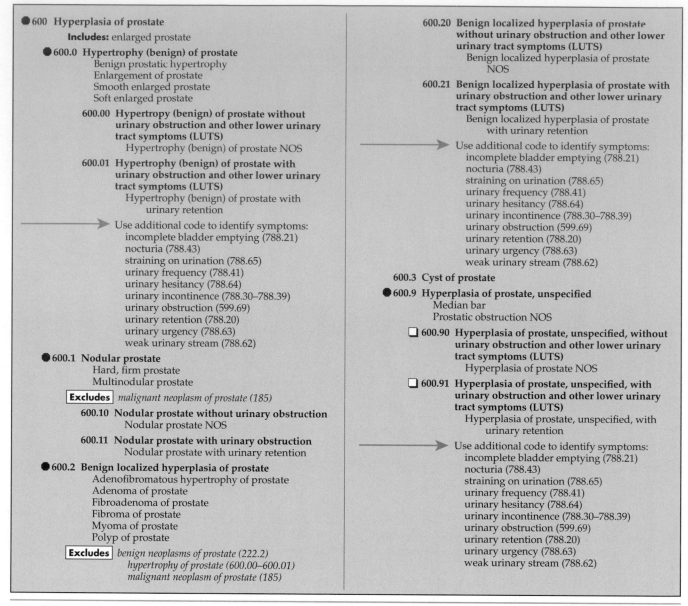

● **600 Hyperplasia of prostate**
   Includes: enlarged prostate
● **600.0 Hypertrophy (benign) of prostate**
   Benign prostatic hypertrophy
   Enlargement of prostate
   Smooth enlarged prostate
   Soft enlarged prostate

   600.00 Hypertropy (benign) of prostate without urinary obstruction and other lower urinary tract symptoms (LUTS)
      Hypertrophy (benign) of prostate NOS

   600.01 Hypertrophy (benign) of prostate with urinary obstruction and other lower urinary tract symptoms (LUTS)
      Hypertrophy (benign) of prostate with urinary retention

   → Use additional code to identify symptoms:
      incomplete bladder emptying (788.21)
      nocturia (788.43)
      straining on urination (788.65)
      urinary frequency (788.41)
      urinary hesitancy (788.64)
      urinary incontinence (788.30–788.39)
      urinary obstruction (599.69)
      urinary retention (788.20)
      urinary urgency (788.63)
      weak urinary stream (788.62)

● **600.1 Nodular prostate**
   Hard, firm prostate
   Multinodular prostate
   Excludes *malignant neoplasm of prostate (185)*

   600.10 Nodular prostate without urinary obstruction
      Nodular prostate NOS

   600.11 Nodular prostate with urinary obstruction
      Nodular prostate with urinary retention

● **600.2 Benign localized hyperplasia of prostate**
   Adenofibromatous hypertrophy of prostate
   Adenoma of prostate
   Fibroadenoma of prostate
   Fibroma of prostate
   Myoma of prostate
   Polyp of prostate
   Excludes *benign neoplasms of prostate (222.2)*
      hypertrophy of prostate (600.00–600.01)
      malignant neoplasm of prostate (185)

   600.20 Benign localized hyperplasia of prostate without urinary obstruction and other lower urinary tract symptoms (LUTS)
      Benign localized hyperplasia of prostate NOS

   600.21 Benign localized hyperplasia of prostate with urinary obstruction and other lower urinary tract symptoms (LUTS)
      Benign localized hyperplasia of prostate with urinary retention

   → Use additional code to identify symptoms:
      incomplete bladder emptying (788.21)
      nocturia (788.43)
      straining on urination (788.65)
      urinary frequency (788.41)
      urinary hesitancy (788.64)
      urinary incontinence (788.30–788.39)
      urinary obstruction (599.69)
      urinary retention (788.20)
      urinary urgency (788.63)
      weak urinary stream (788.62)

600.3 Cyst of prostate
● **600.9 Hyperplasia of prostate, unspecified**
   Median bar
   Prostatic obstruction NOS

   ☐ **600.90 Hyperplasia of prostate, unspecified, without urinary obstruction and other lower urinary tract symptoms (LUTS)**
      Hyperplasia of prostate NOS

   ☐ **600.91 Hyperplasia of prostate, unspecified, with urinary obstruction and other lower urinary tract symptoms (LUTS)**
      Hyperplasia of prostate, unspecified, with urinary retention

   → Use additional code to identify symptoms:
      incomplete bladder emptying (788.21)
      nocturia (788.43)
      straining on urination (788.65)
      urinary frequency (788.41)
      urinary hesitancy (788.64)
      urinary incontinence (788.30–788.39)
      urinary obstruction (599.69)
      urinary retention (788.20)
      urinary urgency (788.63)
      weak urinary stream (788.62)

FIGURE 20-13. Instructions to use additional code(s) for lower urinary tract symptoms (LUTS).

● **601 Inflammatory diseases of prostate**
   Use additional code to identify organism, such as — Use additional code
      Staphylococcus (041.1), or Streptococcus (041.0)

FIGURE 20-14. Instruction is given to use an additional code to identify the organism.

EXERCISE 20-3

Assign codes to the following conditions.

1. Nocturia due to benign prostatic hypertrophy   _____
2. Acute prostatitis due to *Escherichia coli*   _____
3. Scrotal pain and swelling due to epididymitis   _____
4. Hydrocele   _____
5. Phimosis   _____

Disorders of Breast

Breast

Many conditions of the breast described in this chapter are treated in the outpatient setting. Conditions of the breast in a pregnant woman are coded in the obstetrical chapter, or Chapter 11, of the ICD-9-CM code book. Male patients can also have conditions that are classified to the breast. **Mastitis** is inflammation or infection of the breast (Figure 20-15). Swelling, redness, tenderness, and pain may be noted. A breast abscess may form if mastitis is not treated. An abscess may require incision and drainage.

Some patients undergo prophylactic breast removal because they have a strong family history of breast cancer and/or genetic susceptibility or a personal history of breast cancer. After breast reconstruction is performed, complications such as infection, pain, and malfunction or failure of the implant or tissue expander may occur.

EXAMPLE   Patient has diffuse fibroadenosis of both breasts, 610.2 (N60.21, N60.22)

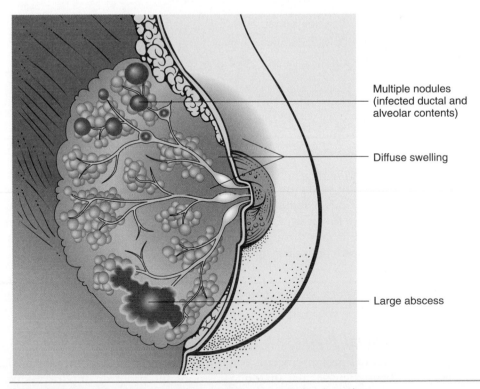

Multiple nodules (infected ductal and alveolar contents)

Diffuse swelling

Large abscess

FIGURE 20-15. Acute mastitis typically occurs during lactation.

EXERCISE 20-4

EXERCISE 20-4

Assign codes to the following conditions.

1. Fibrocystic disease of breast, bilateral _____
2. Nipple discharge, right breast _____
3. Male patient with gynecomastia _____
4. Mastodynia _____

Inflammatory Disease of Female Pelvic Organs

Pelvic Inflammatory Disease

Pelvic inflammatory disease (PID) occurs when vaginal or cervical infection spreads and involves the uterus, fallopian tubes, ovaries, and surrounding tissues. **Salpingitis** is inflammation of the fallopian tubes, which are the most common sites of pelvic inflammation. **Endometritis** is inflammation of the uterus, and **oophoritis** is inflammation of the ovaries. The most prevalent symptoms of these infections include vaginal discharge, pain, and possibly a fever. Complications that may result include infertility, chronic pain, tubal pregnancy, recurrent inflammation, and abscess.

EXAMPLE | Acute and chronic right salpingo-oophoritis, 614.0, 614.1 (N70.03, N70.13).

EXERCISE 20-5

Assign codes to the following conditions.

1. Tubo-ovarian abscess _____
2. Cervicitis _____
3. Bartholin's cyst _____
4. Pelvic adhesions, female _____
5. PID _____

Other Disorders of Female Genital Tract

Endometriosis

Endometriosis is a chronic condition in which endometrial material, the tissue that lines the inside of the uterus, grows outside the uterus and attaches to other organs in the pelvic cavity. Code assignment is based on site of implantation (Figure 20-16). The most common sites are the ovaries and fallopian tubes. Although it is uncommon, endometrial tissue can spread to sites throughout the body to areas such as the lungs. Pain and infertility are the two most common symptoms.

EXAMPLE | Endometriosis of the uterus, 617.0 (N80.0).

Genital Prolapse

Genital prolapse occurs when pelvic organs such as the uterus, bladder, and rectum shift from their normal anatomic positions and protrude into the vagina or press against the wall of the vagina (Figure 20-17). Weakening or damage to the ligaments, muscles,

Umbilicus

Fallopian tube

Peritoneum

Ileum

Ovary

Appendix

Anterior cul-de-sac
and bladder

Uterine
wall

Posterior surface
of uterus and
uterosacral
ligaments

Colon

Posterior
cul-de-sac

Cervix

Perineum

FIGURE 20-16. Possible sites for endometriosis implantation.

and connective tissues that support these organs is the cause of genital prolapse. It occurs commonly in postmenopausal women who have had children. Other contributing factors include genetics, pelvic surgery, and pressures within the abdomen that would weaken the pelvic floor. Different types of prolapse are usually graded on the basis of severity. **Uterine prolapse** is the descent of the uterus and cervix into the vaginal canal. **Cystocele** occurs when the bladder descends and presses into the wall of the vagina. **Urethrocele** results when the urethra presses into the vagina; it usually is reported in conjunction with a cystocele, which is then called a **cystourethrocele**. **Rectocele** is the descent of the rectum and pressing of the rectum against the vaginal wall. **Vaginal vault prolapse** may occur after a hysterectomy has been performed, when the top of the vagina descends into the vault.

EXAMPLE   Vaginal vault prolapse following a hysterectomy, 618.5 (N99.3).

Fistulas

A **fistula** is an abnormal passage or communication between two internal organs, or leading from an organ to the surface of the body (Figure 20-18). A **urethrovaginal fistula** is an abnormal passage between the urethra and the vagina. The bladder has the potential to communicate with the uterus, vagina, and rectum, forming a **vesicouterine fistula**, **vesicovaginal fistula**, and/or **rectovesical fistula**, respectively.

EXAMPLE   Rectovesicovaginal fistula, 619.1 (N82.3).

FIGURE 20-17. Structural abnormalities of the uterus.

Urinary Incontinence

Urinary incontinence can be a significant health problem that interferes with a patient's activities of daily living. This problem is more common among women because of specific features of their anatomy and as the result of childbearing. Incontinence often occurs after radical prostatectomy but usually resolves in time.

Types of incontinence include stress, urge, mixed, and overflow incontinence. **Stress incontinence** is the involuntary loss of small amounts of urine due to increased pressure from coughing, sneezing, or laughing. **Urge incontinence** is the sudden and involuntary loss of large amounts of urine. **Mixed incontinence** is a combination of stress and urge incontinence. **Overflow incontinence** is the constant dribbling of urine. Treatments include diet, Kegel exercises, biofeedback, and bladder training.

EXAMPLE	Neurogenic bladder with stress incontinence, 596.54, 625.6 (N31.9, N39.3).

Cervical and Vulvular Dysplasia

Cervical dysplasia is the abnormal growth of cells on the surface of the cervix. Although not cancer, it is considered a precancerous condition. Cervical dysplasia usually has no symptoms and is discovered on a Pap smear. Dysplasia that is identified on a Pap smear is

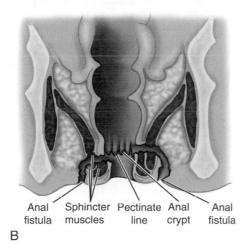

FIGURE 20-18. Various types of fistulas, designated according to site or to organs with which they communicate. **A,** Genitourinary fistulas. **B,** Anal fistulas.

described using the term **squamous intraepithelial lesion** (SIL). These abnormal Pap smear changes may be graded as:

- Low-grade (LSIL)
- High-grade (HSIL)
- Possibly cancerous (malignant)

Dysplasia that is seen on a biopsy of the cervix uses the term **cervical intraepithelial neoplasia** (CIN), and is grouped into the following three categories:

- CIN I—mild dysplasia
- CIN II—moderate to marked dysplasia
- CIN III—severe dysplasia to carcinoma in situ

Vulvar intraepithelial neoplasia (VIN) refers to certain changes that can occur in the skin that covers the vulva. It is similar to CIN or dysplasia of the cervix and can be diagnosed with a biopsy. VIN is grouped into the following three categories:

- VIN I—mild dysplasia
- VIN II—moderate to marked dysplasia
- VIN III—severe dysplasia to carcinoma in situ

If either of these conditions (CIN or VIN) are left untreated, it may result in invasive cancer.

EXAMPLE   Patient was seen in the clinic and her cervical biopsy results showed CIN II, 622.12 (N87.1).

EXERCISE 20-6

Assign codes to the following conditions.

1. Endometriosis of fallopian tube   _____

2. Cystocele with female stress incontinence   _____

3. Corpus luteum cyst   _____

4. Chocolate cyst of the ovary   _____

5. Vaginal stenosis   _____

FACTORS INFLUENCING HEALTH STATUS AND CONTACT WITH HEALTH SERVICES (V CODES/Z CODES)

In the past, V/Z codes have been considered primarily for use in the outpatient setting. This has changed with the addition of more V/Z codes each year. As was discussed in Chapter 8, it may be difficult to locate V/Z codes in the Index. Coders often say, "I did not know there was a V/Z code for that." Refer to Chapter 8 for a listing of common main terms used to locate V/Z codes.

V/Z codes that may be used with diseases of the genitourinary system include the following:

V13.00	Personal history of unspecified urinary disorder
V13.01	Personal history of urinary calculi
V13.02	Personal history of urinary (tract) infection
V13.03	Personal history of nephrotic syndrome
V13.09	Personal history of other disorder of the urinary system
V13.22	Personal history of cervical dysplasia
V18.61	Family history of polycystic kidney
V18.69	Family history of other kidney disease
V18.7	Family history of other genitourinary diseases
V42.0	Organ or tissue replaced by transplant—kidney
V43.5	Organ or tissue replaced by other means—bladder
V44.50	Artificial opening status—cystostomy, unspecified
V44.51	Artificial opening status—cutaneous vesicostomy
V44.52	Artificial opening status—appendicovesicostomy
V44.59	Artificial opening status—other cystostomy
V44.6	Artificial opening status—other artificial opening of urinary tract
V44.7	Artificial vagina
V45.11	Renal dialysis status
V45.12	Noncompliance with renal dialysis
V45.71	Acquired absence of organ—breast and nipple
V45.73	Acquired absence of organ—kidney
V45.74	Acquired absence of organ—other parts of urinary tract
V45.77	Acquired absence of organ—genital organs
V45.83	Other postprocedural status—breast implant removal status
V45.87	Transplanted organ removal status
V47.4	Other problems of internal organs—other urinary problems
V47.5	Other problems of internal organs—other genital problems
V50.2	Routine or ritual circumcision
V50.41	Prophylactic organ removal—breast
V50.42	Prophylactic organ removal—ovary

V51.0	Encounter for breast reconstruction following mastectomy
V52.4	Fitting and adjustment of breast prosthesis and implant
V53.6	Fitting and adjustment of urinary devices
V55.5	Attention to cystostomy
V55.6	Attention to other artificial opening of urinary tract
V55.7	Attention to artificial vagina
V56.0	Encounter for extracorporeal dialysis
V56.1	Encounter for fitting and adjustment of extracorporeal dialysis catheter
V56.2	Encounter for fitting and adjustment of peritoneal dialysis catheter
V56.31	Encounter for adequacy testing for hemodialysis
V56.32	Encounter for adequacy testing for peritoneal dialysis
V56.8	Encounter for other dialysis
V58.44	Aftercare following organ transplant
V58.62	Long-term (current) use of antibiotics
V58.76	Aftercare following surgery of the genitourinary system, NEC
V59.4	Donor—kidney
V67.01	Follow-up vaginal pap smear
V72.31	Routine gynecologic examination
V72.32	Encounter for Papanicolaou cervical smear to confirm finding of recent normal smear following initial abnormal smear
V88.01	Acquired absence of both cervix and uterus
V88.02	Acquired absence of uterus with remaining cervical stump
V88.03	Acquired absence of cervix with remaining uterus

EXAMPLE Adult male is admitted for elective routine circumcision, V50.2, 64.0 (Z41.2, 0VTTXZZ).
The V code indicates that a procedure is going to be performed, but it is not the procedure code. A diagnosis code is not assigned because no medical condition is present.

EXAMPLE Patient is admitted for kidney donation. A laparoscopic left nephrectomy is performed, V59.4, 55.51 (Z52.4, 0TT14ZZ).

EXERCISE 20-7

Assign codes to the following conditions.

1. Status post kidney transplant _____
2. Admission for dialysis for ESRD due to diabetic nephropathy _____
3. Personal history of kidney stones _____
4. Family history of polycystic kidney disease _____
5. Acquired absence of uterus and cervix _____

COMMON TREATMENTS

CONDITION	MEDICATION/TREATMENT
Glomerulonephritis	If due to infection, antibiotics Diuretics, antihypertensives, and diet Serious cases may be treated with corticosteroids and/or Cytoxan
Acute renal failure	Fluid management and treat the underlying cause. Dialysis, if necessary

CONDITION	MEDICATION/TREATMENT
Chronic renal failure	Determine cause. Control blood pressure and diet.
Cystitis	Fluids and possibly antibiotics
Urethritis	Antibiotics
Pyelonephritis	Antibiotics
Calculus of urinary tract	Fluids, pain control, blood pressure control, and antibiotics, if associated infection
Urinary incontinence	Kegel exercises, biofeedback, and medications such as Detrol
Prostatitis	Antibiotics
Benign prostatic hyperplasia	Medications such as tamsulosin hydrochloride (Flomax) and terazosin hydrochloride (Hytrin)
Mastitis	Compresses, massage, fluids, and possibly antibiotics
PID	Antibiotics
Endometriosis	Pain medication and/or hormonal therapy

PROCEDURES

Procedures that may be related to diseases of the genitourinary system can be located in the following chapters of the Procedure Tabular:

10. Operations of the Urinary System (55-59)
11. Operations on the Male Genital Organs (60-64)
12. Operations on the Female Genital Organs (65-71)
15. Operations on the Integumentary System (85-86)

Procedures related to the genitourinary system in ICD-10-PCS can be located in the following tables:

0H0-0HY	Skin and Breast
0T1-0TY	Urinary System
0U1-0UY	Female Reproductive System
0V1-0VW	Male Reproductive System
302-3E1	Administration
5A0-5A2	Extracorporeal Assistance and Performance

Cystoscopy may be the approach used for many procedures involving the urinary tract (Figure 20-19). Code 57.32 is assigned for a diagnostic cystoscopy. Often, another diagnostic or therapeutic procedure, such as biopsy, removal of a stone, dilatation of a stricture, or control of hemorrhage, is performed during a cystoscopic examination. When a procedure is performed in addition to cystoscopy, it is not necessary to code the cystoscopy as it is the approach.

FIGURE 20-19. Cystoscopy.

FIGURE 20-20. Hemodialysis.

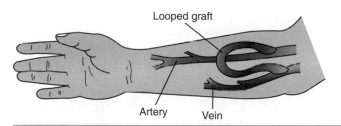

FIGURE 20-21. Arteriovenous graft for dialysis.

> **EXAMPLE**   Bladder lesion with diagnostic transurethral biopsy of the bladder via cystoscope, 596.9, 57.33 (N32.9, 0TBB8ZX).

Dialysis

Dialysis is needed when the kidneys can no longer filter the blood and form urine. Two basic types of dialysis are available. **Hemodialysis** uses a machine called a hemodialyzer to remove wastes from the blood (Figure 20-20). Access is obtained through a surgically created internal (arteriovenous [AV]) fistula that allows blood to pass from the body to the machine for cleansing. Sometimes, an AV graft (Figure 20-21) is used for permanent access. The root operation for creation of an AV fistula is bypass. If treatment must be begun before permanent access is ready or available, temporary access can be obtained through a catheter. Usually, hemodialysis is conducted at dialysis centers, and it is often scheduled 3 times per week. A dialysis session may take 3 to 5 hours to complete. The root operation for hemodialysis is performance.

If the encounter is for dialysis, a V code is assigned as the principal diagnosis. In cases where the patient is receiving treatment in preparation for dialysis (e.g., creation of an arteriovenous fistula), the principal diagnosis will be the medical condition for which the dialysis is required.

> **EXAMPLE**   Patient with ESRD is admitted for hemodialysis, V56.0, 585.6, 39.95 (Z99.2, N18.6, 5A1D00Z).

> **EXAMPLE**   Patient with ESRD and hypertension is admitted for creation of an AV fistula (left radiocephalic fistula using autologous venous tissue). Patient has dialysis on M, W, and F. 403.91, 585.6, V45.11, 39.27 (I12.0, N18.6, Z99.2, 031C09F).

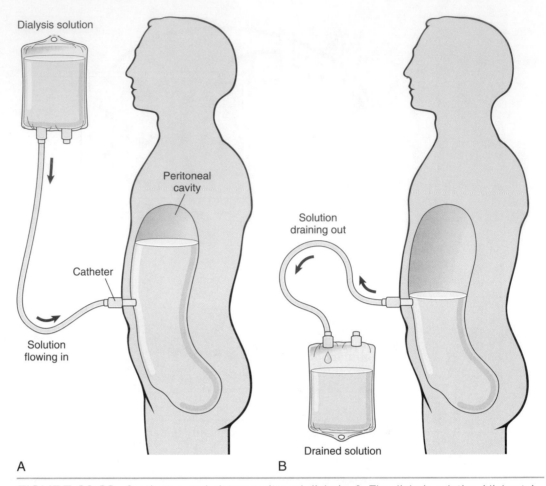

Dialysis solution

Peritoneal cavity

Catheter

Solution flowing in

Solution draining out

Drained solution

A   B

FIGURE 20-22. Continuous ambulatory peritoneal dialysis. **A,** The dialysis solution (dialysate) flows from a collapsible plastic bag through a Tenckhoff catheter into the patient's peritoneal cavity. The empty bag is folded and inserted into undergarments. **B,** After 4 to 8 hours, the bag is unfolded, and the fluid is allowed to drain into it with the help of gravity. The full bag is discarded, and a new bag of fresh dialysate is attached.

Peritoneal dialysis uses the peritoneal membrane in the patient's own body along with a dialysate solution to filter out wastes and excess fluid (Figure 20-22). Dialyzing fluid passes into the peritoneal cavity through a permanent indwelling peritoneal catheter (Tenckhoff catheter) and is then drained from the peritoneal cavity. **Continuous ambulatory peritoneal dialysis** (CAPD) takes about 15 minutes and is performed 3 to 4 times per day and once at night. **Continuous cycling peritoneal dialysis** (CCPD) uses a cycling machine and is performed while the patient sleeps. In some cases, a combination of the two may be needed to achieve the best results. The root operation for peritoneal dialysis is irrigation.

EXAMPLE   Patient with end-stage renal failure has peritoneal dialysis while hospitalized for acute prostatitis, 601.0, 585.6, V45.11, 54.98 (N41.00, N18.6, Z99.2, 3E1M39Z).

Kidney Transplantation

A kidney transplant (Figure 20-23) is one of the most common transplant operations. Prior to performance of a transplant procedure, a thorough pretransplant evaluation is necessary to assess the patient's overall health and identify potential problems to increase the chances of a successful transplant. A couple of different types of kidney transplants may be performed—transplant from a live related donor, transplant from a live nonrelated donor, and

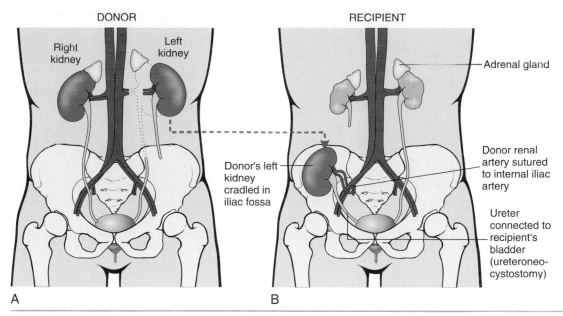

FIGURE 20-23. Kidney transplantation. **A,** Left kidney of the donor is removed for transplant. **B,** The kidney is transplanted to the right pelvis of the recipient.

transplant from a cadaver. Transplants from a living donor are generally scheduled in advance, and the kidney may be transplanted immediately following removal from the donor. The root operation for a kidney transplant is transplantation.

Patients who are on a waiting list for a kidney are notified when a kidney becomes available that is a good match; they must report to the hospital immediately. The transplanted kidney will usually start making urine as soon as the blood starts to flow through it, and most patients feel much better after their surgery has been completed. In most cases, only one kidney is necessary to take over for two failed kidneys. Most of the time, diseased kidneys are left in place.

Prostate Procedures

Prostate procedures are most often performed for benign prostatic hypertrophy or for prostate cancer. A biopsy is usually performed prior to a prostatectomy. Correct procedural code assignment depends on the method of the procedure performed. When **transurethral resection of the prostate** (TURP) is performed, it is not necessary to code the cystoscopy that is performed in the course of the surgical procedure. Cystoscopy is the approach that is used in transurethral procedures. Transurethral ultrasound-guided laser-induced prostatectomy (TULIP) and visual laser ablation of the prostate (VLAP) are two types of laser treatments used for ablation of prostatic tissue. Transurethral microwave thermotherapy (TUMT) and transurethral needle ablation (TUNA) of the prostate use radiofrequency energy to ablate obstructive prostatic tissue; these procedures can be performed in the physician's office. For the prostate procedures, if a biopsy is performed, the root operation is excision, if a prostatectomy with complete removal of the prostate gland is performed, a resection is the root operation, and if an ablation is done, destruction is the root operation.

EXAMPLE | Cancer of the prostate with radical prostatectomy (including bilateral seminal vesicles) with bilateral regional pelvic lymphadenectomy, 185, 60.5, 40.3 (C61, OVTOOZZ, OVT3OZZ, O7BCOZZ).

EXAMPLE   Benign prostatic hypertrophy with urinary obstruction. Endoscopic transurethral ultrasound-guided laser-induced prostatectomy, 600.01, 599.69, 60.21 (N40.1, N13.8, 0VB08ZZ).

Breast Biopsies and Reconstruction

Breast biopsies are performed for diagnostic purposes to determine the nature of a breast abnormality or mass. The root operation for biopsy is excision. A code is used for open biopsy of the breast and for local excision of a lesion of the breast (lumpectomy). In an open biopsy of the breast, a tissue sample is taken for diagnostic examination. In a local excision of the breast, the entire specimen is removed for pathologic examination. It is important to read the operative note and the pathology report to verify how much of the specimen was removed. Physicians may document an excisional biopsy when a lumpectomy is performed.

Sometimes, a needle or **mammographic localization** is necessary to assist the surgeon in identifying the area of breast tissue that must be biopsied or excised. An additional code would be assigned for the localization. This procedure is often performed by a radiologist.

At times, breast biopsy is performed during the same operative episode as a therapeutic procedure or more definitive treatment such as lumpectomy or mastectomy. In these cases, the biopsy is coded in addition to the lumpectomy or the mastectomy. Per Uniform Hospital Discharge Data Set (UHDDS) guidelines for selection of a principal procedure, either lumpectomy or mastectomy would fit the definition of a principal procedure.

Breast reconstructions are often performed following a mastectomy. Reconstruction may be done immediately or as a delayed procedure. The type of reconstruction and the timing of when it is done vary according to the patient's need for radiation and the type of mastectomy that is performed. Reconstruction may also be performed in stages. Implants and tissue expanders are sometimes used to create the breast. Tissue expanders are removed after the skin and muscles have been expanded to accommodate the breast implant or further reconstruction.

Tissue flap procedures use tissue from the abdomen, back, thighs, or buttocks to reconstruct the breast. Several flap procedures are currently used (Figure 20-24); these include the following:

- Transverse rectus abdominis musculocutaneous (TRAM)
- Latissimus dorsi musculocutaneous flap (LDMF)
- Lateral transverse thigh flap
- Nipple—Areola reconstruction
- Deep inferior epigastric perforator (DIEP) flap free
- Superficial inferior epigastric artery (SIEA) flap free
- Gluteal artery perforator (GAP) flap free

A **pedicle flap** involves a flap that remains attached to its original blood supply and tunneling it under the skin to the breast area. A **free flap** involves the cutting of skin, fat, blood vessels, and muscle free from their locations and moving them to the chest area. Blood vessels are connected with the use of a microscope. A free flap takes more time to complete. The root operation for free flap reconstruction is replacement. The root operation for pedicle flap reconstruction is transfer.

EXAMPLE   Patient admitted for bilateral breast reduction due to hypertrophy, 611.1, 85.32 (N62, 0HBV0ZZ).

Removal of Stones

Extracorporeal shock wave lithotripsy (ESWL) is used to break up kidney stones into small particles that can then pass through the urinary tract in the urine. Different devices can be used to transmit shock waves, and usually, x-ray or ultrasound is used to reveal the exact location of the stone. The root operation for ESWL is fragmentation.

A

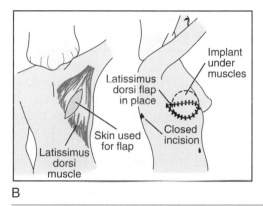

B

FIGURE 20-24. Various flaps used for breast reconstruction.

If the stone is quite large, or the location is such that ESWL is not very effective, a **percutaneous nephrolithotomy** is performed. The root operation for nephrolithotomy is extirpation. The stone is removed by the surgeon with the use of a nephroscope. At times, an ultrasonic or electrohydraulic probe is used to break up the stone, and the fragments are then removed. A nephrostomy tube may have to remain within the kidney during the postoperative phase.

Ureteroscopic stone removal is necessary when a kidney stone has traveled into one of the ureters. The ureteroscope is inserted through the urethra and bladder and into the ureter until the stone can be removed or is broken into pieces.

EXAMPLE	Patient was treated with percutaneous nephrostomy with fragmentation of left kidney stone, 592.0, 55.04 (N20.0, 0TF43ZZ).

EXERCISE 20-8

Assign codes for all diagnoses and procedures.

1. Right solitary renal cyst with right partial laparoscopic nephrectomy _____

2. Endoscopic transurethral needle ablation of prostate (TUNA) in patient with benign prostatic hyperplasia _____

3. Laparoscopically assisted vaginal hysterectomy (LAVH) in patient with endometriosis of the uterus _____

4. Extracorporeal shock wave lithotripsy bladder stone _____

5. Bilateral modified radical mastectomy, and breast reconstruction with latissimus dorsi musculocutaneous flap (LDMF) following prophylactic removal due to strong family history of breast cancer   _____

6. Peritoneal dialysis in patient with ESRD and anemia of chronic renal disease   _____

7. Left kidney transplant in patient with hypertensive renal disease and end-stage renal failure. The patient's spouse was the donor.   _____

8. Left breast cyst with percutaneous breast aspiration   _____

DOCUMENTATION/REIMBURSEMENT/MS-DRGS

Often, coding difficulties are due to lack of documentation. Sometimes pathology and other test results are not available at the time of discharge, or when the physician is dictating the discharge summary or is reporting the final diagnoses.

Definitions and ways a physician uses terms such as "urosepsis" versus "sepsis," and "acute renal insufficiency" versus "acute renal failure" can be problematic and may require a physician query.

Frequently missed complications/comorbidities from this chapter include the following:

- Acute renal failure
- CKD, stages IV and V
- ESRD
- Secondary hyperparathyroidism
- Hydronephrosis
- Calculus of ureter
- Genital tract fistulas

Urosepsis Versus Sepsis

EXAMPLE

Urosepsis compared with sepsis as the principal diagnosis (In ICD-10-CM urosepsis does not have a code, but should be coded to the condition.)

DIAGNOSES	CODES	MS-DRG	RW
Urosepsis	599.0	690	0.7864
Sepsis due to UTI	038.9 (A41.9, N39.0) 995.91	872	1.1545

MS-DRG With and Without MCC/CC

The presence of a complication and/or comorbidity (CC) can make a difference in reimbursement, depending on the principal diagnosis and the MS-DRG assigned. The code for acute renal failure (584.9) is a CC, and the code for acute renal insufficiency (593.9) is not an MCC/CC when it is used as a secondary diagnosis.

EXAMPLE

Patient with pneumonia and acute renal failure (ARF) compared with patient with pneumonia and acute renal insufficiency (ARI)

DIAGNOSES	CODES	MS-DRG	RW
Pneumonia with ARF	486,584.9 (J18.9, N17.9)	194	1.0152
Pneumonia with ARI	486,593.9 (J18.9, N28.9)	195	0.7096

CHAPTER REVIEW EXERCISE

Assign codes for all diagnoses and procedures.

1. Pelvic pain due to interstitial cystitis _____

2. Benign hyperplasia of the prostate with urinary obstruction _____

3. Benign prostatic hypertrophy with urinary obstruction and slight hematuria due to TURP (endoscopic). History of renal calculi _____

4. Complete ureterovaginal prolapse _____

5. Prerenal azotemia _____

6. Vesicoureteral reflux _____

7. Menometrorrhagia with chronic blood loss anemia _____

8. Infertility due to tubal endometriosis _____

9. Hematuria with diagnostic cystoscope performed _____

10. Acute tubular necrosis in patient with labile hypertension _____

11. Berger's disease _____

12. Rectovesical fistula _____

13. Chronic glomerulonephritis due to amyloidosis _____

14. Multinodular prostate _____

15. Infertility due to azoospermia _____

16. Incision and drainage of Bartholin's abscess _____

17. Total abdominal hysterectomy with right salpingo-oophorectomy for symptomatic uterine fibroids and follicular cyst right ovary. Family history of cervical cancer _____

18. Infertility due to dysmucorrhea _____

19. Urethroscrotal fistula _____

20. Nonfunctioning right kidney with laparoscopic nephrectomy _____

21. Postmenopausal bleeding. Diagnostic dilatation and curettage (D&C) of uterus _____

22. Patient with ESRD following transplant nephrectomy who is noncompliant with dialysis sessions _____

23. Descensus of uterus _____

24. Left ureteral stent was placed percutaneously due to obstruction from kidney stone _____

25. Bilateral laparoscopic oophorectomy with salpingectomy due to polycystic ovarian syndrome _____

Write the correct answer(s) in the space(s) provided.

26. Which MS-DRG is reimbursed at a higher rate: MS-DRG 690 or MS-DRG 872?

_____

27. Define fistula.

_____

28. Pyelonephritis involves what organ?

_____

29. Describe the main difference in the female and male genitourinary tract.

_____

30. Define ARF.

_____

CHAPTER GLOSSARY

Acute renal failure: sudden and severe impairment of renal function characterized by oliguria, increased serum urea, and acidosis.

Benign prostatic hyperplasia: condition resulting in enlargement of the prostate gland; usually occurs in men older than 50 years of age.

Benign prostatic hypertrophy: condition resulting in enlargement of the prostate gland; usually occurs in men older than 50 years of age.

Calculus: a stone. Calculi, which vary in size, can develop anywhere in the urinary tract.

Cervical dysplasia: abnormal growth of cells on the surface of the cervix.

Cervical intraepithelial neoplasia (CIN): dysplasia that is seen on a biopsy of the cervix.

Continuous ambulatory peritoneal dialysis: type of peritoneal dialysis that takes about 15 minutes and is performed 3 to 4 times per day and once at night.

Continuous cycling peritoneal dialysis: type of peritoneal dialysis that uses a cycling machine and is performed while the patient sleeps.

Cystitis: lower tract infection that affects the bladder.

Cystocele: when the bladder descends and presses into the wall of the vagina.

Cystoscopy: approach used for many procedures of the urinary tract.

Cystourethrocele: a urethrocele in conjunction with a cystocele.

Endometriosis: a chronic condition in which endometrial material, the tissue that lines the inside of the uterus, grows outside the uterus and attaches to other organs in the pelvic cavity.

Endometritis: inflammation of the uterus.

Extracorporeal shock wave lithotripsy: used to break up kidney stones into small particles that can then pass through the urinary tract into the urine.

Fistula: abnormal passage or communication between two internal organs, or leading from an organ to the surface of the body.

Free flap: involves the cutting of skin, fat, blood vessels, and muscle free from its location and moving it to the chest area.

Genital prolapse: when pelvic organs such as the uterus, bladder, and rectum shift from their normal anatomic positions and protrude into the vagina or press against the wall of the vagina.

Glomerulonephritis: inflammation of the glomeruli of the kidneys.

Hematuria: the presence of blood in the urine.

Hemodialysis: process that uses a machine called a hemodialyzer to remove wastes from the blood.

Hydronephrosis: abnormal dilatation of the renal pelvis caused by pressure from urine that cannot flow past an obstruction in the urinary tract.

Hydroureter: accumulation of urine in the ureters.

Lactation: the secretion of milk from mammary glands.

Mammographic localization: procedure that may be necessary to assist the surgeon in identifying the area of breast tissue that must be biopsied or excised.

Mastitis: inflammation or infection of the breast.

Mixed incontinence: combination of stress and urge incontinence.

Nephrolithiasis: kidney stone.

Nephrotic syndrome: condition marked by proteinuria (protein in the urine), low levels of protein in the blood, hypercholesterolemia, and swelling of the eyes, feet, and hands.

Oophoritis: inflammation of the ovaries.

Overflow incontinence: the constant dribbling of urine.

Pedicle flap: involves identifying a flap that remains attached to its original blood supply and tunneling it under the skin to a particular area such as the breast.

Pelvic inflammatory disease: when vaginal or cervical infections spread and involve the uterus, fallopian tubes, ovaries, and surrounding tissues.

Percutaneous nephrolithotomy: procedure in which the surgeon uses a nephroscope to remove a stone. At times, an ultrasonic or electrohydraulic probe is used to break up the stone, and the fragments are then removed.

Peritoneal dialysis: when the peritoneal membrane in the patient's own body is used with a dialysate solution to filter out the wastes and excess fluids.

Prostate-specific antigen (PSA): protein produced by the prostate gland.

Prostatitis: inflammation of the prostate that can be acute and/or chronic in nature and is due to a bacterium or inflammation that is not caused by a bacterial infection.

Proteinuria: protein in urine.

Pyelonephritis: upper tract infection that involves the kidneys.

Rectocele: descent of the rectum and pressing of the rectum against the vaginal wall.

Rectovesical fistula: a communication between the bladder and the rectum.

Renal colic: intense pain associated with the body's efforts to try to force the stone through the ureters.

Salpingitis: inflammation of the fallopian tubes, which are the most common site of pelvic inflammation.

Squamous intraepithelial lesion (SIL): dysplasia of the cervix that is identified on a Pap smear.

Stress incontinence: involuntary loss of small amounts of urine due to increased pressure resulting from coughing, sneezing, or laughing.

Transurethral resection of the prostate: endoscopic removal of prostate tissue.

Ureterolithiasis: ureter stone.

Urethritis: infection of the urethra.

Urethrocele: when the urethra presses into the vagina.

Urethrovaginal fistula: abnormal passage between the urethra and the vagina.

Urge incontinence: sudden and involuntary loss of large amounts of urine.

Urinary tract infection: general term used to describe infection in any area of the urinary tract.

Urolithiasis: a stone in the urinary tract.

Uterine prolapse: descent of the uterus and the cervix into the vaginal canal.

Vaginal vault prolapse: condition that may occur following a hysterectomy, when the top of the vagina descends.

Vesicouterine fistula: communication between the bladder and the uterus.

Vesicovaginal fistula: communication between the bladder and the vagina.

Vulvar intraepithelial neoplasia (VIN): certain changes that can occur in the skin that covers the vulva.

REFERENCES

1. American Hospital Association. *Coding Clinic for ICD-9-CM* 2002:3Q:p21-22. ARF due to dehydration and treated with IV hydration only.
2. American Hospital Association. *Coding Clinic for ICD-9-CM* 2005:4Q:p77-79. Chronic kidney disease.
3. American Hospital Association. *Coding Clinic for ICD-9-CM* 1995:3Q:p8. Hematuria secondary to renal stones.
4. American Hospital Association. *Coding Clinic for ICD-9-CM* 1999:2Q:p15-16. Urinary tract infection not specified with acute cystitis.
5. American Hospital Association. *Coding Clinic for ICD-9-CM* 1996:2Q:p7. Chronic recurrent urinary tract infection w/o urinary symptoms.
6. From Frazier ME, Drzymkowski JW. Essentials of Human Diseases and Conditions, 3rd ed. St. Louis, Saunders, 2004, Table 11-1, p 504.
7. American Hospital Association. *Coding Clinic for ICD-9-CM* 1991:1Q:p11. Renal colic due to ureteral calculus.

21

Complications of Pregnancy, Childbirth, and the Puerperium

(ICD-9-CM Chapter 11, Codes 630-679, and ICD-10-CM Chapter 15, Codes O00-O9A)

CHAPTER OUTLINE

ICD-9-CM Official Guidelines for Coding and Reporting
ICD-10-CM Official Guidelines for Coding and Reporting
Guideline Differences Between ICD-9-CM and ICD-10-CM
Major Differences Between ICD-9-CM and ICD-10-CM
Anatomy and Physiology
> Common Pregnancy Definitions

Conditions of Pregnancy, Childbirth, and Puerperium
> Ectopic and Molar Pregnancy
> Coding of Pregnancy
> Guidelines for Obstetric Cases
> Abortions

Factors Influencing Health Status and Contact with Health Services (V codes/Z codes)
Common Treatments
Procedures
> Labor
> Delivery
> Cesarean Section

Documentation/Reimbursement/MS-DRGs
Chapter Review Exercise
Chapter Glossary

LEARNING OBJECTIVES

1. Apply and assign the correct ICD-9-CM and ICD-10-CM codes in accordance with Official Guidelines for Coding and Reporting
2. Identify major differences between ICD-9-CM and ICD-10-CM related to complications of pregnancy, childbirth, and the puerperium
3. Identify pertinent anatomy and physiology of pregnancy, childbirth, and the puerperium
4. Recognize conditions and complications of pregnancy, childbirth, and the puerperium
5. Assign the correct V codes and procedure codes related to pregnancy, childbirth, and the puerperium

6. Identify common treatments, medications, laboratory values, and diagnostic tests
7. Explain the importance of documentation in relation to MS-DRGs for reimbursement

**ABBREVIATIONS/
ACRONYMS**

AROM artificial rupture of membranes

CPD cephalopelvic disproportion

D&C dilatation and curettage

EDC estimated date of confinement

EMS emergency medical services

hCG human chorionic gonadotropin

ICD-9-CM *International Classification of Diseases, 9th Revision, Clinical Modification*

ICD-10-CM *International Classification of Diseases, 10th Revision, Clinical Modification*

ICD-10-PCS *International Classification of Diseases, 10th Revision, Procedure Coding System*

IOL induction of labor

LGA large for gestational age

LTCS low transverse cesarean section

MS-DRG Medicare Severity diagnosis-related group

NST nonstress test

OB obstetrics

PIH pregnancy-induced hypertension

POCs products of conception

PROM premature rupture of membranes

PTA prior to admission

PTL preterm labor

SVD spontaneous vaginal delivery

UTI urinary tract infection

VBAC vaginal birth after cesarean section

ICD-9-CM	
Official Guidelines for Coding and Reporting	Please refer to the companion Evolve website for the most current guidelines.
	As there are many guidelines governing the coding and reporting of pregnancy, this chapter will follow a slightly different format than previous chapters, with the ICD-9-CM guidelines being interspersed throughout the chapter.

Apply the General Coding Guidelines as found in Chapter 5 and the Procedural Guidelines as found in Chapter 6.

ICD-10-CM	
Official Guidelines for Coding and Reporting	Please refer to the companion Evolve website for the most current guidelines.

15. Chapter 15: Pregnancy, Childbirth, and the Puerperium (O00-*O9A*)
 a. **General Rules for Obstetric Cases**
  1) **Codes from chapter 15 and sequencing priority**
   Obstetric cases require codes from chapter 15, codes in the range O00-O9A, Pregnancy, Childbirth, and the Puerperium. Chapter 15 codes have sequencing priority over codes from other chapters. Additional codes from other chapters may be used in conjunction with chapter 15 codes to further specify conditions. Should the provider document that the pregnancy is incidental to the encounter, then code Z33.1, Pregnant state, incidental, should be used in place of any chapter 15 codes. It is the provider's responsibility to state that the condition being treated is not affecting the pregnancy.
  2) **Chapter 15 codes used only on the maternal record**
   Chapter 15 codes are to be used only on the maternal record, never on the record of the newborn.
  3) **Final character for trimester**
   The majority of codes in Chapter 15 have a final character indicating the trimester of pregnancy. The timeframes for the trimesters are indicated at the beginning of the chapter. If trimester is not a component of a code it is because the condition always occurs in a specific trimester, or the concept of trimester of pregnancy is not applicable. Certain codes have characters for only certain trimesters because the condition does not occur in all trimesters, but it may occur in more than just one.

Assignment of the final character for trimester should be based on the **provider's documentation of the** trimester **(or number of weeks)** for the current admission/encounter. This applies to the assignment of trimester for pre-existing conditions as well as those that develop during or are due to the pregnancy.

The provider's documentation of the number of weeks may be used to assign the appropriate code identifying the trimester.

Whenever delivery occurs during the current admission, and there is an "in childbirth" option for the obstetric complication being coded, the "in childbirth" code should be assigned.

4) **Selection of trimester for inpatient admissions that encompass more than one trimesters**
In instances when a patient is admitted to a hospital for complications of pregnancy during one trimester and remains in the hospital into a subsequent trimester, the trimester character for the antepartum complication code should be assigned on the basis of the trimester when the complication developed, not the trimester of the discharge. If the condition developed prior to the current admission/encounter or represents a pre-existing condition, the trimester character for the trimester at the time of the admission/encounter should be assigned.

5) **Unspecified trimester**
Each category that includes codes for trimester has a code for "unspecified trimester." The "unspecified trimester" code should rarely be used, such as when the documentation in the record is insufficient to determine the trimester and it is not possible to obtain clarification.

6) *Fetal Extensions*
Where applicable, a 7th character is to be assigned for certain categories (O31, O32, O33.3-O33.6, O35, O36, O40, O41, O60.1, O60.2, O64, and O69) to identify the fetus for which the complication code applies.
Assign 7th character "0":
  • **For single gestations**
  • **When the documentation in the record is insufficient to determine the fetus affected and it is not possible to obtain clarification.**
  • **When it is not possible to clinically determine which fetus is affected.**

b. **Selection of OB Principal or First-listed Diagnosis**
1) **Routine outpatient prenatal visits**
For routine outpatient prenatal visits when no complications are present, a code from category Z34, Encounter for supervision of normal pregnancy, should be used as the first-listed diagnosis. These codes should not be used in conjunction with chapter 15 codes.

2) **Prenatal outpatient visits for high-risk patients**
For routine prenatal outpatient visits for patients with high-risk pregnancies, a code from category O09, Supervision of high-risk pregnancy, should be used as the first-listed diagnosis. Secondary chapter 15 codes may be used in conjunction with these codes if appropriate.

3) **Episodes when no delivery occurs**
In episodes when no delivery occurs, the principal diagnosis should correspond to the principal complication of the pregnancy which necessitated the encounter. Should more than one complication exist, all of which are treated or monitored, any of the complications codes may be sequenced first.

4) **When a delivery occurs**
When a delivery occurs, the principal diagnosis should correspond to the main circumstances or complication of the delivery. In cases of cesarean delivery, the selection of the principal diagnosis should be the condition established after study that was responsible for the patient's admission. If the patient was admitted with a condition that resulted in the performance of a cesarean procedure, that condition should be selected as the principal diagnosis. If the reason for the admission/encounter was unrelated to the condition resulting in the cesarean delivery, the condition related to the reason for the admission/encounter should be selected as the principal diagnosis.

5) **Outcome of delivery**
A code from category Z37, Outcome of delivery, should be included on every maternal record when a delivery has occurred. These codes are not to be used on subsequent records or on the newborn record.

c. Pre-existing conditions versus conditions due to the pregnancy

Certain categories in Chapter 15 distinguish between conditions of the mother that existed prior to pregnancy (pre-existing) and those that are a direct result of pregnancy. When assigning codes from Chapter 15, it is important to assess if a condition was pre-existing prior to pregnancy or developed during or due to the pregnancy in order to assign the correct code.

Categories that do not distinguish between pre-existing and pregnancy-related conditions may be used for either. It is acceptable to use codes specifically for the puerperium with codes complicating pregnancy and childbirth if a condition arises postpartum during the delivery encounter.

d. Pre-existing hypertension in pregnancy

Category O10, Pre-existing hypertension complicating pregnancy, childbirth and the puerperium, includes codes for hypertensive heart and hypertensive chronic kidney disease. When assigning one of the O10 codes that includes hypertensive heart disease or hypertensive chronic kidney disease, it is necessary to add a secondary code from the appropriate hypertension category to specify the type of heart failure or chronic kidney disease.

See Section I.C.9. Hypertension.

e. Fetal Conditions Affecting the Management of the Mother

1) Codes from categories O35 and O36

Codes from categories O35, Maternal care for known or suspected fetal abnormality and damage, and O36, Maternal care for other fetal problems, are assigned only when the fetal condition is actually responsible for modifying the management of the mother, i.e., by requiring diagnostic studies, additional observation, special care, or termination of pregnancy. The fact that the fetal condition exists does not justify assigning a code from this series to the mother's record.

2) In utero surgery

In cases when surgery is performed on the fetus, a diagnosis code from category O35, Maternal care for known or suspected fetal abnormality and damage, should be assigned identifying the fetal condition. Assign the appropriate procedure code for the procedure performed.

No code from Chapter 16, the perinatal codes, should be used on the mother's record to identify fetal conditions. Surgery performed in utero on a fetus is still to be coded as an obstetric encounter.

f. HIV Infection in Pregnancy, Childbirth and the Puerperium

During pregnancy, childbirth or the puerperium, a patient admitted because of an HIV-related illness should receive a principal diagnosis from subcategory O98.7-, Human immunodeficiency [HIV] disease complicating pregnancy, childbirth and the puerperium, followed by the code(s) for the HIV-related illness(es).

Patients with asymptomatic HIV infection status admitted during pregnancy, childbirth, or the puerperium should receive codes of O98.7- and Z21, Asymptomatic human immunodeficiency virus [HIV] infection status.

g. Diabetes mellitus in pregnancy

Diabetes mellitus is a significant complicating factor in pregnancy. Pregnant women who are diabetic should be assigned a code **from category** O24, Diabetes mellitus in pregnancy, childbirth, and the puerperium, first, followed by the appropriate diabetes code(s) (E08-E13) from Chapter 4.

h. Long term use of insulin

Code Z79.4, Long-term (current) use of insulin, should also be assigned if the diabetes mellitus is being treated with insulin.

i. Gestational (pregnancy induced) diabetes

Gestational (pregnancy induced) diabetes can occur during the second and third trimester of pregnancy in women who were not diabetic prior to pregnancy. Gestational diabetes can cause complications in the pregnancy similar to those of pre-existing diabetes mellitus. It also puts the woman at greater risk of developing diabetes after the pregnancy. Codes for gestational diabetes are in subcategory O24.4, Gestational diabetes mellitus. No other code from category O24, Diabetes mellitus in pregnancy, childbirth, and the puerperium, should be used with a code from O24.4

The codes under subcategory O24.4 include diet controlled and insulin controlled. If a patient with gestational diabetes is treated with both diet and insulin, only the code for insulin-controlled is required. Code Z79.4, Long-term (current) use of insulin, should not be assigned with codes from subcategory O24.4.

An abnormal glucose tolerance in pregnancy is assigned a code from subcategory O99.81, Abnormal glucose complicating pregnancy, childbirth, and the puerperium.

j. Sepsis and septic shock complicating abortion, pregnancy, childbirth and the puerperium
When assigning a chapter 15 code for sepsis complicating abortion, pregnancy, childbirth, and the puerperium, a code for the specific type of infection should be assigned as an additional diagnosis. If severe sepsis is present, a code from subcategory R65.2, Severe sepsis, and code(s) for associated organ dysfunction(s) should also be assigned as additional diagnoses.

k. Puerperal sepsis
Code O85, Puerperal sepsis, should be assigned with a secondary code to identify the causal organism (e.g., for a bacterial infection, assign a code from category B95-B96, Bacterial infections in conditions classified elsewhere). A code from category A40, Streptococcal sepsis, or A41, Other sepsis, should not be used for puerperal sepsis. If applicable, use additional codes to identify severe sepsis (R65.2-) and any associated acute organ dysfunction.

l. Alcohol and tobacco use during pregnancy, childbirth and the puerperium
1) Alcohol use during pregnancy, childbirth and the puerperium
Codes under subcategory O99.31, Alcohol use complicating pregnancy, childbirth, and the puerperium, should be assigned for any pregnancy case when a mother uses alcohol during the pregnancy or postpartum. A secondary code from category F10, Alcohol related disorders, should also be assigned **to identify the manifestations of the alcohol use**.

2) Tobacco use during pregnancy, childbirth and the puerperium
Codes under subcategory O99.33, Smoking (tobacco) complicating pregnancy, childbirth, and the puerperium, should be assigned for any pregnancy case when a mother uses any type of tobacco product during the pregnancy or postpartum. A secondary code from category F17, Nicotine dependence, or code Z72.0, Tobacco use, should also be assigned **to identify the type of nicotine dependence**.

m. Poisoning, toxic effects, adverse effects and underdosing in a pregnant patient
A code from subcategory O9A.2, Injury, poisoning and certain other consequences of external causes complicating pregnancy, childbirth, and the puerperium, should be sequenced first, followed by the appropriate poisoning, toxic effect, adverse effect or underdosing code, and then the additional code(s) that specifies the condition caused by the poisoning, toxic effect, adverse effect or underdosing.
See Section I.C.19. Adverse effects, poisoning, underdosing and toxic effects.

n. Normal Delivery, Code O80
1) Encounter for full term uncomplicated delivery
Code O80 should be assigned when a woman is admitted for a full-term normal delivery and delivers a single, healthy infant without any complications antepartum, during the delivery, or postpartum during the delivery episode. Code O80 is always a principal diagnosis. It is not to be used if any other code from chapter 15 is needed to describe a current complication of the antenatal, delivery, or perinatal period. Additional codes from other chapters may be used with code O80 if they are not related to or are in any way complicating the pregnancy.

2) Uncomplicated delivery with resolved antepartum complication
Code O80 may be used if the patient had a complication at some point during the pregnancy, but the complication is not present at the time of the admission for delivery.

3) Outcome of delivery for O80
Z37.0, Single live birth, is the only outcome of delivery code appropriate for use with O80.

o. The Peripartum and Postpartum Periods
1) Peripartum and Postpartum periods
The postpartum period begins immediately after delivery and continues for six weeks following delivery. The peripartum period is defined as the last month of pregnancy to five months postpartum.

2) Peripartum and postpartum complication
A postpartum complication is any complication occurring within the six-week period.

3) Pregnancy-related complications after 6 week period
Chapter 15 codes may also be used to describe pregnancy-related complications after the peripartum or postpartum period if the provider documents of that a condition is pregnancy related.

4) Admission for routine postpartum care following delivery outside hospital
When the mother delivers outside the hospital prior to admission and is admitted for routine postpartum care and no complications are noted, code Z39.0, Encounter for care and examination of mother immediately after delivery, should be assigned as the principal diagnosis.

5) Pregnancy associated cardiomyopathy
Pregnancy associated cardiomyopathy, code O90.3, is unique in that it may be diagnosed in the third trimester of pregnancy but may continue to progress months after delivery. For this reason, it is referred to as peripartum cardiomyopathy. Code O90.3 is only for use when the cardiomyopathy develops as a result of pregnancy in a woman who did not have pre-existing heart disease.

p. Code O94, Sequelae of complication of pregnancy, childbirth, and the puerperium

1) Code O94
Code O94, Sequelae of complication of pregnancy, childbirth, and the puerperium, is for use in those cases when an initial complication of a pregnancy develops a sequelae requiring care or treatment at a future date.

2) After the initial postpartum period
This code may be used at any time after the initial postpartum period.

3) Sequencing of Code O94
This code, like all late effect codes, is to be sequenced following the code describing the sequelae of the complication.

q. Abortions

1) Abortion with Liveborn Fetus
When an attempted termination of pregnancy results in a liveborn fetus, assign a code from subcategory O60.1, Preterm labor with preterm delivery, and a code from category Z37, Outcome of Delivery. The procedure code for the attempted termination of pregnancy should also be assigned.

2) Retained Products of Conception following an abortion
Subsequent encounters for retained products of conception following a spontaneous abortion or elective termination of pregnancy are assigned the appropriate code from category O03, Spontaneous abortion, or **codes O07.4, Failed attempted termination of pregnancy without complication and** Z33.2, Encounter for elective termination of pregnancy. This advice is appropriate even when the patient was discharged previously with a discharge diagnosis of complete abortion.

r. *Abuse in a pregnant patient*
For suspected or confirmed cases of abuse of a pregnant patient, a code(s) from subcategories O9A.3, Physical abuse complicating pregnancy, childbirth, and the puerperium, O9A.4, Sexual abuse complicating pregnancy, childbirth, and the puerperium, and O9A.5, Psychological abuse complicating pregnancy, childbirth, and the puerperium, should be sequenced first, followed by the appropriate codes (if applicable) to identify any associated current injury due to physical abuse, sexual abuse, and the perpetrator of abuse.
See Section I.C.19.f. Adult and child abuse, neglect and other maltreatment.

Apply the General Coding Guidelines as found in Chapter 5 and the Procedural Guidelines as found in Chapter 7.

GUIDELINE DIFFERENCES BETWEEN ICD-9-CM AND ICD-10-CM

■ The final character in most codes in this chapter of ICD-10-CM indicates the trimester of pregnancy, not the episode of care. Trimesters are defined at the beginning of Chapter 15. They are as follows:

- First trimester—less than 14 weeks 0 days
- Second trimester—14 weeks 0 days to less than 28 weeks 0 days
- Third trimester—28 weeks 0 days until delivery
- Supervision of care for high-risk pregnancy has been moved to this chapter.
- Guidelines added for preexisting conditions versus conditions due to the pregnancy have been added to ICD-10-CM.
- Guidelines for the use of alcohol and tobacco in pregnancy have been added to ICD-10-CM.
- Guidelines for adverse effects and underdosing in a pregnant patient have been added to ICD-10-CM.
- A guideline for pregnancy-associated cardiomyopathy has been added to ICD-10-CM.
- Many of the guidelines for abortion have been removed from ICD-10-CM due to either episode-of-care issues or due to the fact that elective, legal, and therapeutic abortions are no longer classified here.

MAJOR DIFFERENCES BETWEEN ICD-9-CM AND ICD-10-CM

- Code extensions have been added to identify a specific fetus affected by obstetric conditions.
- Elective, legal, or therapeutic abortions are not classified to abortion codes (code to Z33.2, Encounter for elective termination of pregnancy).
- The reason for obstruction is incorporated into obstructed labor codes.
- Documentation of the presence or absence of proteinuria is important.

ANATOMY AND PHYSIOLOGY

The organs of the female reproductive system include the ovaries, fallopian tubes, uterus, vagina, and cervix (Figure 21-1). These organs aid in reproduction and supply hormones that aid in the development of secondary female sex characteristics such as body hair and breasts.

The **vulva** is the external covering to the vagina. The **labia** surround the vaginal opening. The vagina is a muscular tube that extends from the vaginal opening to the uterus.

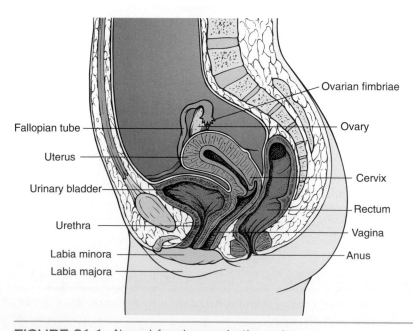

FIGURE 21-1. Normal female reproductive system.

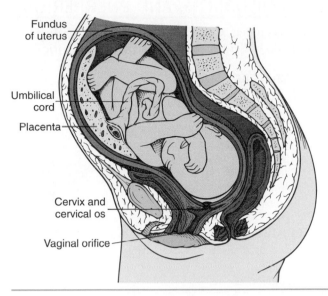

FIGURE 21-2. Normal uterine pregnancy.

The **vagina** serves three purposes: It is the receptacle for sperm during intercourse, it serves as the birth canal for childbirth, and it rids the body of menstrual blood during menstruation.

The **cervix** is the neck of the uterus and serves as an outlet from the uterus. The **uterus** is a muscular organ that serves as an incubator for the developing fetus. The wall of the uterus is composed of three layers. The inner layer, the endometrium, is where an egg grows if fertilized.

The **ovaries** produce female hormones and eggs. If the egg is fertilized and becomes a fetus, all the other female organs assist in development and expulsion of the fetus. When an egg becomes mature and is ready for fertilization, it travels through the **fallopian tube** to the uterus. The purpose of the fallopian tube is to deliver the mature egg to the uterus for fertilization. See Figure 21-2 for the anatomy of a normal uterine pregnancy.

To confirm a pregnancy, a woman's blood or urine may be tested for human chorionic gonadotropin (hCG). In the early months of pregnancy, secretion of hCG occurs at a high level.

Common Pregnancy Definitions

Antepartum: before delivery
Elderly obstetric patient: 35 years or older at date of delivery
Gravid: pregnant
Habitual aborter: a woman who miscarries at least three consecutive times
Lactation: process of milk production
Multigravida or **multiparity:** two or more pregnancies
Postpartum: after delivery
Postterm pregnancy: pregnancy longer than 40 weeks up to 42 weeks
Precipitate labor: rapid labor and delivery
Pregestational: condition present prior to pregnancy
Prenatal: before birth
Primigravida: first pregnancy
Prolonged pregnancy: beyond 42 weeks of pregnancy
Puerperium: time from delivery through first 6 weeks post partum
Stillbirth: dead at birth
Young obstetric patient: younger than 16 years at date of delivery

CONDITIONS OF PREGNANCY, CHILDBIRTH, AND PUERPERIUM

Complications of Pregnancy, Childbirth, and the Puerperium (630-679), Chapter 11 in the ICD-9-CM code book, is divided into the following categories:

CATEGORY	SECTION TITLE
630-633	Ectopic and Molar Pregnancy
634-639	Other Pregnancy With Abortive Outcome
640-649	Complications Mainly Related to Pregnancy
650-659	Normal Delivery, and Other Indications for Care in Pregnancy, Labor, and Delivery
660-669	Complications Occurring Mainly in the Course of Labor and Delivery
670-677	Complications of the Puerperium
678-679	Other Maternal and Fetal Complications

Pregnancy, Childbirth, and the Puerperium (O00-O9A), Chapter 15 in the ICD-10-CM code book, is divided into the following categories:

CATEGORY	SECTION TITLE
O00-O08	Pregnancy with Abortive Outcome
O09	Supervision of High-Risk Pregnancy
O10-O16	Edema, Proteinuria, and Hypertensive Disorders in Pregnancy, Childbirth, and the Puerperium
O20-O29	Other Maternal Disorders Predominantly Related to Pregnancy
O30-O48	Maternal Care Related to the Fetus and Amniotic Cavity and Possible Delivery Problems
O60-O77	Complications of Labor and Delivery
O80-O82	Encounter for Delivery
O85-O92	Complications Predominantly Related to the Puerperium
O94-O9A	Other Obstetric Conditions, Not Elsewhere Classified

Ectopic and Molar Pregnancy

Ectopic pregnancies usually occur when the egg is implanted outside the cavity of the uterus, most commonly in the fallopian tube (Figure 21-3). This type of pregnancy occurs in 1 of every 50 pregnancies. Pelvic infections may predispose a woman to having ectopic pregnancies. Molar pregnancies are rare and occur in 1 in 1000 pregnancies. In a **molar pregnancy**, the embryo does not form at all or is malformed. The early placenta develops

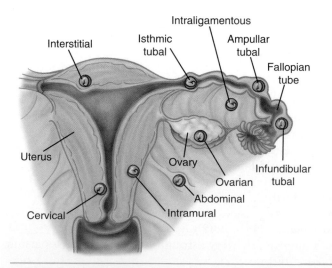

FIGURE 21-3. Diagram showing locations of ectopic (extrauterine) pregnancy.

A   B

FIGURE 21-4. Hydatidiform mole.

into a mass of cysts within a hydatidiform mole (Figure 21-4). Occasionally, a molar pregnancy can turn into a rare, pregnancy-related form of cancer.

EXAMPLE   Patient presents to her physician's office with a pregnancy in the 10th week. She comes in because she is experiencing dark brown vaginal bleeding. The physician identifies a molar pregnancy. The patient is admitted to the hospital for suction curettage to remove the molar tissue.
    Codes: 631.8, Abnormal products of conception (O02.0)
                69.59, Other aspiration curettage of uterus (10D17ZZ)

It is appropriate to use codes from 639 (O08.–) to describe any complications that may occur during an ectopic or molar pregnancy. According to the general rule for obstetric cases, additional codes from other chapters may be used in conjunction with Chapter 11 codes to further specify conditions.

EXAMPLE   Patient is admitted to the hospital with a tubal pregnancy without intrauterine pregnancy. After the tubal pregnancy is removed, the patient develops a urinary tract infection (UTI).
    Codes: 633.10, Tubal pregnancy without intrauterine pregnancy (O00.1)
                639.8, Other specified complications following abortion or ectopic and molar pregnancy (O08.83)
                599.0, Urinary tract infection

EXERCISE 21-1

Assign codes to the following conditions.

1. Ruptured ectopic pregnancy   _____
2. Vesicular mole   _____
3. Ectopic pregnancy of the fallopian tube followed by oliguria _____

Coding of Pregnancy

A normal pregnancy (Figure 21-5) usually lasts anywhere from 37 to 40 weeks. These weeks are counted from the beginning of the last menstrual cycle. A normal pregnancy has three trimesters, counted from the first day of the last menstrual period. They are defined as follows:

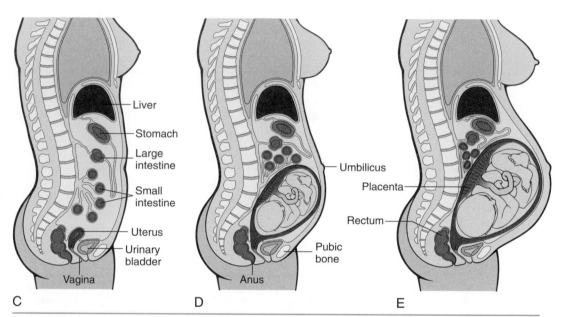

FIGURE 21-5. A, Implantation of the embryo in the endometrium. **B,** The placenta and membranes (chorion and amnion). **C–E,** Sagittal sections of pregnancy. **C,** Nonpregnant woman. **D,** Woman who is 20 weeks pregnant. **E,** Woman who is 30 weeks pregnant.

First trimester—less than 14 weeks 0 days

Second trimester—14 weeks 0 days to less than 28 weeks 0 days

Third trimester—28 weeks 0 days until delivery

When a pregnancy lasts longer than 40 weeks (post-term), complications can occur; and therefore this is no longer considered a normal pregnancy.

Labor is the process of expelling the products of conception from the uterus through the vagina to the outside world. There are four stages of labor:

- First stage—dilation

  Begins with cervical dilation and regular uterine contraction and ends when the patient is completely dilated and **effaced** (shortening or thinning of the cervix has occurred). The average length of time for this process is 10 to 14 hours.

- Second stage—expulsion

  Begins with complete dilation and effacement of the cervix and ends with the birth of the baby. The average length of time for this process is 1 to 4 hours.

- Third stage—placenta
  Begins with the birth of the baby and ends with the delivery of the placenta. The average length of time for this process is from 5 to 15 minutes.
- Fourth stage—return to normal
  Begins with the delivery of the placenta and ends 1 to 2 hours after delivery, when uterine tone is established.

All deliveries require an outcome of delivery code on the mother's record. The outcome of delivery is the code used to describe the number of newborns delivered and their status, i.e., live or stillborn. The outcome of delivery code is a V code that is found in the Alphabetic Index under the main term "outcome of delivery." **It is important to note that if code 650 is selected, it cannot be used with any other code in the range of 630-676.**

When codes are selected for complications of pregnancy, childbirth, and the puerperium, a variety of main terms in the Index may be accessed. If the condition is affecting the pregnancy, the Index term is "Pregnancy." Likewise, if the condition is affecting the **labor** of the patient, the Index term selected may be "Labor," and the Index may direct the coder to *see also* "Delivery." The Alphabetic Index may be checked directly for a condition (Figure 21-6).

Other main terms in the Alphabetic Index that may be used to locate pregnancy-related codes include the following:

- Failure
- Arrest
- Presentation
- Laceration
- Puerperal
- Labor
- Pregnancy
- Delivery

Vomiting 787.03
  with nausea 787.01
  allergic 535.4
  asphyxia 933.1
  bilious (cause unknown) 787.0
    following gastrointestinal surgery
      564.3
  blood (*see also* Hematemesis) 578.0
  causing asphyxia, choking, or suffoca-
    tion (*see also* Asphyxia, food)
      933.1
  cyclical 536.2
    psychogenic 306.4
  epidemic 078.82
  fecal matter 569.89
  following gastrointestinal surgery
      564.3
  functional 536.8
    psychogenic 306.4
  habit 536.2
  hysterical 300.11
  nervous 306.4
  neurotic 306.4
  newborn 779.3
  of or complicating pregnancy 643.9
    due to
      organic disease 643.8
      specific cause NEC 643.8
    early - *see* Hyperemesis, gravidarum
    late (after 22 completed weeks of
      gestation) 643.2
  pernicious or persistent 536.2
    complicating pregnancy - *see* Hyper-
      emesis, gravidarum

FIGURE 21-6. Alphabetic Index entry for vomiting in early pregnancy.

EXERCISE 21-2

Answer the following questions.

1. The duration of a normal pregnancy is

   _____

2. Can code 650 be used with 660.71?

   _____

3. What are the three most common areas of the Alphabetic Index to look under for codes related to Chapter 16?

   1. _____

   2. _____

   3. _____

4. What are the organs of the female reproductive system?   _____

5. To confirm a pregnancy, what is tested for from a woman's blood or urine?

   _____

6. If a woman is pregnant for the first time at age 36, what would be another term for her?

   _____

7. If a woman delivers at 41 weeks, what would this be considered?   _____

8. How long does the puerperium last?   _____

Identify the main term(s) that would be used to locate the following in the Alphabetic Index.

9. Obstructed labor   _____

10. First-degree perineal laceration delivered single liveborn vaginally   _____

11. Arrested labor   _____

12. Fever due to amnionitis during labor   _____

13. Twin pregnancy   _____

14. Oligohydramnios   _____

15. Premature rupture of membranes   _____

16. Primary uterine inertia   _____

17. Postpartum hemorrhage   _____

18. Breech delivery   _____

19. Prolonged labor   _____

20. Precipitous delivery   _____

Guidelines for Obstetric Cases

General Rules for Obstetric Cases

11. **Chapter 11: Complications of Pregnancy, Childbirth, and the Puerperium (630-679)**
    a. **General Rules for Obstetric Cases**
       1) **Codes from chapter 11 and sequencing priority**
          Obstetric cases require codes from chapter 11, codes in the range 630-679, Complications of Pregnancy, Childbirth, and the Puerperium. Chapter 11 codes have sequencing priority over codes from other chapters. Additional codes from other chapters may be used in conjunction with chapter 11 codes to further specify conditions. Should the provider document that the pregnancy is incidental to the encounter, then V22.2 should be used in place of any chapter 11 codes. It is the provider's responsibility to state that the condition being treated is not affecting the pregnancy.

In most cases, when a patient is pregnant, a code from Chapter 11 must be assigned regardless of what condition the patient presents with. The exception to this rule would occur when a physician documents that the pregnancy is incidental to the reason for this encounter. Almost ALWAYS, codes from the pregnancy chapter are to be assigned. This does not mean that codes from other chapters cannot be used to more fully describe a condition. The codes from Chapter 11 have sequencing priority.

EXAMPLE   Patient presents to physician office with pain and burning on urination. The physician documents that the patient is 26 weeks pregnant and has a UTI. Codes would be as follows: 646.63, Infections of the genitourinary tract in pregnancy (O23.42) 599.0, UTI.

EXAMPLE   A patient with gastroenteritis is seen in the Emergency Room (ER). The ER physician documents that the pregnancy is incidental to her gastroenteritis. Codes would be as follows: 558.9, Gastroenteritis (K52.9) V22.2, Pregnancy state, incidental (Z33.1).

2) Chapter 11 codes used only on the maternal record
Chapter 11 codes are to be used only on the maternal record, never on the record of the newborn.

It can be confusing as to what can be reported on the mother's chart and what can be reported on the newborn's chart. If possible it may be helpful to code both charts at the same time.

In the example above, if a pregnant woman has a UTI that in turn affects the care of the newborn, the code 646.6X (O23.90) would not be used on the newborn chart. The code 760.1 (P00.1) would be assigned to the newborn chart and is found in the Index. See Figure 21-7 for an example of a condition that may complicate pregnancy.

Codes that are assigned to the newborn are discussed in Chapter 17.

3) Chapter 11 fifth-digits
Categories 640-648, 651-676 have required fifth-digits, which indicate whether the encounter is antepartum, postpartum and whether a delivery has also occurred.

The fifth digits to be used with the codes listed above from Chapter 11 are as follows:
- 0   Unspecified as to episode of care or not applicable
- 1   Delivered, with or without mention of antepartum condition
- 2   Delivered, with mention of postpartum complication
- 3   Antepartum condition or complication
- 4   Postpartum condition or complication

urinary (tract) NEC 599.0
  with
    abortion – *see* Abortion, by type,
     with urinary tract infection
    ectopic pregnancy (*see also*
     categories 633.0-633.9) 639.8
    molar pregnancy (*see also* categories
     630-632) 639.8
  candidal 112.2
  complicating pregnancy, childbirth, or
    puerperium 646.6
    affecting fetus or newborn 760.1
    asymptomatic 646.5
     affecting fetus or newborn 760.1

FIGURE 21-7. A urinary tract infection is an example of a condition that may complicate pregnancy.

The fifth digit of 0 would rarely be used, because in most cases, it is known whether this is an antepartum problem, a postpartum problem, or a delivery.

When the patient comes in to deliver, the fifth digit of 1 or 2 is used. If a patient presents prior to delivery, then the fifth digit of 3 would be used; likewise, if the patient presents after delivery, the fifth digit of 4 is selected.

The following combinations of fifth digit codes are NOT valid and should not be used:

- 0 with 1, 2, 3, or 4
- 1 with 0, 3, or 4
- 2 with 0, 3, or 4
- 3 with 0, 1, 2, or 4
- 4 with 0, 1, 2, or 3

> **4) Fifth-digits, appropriate for each code**
> The fifth-digits, which are appropriate for each code number, are listed in brackets under each code (Figure 21-8). The fifth-digits on each code should all be consistent with each other. That is, should a delivery occur all of the fifth-digits should indicate the delivery.

EXAMPLE
A patient is admitted in labor and she delivers a 7-lb baby boy. After vaginal delivery, she hemorrhages. The physician documents that the hemorrhage is due to a retained placenta, 666.02, V27.0, 73.59 (O72.0, Z37.0, 10E0XZZ).

EXAMPLE
A patient is admitted in labor and delivers a 7-lb baby boy vaginally. The physician requests a social work consult because this mother has struggled with depression prior to and during this pregnancy, 648.41, 311, V27.0, 73.59 (O99.344, F32.9, 10E0XZZ, Z37.0).

COMPLICATIONS MAINLY RELATED TO PREGNANCY (640–649)

Includes: the listed conditions even if they arose or were present during labor, delivery, or the puerperium

The following fifth-digit subclassification is for use with categories 640–649 to denote the current episode of care:

- 0 **unspecified as to episode of care or not applicable**
- 1 **delivered, with or without mention of antepartum condition**
  Antepartum condition with delivery
  Delivery NOS (with mention of antepartum complication during current episode of care)
  Intrapartum
   obstetric condition (with mention of antepartum complication during current episode of care)
  Pregnancy, delivered (with mention of antepartum complication during current episode of care)
- 2 **delivered, with mention of postpartum complication**
  Delivery with mention of puerperal complication during current episode of care
- 3 **antepartum condition or complication**
  Antepartum obstetric condition, not delivered during the current episode of care
- 4 **postpartum condition or complication**
  Postpartum or puerperal obstetric condition or complication following delivery that occurred:
  during previous episode of care
  outside hospital, with subsequent admission for observation or care

Fifth digits →

● **640 Hemorrhage in early pregnancy**
  Requires fifth digit; valid digits are in [brackets] under each code. See beginning of section 640–648 for definitions.
  Includes: hemorrhage before completion of 22 weeks' gestation
● **640.0 Threatened abortion**
  [0,1,3]
● □ **640.8 Other specified hemorrhage in early pregnancy**
  [0,1,3]
● □ **640.9 Unspecified hemorrhage in early pregnancy**
  [0,1,3]

Appropriate fifth digits enclosed in brackets

● **641 Antepartum hemorrhage, abruptio placentae, and placenta previa**
  Requires fifth digit; valid digits are in [brackets] under each code. See beginning of section 640–648 for definitions.
● **641.0 Placenta previa without hemorrhage**
  [0,1,3] Low implantation of placenta without hemorrhage
           Placenta previa noted:
            during pregnancy without hemorrhage
            before labor (and delivered by cesarean delivery) without hemorrhage
● **641.1 Hemorrhage from placenta previa**
  [0,1,3] Low-lying placenta NOS or with hemorrhage (intrapartum)
           Placenta previa:
            incomplete NOS or with hemorrhage (intrapartum)
            marginal NOS or with hemorrhage (intrapartum)
            partial NOS or with hemorrhage (intrapartum)
            total NOS or with hemorrhage (intrapartum)
  Excludes hemorrhage from vasa previa (663.5)

FIGURE 21-8. Fifth digits used in pregnancy codes and designation of the appropriate fifth digit for use with specific codes are enclosed in brackets.

Answer the questions and assign codes to the following conditions.

1. Patient presents with acute sinusitis. She is 8 weeks pregnant. Physician documents that the pregnancy is incidental to her acute sinusitis. _____

2. Patient has a postpartum hemorrhage; she delivered 5 days PTA. _____

3. Patient vaginally delivered at 35 weeks; single liveborn infant _____

4. Patient presents with PIH at 32 weeks; she is treated and sent home. _____

5. Patient presents in labor; she had a previous cesarean section and delivered on this admit with no complications; vaginal delivery of single liveborn _____

6. Patient is given pitocin to induce labor for post-dates (41 weeks); induction is unsuccessful and she is sent home. _____

7. Patient presents with premature rupture of membranes and delivers a healthy newborn vaginally. _____

8. Can a fifth digit of 4 be used with code 660.1? _____

9. If the mother of a newborn has diabetes, is the code 648.01 used on the newborn chart? _____

10. Is it possible to code 650 and 652.51 together? _____

11. Are these two codes allowed to be used together: 648.24 and 648.02? _____

Selection of OB Principal or First-Listed Diagnosis

> **b. Selection of OB Principal or First-listed Diagnosis**
> **1) Routine outpatient prenatal visits**
> For routine outpatient prenatal visits when no complications are present codes V22.0, Supervision of normal first pregnancy, and V22.1, Supervision of other normal pregnancy, should be used as the first-listed diagnoses. These codes should not be used in conjunction with chapter 11 codes.

EXAMPLE The patient is seen in her first trimester for a routine prenatal visit. She also has a 2-year-old daughter, V22.1 (Z34.81).

EXAMPLE The patient is seen in her first trimester for a routine prenatal visit. The physician documents that she has iron deficiency anemia, 648.23, 280.9 (O99.011, D50.9).

> **2) Prenatal outpatient visits for high-risk patients**
> For prenatal outpatient visits for patients with high-risk pregnancies, a code from category V23, Supervision of high-risk pregnancy, should be used as the principal or first-listed diagnosis. Secondary chapter 11 codes may be used in conjunction with these codes if appropriate.

For a patient at high risk, first-listed diagnoses should be selected from the V23 category for outpatient prenatal visits. ICD-9-CM has separate codes for different high-risk categories such as infertility, history of abortion, multiparity, history of preterm labor, poor reproductive history, insufficient prenatal care, elderly primigravida or multigravida, and young primigravida or multigravida. The *Merck Manual* reports that "high-risk" pregnancy has no formal or universally accepted definition, but it goes on to list the following risk factors:

- Weight of mother less than 100 lb
- Obese mother
- Short stature of mother
- Structural abnormalities such as double uterus or incompetent cervix
- Disorders of a mother that are present prior to pregnancy, such as heart disease, high blood pressure, and seizure.

There are instructional notes under code V23.4X that direct the coder that a patient with a history of conditions classifiable to 630-676 may fall into this category.

EXAMPLE

> A pregnant patient in the first trimester presents for a routine prenatal visit. During her previous pregnancy, she had early pregnancy vomiting and the physician documents high-risk pregnancy, V23.49 (O09.891).

It is also important to note that unlike the codes from category V22 (Z34), the codes from V23 (O09) can be used in conjunction with other codes from Chapter 11.

EXAMPLE

> A gravid patient in the first trimester presents for a routine prenatal visit. This patient had preeclampsia on her previous pregnancy and the physician documents high-risk pregnancy. She has blood work taken on this visit and is found to be anemic. The physician prescribes an iron supplement, V23.49, 648.23, 285.9 (O09.891, O99.011, D64.9).

> **3) Episodes when no delivery occurs**
> In episodes when no delivery occurs, the principal diagnosis should correspond to the principal complication of the pregnancy, which necessitated the encounter. Should more than one complication exist, all of which are treated or monitored, any of the complications codes may be sequenced first.

At times, a pregnant woman may have to be admitted to the hospital prior to delivery and sent home before delivery occurs. In these cases, the principal diagnosis is the reason the patient was admitted to the hospital.

Some common causes of admission to the hospital prior to delivery include:

- **Preeclampsia** is a condition characterized by hypertension, edema, and/or proteinuria. This may also be called toxemia of pregnancy. Signs and symptoms usually appear in the last half of the pregnancy and are usually unknown to the patient. In more severe cases, the patient may experience headaches or visual disturbances. In very severe cases, the patient may develop HELLP syndrome (H = hemolysis, EL = elevated liver enzymes, LP = low platelets).
- **Hyperemesis gravidarum** is commonly known as a severe form of morning sickness. This is characterized by unrelenting vomiting and nausea.
- **Premature labor** is labor that occurs before the 37th week of pregnancy. It is characterized by contractions, back ache, blood or watery fluid from the vagina, and menstrual-like cramps. Premature labor may result in the birth of a premature baby.
- **Incompetent cervix** is when the cervix starts to open before the baby is ready to be born. This is usually caused by pressure from the baby on the cervix. A cervix that is incompetent or weakened can be due to previous surgery on the cervix, damage during a difficult birth, or trauma from an abortion or miscarriage.

EXAMPLE

> A pregnant patient in the first trimester presents to the ER with dehydration related to hyperemesis gravidarum. The physician in the ER discovers that the patient has pregnancy-induced hypertension. The patient is admitted, 643.13, 642.33, 276.51 (O21.1, O13.1).

> **4) When a delivery occurs**
> When a delivery occurs, the principal diagnosis should correspond to the main circumstances or complication of the delivery. In cases of cesarean delivery, the selection of the principal diagnosis should be the condition established after study that was responsible for the patient's admission. If the patient was admitted with a condition that resulted in the performance of a cesarean procedure, that condition should be selected as the principal diagnosis. If the reason for the admission/encounter was unrelated to the condition resulting in the cesarean delivery, the condition related to the reason for the admission/encounter should be selected as the principal diagnosis, even if a cesarean was performed.

EXAMPLE A patient is admitted to the hospital in labor. She is 40 years old in her third trimester, and labor proceeds uneventfully. This is her sixth pregnancy, and the baby weighs 11 lb. She is delivered by a physician, who performs a midline episiotomy. Physician documents LGA, 656.61, 659.61, V27.0, 73.6 (O36.63x0, O09.523, Z37.0, 0W8NXZZ).

EXAMPLE A patient is admitted to the hospital for severe preeclampsia. She is 36 weeks pregnant. A low transverse cervical cesarean section (LTCS) is performed immediately, and she delivers a healthy baby boy, 642.51, 644.21, V27.0, 74.1 (O14.13, O60.14x0, Z37.0, 10D00Z1).

> **5) Outcome of delivery**
> An outcome of delivery code, V27.0-V27.9, should be included on every maternal record when a delivery has occurred. These codes are not to be used on subsequent records or on the newborn record.

EXAMPLE Healthy 40-year-old primigravida presents to the hospital at 37 weeks and delivers twins vaginally, 651.01, 659.51, V27.2, V91.00, 73.59 (O30.003, O09.513, Z37.2, 10E0XZZ).

EXAMPLE A pregnant woman at 39 weeks presents to the hospital for delivery of known quadruplets. She is taken to the Operating Room for a cesarean section (LTCS). As the babies are delivered, it is discovered that one has died in utero, 651.21, 656.41, V27.6, V91.20, 74.1 (O30.203, O36.4xx0, Z37.62, 10D00Z1).

EXERCISE 21-4

Assign codes to the following conditions.

1. Patient is a primigravida and is being seen in the obstetrics (OB) office for a routine pregnancy visit. _____

2. Patient with a history of preterm labor is seen in the OB office for a routine pregnancy visit. _____

3. Can a V22.0 code be used with a 648.23 code at an outpatient visit? _____

4. An obese pregnant woman presents to the hospital with extremely high blood pressure. The physician documents mild preeclampsia. She is put on medications and sent home. _____

5. A pregnant woman presents to the hospital in preterm labor at 34 weeks; she is treated with tocolysis for 3 days and is sent home on bed rest. _____

6. A pregnant woman presents to the hospital with gestational diabetes; she delivers a single liveborn vaginally.

_____

7. A pregnant woman presents to the hospital in labor with a diagnosis of severe preeclampsia. She has smoked this entire pregnancy. She is 35 weeks pregnant and delivers a baby girl vaginally.

_____

8. A pregnant woman presents to the hospital in labor at 32 weeks. After 2 weeks of treatment with tocolytics, she goes into heavy labor. Her cervix has failed to dilate, and a low transverse cesarean section is performed. She delivers a healthy baby boy.

_____

9. A pregnant woman at 30 weeks presents to the hospital in labor; she has a twin pregnancy and vaginally delivers two baby girls.

_____

10. A 15-year-old girl presents to the hospital in labor. She has a known twin pregnancy. A low cervical cesarean section is performed. One of the twins is stillborn.

_____

Fetal Conditions Affecting the Management of the Mother

c. **Fetal Conditions Affecting the Management of the Mother**
   1) **Codes from categories 655 and 656**
      Codes from categories 655, Known or suspected fetal abnormality affecting management of the mother, and 656, Other **known or suspected** fetal and placental problems affecting the management of the mother, are assigned only when the fetal condition is actually responsible for modifying the management of the mother, i.e., by requiring diagnostic studies, additional observation, special care, or termination of pregnancy. The fact that the fetal condition exists does not justify assigning a code from this series to the mother's record.
      See I.C.18.d. for suspected maternal and fetal conditions not found.

EXAMPLE Fetal chromosomal abnormality with elective termination of pregnancy, with insertion of laminaria and vacuum aspiration curettage of uterus, with complete extraction of products of conception, 635.92, 655.13, 69.93, 69.51 (Z33.2, O35.1xx0, 10A07ZW, 10A07Z6).

EXAMPLE Mother presents for delivery. The physician documents that the baby appears large for dates (LGA [large for gestational age]). The mother vaginally delivers a 7 lb baby girl without any complications, 650, V27.0 (O80, Z37.0).
   In this case, the LGA code would not be used because it does not affect the management of the mother.

   2) **In utero surgery**
      In cases when surgery is performed on the fetus, a diagnosis code from category 655, Known or suspected fetal abnormalities affecting management of the mother, should be assigned identifying the fetal condition. Procedure code 75.36, Correction of fetal defect, should be assigned on the hospital inpatient record.
      No code from Chapter 15, the perinatal codes, should be used on the mother's record to identify fetal conditions. Surgery performed in utero on a fetus is still to be coded as an obstetric encounter.

EXAMPLE
> A fetus is known to have spina bifida. The parents find a surgeon trained in operating in utero and have this problem corrected prior to birth. Codes: 655.03, Central nervous system malformation in fetus (O35.0xx0), 75.36 (10Q00ZE), Open correction of fetal defect.

HIV Infection in Pregnancy, Childbirth, and the Puerperium

> **d. HIV Infection in Pregnancy, Childbirth and the Puerperium**
> During pregnancy, childbirth or the puerperium, a patient admitted because of an HIV-related illness should receive a principal diagnosis of 647.6X, Other specified infectious and parasitic diseases in the mother classifiable elsewhere, but complicating the pregnancy, childbirth or the puerperium, followed by 042 and the code(s) for the HIV-related illness(es).
> Patients with asymptomatic HIV infection status admitted during pregnancy, childbirth, or the puerperium should receive codes of 647.6X and V08.

EXAMPLE
> A 32-year-old female who is 23 weeks pregnant with known AIDS is admitted with severe diarrhea determined to be caused by cryptosporidium. She is treated with IV fluids, 647.63, 042, 007.4 (O98.712, B20, A07.2).

Patients with asymptomatic HIV infection status admitted during pregnancy, childbirth, or the puerperium should receive codes of 647.6X and V08.

EXAMPLE
> A 23-year-old gravid female is admitted in preterm labor at 35 weeks. She has had an uneventful pregnancy, except for the fact that she has an asymptomatic human immunodeficiency virus (HIV) infection. She vaginally delivers a 7 lb 2 oz baby, 644.21, 647.61, V08, V27.0, 73.59 (O60.14x0, O98.713, Z37.0, Z21, 10E0XZZ).

Current Conditions Complicating Pregnancy

> **e. Current Conditions Complicating Pregnancy**
> Assign a code from subcategory 648.X for patients that have current conditions when the condition affects the management of the pregnancy, childbirth, or the puerperium. Use additional secondary codes from other chapters to identify the conditions, as appropriate.

The important concept in this guideline is to assign a code from this category when the condition affects the management of pregnancy, childbirth, or the puerperium. In some cases, the presentation of the fetus complicates the delivery (Figure 21-9). Some common conditions that may occur at the time of delivery:

■ Lacerations of the cervix are a common occurrence during delivery
■ Prolonged labor or failure to progress
■ Cephalopelvic disproportion
■ Uterine bleeding
■ Abnormal presentation of the fetus
■ Umbilical cord prolapsed
■ Umbilical cord compression
■ Post-term pregnancy

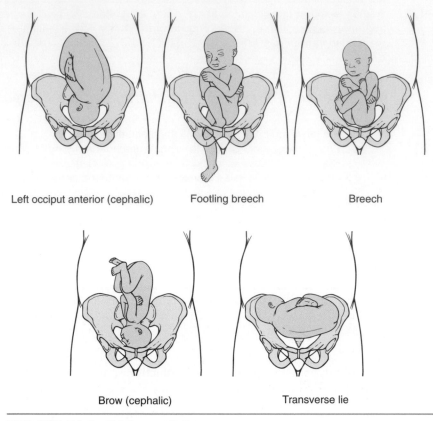

Left occiput anterior (cephalic)   Footling breech   Breech

Brow (cephalic)   Transverse lie

FIGURE 21-9. Fetal presentations.

EXAMPLE

A 33-year-old presents at 40 weeks in labor. She has had an uneventful pregnancy, except for slight anemia that is still being treated with iron. She has an uncomplicated vaginal delivery of a 6 lb baby girl, 648.21, 285.9, V27.0, 73.59 (O99.013, D64.9, Z37.0, 10E0XZZ).

EXAMPLE

A 15-year-old pregnant primigravida presents in active labor. She has no past history, except for several bouts of asthma as a toddler. She had an uncomplicated delivery of a healthy baby boy, 659.81, V27.0, 73.59 (O09.613, Z37.0, 10E0XZZ).

Diabetes in Pregnancy

f. Diabetes mellitus in pregnancy
Diabetes mellitus is a significant complicating factor in pregnancy. Pregnant women who are diabetic should be assigned code 648.0x, Diabetes mellitus complicating pregnancy, and a secondary code from category 250, Diabetes mellitus, or category 249, Secondary diabetes, to identify the type of diabetes.

Code V58.67, Long-term (current) use of insulin, should also be assigned if the diabetes mellitus is being treated with insulin.

EXAMPLE

Patient is admitted to hospital in diabetic ketoacidosis. The admitting physician documents that the patient is 12 weeks pregnant with a history of type I diabetes. She is treated with sliding scale insulin, 648.03, 250.13, V58.67 (O24.011, E10.10, Z79.4).

g. Gestational diabetes

Gestational diabetes can occur during the second and third trimester of pregnancy in women who were not diabetic prior to pregnancy. Gestational diabetes can cause complications in the pregnancy similar to those of pre-existing diabetes mellitus. It also puts the woman at greater risk of developing diabetes after the pregnancy. Gestational diabetes is coded to 648.8x, Abnormal glucose tolerance. Codes 648.0x and 648.8x should never be used together on the same record.

Code V58.67, Long-term (current) use of insulin, should also be assigned if the gestational diabetes is being treated with insulin.

EXAMPLE A patient is admitted to the hospital in labor at 39 weeks. She has had a relatively uneventful pregnancy except for gestational diabetes that was diet-controlled. She vaginally delivers a healthy 7 lb baby girl, 648.81, V27.0, 73.59 (O24.410, Z37.0, 10E0XZZ).

Normal Delivery

h. Normal Delivery, Code 650
   1) Normal delivery
      Code 650 is for use in cases when a woman is admitted for a full-term normal delivery and delivers a single, healthy infant without any complications antepartum, during the delivery, or postpartum during the delivery episode. Code 650 is always a principal diagnosis. It is not to be used if any other code from chapter 11 is needed to describe a current complication of the antenatal, delivery, or perinatal period. Additional codes from other chapters may be used with code 650 if they are not related to or are in any way complicating the pregnancy.

EXAMPLE Patient is admitted to the hospital in labor. She is 40 weeks pregnant. She has had an uneventful pregnancy and vaginally delivers a 7 lb 2 oz baby boy. The doctor performs an episiotomy followed by suturing during delivery, 650, V27.0, 73.6 (O80, Z37.0, 0W8NXZZ).

EXAMPLE Patient is admitted to the hospital in labor. She is 40 weeks pregnant. She has had an uneventful pregnancy and vaginally delivers a 7 lb 2 oz baby boy. The doctor performs an episiotomy and the baby is delivered with the use of a vacuum extractor, 669.51, V27.0, 72.71 (O75.9, Z37.0, 10D07Z6, 0W8NXZZ).

The use of a vacuum extractor in the above example prohibits the use of code 650 for this delivery.

EXAMPLE Patient is admitted to the hospital in labor. She is 40 weeks pregnant, has had an uneventful pregnancy, and vaginally delivers a 7 lb 2 oz baby boy. The doctor performs an episiotomy with a first-degree extension with repair, 664.01, V27.0, 75.69, 73.6 (O70.0, Z37.0, 0HQ9XZZ).

As in the previous example, the first-degree extension in this example prohibits the use of 650 (O80). When an extension of an episiotomy occurs, both the episiotomy and laceration repair are coded.

   2) Normal delivery with resolved antepartum complication
      Code 650 may be used if the patient had a complication at some point during her pregnancy, but the complication is not present at the time of the admission for delivery.

EXAMPLE

Patient is admitted to the hospital in labor. She is 40 weeks pregnant. She had a UTI early on in her pregnancy and was treated appropriately. She delivers a 7 lb 2 oz baby boy by spontaneous vaginal delivery, 650, V27.0, 73.59 (O80, Z37.0, 10E0XZZ).

EXAMPLE

Patient is 40 weeks pregnant. The physician documents that chlamydia was discovered early on in the pregnancy, and the patient now tests negative. Patient has a spontaneous vaginal delivery of an 8 lb baby girl, 650, V27.0, 73.59 (O80, Z37.0, 10E0XZZ).

> **3) V27.0, Single liveborn, outcome of delivery**
> V27.0, Single liveborn, is the only outcome of delivery code appropriate for use with 650.

EXAMPLE

Patient is admitted to the hospital at term in labor. She has had an uneventful pregnancy and goes on to a spontaneous vaginal delivery of twin boys, 651.01, V27.2, 73.59 (O30.003, Z37.2, 10E0XZZ).

EXERCISE 21-5

Answer the following and assign codes to the following conditions.

1. The patient had a low transverse cesarean section due to the baby being large for dates. _____

2. The patient was induced as the baby was suspected to have spina bifida; she vaginally delivered a 5 lb baby boy. _____

3. Pregnant woman is admitted to the hospital with *Pneumocystis carinii* pneumonia and known AIDS; she is treated with high-dose antibiotics and is discharged. _____

4. The patient has been dependent on methadone for the entire pregnancy. She delivers a baby girl on this admit. She has no complications during delivery and has a normal, spontaneous vaginal birth. _____

5. The patient presents for delivery. She is a known type II diabetic, treated with *insulin* at the onset of pregnancy. She delivers a large for dates baby via cesarean section. _____

6. Pregnant woman presents to doctor's office with complaints of blurred vision. Testing is done, and the diagnosis of gestational diabetes is made. _____

7. Pregnant woman had pneumonia early in her pregnancy. She presents to the hospital in labor with no other complaints. She vaginally delivers a healthy baby. _____

8. Can code 650 be used as a secondary diagnosis? _____

9. What is the only outcome of delivery that can be used with 650? _____

10. If surgery is performed in utero, is this coded on the baby's chart or on the mother's chart? _____

Postpartum and Peripartum Periods

> i. **The Postpartum and Peripartum Periods**
>   1) **Postpartum and peripartum periods**
>   The postpartum period begins immediately after delivery and continues for six weeks following delivery. The peripartum period is defined as the last month of pregnancy to five months postpartum.

EXAMPLE Patient is admitted to hospital for mastitis. She is 5 weeks postpartum and is given a course of intravenous (IV) antibiotics, 675.24 (O91.22).

Mastitis would be a common postpartum complication.

EXAMPLE Patient is admitted to the hospital 3 weeks postpartum. She is having pain in her lower right leg and is given a diagnosis of deep vein thrombosis. The patient is treated with IV heparin, 671.44, 453.42 (O87.1, I82.4Z1).

> 2) **Postpartum complication**
>   A postpartum complication is any complication occurring within the six-week period.

EXAMPLE A patient is admitted to the hospital 4 weeks postpartum with a high fever. The physician suspects endometritis. The patient is treated with IV antibiotics, 670.14, 615.9 (O86.12).

> 3) **Pregnancy-related complications after 6 week period**
>   Chapter 11 codes may also be used to describe pregnancy-related complications after the six-week period should the provider document that a condition is pregnancy related.

EXAMPLE Patient is admitted to the hospital with postpartum cholecystitis. She delivered 12 weeks prior to this presentation, 674.84, 575.10 (O99.63, K81.9).
In this case, the physician documented that this was a postpartum condition; therefore, it was coded as such even though it occurred beyond the 6-week time period.

> 4) **Postpartum complications occurring during the same admission as delivery**
>   Postpartum complications that occur during the same admission as the delivery are identified with a fifth digit of "2." Subsequent admissions/encounters for postpartum complications should be identified with a fifth digit of "4."

EXAMPLE Patient was admitted in labor. She had an uneventful pregnancy and had a spontaneous vaginal delivery of a healthy baby girl. The patient developed fever and back pain after delivery, and it was determined that she had a UTI. She was started on antibiotics and was sent home, 646.62, 599.0, V27.0, 73.59 (O86.20 Z37.0, 10E0XZZ).

> **5) Admission for routine postpartum care following delivery outside hospital**
> When the mother delivers outside the hospital prior to admission and is admitted for routine postpartum care and no complications are noted, code V24.0, Postpartum care and examination immediately after delivery, should be assigned as the principal diagnosis.

EXAMPLE

Patient delivers baby in the car on the way to the hospital. She is admitted through the ER for examination, V24.0 (Z39.0).

> **6) Admission following delivery outside hospital with postpartum conditions**
> A delivery diagnosis code should not be used for a woman who has delivered prior to admission to the hospital. Any postpartum conditions and/or postpartum procedures should be coded.

EXAMPLE

A patient pregnant with her fourth child calls Emergency Medical Services (EMS) to inform them that she is home alone and is about to deliver. By the time EMS arrives, the woman has already delivered a healthy baby girl. She is transported to the hospital for postpartum care.

Upon arrival to the hospital, the patient is examined by the obstetrician, who manually removes the retained placenta and repairs the first-degree perineal laceration, 664.04, 667.04, 75.4, 75.69 (O73.0, O70.0, 10D17ZZ, 0HQ9XZZ).

> **7) Puerperal sepsis**
> Code 670.2x, Puerperal sepsis, should be assigned with a secondary code to identify the causal organism (e.g., for a bacterial infection, assign a code from category 041, Bacterial infections in conditions classified elsewhere and of unspecified site). A code from category 038, Septicemia, should not be used for puerperal sepsis. Do not assign code 995.91, Sepsis, as code 670.2x describes the sepsis. If applicable, use additional codes to identify severe sepsis (995.92) and any associated acute organ dysfunction.

EXAMPLE

A 38 week primigravida spontaneously delivers an SGA baby. Following delivery the obstetrician manually removes fragments of the retained placenta. On the second day after delivery, the patient develops a fever and foul-smelling discharge. Antibiotics are initiated and puerperal sepsis is documented, 667.12, 670.22, V27.0, 73.59, 75.4 (O73.1, O85, Z37.0, 10D17ZZ, 10E0XZZ).

Late Effect of Complication of Pregnancy

> **j. Code 677, Late effect of complication of pregnancy**
> **1) Code 677**
> Code 677, Late effect of complication of pregnancy, childbirth, and the puerperium is for use in those cases when an initial complication of a pregnancy develops a sequelae requiring care or treatment at a future date.
> **2) After the initial postpartum period**
> This code may be used at any time after the initial postpartum period.
> **3) Sequencing of Code 677**
> This code, like all late effect codes, is to be sequenced following the code describing the sequelae of the complications.

EXAMPLE

The patient presents to the physician's office complaining of painful intercourse. She is 6 months postpartum. The obstetrician determines that the patient is suffering from a late effect of the repair of the perineum, 625.0, 677, E8784, E878.4 (N94.1, O94, Y83.8).

EXERCISE 21-6

Answer the following questions and assign codes to the following conditions.

1. True or False. The late effect of complication of pregnancy code, 677, should be sequenced first.

    _____

2. When can the late effect of complication of pregnancy code, 677, start to be used?

    _____

3. How long does the postpartum period last?

    _____

4. A woman delivers a 5-lb baby in her home. She is brought by _____ paramedics to the hospital, where they find that she has a first-degree perineal laceration. This is repaired, and the patient is admitted.

5. A woman delivers in her car in the parking lot of the hospital. _____ She is admitted for routine postpartum care.

6. A woman is admitted 6 weeks after a cesarean delivery with _____ infection of the cesarean wound.

7. A woman delivered 5 weeks ago. She is admitted for an _____ abscess of the breast.

8. A patient presents with abdominal pain 3 months after the _____ birth of her first baby. The physician documents that she has cholelithiasis that is related to her pregnancy.

9. Two weeks after delivery, a woman has terrible pain in her _____ leg. Her physician diagnoses her with a superficial thrombophlebitis of the leg.

10. Five months after delivery of her firstborn, an obese woman _____ is diagnosed with postpartum cardiomyopathy.

Abortions

Abortion is the termination of a pregnancy by natural causes or by medical intervention.

Types of Abortion

Complete abortion is an abortion in which all the products of conception are expelled.

Elective abortion is the elective termination of pregnancy.

Incomplete abortion is an abortion in which not all of the products of conception are expelled.

Inevitable abortion occurs when symptoms are present, and a miscarriage will happen.

Miscarriage is spontaneous termination of a pregnancy before the fetus has reached 20 weeks.

Missed abortion is a pregnancy with fetal demise before 20 weeks, when no products of conception are expelled.

Spontaneous abortion is the loss of a fetus due to natural causes; it is also known as a miscarriage.

Therapeutic abortion is an abortion performed when the pregnancy is endangering the mother's health, or when the fetus has a condition that is incompatible with life.

Threatened abortion occurs when symptoms are present that indicate that a miscarriage is possible.

k. Abortions

1) Fifth-digits required for abortion categories

Fifth-digits are required for abortion categories 634-637. Fifth digit assignment is based on the status of the patient at the beginning (or start) of the encounter. Fifth-digit 1, incomplete, indicates that all the products of conception have not been expelled from the uterus. Fifth-digit 2, complete, indicates that all products of conception have been expelled from the uterus.

The fifth digit for categories 634-637 identifies the stage of the abortion; these are as follows:

- 0 unspecified
- 1 incomplete
- 2 complete

EXAMPLE | Patient presents to the hospital with known pregnancy. She is in her 11th week and is now complaining of severe back pain and vaginal bleeding. The physician examines the patient and determines that she has suffered an incomplete abortion. A dilation and curettage (D&C) is performed, and the patient is discharged, 634.91, 69.02 (003.4, 10D17ZZ).

EXAMPLE | Pregnant patient presents to the hospital with vaginal bleeding and abdominal cramps. She is evaluated in the ER and is found to have a UTI. It is also determined that she has suffered a complete miscarriage. The patient is monitored for several hours and is discharged on a course of antibiotics, 634.72, 599.0 (003.88).

2) Code from categories 640-648 and 651-659

A code from categories 640-648 and 651-659 may be used as additional codes with an abortion code to indicate the complication leading to the abortion.

Fifth digit 3 is assigned with codes from these categories when used with an abortion code because the other fifth digits will not apply. Codes from 660-669 series are not to be used for complications of abortion.

EXAMPLE | Spontaneous abortion at 12 weeks, incomplete, in patient with gestational hypertension. D&C was performed, 634.91, 642.33, 69.02 (003.4, 013.1, 10D17ZZ).

3) Code 639 for complications

Code 639 is to be used for all complications following abortion. Code 639 cannot be assigned with codes from categories 634-638.

EXAMPLE | Patient had a spontaneous abortion 2 weeks ago. She presents to the hospital with a high fever, hypotension, and chills. Sepsis is suspected and she is admitted, 639.0, 038.9, 995.91 (003.87).

4) Abortion with Liveborn Fetus

When an attempted termination of pregnancy results in a liveborn fetus assign code 644.21, Early onset of delivery, with an appropriate code from category V27, Outcome of Delivery. The procedure code for attempted termination of pregnancy should also be assigned.

EXAMPLE   A woman is admitted at 22 weeks for insertion of a laminaria for termination of pregnancy. She delivers a liveborn fetus, 644.21, V27.0, 69.93 (O60.12x0, Z37.0, 10E0XZZ, 10A07ZW).

> **5) Retained Products of Conception following an abortion**
> Subsequent admissions for retained products of conception following a spontaneous or legally induced abortion are assigned the appropriate code from category 634, Spontaneous abortion, or 635 Legally induced abortion, with fifth digit of "1" (incomplete). This advice is appropriate even when the patient was discharged previously with a discharge diagnosis of complete abortion.

EXAMPLE   Retained products of conception after spontaneous abortion at 8 weeks' gestation. The products of conception were initially passed at home 2 days ago. D&C was performed, 634.91, 69.02 (O03.4, 10D17ZZ).

EXERCISE 21-7

Assign codes to the following conditions.

1. Woman is admitted to the hospital after having a miscarriage. The physician performs a suction curettage to remove the products of conception. It is believed that the miscarriage occurred in association with placenta previa.   _____

2. Patient presents to the hospital for an elective abortion. After the abortion is performed by suction curettage, she spikes a high fever and is diagnosed with endometritis.   _____

3. Patient with missed abortion was admitted to the hospital for a therapeutic abortion by D&C.   _____

4. Patient presents to the hospital for an elective abortion because the fetus is hydrocephalic. An aspiration curettage is performed.   _____

5. Patient presents to the hospital with hemorrhage after a self-induced abortion. Physician performs a D&C to control hemorrhage. Products of conception completely aborted prior to admission.   _____

FACTORS INFLUENCING HEALTH STATUS AND CONTACT WITH HEALTH SERVICES (V CODES/Z CODES)

In the past, V/Z codes have been considered for use primarily in the outpatient setting. This has changed with the addition of more V/Z codes each year. As was discussed in Chapter 8, it is difficult to locate V/Z codes in the Index. Coders will often say, "I did not know there was a V/Z code for that."

Refer to Chapter 8 for a listing of common main terms used to locate V/Z codes. V/Z codes that may be used during pregnancy, childbirth, and the puerperium include the following:

V02.51	Carrier or suspected carrier of Group B *Streptococcus*
V22.0	Supervision of normal first pregnancy
V22.1	Supervision of other normal pregnancy
V22.2	Pregnant state, incidental

V23.0	Pregnancy with history of infertility
V23.1	Pregnancy with history of trophoblastic disease
V23.2	Pregnancy with history of abortion
V23.3	Grand multiparity
V23.41	Pregnancy with history of preterm labor
V23.49	Pregnancy with poor obstetric history
V23.5	Pregnancy with other poor reproductive history
V23.7	Insufficient prenatal care
V23.81	Elderly primigravida
V23.82	Elderly multigravida
V23.83	Young primigravida
V23.84	Young multigravida
V24.0	Postpartum care and examination immediately after delivery
V24.1	Postpartum care and examination of lactating mother
V24.2	Routine postpartum follow-up
V25.04	Counseling and instruction in natural family planning to avoid pregnancy
V25.2	Admission for sterilization
V26.21	Fertility testing
V26.41	Procreative counseling and advice using natural family planning
V26.49	Other procreative management, counseling, and advice
V26.81	Encounter for assisted reproductive fertility procedure
V26.89	Other specified procreative management
V27.0	Single liveborn
V27.1	Single stillborn
V27.2	Twins
V27.3	Twins, one liveborn and one stillborn
V27.4	Twins, both stillborn
V27.5	Other multiple birth, all liveborn
V27.6	Other multiple birth, some liveborn
V27.7	Other multiple birth, all stillborn
V27.9	Unspecified outcome of delivery
V28.0	Encounter for screening for chromosomal anomalies by amniocentesis
V28.1	Encounter for screening for raised alpha-fetoprotein levels in amniotic fluid
V28.2	Encounter for other screening based on amniocentesis
V28.3	Encounter for screening for malformation using ultrasonics
V28.4	Encounter for screening for fetal growth retardation using ultrasonics
V28.5	Encounter for screening of isoimmunization
V28.6	Encounter for screening for *Streptococcus* B
V28.8	Encounter for other specified antenatal screening
V28.9	Encounter for unspecified antenatal screening
V45.51	Presence of intrauterine contraceptive device
V45.52	Presence of subdermal contraceptive implant
V45.59	Presence of other contraceptive device
V72.40	Pregnancy examination or test, pregnancy unconfirmed
V72.41	Pregnancy examination or test, negative result
V72.42	Pregnancy examination or test, positive result
V89.01	Suspected problems with amniotic cavity and membrane not found
V89.02	Suspected placental problems not found
V89.03	Suspected fetal anomaly not found
V89.04	Suspected problem with fetal growth not found
V89.05	Suspected cervical shortening not found
V89.09	Other suspected maternal and fetal condition not found

EXAMPLE Patient presents to obstetrician's office for routine prenatal checkup. She is 12 weeks along. This is her first pregnancy and she is 40 years old, V23.81 (O09.511).

EXERCISE 21-8

Assign codes for all diagnoses and procedures.

1. Patient is induced by pitocin for postdate pregnancy (41 weeks). She delivers a 6 lb 4 oz baby vaginally.

   _____

2. Elderly multigravida presents in labor. After 20 hours of labor, an LTCS is performed because of failure to progress. She delivers a normal newborn.

   _____

3. A 22-year-old primigravida presents for induction. She is known to have oligohydramnios. Pitocin is administered, and she goes on to vaginally deliver an SGA normal newborn. The physician performs an episiotomy to facilitate delivery, and a second-degree extension is repaired.

   _____

4. Patient presents in active labor. She is in her 38th week of pregnancy. She labors for 8 hours, after which the physician decides to perform a C-section because of CPD. A normal newborn is delivered.

   _____

5. Patient presents with severe preeclampsia. She is taken directly to the Operating Room, where an LTCS is performed. She delivers a normal newborn.

   _____

COMMON TREATMENTS

CONDITION	MEDICATION/TREATMENT
Narcotics for Labor Pain	Stadol (butorphanol), fentanyl
	Demerol (meperidine) Nubain (nalbuphine)
	Used for decreasing pain
Anesthesia for Labor Pain	Epidural is a regional anesthetic injected into the epidural space
	Spinal is also a regional anesthetic which is injected into the cerebrospinal fluid
Drugs for Inducing Labor	Pitocin is a synthetic oxytocin which is a natural hormone produced by a woman's body to cause the uterus to contract
	Cervidil (dinoprostone) is vaginally inserted and used for ripening of the cervix
Drugs Used to Inhibit Labor	Beta agonists (terbutaline, ritodrine, isoxsuprine), magnesium sulfate

PROCEDURES

Procedures that may be related to pregnancy and childbirth may be located in the following chapter of the Procedure Tabular:

Chapter 13   Obstetrical Procedures (72-75)

Procedures that may be related to complications of pregnancy, childbirth, and the puerperium in ICD-10-PCS may be found in the following tables:

Obstetrics   102-10Y
Female Reproductive System   0U1-0UY

FIGURE 21-10. Cephalic presentation ("crowning") of the fetus during delivery from the vaginal (birth) canal during a normal delivery.

Perineum

Labor

Labor can be induced in a variety of ways. Often, artificial rupture of the membranes (AROM) is performed to start labor. Pitocin induction may also be used. Pitocin is a drug used for medical induction of labor.

A nonstress test (NST) is performed to confirm the health of the baby. A mother is hooked up to a fetal monitor and the test is performed without giving the mother medications. The test records the baby's heart rate while moving. This test may be performed throughout the pregnancy if the mother has medical conditions or if the pregnancy is considered high risk. Results of these tests are recorded as "reactive," meaning the baby moved and the heart rate increased appropriately, or "nonreactive," which means that either the baby did not move or the heart rate did not increase enough when the baby did move.

When the NST is abnormal, another test is performed. This test is called a CST, or a contraction stress test. In this test, which is done during fetal monitoring, a drug (Pitocin) may be administered to initiate contractions. The purpose is to see how the baby will handle the stress of labor. The baby's heart should speed up during a contraction; if this does not happen during this test, problems may occur during labor.

Amnioinfusion is the insertion of normal saline or lactated Ringer's solution into the amniotic sac. The injection may be done transabdominally or transcervically. This procedure is performed for a variety of reasons, such as oligohydramnios, variable decelerations, and thick meconium. The volume of amniotic fluid is increased, which increases the likelihood of better outcomes of delivery.

Delivery

In a normal pregnancy with no complications, a code of 73.59 (10E0XZZ) may be assigned for manually assisted delivery (Figure 21-10). Forceps and vacuum extraction may be used in cases in which the baby does not spontaneously deliver and assistance is needed (Figure 21-11).

Episiotomy is performed to facilitate delivery. The root operation in ICD-10-PCS for an episiotomy is division of the female perineum. The physician makes a cut in the perineum to make room for the baby's head to emerge. Repair of an episiotomy is included in the code for episiotomy. If a forceps delivery and an episiotomy are performed, a combination code may be used; a combination code may also be used for a vacuum extraction and an episiotomy. Sometimes, an episiotomy will extend and will become a laceration. If this happens, codes for both episiotomy and laceration repair are required. The degree of perineal laceration is coded under the diagnostic category of 664.0X-664.3X. If more than one degree is mentioned, only the highest degree should be assigned.

FIGURE 21-11. Forceps delivery.

Cesarean Section

A cesarean section (C-section) is an operation that is performed to deliver a baby through an incision in the abdomen. The root operation in ICD-10-PCS for a cesarean section is extraction of products of conception. This procedure is performed for a variety of reasons:

■ *Cephalopelvic disproportion (CPD):* This is when the baby's head is too large to fit through the birth canal.
■ *Prolapsed cord:* The cord is being delivered before the baby
■ *Fetal distress:* Distress of the fetus during labor or before, noted by low oxygen levels or the presence of meconium
■ *Conditions of the mother:* Such as hypertension or active herpes

Three main types of cesarean operations are performed: (1) *low transverse,* which is done via a horizontal incision in the lower uterus; (2) *low vertical,* which is done via a vertical incision in the lower uterus; and (3) *classical,* which involves a vertical incision in the main body of the uterus. The most commonly performed type is the low transverse (LTCS).

Vaginal birth after cesarean section (VBAC) occurs when a woman delivers vaginally after having delivered previously via cesarean section. At one point in time, it was believed that it was unsafe for a woman who had delivered via C-section to deliver vaginally. Many variables go into deciding whether a VBAC is a safe option; however, it is being performed more and more frequently.

DOCUMENTATION/REIMBURSEMENT/MS-DRGs

Often, coding difficulties are due to lack of documentation. Sometimes pathology and other test results are not available at the time of discharge or when the physician is dictating the discharge summary or is reporting the final diagnoses.

The most common MS-DRGs for deliveries include the following:

MS-DRG	RW
766 C-section without CC/MCC	0.7995
765 C-section with CC/MCC	1.1269
775 Vaginal delivery without complicating dx	0.5256
774 Vaginal delivery with complicating dx	0.6848
767 Vaginal delivery with sterilization and/or D&C	0.9111

CHAPTER REVIEW EXERCISE

Assign codes for all diagnoses and procedures.

1. Breech presentation with obstructed labor; delivery by cesarean section (LTCS); single liveborn   _____

2. Patient admitted 2 weeks post delivery with postpartum depression   _____

3. Patient delivers 12-lb baby (LGA), requiring an episiotomy.   _____

4. Patient is admitted to the hospital for delivery; she is being treated with methadone for heroin dependence; vaginal delivery of single liveborn   _____

5. Patient with a history of preterm labor and previous cesarean section is admitted in labor; she has a vaginal birth after cesarean (VBAC) of single liveborn.   _____

6. Patient is admitted to hospital for HELLP (hemolytic anemia, elevated liver enzymes, and low platelet count) syndrome; she is taken to the Operating Room for delivery by cesarean section (LTCS) of single liveborn.   _____

7. Patient is admitted to the hospital in preterm labor; she is 35 weeks pregnant; three days after admission, the patient vaginally delivers a small for gestational age (SGA) baby.   _____

8. Patient presents to physician's office for a routine obstetric visit; she had a spontaneous abortion 1 year ago.   _____

9. Patient is admitted to the hospital at 33 weeks; she has a twin pregnancy and has a spontaneous vaginal delivery (SVD) of liveborn twins; the evening after delivery, she hemorrhages.   _____

10. Patient is pregnant and has known uterine fibroids; the fibroids are so large that the physician recommends an abortion; patient presents to hospital for abortion to be performed by aspiration curettage.   _____

11. The patient was treated for a sprained wrist. Incidentally, the patient is 10 weeks pregnant.   _____

12. Urinary tract infection in patient who delivered 1 week ago   _____

13. This mother delivered liveborn twins vaginally during her hospital stay. The outcome of delivery is coded on the mother's record.   _____

14. The patient was admitted for treatment of hyperemesis gravidarum. The patient is 12 weeks pregnant.   _____

15. The patient has a high-risk pregnancy and two previous miscarriages.   _____

16. The patient is 16 weeks pregnant, and her condition is complicated by diabetes mellitus, type 2, which is uncontrolled.   _____

17. The patient is admitted with HIV and *Pneumocystis carinii* pneumonia (PCP) and is 35 weeks pregnant.   _____

18. The patient is 19 weeks pregnant and has hypothyroidism.   _____

19. The patient delivered a baby 6 days ago. She is now being admitted because of dehiscence of her cesarean wound. The wound was sutured.   _____

20. Urinary tract infection in a patient who is 30 weeks pregnant   _____

CHAPTER GLOSSARY

Abortion: termination of a pregnancy by natural causes or by medical intervention.

Amnioinfusion: the insertion of normal saline or lactated Ringer's solution into the amniotic sac.

Antepartum: time from conception until delivery or childbirth with regard to the mother.

Cervix: the neck of the uterus that serves as an outlet from the uterus.

Complete abortion: abortion in which all the products of conception are expelled.

Ectopic: type of pregnancy that occurs when the egg is implanted outside the cavity of the uterus.

Effaced: cervical thinning.

Elderly obstetric patient: 35 years or older at date of delivery.

Elective abortion: the elective termination of pregnancy.

Endometritis: inflammation of the uterus.

Fallopian tube: delivers the mature egg to the uterus for fertilization.

Gravid: pregnant.

Habitual aborter: a woman who miscarries at least three consecutive times.

Hyperemesis gravidarum: excessive vomiting in pregnancy.

Incompetent cervix: cervix begins to open before baby is ready to be born.

Incomplete abortion: abortion in which not all of the products of conception are expelled.

Inevitable abortion: abortion that occurs when symptoms are present and a miscarriage will happen.

Labia: surrounds the vaginal opening.

Labor: process by which the products of conception are expelled from the uterus.

Lactation: process of milk production.

Miscarriage: spontaneous termination of pregnancy before the fetus has reached 20 weeks.

Missed abortion: pregnancy with fetal demise before 20 weeks; products of conception are not expelled.

Molar pregnancy: fertilized ovum is converted to a mole.

Multigravida: a woman with two or more pregnancies.

Multiparity: a woman with two or more pregnancies.

Ovaries: produce female hormones and eggs.

Postpartum: after delivery or childbirth.

Postterm pregnancy: pregnancy longer than 40 weeks up to 42 weeks.

Precipitate labor: rapid labor and delivery.

Preeclampsia: pregnancy complication characterized by hypertension, edema, and/or proteinuria.

Pregestational: condition present prior to pregnancy.

Premature labor: labor that occurs before the 37th week of pregnancy.

Prenatal: before birth.

Primigravida: first pregnancy.

Prolonged pregnancy: beyond 42 weeks of pregnancy.

Puerperium: time from delivery through the first 6 weeks postpartum.

Spontaneous abortion: loss of a fetus due to natural causes; also known as *miscarriage*.

Stillbirth: born dead.

Therapeutic abortion: abortion performed when the pregnancy is endangering the mother's health, or when the fetus has a condition that is incompatible with life.

Threatened abortion: abortion that occurs when symptoms are present that indicate the possibility of a miscarriage.

Uterus: a muscular organ that serves as an incubator for the developing fetus.

Vagina: a muscular tube that extends from the vaginal opening to the uterus.

Vulva: the external covering to the vagina.

Young obstetric patient: younger than 16 years at date of delivery.

22

Congenital Anomalies and Perinatal Conditions

(ICD-9-CM Chapter 14, Codes 740-759, and Chapter 15, Codes 760-779, and ICD-10-CM Chapter 16, Codes P00-P96, and Chapter 17, Codes Q00-Q99)

CHAPTER OUTLINE

ICD-9-CM Official Guidelines for Coding and Reporting
ICD-10-CM Official Guidelines for Coding and Reporting
Guideline Differences Between ICD-9-CM and ICD-10-CM
Major Differences Between ICD-9-CM and ICD-10-CM
Disease Conditions
    Congenital Anomalies
    Coding the Birth of an Infant
    Maternal Causes of Perinatal Morbidity and Mortality
    Other Conditions Originating in the Perinatal Period
    Observation and Evaluation of Newborns
Factors Influencing Health Status and Contact with Health Services (V Codes/Z Codes)
Documentation/Reimbursement/MS-DRGs
Chapter Review Exercise
Chapter Glossary
References

LEARNING OBJECTIVES

1. Apply and assign the correct ICD-9-CM and ICD-10-CM codes in accordance with Official Guidelines for Coding and Reporting
2. Identify major differences between ICD-9-CM and ICD-10-CM related to congenital anomalies and perinatal conditions
3. Identify congenital anomalies and perinatal conditions
4. Assign the correct V/Z codes and procedure codes to congenital anomalies and perinatal conditions
5. Identify common treatments, medications, laboratory values, and diagnostic tests
6. Explain the importance of documentation as it relates to MS-DRGs for reimbursement

ABBREVIATIONS/ ACRONYMS

AGA appropriate for gestational age

BPD bronchopulmonary dysplasia

CHD congenital heart disease

ICD-9-CM *International Classification of Diseases, 9th Revision, Clinical Modification*

ICD-10-CM *International Classification of Diseases, 10th Revision, Clinical Modification*

ICD-10-PCS *International Classification of Diseases, 10th*

Revision, Procedure Coding System

IUGR intrauterine growth retardation

LGA large for gestational age

MSAFP maternal serum alpha-fetoprotein

MS-DRG Medicare Severity diagnosis-related group

NICU neonatal intensive care unit

PDA patent ductus arteriosus

PKU phenylketonuria

PPH primary pulmonary hypertension

RDS respiratory distress syndrome

SGA small for gestational age

TOF tetralogy of Fallot

TTN transitory tachypnea of the newborn

VSD ventricular septal defect

ICD-9-CM

Official Guidelines for Coding and Reporting

Please refer to the companion Evolve website for the most current guidelines.

14. Chapter 14: Congenital Anomalies (740-759)

a. Codes in categories 740-759, Congenital Anomalies

Assign an appropriate code(s) from categories 740-759, Congenital Anomalies, when an anomaly is documented. A congenital anomaly may be the principal/first listed diagnosis on a record or a secondary diagnosis.

When a congenital anomaly does not have a unique code assignment, assign additional code(s) for any manifestations that may be present.

When the code assignment specifically identifies the congenital anomaly, manifestations that are an inherent component of the anomaly should not be coded separately. Additional codes should be assigned for manifestations that are not an inherent component.

Codes from Chapter 14 may be used throughout the life of the patient. If a congenital anomaly has been corrected, a personal history code should be used to identify the history of the anomaly. Although present at birth, a congenital anomaly may not be identified until later in life. Whenever the condition is diagnosed by the physician, it is appropriate to assign a code from codes 740-759.

For the birth admission, the appropriate code from category V30, Liveborn infants, according to type of birth should be sequenced as the principal diagnosis, followed by any congenital anomaly codes, 740-759.

EXAMPLE

Patient is a 30-year-old male with a bicuspid aortic valve, 746.4 (Q23.1).

EXAMPLE

Infant was delivered by vaginal delivery and examination shows hypospadias, V30.00, 752.61 (Z38.00, Q54.9).

---

15. Chapter 15: Newborn (Perinatal) Guidelines (760-779)

For coding and reporting purposes the perinatal period is defined as before birth through the 28th day following birth. The following guidelines are provided for reporting purposes. Hospitals may record other diagnoses as needed for internal data use.

a. General Perinatal Rules

1) Chapter 15 Codes

They are never for use on the maternal record. Codes from Chapter 11, the obstetric chapter, are never permitted on the newborn record. Chapter 15 code may be used throughout the life of the patient if the condition is still present.

2) Sequencing of perinatal codes

Generally, codes from Chapter 15 should be sequenced as the principal/first-listed diagnosis on the newborn record, with the exception of the appropriate V30 code for the birth episode, followed by codes from any other chapter that provide additional detail. The "use additional code" note at the beginning of the chapter supports this guideline. If the index does not provide a specific code for a perinatal condition, assign code 779.89, Other specified conditions originating in the perinatal period, followed by the code from another chapter that specifies the condition. Codes for signs and symptoms may be assigned when a definitive diagnosis has not been established.

EXAMPLE An infant was delivered in the hospital via cesarean section. On discharge, the infant was examined and appeared completely healthy with the exception of neonatal jaundice. A bilirubin count should be performed in 2 days, V30.01, 774.6 (Z38.01, P59.9).

3) Birth process or community acquired conditions

If a newborn has a condition that may be either due to the birth process or community acquired and the documentation does not indicate which it is, the default is due to the birth process and the code from Chapter 15 should be used. If the condition is community-acquired, a code from Chapter 15 should not be assigned.

4) Code all clinically significant conditions

All clinically significant conditions noted on routine newborn examination should be coded. A condition is clinically significant if it requires:

- clinical evaluation; or
- therapeutic treatment; or
- diagnostic procedures; or
- extended length of hospital stay; or
- increased nursing care and/or monitoring; or
- has implications for future health care needs

Note: The perinatal guidelines listed above are the same as the general coding guidelines for "additional diagnoses", except for the final point regarding implications for future health care needs. Codes should be assigned for conditions that have been specified by the provider as having implications for future health care needs. Codes from the perinatal chapter should not be assigned unless the provider has established a definitive diagnosis.

b. Use of codes V30-V39

When coding the birth of an infant, assign a code from categories V30-V39, according to the type of birth. A code from this series is assigned as a principal diagnosis, and assigned only once to a newborn at the time of birth.

EXAMPLE The infant was born via vaginal delivery and suffered a fractured clavicle caused by the delivery, V30.00, 767.2 (Z38.00, P13.4).

c. Newborn transfers

If the newborn is transferred to another institution, the V30 series is not used at the receiving hospital.

EXAMPLE The infant was born via cesarean section at Hospital Anytown and was transferred to Hospital Everytown for treatment in the NICU for hyaline membrane disease.
Hospital Anytown, V30.01, 769 (Z38.01, P22.0).
Hospital Everytown, 769 (P22.0).

d. Use of category V29

1) Assigning a code from category V29

Assign a code from category V29, Observation and evaluation of newborns and infants for suspected conditions not found, to identify those instances when a healthy newborn is evaluated for a suspected condition that is determined after study not to be present. Do not use a code from category V29 when the patient has identified signs or symptoms of a suspected problem; in such cases, code the sign or symptom.

A code from category V29 may also be assigned as a principal code for readmissions or encounters when the V30 code no longer applies. Codes from category V29 are for use only for healthy newborns and infants for which no condition after study is found to be present.

2) V29 code on a birth record

A V29 code is to be used as a secondary code after the V30, Outcome of delivery, code.

EXAMPLE A male infant was born by a precipitous vaginal delivery and was observed for a spontaneous pneumothorax. Chest x-ray was negative, V30.00, V29.2 (Z38.00, P03.9).

e. Use of other V codes on perinatal records

V codes other than V30 and V29 may be assigned on a perinatal or newborn record. The codes may be used as a principal or first-listed diagnosis for specific types of encounters or for readmissions or encounters when the V30 code no longer applies.

See Section 1.C.18 for information regarding the assignment of V codes.

EXAMPLE 10-day-old infant is seen in pediatrician's office for routine well baby care, V20.2.

f. Maternal Causes of Perinatal Morbidity

Codes from categories 760-763, Maternal causes of perinatal morbidity and mortality, are assigned only when the maternal condition has actually affected the fetus or newborn. The fact that the mother has an associated medical condition or experiences some complication of pregnancy, labor or delivery does not justify the routine assignment of codes from these categories to the newborn record.

EXAMPLE A baby tested positive for cocaine. The mother had used cocaine on the day prior to vaginal delivery, V30.00, 760.75 (Z38.00, P04.41).

g. Congenital Anomalies in Newborns

For the birth admission, the appropriate code from category V30, Liveborn infants according to type of birth, should be used, followed by any congenital anomaly codes, categories 740-759. Use additional secondary codes from other chapters to specify conditions associated with the anomaly, if applicable.

Also, see Section 1.C.14 for information on the coding of congenital anomalies.

EXAMPLE A female twin infant was delivered via cesarean section with congenital left hip dislocation. The twin male infant was stillborn, V32.01, 754.30 (Z38.31, Q65.02).

h. Coding Additional Perinatal Diagnoses

1) Assigning codes for conditions that require treatment

Assign codes for conditions that require treatment or further investigation, prolong the length of stay, or require resource utilization.

EXAMPLE | Gestational diabetes resulting in hypoglycemia of a newborn female infant born in the parking lot via vaginal delivery, V30.1, 775.0 (Z38.1, P70.4).

2) Codes for conditions specified as having implications for future health care needs
Assign codes for conditions that have been specified by the provider as having implications for future health care needs.
Note: This guideline should not be used for adult patients.

EXAMPLE | A male infant was born via vaginal delivery. The clinician will evaluate and review treatment options for his undescended right testicle at the 6-week appointment, V30.00, 752.51 (Z38.00, Q53.10).

3) Codes for newborn conditions originating in the perinatal period
Assign a code for newborn conditions originating in the perinatal period (categories 760-779), as well as complications arising during the current episode of care classified in other chapters, only if the diagnoses have been documented by the responsible provider at the time of transfer or discharge as having affected the fetus or newborn.

i. Prematurity and Fetal Growth Retardation
Providers utilize different criteria in determining prematurity. A code for prematurity should not be assigned unless it is documented. The 5th digit assignment for codes from category 764 and subcategories 765.0 and 765.1 should be based on the recorded birth weight and estimated gestational age.
A code from subcategory 765.2, Weeks of gestation, should be assigned as an additional code with category 764 and codes from 765.0 and 765.1 to specify weeks of gestation as documented by the provider in the record.

EXAMPLE | A premature infant was born in the hospital via vaginal delivery. The infant weighed 4 pounds and was 33 weeks gestational age, V30.00, 765.17, 765.27 (Z38.00, P07.17, P07.32).

j. Newborn sepsis
Code 771.81, Septicemia [sepsis] of newborn, should be assigned with a secondary code from category 041, Bacterial infections in conditions classified elsewhere and of unspecified site, to identify the organism. A code from category 038, Septicemia, should not be used on a newborn record. Do not assign code 995.91, Sepsis, as code 771.81 describes the sepsis. If applicable, use additional codes to identify severe sepsis (995.92) and any associated acute organ dysfunction.

Apply the General Coding Guidelines as found in Chapter 5 and the Procedural Guidelines as found in Chapter 6.

ICD-10-CM

Official Guidelines for Coding and Reporting

Please refer to the companion Evolve website for the most current guidelines.
16. Chapter 16: Newborn (Perinatal) Guidelines (P00-P96)
For coding and reporting purposes the perinatal period is defined as before birth through the 28th day following birth. The following guidelines are provided for reporting purposes
a. General Perinatal Rules
1) Use of Chapter 16 Codes
Codes in this chapter are <u>never</u> for use on the maternal record. Codes from Chapter 15, the obstetric chapter, are never permitted on the newborn record. Chapter 16 **codes** may be used throughout the life of the patient if the condition is still present.

2) Principal Diagnosis for Birth Record

When coding the birth episode in a newborn record, assign a code from category Z38, Liveborn **infants** according to place of birth and type of delivery, as the principal diagnosis. A code from category Z38 is assigned only once, to a newborn at the time of birth. If a newborn is transferred to another institution, a code from category Z38 should not be used at the receiving hospital.

A code from category Z38 is used only on the newborn record, not on the mother's record.

3) Use of Codes from other Chapters with Codes from Chapter 16

Codes from other chapters may be used with codes from chapter 16 if the codes from the other chapters provide more specific detail. Codes for signs and symptoms may be assigned when a definitive diagnosis has not been established. If the reason for the encounter is a perinatal condition, the code from chapter 16 should be sequenced first.

4) Use of Chapter 16 Codes after the Perinatal Period

Should a condition originate in the perinatal period, and continue throughout the life of the patient, the perinatal code should continue to be used regardless of the patient's age.

5) Birth process or community acquired conditions

If a newborn has a condition that may be either due to the birth process or community acquired and the documentation does not indicate which it is, the default is due to the birth process and the code from Chapter 16 should be used. If the condition is community-acquired, a code from Chapter 16 should not be assigned.

6) Code all clinically significant conditions

If a newborn has a condition that may be either due to the birth process or community acquired and the all clinically significant conditions noted on routine newborn examination should be coded. A condition is clinically significant if it requires:

- clinical evaluation; or
- therapeutic treatment; or
- diagnostic procedures; or
- extended length of hospital stay; or
- increased nursing care and/or monitoring; or
- has implications for future health care needs

Note: The perinatal guidelines listed above are the same as the general coding guidelines for "additional diagnoses", except for the final point regarding implications for future health care needs. Codes should be assigned for conditions that have been specified by the provider as having implications for future health care needs.

b. Observation and Evaluation of Newborns for Suspected Conditions not Found

Assign a code from categories P00-P04 to identify those instances when a healthy newborn is evaluated for a suspected condition that is determined after study not to be present. Do not use a code from categories P00-P04 when the patient has identified signs or symptoms of a suspected problem; in such cases, code the sign or symptom.

c. Coding Additional Perinatal Diagnoses

1) Assigning codes for conditions that require treatment

Assign codes for conditions that require treatment or further investigation, prolong the length of stay, or require resource utilization.

2) Codes for conditions specified as having implications for future health care needs

Assign codes for conditions that have been specified by the provider as having implications for future health care needs.

Note: This guideline should not be used for adult patients.

d. Prematurity and Fetal Growth Retardation

Providers utilize different criteria in determining prematurity. A code for prematurity should not be assigned unless it is documented. Assignment of codes in categories P05, Disorders of newborn related to slow fetal growth and fetal malnutrition, and P07, Disorders of newborn related to short gestation and low birth weight, not elsewhere classified, should be based on the recorded birth weight and estimated gestational age. Codes from category P05 should not be assigned with codes from category P07.

When both birth weight and gestational age are available, two codes from category P07 should be assigned, with the code for birth weight sequenced before the code for gestational age.

e. Low birth weight and immaturity status

Codes from **category P07, Disorders of newborn related to short gestation and low birth weight, not elsewhere classified, are for use for a child or adult who was premature** or had a low birth weight as a newborn and this is affecting the patient's current health status.

See Section I.C.21. Factors influencing health status and contact with health services, Status.

f. Bacterial Sepsis of Newborn

Category P36, Bacterial sepsis of newborn, includes congenital sepsis. If a perinate is documented as having sepsis without documentation of congenital or community acquired, the default is congenital and a code from category P36 should be assigned. If the P36 code includes the causal organism, an additional code from category B95, Streptococcus, Staphylococcus, and Enterococcus as the cause of diseases classified elsewhere, or B96, Other bacterial agents as the cause of diseases classified elsewhere, should not be assigned. If the P36 code does not include the causal organism, assign an additional code from category B96. If applicable, use additional codes to identify severe sepsis (R65.2-) and any associated acute organ dysfunction.

g. Stillbirth

Code P95, Stillbirth, is only for use in institutions that maintain separate records for stillbirths. No other code should be used with P95. Code P95 should not be used on the mother's record.

17. Chapter 17: Congenital malformations, deformations, and chromosomal abnormalities (Q00-Q99)

Assign an appropriate code(s) from categories Q00-Q99, Congenital malformations, deformations, and chromosomal abnormalities when a malformation/deformation or chromosomal abnormality is documented. A malformation/deformation/or chromosomal abnormality may be the principal/**first-listed** diagnosis on a record or a secondary diagnosis.

When a malformation/deformation/or chromosomal abnormality does not have a unique code assignment, assign additional code(s) for any manifestations that may be present.

When the code assignment specifically identifies the malformation/deformation/or chromosomal abnormality, manifestations that are an inherent component of the anomaly should not be coded separately. Additional codes should be assigned for manifestations that are not an inherent component.

Codes from Chapter 17 may be used throughout the life of the patient. If a congenital malformation or deformity has been corrected, a personal history code should be used to identify the history of the malformation or deformity. Although present at birth, malformation/deformation/or chromosomal abnormality may not be identified until later in life. Whenever the condition is diagnosed by the physician, it is appropriate to assign a code from codes Q00-Q99.

For the birth admission, the appropriate code from category Z38, Liveborn infants, according to place of birth and type of delivery, should be sequenced as the principal diagnosis, followed by any congenital anomaly codes, Q00-Q99.

Apply the General Coding Guidelines as found in Chapter 5 and the Procedural Guidelines as found in Chapter 7.

GUIDELINE DIFFERENCES BETWEEN ICD-9-CM AND ICD-10-CM

- New Z codes appear in ICD-10-CM for low birth weight and immaturity status. These codes can be used on both children and adult records when they may affect the patient's current health status.
- Stillbirth code P95 cannot be used with any additional codes and is only used in hospitals that maintain separate records for stillborns.

MAJOR DIFFERENCES BETWEEN ICD-9-CM AND ICD-10-CM

The following code changes have occurred in ICD-10-CM:

- Different codes are used for "light for gestational age" and "small for gestational age."
- Birthweight should be sequenced before gestational age.
- Codes for assigning birth trauma have been expanded.
- Code changes identify slow fetal growth and malnutrition.
- Codes identify low birth weight not due to slow fetal growth or malnutrition.
- The term "fetus" has been removed from many titles.

EXERCISE 22-1

Answer the questions and assign codes to the following conditions.

1. A congenital anomaly is always listed second on a newborn record.
   A. True
   B. False

2. A congenital anomaly code can be assigned to an adult record.
   A. True
   B. False

3. Codes from Chapter 11 can be used on the newborn record.
   A. True
   B. False

4. Chapter 15 codes can be used anytime throughout the life of the patient.
   A. True
   B. False

5. Code 762.7 belongs on the mother's record.
   A. True
   B. False

6. If a newborn has a condition that has implications for future healthcare needs, that condition may be coded. The same is true for the adult population.
   A. True
   B. False

7. When a newborn is transferred to another hospital, the principal diagnosis should be a code from the V30 series.
   A. True
   B. False

8. V29 can be assigned as a principal diagnosis.
   A. True
   B. False

9. A coder should assign a code for prematurity on the basis of weeks and/or weight in grams.
   A. True
   B. False

10. If the mother of a newborn has hypertension, code 760.0 is assigned.
    A. True
    B. False

11. When the code 775.5 is used and the baby is dehydrated, _____ would it also be appropriate to use code 276.51?

12. If it is not clearly documented on the infant's chart whether a condition is community acquired or is due to the birth process, which is the default? _____

13. What makes a condition clinically significant? _____

14. What category of codes is used as the principal diagnosis for newborns? _____

15. If the Index does not provide a specific code for a perinatal condition, which code should be assigned? _____

16. When a baby is born extremely prematurely at 25 weeks' gestation and has a birth weight of 950 grams, what code or codes are assigned? _____

17. When a newborn has a diagnosis of sepsis, what code or codes are assigned? _____

18. What is the definition of "congenital"? _____

19. The principal diagnosis code for a single newborn who is delivered by a cesarean section is _____

20. How long does the perinatal period last? _____

DISEASE CONDITIONS

Congenital Anomalies, Chapter 14, and Perinatal Conditions, Chapter 15 (740-759 and 760-779) in the ICD-9-CM code book, are divided into the following categories:

CATEGORY	SECTION TITLES
740-759	Congenital Anomalies
760-763	Maternal Causes of Perinatal Morbidity and Mortality
764-779	Other Conditions Originating in the Perinatal Period

Certain Conditions Originating in the **Perinatal Period** (P00-P96), Chapter 16 in the ICD-10-CM code book, and Congenital Malformations, Deformations, and Chromosomal Abnormalities (Q00-Q99), Chapter 17, is divided into the following categories:

CATEGORY	SECTION TITLES
P00-P04	Newborn Affected by Maternal Factors and by Complications of Pregnancy, Labor, and Delivery
P05-P08	Disorders Related to Length of Gestation and Fetal Growth
P09	Abnormal Findings on Neonatal Screening
P10-P15	Birth Trauma
P19-P29	Respiratory and Cardiovascular Disorders Specific to the Perinatal Period
P35-P39	Infections Specific to the Perinatal Period
P50-P61	Hemorrhagic and Hematological Disorders of Newborn
P70-P74	Transitory Endocrine and Metabolic Disorders Specific to Newborn
P76-P78	Digestive System Disorders of Newborn
P80-P83	Conditions Involving the Integument and Temperature Regulation of Newborn
P84	Other Problems with Newborn
P90-P96	Other Disorders Originating in the Perinatal Period
Q00-Q07	Congenital Malformations of the Nervous System
Q10-Q18	Congenital Malformations of the Eye, Ear, Face, and Neck
Q20-Q28	Congenital Malformations of the Circulatory System
Q30-Q34	Congenital Malformations of the Respiratory System
Q35-Q37	Cleft Lip and Cleft Palate
Q38-Q45	Other Congenital Malformations of the Digestive System
Q50-Q56	Congenital Malformations of Genital Organs
Q60-Q64	Congenital Malformations of the Urinary System
Q65-Q79	Congenital Malformations and Deformations of the Musculoskeletal System
Q80-Q89	Other Congenital Malformations
Q90-Q99	Chromosomal Abnormalities, Not Elsewhere Classified

SPINA BIFIDA
Posterior vertebral arches
have not fused; there is no
herniation of the spinal cord
or meninges

MENINGOCELE
External protruding sac
contains meninges and CSF

MYELOMENINGOCELE
External sac contains
meninges, CSF, and the
spinal cord

FIGURE 22-1. Congenital spinal cord defects.

Congenital Anomalies

A **congenital anomaly** is an abnormal condition that is present at birth. Sometimes, conditions that a person is born with do not appear until later in life. Some conditions are congenital by definition, such as Meckel's diverticulum. This condition is present at birth but may not manifest until later in life. Congenital anomalies may be located in the Alphabetic Index under the specific condition or anomaly and/or deformity.

Spina bifida is a disorder that involves incomplete development of the brain, spinal cord, and/or their protective coverings (Figure 22-1). It occurs in 1 in every 2000 births in the United States. Pregnant women can be tested with a blood test called MSAFP (maternal serum alpha-fetoprotein) to screen for spina bifida. This disorder occurs during the first month of pregnancy and is caused by the spine of the fetus not closing properly. This results in permanent nerve damage to various degrees, even though the opening can be closed in utero or after birth. Three types of spina bifida have been identified: (1) myelomeningocele, which is the most severe form; the spinal cord and the meninges protrude from the opening in the spine; (2) meningocele, which is the most rare form; the spinal cord is normally developed, but the meninges protrudes through the opening; and (3) occulta, which is the mildest form; one or more vertebrae are malformed; this type usually involves no treatment.

Children with spina bifida often have bowel and bladder complications and hydrocephalus (Figure 22-2). Spina bifida has no cure because nerve tissue cannot be repaired. Treatment is rendered according to the severity of the condition. Children born with spina bifida are usually treated through surgery that is performed to close the opening within 24 hours of birth. If a child is born with the most severe type, he or she often has **hydrocephalus**; this is treated by inserting a **ventricular shunt** into the brain to drain accumulating fluid (Figure 22-3). Another complication of a severe case of spina bifida is a tethered spinal cord. A tethered spinal cord is a cord that does not move up and down during movement, as it is designed to do. If a child has severe pain, surgery may be performed to untether the spinal cord.

Some children are born with syndromes that manifest with a series of anomalies. If the syndrome is not specifically indexed in ICD-9-CM, then a code should be assigned for each presenting manifestation of the syndrome, as well as 759.89.

EXAMPLE A child with Cockayne's Syndrome is seen by a physician who documents that the patient has mental retardation, retinal atrophy, and microcephaly, 759.89, 319, 362.60, 742.1 (Q87.1). In ICD-10-CM the syndrome is indexed.

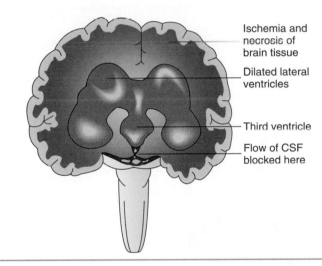

FIGURE 22-2. Hydrocephalus.

EXAMPLE

Baby born by cesarean section is found to have spina bifida with hydrocephalus, V30.01, 741.00 (Z38.01, Q05.4).

Tetralogy of Fallot

Tetralogy of Fallot (Figure 22-4) is a congenital heart defect that manifests with four key features: (1) a hole between the ventricles (ventral septal defect [VSD]); (2) pulmonary stenosis; (3) aorta lying directly over the hole; and (4) thick, muscled right ventricle (hypertrophy). The treatment recommended for this condition is surgery. Often, surgery requires two stages. The first stage occurs when the infant is first born; a little later, after growth has occurred, the second stage is performed. Patients who have undergone repair often are at greater risk for arrhythmia; sometimes, additional surgery is required later in life. The operation performed to treat this condition is called the **Blalock-Taussig procedure**.

EXAMPLE

VSD is diagnosed in a baby, along with pulmonary stenosis and hypertrophy of the right ventricle, as well as dextroposition of the aorta. The baby is seen by a surgeon for total repair of a ventral septal defect, 745.2, 35.81 (Q21.3, 02QM0ZZ).

Ventriculoatrial shunt

Ventriculoperitoneal shunt

FIGURE 22-3. Shunting procedures for hydrocephalus. **Ventriculoperitoneal shunt** is the preferred procedure.

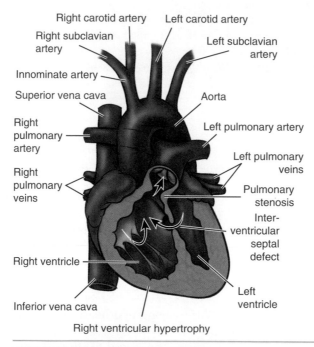

FIGURE 22-4. Tetralogy of Fallot.

Cleft Lip and Cleft Palate

A **cleft lip/palate** is an opening in the lip or palate of an infant that occurs in utero.
Three different types of clefts can occur on one or both sides of the mouth:
1. Cleft lip without a cleft palate (Figure 22-5)
2. Cleft palate without a cleft lip
3. Cleft lip and cleft palate together

FIGURE 22-5. Unilateral cleft lip.

FIGURE 22-6. Photograph of $3\frac{1}{2}$-year-old girl with typical facial appearance of Down's syndrome.

Approximately 1 in 600 babies is born with a cleft. Surgery is performed to repair the cleft; often, surgery is completed in several stages. The first surgery is usually done when a baby is 10 weeks of age or older and weighs at least 10 pounds. The cleft lip/palate diagnosis code may be assigned as many times as surgery is performed to correct this defect, per *Coding Clinic* (1996:1Q:p14).[1]

EXAMPLE | The child was admitted for repair of upper cleft lip and soft and hard palate. A repair of both the hard and soft palate and lip is performed by external approach, 749.24, 27.62, 27.54 (Q37.4, OCQ0XZZ, OCQ2XZZ, OCQ3XZZ).

Meckel's Diverticulum

Meckel's diverticulum occurs during the fifth week of fetal development. This is a small pouch on the wall of the small bowel that contains ectopic tissue. It occurs in about 2% of the population, and most people who have this condition have no problems. Complications of Meckel's diverticulum include hematochezia in children and obstruction or diverticulitis in adults. Treatment varies but may require only observation and treatment of symptoms or surgery to remove the diverticulum.

EXAMPLE | A 60-year-old woman presents to the hospital with severe abdominal pain. A scan is performed, and Meckel's diverticulum is discovered. The surgeon is called in and performs an open ileal resection, 751.0, 45.62 (Q43.0, ODTB0ZZ).

Chromosomal Anomalies

One in 200 babies is born with a chromosomal abnormality. Each egg and sperm cell contains 23 chromosomes. When they unite, 23 pairs or 46 chromosomes are created. If a baby is born with too many, too few, or broken or rearranged chromosomes, birth defects may occur. A chromosomal abnormality with three instead of two of a specific chromosome is called a **trisomy**. In most cases when this occurs, the pregnancy ends in a miscarriage.

Down's syndrome (Figure 22-6), the most common chromosomal abnormality, is also known as trisomy 21. Babies with Down's syndrome have an extra chromosome 21. Children with Down's syndrome can have a combination of birth defects. Some of these are characteristic facial features, mental retardation, and heart defects. No cure is known for Down's syndrome; however, the older the mother is, the greater is the risk; research suggests that folic acid can help to prevent this condition. Physicians can test for this condition during pregnancy with a test called chorionic villus sampling (CVS). A tiny sample of tissue is taken from the placenta of the mother for this test, which is performed transcervically or transvaginally. CVS can also be used to test for other disorders.

EXAMPLE | Patient with Down's syndrome, 758.0 (Q90.9).

Klinefelter's syndrome is a sex chromosome disorder that occurs only in males in which the individual has an extra X chromosome. Most commonly, the child is born with 47 chromosomes in each cell, rather than 46. Symptoms of this condition generally do not appear until puberty. Individuals have low levels of testosterone and small testicles and may exhibit behavior problems.

EXAMPLE | Patient diagnosed with Klinefelter's syndrome, 758.7 (Q98.4).

Marfan's Syndrome

Marfan's syndrome (Figure 22-7), which is caused by a gene mutation, is an inherited condition that affects the connective tissue. Because connective tissue is found throughout the body, Marfan's may affect many body systems. Often, patients with Marfan's have skeletal defects such as spider-like fingers, pectus excavatum, and curvature of the spine. They also may have cardiovascular problems such as aortic regurgitation or prolapse of the mitral valve. *Coding Clinic* (1993:3Q:p11)[2] addresses the assignment of codes for Marfan's syndrome. Conditions that are inherent in this syndrome are not coded separately. When an adult presents for heart surgery to correct conditions associated with Marfan's, 759.82 (Q87.418) is assigned as the principal diagnosis.

EXAMPLE | Aortic regurgitation in a patient with Marfan's syndrome, 759.82 (Q87.418, I35.1).

EXERCISE 22-2

Assign codes to the following conditions.

1. Unilateral, complete cleft lip _____
2. Tongue tie _____
3. Primary pulmonary hypertension of the newborn _____
4. Patent ductus arteriosus (PDA) of the newborn _____
5. Ventricular septal defect (VSD) of the newborn _____
6. Preauricular cyst _____
7. Transposition of the great vessels _____
8. Ptosis of the eyelid present at birth _____
9. Microcephalus _____
10. Arnold-Chiari syndrome type II _____
11. Cerebral cyst present at birth _____
12. Supernumerary ear _____
13. Brachial cleft cyst _____
14. Hypospadias _____
15. Micro-penis _____

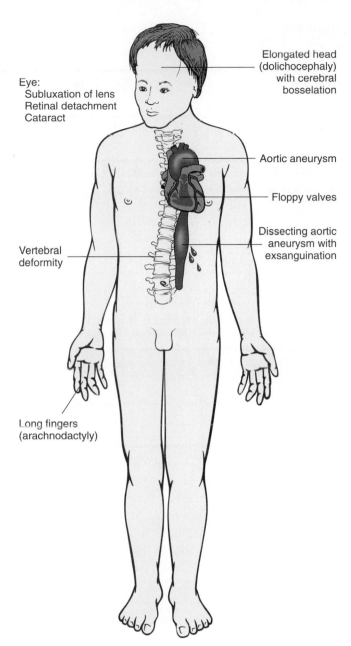

FIGURE 22-7. Typical features of Marfan's syndrome.

Coding the Birth of an Infant

All newborn charts must contain a code from V30-V39 (Z38.−) for the principal diagnosis on the baby's birth record. This V code is only used one time. If the baby is transferred to another facility, these sets of V codes are not used and the reason for admission at that facility is the principal diagnosis.

These V codes have both fourth and fifth digits available.

Fourth Digits

    0 Born in hospital

    1 Born before admission to hospital

    2 Born outside hospital and not hospitalized

Fifth Digits

    These fifth digits are for use **only** with the fourth digit of .0, Born in the hospital:

    0 Delivered without mention of cesarean delivery

    1 Delivered by cesarean delivery

These digits help identify where the baby was born and whether a cesarean delivery was performed.

EXAMPLE	Single liveborn, born in hospital, via cesarean section, V30.01 (Z38.01).

EXAMPLE	Twin, mate liveborn, delivered vaginally in hospital, V31.00 (Z38.30).

EXAMPLE	Single liveborn delivered by cesarean section at Hospital A. The infant was transferred to Hospital B because of bladder exstrophy.
	    Hospital A V30.01, 753.5 (Z38.01, Q64.10)
	    Hospital B 753.5 (Q64.10)

Maternal Causes of Perinatal Morbidity and Mortality

As is stated in the guidelines, these conditions are assigned only if and when the maternal condition has actually affected the fetus or the newborn. Just because a mother has a condition does not necessarily mean that it affects the newborn.

EXAMPLE	Mother used heroin during this pregnancy. Upon vaginal delivery, it is noted that the baby is jittery and is experiencing symptoms of withdrawal, V30.00, 779.5 (Z38.00, P96.1).

EXERCISE 22-3

Answer the following questions.

1. Mother had a urinary tract infection (UTI) during the pregnancy; this was treated, and no effect on the fetus was observed. Should code 760.1 be added to the baby's chart?   _____

2. Mother had an automobile accident. She needed to undergo immediate surgery to correct the open fracture of her arm. It was decided that a cesarean section should be performed and the baby delivered prior to repair of the fracture. Should code 760.5 be added to the baby's chart?   _____

3. A baby is born with spina bifida, and the mother had taken statins during pregnancy. Should code 760.78 be used on the baby's chart? See *Coding Clinic* (2005:4Q:p82-83).[3]   _____

4. A baby is born to a mother who used cocaine during the pregnancy. The baby experiences no signs of withdrawal but has a positive drug screen. Should 760.75 be used on this baby's chart? See *Coding Clinic* (1992:2Q:p12).[4]   _____

5. A newborn is delivered via vacuum extractor. A large hematoma is located on the scalp. Should 763.3 be coded?   _____

Other Conditions Originating in the Perinatal Period

Prematurity, Low Birth Weight

Fifth digits are required for categories 764.XX (Slow fetal growth and fetal malnutrition), 765.0X, and 765.1X (Extreme immaturity and other preterm infants). Prematurity must be documented by the provider. Fifth digits should be assigned on the basis of recorded birth weight and gestational age. Additionally, a code for weeks of gestation (765.2X) should be assigned to categories 764.XX and 765.0X and 765.1X. The "Number of gestational weeks" code may be assigned when the provider has documented that prematurity is a contributing factor to a current condition.

EXAMPLE

> The physician documented that the baby was small for gestational age (SGA). The baby weighed 1850 grams. The infant was born in the hospital by vaginal delivery, V30.00, 764.07, 765.20 (Z38.00, P05.17).

The guidelines state that all clinically significant conditions noted on routine newborn examination should be coded. These follow the same general guidelines for assigning secondary diagnoses except for the guideline regarding implications for future healthcare needs.

A condition is clinically significant if it requires the following:

- Clinical evaluation, or
- Therapeutic treatment, or
- Diagnostic procedures, or
- Extended length of hospital stay, or
- Increased nursing care and/or monitoring; or if it has
- Implications for future healthcare needs (applies to newborn only)

When coding secondary diagnoses from other chapters on a newborn's chart, guidelines state that code 779.89 should also be assigned. If there is no specific code from the Congenital anomalies and perinatal condition chapter to describe the condition, disease, or complication of the newborn, then a code from other chapters should be used as well as code 779.89.

EXAMPLE

> Infant was delivered by Cesarean section. Physician notes hemangioma of skin of torso. Will re-evaluate at 6-week check up, V30.01, 779.89, 228.01 (Z38.01, D18.01).

Fetal Distress

Fetal distress occurs when the fetus develops a problem before or during labor. No exact consensus has been reached as to what constitutes fetal distress, but the term often refers to **hypoxia** (insufficient oxygen in blood), **bradycardia** (slow heartbeat), **tachycardia** (fast heartbeat), fetal acidosis, and/or the presence of thick meconium.

EXAMPLE

> Fetal distress first noted during labor, infant born vaginally, V30.00, 768.3 (Z38.00, P84).

EXAMPLE

> Fetal hypoxia in infant born by C-section, V30.01, 770.88 (Z38.01, P84).

EXAMPLE

> Abnormal fetal heart rate or rhythm during labor, infant delivered by C-section, V30.01, 763.82 (Z38.01, P03.811).

Apgar Scores

All babies are assessed after birth by what is known as an **Apgar** test (Figure 22-8). This test is usually given twice—once at 1 minute and again at 5 minutes. If problems are noted with the baby, the test may be done a third time. It is good to be familiar with this test because a low Apgar score is often indicative of problems.

Five factors are used for evaluation; the baby is given a score of 0 to 2 for each factor. These consist of the following:

1. Heart (pulse)
2. Breathing (rate and effort)
3. Activity and muscle tone

APGAR SCORING CHART

SIGN	0	1	2
Heart rate	Absent	Below 100	Over 100
Respiratory effort	Absent	Slow, irregular	Good, crying
Muscle tone	Limp	Some flexion of extremities	Active motion
Response to catheter in nostril (tested after oropharynx is clear)	No response	Grimace	Cough or sneeze
Color	Blue, pale	Body pink, extremities blue	Completely pink

FIGURE 22-8. Apgar scoring chart.

4. Grimace (reflex irritability)
5. Appearance (skin coloration)

If a baby scores 7 or above at 1 minute after birth, the baby is considered healthy. If a score between 4 and 6 is recorded at 1 minute, usually the baby needs immediate care with oxygen or suctioning.

Respiratory Problems After Birth

If a baby is born by cesarean section, a pediatrician may be asked to be present for the birth. If an abnormal heart rate occurs during labor, or any indications suggest that the baby might be in trouble, a pediatrician may be called and is asked to be present for the delivery. Documentation by the physician should note any abnormal conditions.

Transitory Tachypnea of Newborn (TTN). This is a respiratory problem that is likely due to retained lung fluid. It usually resolves in 24 to 48 hours. The baby may be treated with oxygen.

Apnea of the Newborn. This tends to occur in premature infants and is defined as a pause in breathing for longer than 15 seconds that can result in cyanosis.

Respiratory Distress Syndrome (RDS). This syndrome rarely affects full-term infants. It is caused by lack of lung surfactant. Surfactant is a chemical that keeps the air sacs from collapsing. The more premature the baby is, the greater is the chance of RDS. Treatment for mild cases consists of oxygen. Patients with more severe disease must be ventilated; sometimes, an artificial lung surfactant is placed in the lungs of an infant who is at high risk, to try to prevent RDS.

EXAMPLE | Respiratory distress syndrome in liveborn infant that was delivered vaginally, V30.00, 769 (Z38.00, P22.0).

Bronchopulmonary Dysplasia (BPD)

Bronchopulmonary dysplasia (BPD) is a chronic lung disease that develops in babies during the first 4 weeks after birth. It occurs most often in premature babies, that is, those weighing less than 1500 grams. Sometimes, the ventilator that is keeping a baby alive may cause BPD. BPD may also be caused by infections, such as pneumonia.

EXAMPLE | A 4-week-old infant is diagnosed with bronchopulmonary dysplasia. Infant was on a ventilator following birth, 770.7 (P27.1).

Meconium Aspiration Syndrome

Meconium is the fecal matter within a baby's intestines before birth. Normally, it is expelled after birth, but if problems occur during labor, the baby may expel meconium into the amniotic fluid. Meconium may be inhaled by the baby while within the uterus or during birth. Inhalation of meconium occurs most often in postterm babies.

A physician may suspect aspiration if the newborn is covered with meconium, or if thick meconium is found in the amniotic fluid. Aspiration of meconium can result in major problems for the newborn.

A variety of codes may be used to indicate the different ways in which meconium may be found.

- 779.84, Meconium staining (P96.83)
- 763.84, Meconium passage during delivery (P03.82)
- 770.11, Meconium aspiration without respiratory symptoms (P24.00)
- 770.12, Meconium aspiration with respiratory symptoms (P24.01)
- 770.10, Fetal and newborn aspiration, unspecified (P24.9)

Hemolytic Disease of Fetus or Newborn Due to Isoimmunization and Other Perinatal Jaundice

Many newborns have jaundice. Jaundice results from too many red blood cells and the breakdown of these cells into bilirubin. A large amount of bilirubin causes the skin to take on a yellow color. The most common type of jaundice is physiological jaundice. Other factors may cause jaundice, but the next most common cause is Rh or ABO incompatibility. ABO incompatibility affects newborns who have mothers with a blood type of O and babies whose blood type is A, B, or AB.

Coombs' test may be performed on newborns who are jaundiced. This is done to look for possible causes of **hemolysis** (the breaking down of red blood cells). Two common forms of hemolysis in the newborn are Rh incompatibility and ABO incompatibility. Rh incompatibility occurs when an Rh-negative (anti-Rh antibodies in blood) mom gives birth to an Rh-positive baby. If any maternal and fetal blood gets mixed during pregnancy or the birth process, the mother's Rh-negative antibodies will attack the baby's Rh-positive RBCs and destroy them. ABO incompatibility is very similar in mechanism. Often, documentation in the chart indicates that routine cord blood tests show ABO incompatibility. The coder must verify whether Coombs' test results were positive in order to assign this code. If cord blood shows ABO incompatibility and Coombs' test results are positive, code 773.1 should be assigned according to *Coding Clinic* (1992:3Q:p8-9).[5]

Most often, jaundice is treated by putting a baby under "bili" lights. Phototherapy code 99.83 is used for this treatment. In very mild cases, a mother is instructed to put the baby in a sunlit window. In very severe cases, a transfusion may be required.

EXAMPLE

Newborn with Rh incompatibility. Infant was delivered vaginally, V30.00, 773.0 (Z38.00, P55.0).

Infection in the Perinatal Period

Newborn Sepsis. To locate infections of the newborn in the Index, it is best to look under the main term for the infection, and then to look for a subterm of newborn, fetal, or congenital.

For example, newborn sepsis codes to 771.81 (P36.9). It is also important to assign a code from category 041 to identify the organism responsible for the infection. The guidelines state that code 995.9x, SIRS (systemic inflammatory response syndrome), is not to be used on a newborn record, nor should the code 038.xx be used for septicemia.

The guidelines also state that if a newborn has a condition that may be due to the birth process or may be community acquired, and the documentation is not clear regarding the underlying cause, the default is to a code from Chapter 15, the congenital condition.

EXAMPLE | A 7-day-old infant presents to the physician's office with pneumonia, 770.0 (P23.9).

Observation and Evaluation of Newborns

Often, a newborn is evaluated for a condition that may be suspected but is then ruled out. In cases in which this happens, it is appropriate to assign a code from the V29 (P00.–) category as a diagnosis in support of the testing and treatment that is being performed. Sometimes, a mother is running a fever during labor, and the physician must make sure that the infant does not have an infection. The physician orders tests, observation, and/or treatment until this condition can be ruled out. If the newborn is experiencing signs or symptoms, then a code from category V29 is not to be used. Likewise, a V29 (P00.–) code may be assigned as the principal diagnosis code for readmission when a condition is suspected and is subsequently ruled out. It is important to remember that this code can be used only during the neonatal period (the first 28 days of life).

EXAMPLE | Newborn delivered vaginally and is given antibiotics due to mother being diagnosed with chorioamnionitis, V30.00, V29.0 (Z38.00, P02.7).

FACTORS INFLUENCING HEALTH STATUS AND CONTACT WITH HEALTH SERVICES (V CODES/Z CODES)

In the past, V/Z codes were primarily considered for use in the outpatient setting. This has changed with the addition of more V/Z codes each year. As was discussed in Chapter 8, it may be difficult to locate V/Z codes in the Index. Coders often say, "I did not know there was a V/Z code for that."

Refer to Chapter 8 for a listing of common main terms used to locate V/Z codes.

V13.61	Personal history of (corrected) hypospadias
V13.62	Personal history of other (corrected) congenital malformations of genitourinary system
V13.63	Personal history of (corrected) congenital malformations of the nervous system
V13.64	Personal history of (corrected) congenital malformations of the eye, ear, face and neck
V13.65	Personal history of (corrected) congenital malformations of heart and circulatory system
V13.66	Personal history of (corrected) congenital malformations of respiratory system
V13.67	Personal history of (corrected) congenital malformations of digestive system
V13.68	Personal history of (corrected) congenital malformations of integument, limbs, and musculoskeletal system
V13.69	Personal history of other (corrected) congenital malformations
V20.0	Foundling
V20.1	Other healthy infant or child receiving care
V20.2	Routine infant or child health check
V21.0	Period of rapid growth in childhood
V21.2	Other adolescence
V21.30	Low birth weight status, unspecified
V21.31	Low birth weight status, less than 500 grams
V21.32	Low birth weight status, 500-999 grams
V21.33	Low birth weight status, 1000-1499 grams
V21.34	Low birth weight status, 1500-1999 grams
V21.35	Low birth weight status, 2000-2500 grams
V21.8	Other specified constitutional states in development

V21.9	Unspecified constitutional state in development
V30.xx	Single liveborn
V31.xx	Twin, mate liveborn
V32.xx	Twin, mate stillborn
V33.xx	Twin, unspecified
V34.xx	Other multiple, mates all liveborn
V35.xx	Other multiple, mates all stillborn
V36.xx	Other multiple, mates live and stillborn
V37.xx	Other multiple, unspecified
V64.00	Vaccination not carried out, unspecified reason
V64.01	Vaccination not carried out because of acute illness
V64.02	Vaccination not carried out because of chronic illness or condition
V64.03	Vaccination not carried out because of immune compromised state
V64.04	Vaccination not carried out because of caregiver refusal
V64.05	Vaccination not carried out because of patient refusal
V64.07	Vaccination not carried out for religious reasons
V64.08	Vaccination not carried out because patient had disease being vaccinated against
V64.09	Vaccination not carried out for other reason
V72.11	Encounter for hearing examination following failed hearing screening
V77.3	Special screening for Phenylketonuria (PKU)
V82.3	Special screening for congenital dislocation of hip

EXAMPLE Patient was born with tetralogy of Fallot that was repaired immediately after birth, V13.65 (no corresponding ICD-10-CM code).

DOCUMENTATION/REIMBURSEMENT/MS-DRGs

Often, coding difficulties are due to lack of documentation. Sometimes pathology and other test results are not available at the time of discharge or when the physician is dictating the discharge summary or is reporting the final diagnoses.

Frequently missed complications/comorbidities from congenital anomalies and perinatal conditions include:

- Congenital deformities of the brain
- Tetralogy of Fallot
- Congenital anomalies of the pulmonary artery
- Congenital pneumonia
- Meconium aspiration with respiratory symptoms
- Necrotizing enterocolitis
- Chronic respiratory disease arising in the perinatal period
- Convulsions of the newborn
- Ventricular septal defect
- Renal agenesis and dysgenesis
- Polycystic kidney disease
- Exstrophy of urinary bladder
- Osteogenesis imperfect
- Apnea of the newborn
- Congenital anemia
- Drug withdrawal syndrome in newborn

NEWBORN MS-DRGS	RW	DRG TITLE
789	1.4877	Died or transferred
790	4.9058	Extreme immaturity or RDS
791	3.3505	Premature with major problems
792	2.0216	Premature without major problems
793	3.4417	Full-term neonate with major problems
794	1.2181	Neonate with other significant problems
795	0.1649	Normal newborn

As is evident from the MS-DRGs listed here, correct capture of the discharge disposition is very important, as is following the perinatal guidelines to capture all newborn conditions. It also is important to watch for documentation of prematurity and low birth weight.

	CODE	MS-DRGS	RW
Normal newborn	V30.00 (Z38.00)	795	0.1649
Newborn with meconium during delivery	V30.00 (Z38.00) 763.84 (P03.82)	794	1.2181
Newborn with aspiration of clear amniotic fluid with respiratory symptoms	V30.00 (Z38.00) 770.14 (P24.10)	793	3.4417
Premature newborn Delivered at 29 weeks weighing 1500 grams	V30.00 (Z38.00) 765.16 (P07.16) 765.25 (P07.31)	792	2.0216
Newborn with respiratory distress syndrome	V30.00 (Z38.00) 769 (P22.0)	790	4.9058

CHAPTER REVIEW EXERCISE

Where applicable, assign codes for diagnoses, procedures, V/Z codes, and external cause codes.

1. Newborn delivered by cesarean section _____

2. Twins born in the parking lot of the hospital _____

3. Baby was born at 2500 grams; physician documented "small for dates"; delivered vaginally _____

4. Newborn at 43 weeks' gestation, vaginal delivery _____

5. Newborn with IUGR (intrauterine growth retardation); delivered vaginally _____

6. Newborn fractured clavicle during birth process; vaginal delivery _____

7. TTN (transitory tachypnea of the newborn); infant delivered by emergency C-section _____

8. 7-day-old with thrush; seen in physician office _____

9. Transfer from community hospital for treatment of interstitial pulmonary fibrosis of prematurity in a newborn _____

10. Baby is admitted 5 days after birth for jaundice due to breast feeding _____

11. 7-day-old infant with infection of the navel cord _____

12. Newborn with a hydrocele following vaginal delivery _____

13. Baby delivered by cesarean section in respiratory failure and immediately transferred to NICU (neonatal intensive care unit) _____

14. Newborn aspirated meconium during vaginal delivery _____

15. Neonatal bradycardia following C-section _____

16. Newborn with fetal alcohol syndrome delivered vaginally _____

17. Newborn delivered vaginally; suspected of having pneumonia; chest x-ray is performed, revealing no diagnosis _____

18. Newborn with hypoglycemia, whose mother has diabetes, delivered vaginally   _____

19. Newborn with apnea following vaginal delivery   _____

20. Newborn delivered vaginally in the hospital; failed hearing test   _____

CHAPTER GLOSSARY

Apgar: test used to measure the condition of a newborn at birth.

Blalock-Taussig procedure: procedure used to treat patients with tetralogy of Fallot who have insufficient pulmonary arterial flow.

Bradycardia: slow heart rate.

Bronchopulmonary dysplasia: chronic lung disease that develops in babies during the first 4 weeks after birth.

Cleft lip/palate: opening in the lip or palate of an infant that occurs in utero.

Congenital anomaly: an abnormal condition present at birth.

Hemolysis: the breaking down of red blood cells.

Hydrocephalus: cerebrospinal fluid collection in the skull.

Hypoxia: insufficient oxygen in the blood.

Klinefelter's syndrome: a sex chromosome disorder that occurs in males and is caused by an extra X chromosome.

Marfan's syndrome: an inherited condition that affects connective tissue and is caused by gene mutation.

Meconium: material in the intestine of a fetus.

Perinatal period: before birth through the first 28 days of life.

Spina bifida: a disorder that involves incomplete development of the brain, spinal cord, and/or their protective coverings.

Tachycardia: fast heartbeat.

Trisomy: extra chromosome.

REFERENCES

1. American Hospital Association. *Coding Clinic for ICD-9-CM* 1996:1Q:p14. Revision of bilateral cleft lip and palate repair.
2. American Hospital Association. *Coding Clinic for ICD-9-CM* 1993:3Q:p11. Marfan syndrome in adult w/associated conditions.
3. American Hospital Association. *Coding Clinic for ICD-9-CM* 2005:4Q:p82-83. Noxious influences affecting fetus or newborn.
4. American Hospital Association. *Coding Clinic for ICD-9-CM* 1992:2Q:p12. Newborn delivered by cocaine abuser/dependent mother.
5. American Hospital Association. *Coding Clinic for ICD-9-CM* 1992:3Q:p8-9. ABO incompatibility w/negative Coombs test.

Injuries and E Codes

(ICD-9-CM Chapter 17, Codes 800-995, and External Causes, E800-E999, and ICD-10-CM Chapters 19 and 20, Codes S00-Y99)

LEARNING OBJECTIVES

1. Apply and assign the correct ICD-9-CM and ICD-10-CM codes in accordance with Official Guidelines for Coding and Reporting
2. Identify major differences between ICD-9-CM and ICD-10-CM related to injuries and E codes
3. Identify the various types of injuries

4. Assign the correct V/Z codes, E/External Cause codes, and procedure codes related to injuries
5. Identify common treatments, medications, and diagnostic tests
6. Explain the importance of documentation in relation to MS-DRGs for reimbursement

ABBREVIATIONS/ ACRONYMS

AKA above-knee amputation

ATV all-terrain vehicle

CHI closed head injury

CT computerized tomography

FB foreign body

ICD-9-CM *International Classification of Diseases, 9th Revision, Clinical Modification*

ICD-10-CM *International Classification of Diseases, 10th Revision, Clinical Modification*

ICD-10-PCS *International Classification of Diseases, 10th Revision, Procedure Coding System*

LOC loss of consciousness

MRI magnetic resonance imaging

MS-DRG Medicare Severity diagnosis-related group

MVA motor vehicle accident

OIG Office of the Inspector General

OR Operating Room

ORIF open reduction with internal fixation

SCI spinal cord injury

SLAP superior labrum anterior-posterior

TBI traumatic brain injury

ICD-9-CM

Official Guidelines for Coding and Reporting

Please refer to the companion Evolve website for the most current guidelines.
17. Chapter 17: Injury and Poisoning (800-999)
  a. Coding of Injuries
  When coding injuries, assign separate codes for each injury unless a combination code is provided, in which case the combination code is assigned. Multiple injury codes are provided in ICD-9-CM, but should not be assigned unless information for a more specific code is not available. These traumatic injury codes are not to be used for normal, healing surgical wounds or to identify complications of surgical wounds.
  The code for the most serious injury, as determined by the provider and the focus of treatment, is sequenced first.
  1) Superficial injuries
  Superficial injuries such as abrasions or contusions are not coded when associated with more severe injuries of the same site.

EXAMPLE   Abrasion with laceration to the left knee, 891.0, E928.9 (S81.012A, X58.xxxA).

Usually, when initial injuries are coded, E code(s) would describe the injury and place of occurrence. Because of the limited information given in these examples, it may not be possible to assign E code(s).

  2) Primary injury with damage to nerves/blood vessels
  When a primary injury results in minor damage to peripheral nerves or blood vessels, the primary injury is sequenced first with additional code(s) from categories 950-957, Injury to nerves and spinal cord, and/or 900-904, Injury to blood vessels. When the primary injury is to the blood vessels or nerves, that injury should be sequenced first.

EXAMPLE   Minor laceration of splenic artery and fracture of right little finger due to trauma from being kicked and falling during a football game. Suture of laceration of splenic artery, 902.23, 816.00, E917.5, E849.4, E007.0, 39.31 (S35.291A, S62.606A, W50.1xxA, Y92.321, 04Q40ZZ).

b. Coding of Traumatic Fractures

The principles of multiple coding of injuries should be followed in coding fractures. Fractures of specified sites are coded individually by site in accordance with both the provisions within categories 800-829 and the level of detail furnished by medical record content. Combination categories for multiple fractures are provided for use when there is insufficient detail in the medical record (such as trauma cases transferred to another hospital), when the reporting form limits the number of codes that can be used in reporting pertinent clinical data, or when there is insufficient specificity at the fourth-digit or fifth-digit level. More specific guidelines are as follows:

1) Acute Fractures vs. Aftercare

Traumatic fractures are coded using the acute fracture codes (800-829) while the patient is receiving active treatment for the fracture. Examples of active treatment are: surgical treatment, emergency department encounter, and evaluation and treatment by a new physician.

EXAMPLE The patient suffered a blow-out fracture 1 week ago and is now being referred to a specialist for consultation, 802.6, E887 (S02.3xxA, X58.xxxA).

Fractures are coded using the aftercare codes (subcategories V54.0, V54.1, V54.8, or V54.9) for encounters after the patient has completed active treatment of the fracture and is receiving routine care for the fracture during the healing or recovery phase. Examples of fracture aftercare are: cast change or removal, removal of external or internal fixation device, medication adjustment, and follow up visits following fracture treatment.

EXAMPLE The patient is seen in follow-up for healing blow-out fracture, V54.19 (S02.3xxD, X58.xxxD).

Care for complications of surgical treatment for fracture repairs during the healing or recovery phase should be coded with the appropriate complication codes.

Care of complications of fractures, such as malunion and nonunion, should be reported with the appropriate codes.

Pathologic fractures are not coded in the 800-829 range, but instead are assigned to subcategory 733.1. *See Section I.C.13.a for additional information.*

2) Multiple fractures of same limb

Multiple fractures of same limb classifiable to the same three-digit or four-digit category are coded to that category.

EXAMPLE Fractures of multiple metacarpal bones of the right hand, 815.09, E887 (S62.309A, X58.xxxA).

3) Multiple unilateral or bilateral fractures of same bone

Multiple unilateral or bilateral fractures of same bone(s) but classified to different fourth-digit subdivisions (bone part) within the same three-digit category are coded individually by site.

EXAMPLE Closed fracture of right surgical neck of humerus and left open fracture of anatomic neck of humerus, 812.12, 812.01, E887 (S42.292B, S42.211A, X58.xxxA).

> **4) Multiple fracture categories 819 and 828**
> Multiple fracture categories 819 and 828 classify bilateral fractures of both upper limbs (819) and both lower limbs (828), but without any detail at the fourth-digit level other than open and closed type of fractures.
> **5) Multiple fractures sequencing**
> Multiple fractures are sequenced in accordance with the severity of the fracture. The provider should be asked to list the fracture diagnoses in the order of severity.

EXAMPLE   The patient had a fractured parietal bone of the skull and fracture of the left fifth rib, 800.00, 807.01, E887 (S02.0xxA, S22.32xA, X58.xxxA).

EXTERNAL CAUSES

As with V codes, detailed guidelines have been put forth for the use of E codes. In ICD-9-CM the Index for E codes is located after the Alphabetic Index for diseases. Codes are located by using the Index and then verifying the appropriate E code in the Tabular. The Tabular List for E codes is found after the V code Tabular. The assignment of E codes may depend on facility policy and particular state requirements. For example, the assignment of E codes could be helpful in determining the number of head injuries that occur as the result of bicycle accidents. These data may be used to support bicycle helmet programs in a particular city or state. Codes for external causes are never used as a principal diagnosis; E codes are always assigned as an additional code. E codes identify the cause of an injury, adverse effects or poisoning, and the intent and place of occurrence. E codes for an adverse effect or poisoning can be found in the Table of Drugs and Chemicals. It may be necessary to assign more than one E code to fully describe the event.

According to the guidelines, E codes only need to be assigned for the initial visit (except when acute fracture codes are still applicable). Insufficient documentation can make it difficult to assign E codes and especially place of occurrence E codes. Although a place of occurrence code, E849.9, is in the code book to designate an unspecified place, the guidelines state not to use an E code if the place of occurrence is not stated. It takes practice to figure out which main terms to look up in the Alphabetic Index.

EXAMPLE   Concussion due to accidental fall down steps at home, 850.9, E880.9, E849.0 (S06.0x9A, W10.9xxA, Y92.00, Y99.8).

The E code guidelines are used for injuries, poisonings, adverse affects, complications of surgical and medical care, and other late effects. Because these conditions are covered in the next three chapters, the E code guidelines have been addressed in their respective chapters and numbering/lettering may not be sequential.

> **19. Supplemental Classification External Causes Injury and Poisoning (E-codes, E800-E999)**
> Introduction: These guidelines are provided for those who are currently collecting E codes in order that there will be standardization in the process. If your institution plans to begin collecting E codes, these guidelines are to be applied. The use of E codes is supplemental to the application of ICD-9-CM diagnosis codes.
> External causes of injury and poisoning codes (categories E000 and E800-E999) are intended to provide data for injury research and evaluation of injury prevention strategies. Activity codes (categories E001-E030) are intended to be used to describe the activity of a person seeking care for injuries as well as other health conditions, when the injury or other health condition resulted from an activity or the activity contributed to a condition. E codes capture how the injury, poisoning, or adverse effect happened (cause), the intent (unintentional or accidental; or intentional, such as suicide or assault), the person's status (e.g. civilian, military), the associated activity and the place where the event occurred.

Some major categories of E codes include:
- transport accidents
- poisoning and adverse effects of drugs, medicinal substances and biologicals
- accidental falls
- accidents caused by fire and flames
- accidents due to natural and environmental factors
- late effects of accidents, assaults or self injury
- assaults or purposely inflicted injury
- suicide or self inflicted injury

These guidelines apply for the coding and collection of E codes from records in hospitals, outpatient clinics, emergency departments, other ambulatory care settings and provider offices, and nonacute care settings, except when other specific guidelines apply.

The Supplementary Classification of E codes is divided into the following categories:

CATEGORY	SECTION TITLES
E800-E807	Railway Accidents
E810-E819	Motor Vehicle Traffic Accidents
E820-E825	Motor Vehicle Nontraffic Accidents
E826-E829	Other Road Vehicle Accidents
E830-E838	Water Transport Accidents
E840-E845	Air and Space Transport Accidents
E846-E848	Vehicle Accidents, Not Elsewhere Classifiable
E849	Place of Occurrence
E850-E858	Accidental Poisoning by Drugs, Medicinal Substances, and Biologicals
E860-E869	Accidental Poisoning by Other Solid and Liquid Substances, Gases, and Vapors
E870-E876	Misadventures of Patients During Surgical and Medical Care
E878-E879	Surgical and Medical Procedure as the Cause of Abnormal Reaction of Patient or Later Complication, Without Mention of Misadventure at the Time of Procedure
E880-E888	Accidental Falls
E890-E899	Accidents Caused by Fire and Flames
E900-E909	Accidents Due to Natural and Environmental Factors
E910-E915	Accidents Caused by Submersion, Suffocation, and Foreign Bodies
E916-E928	Other Accidents
E929	Late Effects of Accidental Injury
E930-E949	Drugs, Medicinal and Biological Substances Causing Adverse Effects in Therapeutic Use
E950-E959	Suicide and Self-inflicted Injury
E960-E969	Homicide and Injury Purposely Inflicted by Other Persons
E970-E978	Legal Intervention
E980-E989	Injury Undetermined Whether Accidentally or Purposely Inflicted
E990-E999	Injury Resulting from Operations of War

a. General E Code Coding Guidelines
   1) Used with any code in the range of 001-*V91*

An E code from categories E800-E999 may be used with any code in the range of 001-**V91**, which indicates an injury, poisoning, or adverse effect due to an external cause.

An activity E code (categories E001-E030) may be used with any code in the range of 001-**V91** that indicates an injury, or other health condition that resulted from an activity, or the activity contributed to a condition.

The activity codes are not applicable to poisonings, adverse effects, misadventures or late effects. **Do not assign E030, Unspecified activity, if the activity is not stated.**

2) Assign the appropriate E code for all initial treatments

Assign the appropriate E code for the initial encounter of an injury, poisoning, or adverse effect of drugs, not for subsequent treatment.

External cause of injury codes (E-codes) may be assigned while the acute fracture codes are still applicable.

See Section 1.C.17.b.1 for coding of acute fractures.

EXAMPLE

Injury of left knee due to twisting movement while playing basketball at the YMCA gym, 959.7, E927.0, E849.4, E007.6, E000.8 (S89.92xA, Y93.67, Y92.310, Y99.8).

3) Use the full range of E codes

Use the full range of E codes (E800-E999) to completely describe the cause, the intent and the place of occurrence, if applicable, for all injuries, poisonings, and adverse effects of drugs.

See a.1.), j.), and k.) in this section for information on the use of status and activity E codes.

EXAMPLE

Injury of left wrist and dislocation of right elbow from fall on escalator in public building. Dislocation was reduced, 832.00, 959.3, E880.0, E849.6, 79.72 (S53.104A, S69.92xA, W10.0xxA, Y92.29, 0RSLXZZ).

4) Assign as many E codes as necessary

Assign as many E codes as necessary to fully explain each cause. If only one E code can be recorded, assign the E code most related to the principal diagnosis.

5) The selection of the appropriate E code

The selection of the appropriate E code is guided by the Index to External Causes, which is located after the alphabetical index to diseases and by Inclusion and Exclusion notes in the Tabular List.

6) E code can never be a principal diagnosis

An E code can never be a principal (first listed) diagnosis.

Usually, E codes are reported in a specific designated area within a computer system or on an abstracting form. A limited number of fields may be available for reporting of E codes. When this occurs, the coder will need to refer to these guidelines to aid in the selection of the most important E codes. Facility policy may also provide instruction.

7) External cause code(s) with systemic inflammatory response syndrome (SIRS)

An external cause code is not appropriate with a code from subcategory 995.9, unless the patient also has another condition for which an E code would be appropriate (such as an injury, poisoning, or adverse effect of drugs.

8) Multiple Cause E Code Coding Guidelines

More than one E-code is required to fully describe the external cause of an illness, injury or poisoning. The assignment of E-codes should be sequenced in the following priority:

If two or more events cause separate injuries, an E code should be assigned for each cause. The first listed E code will be selected in the following order:

E codes for child and adult abuse take priority over all other E codes.

See Section I.C.19.e., Child and Adult abuse guidelines.

E codes for terrorism events take priority over all other E codes except child and adult abuse.

E codes for cataclysmic events take priority over all other E codes except child and adult abuse and terrorism.

E codes for transport accidents take priority over all other E codes except cataclysmic events, child and adult abuse and terrorism.

Activity and external cause status codes are assigned following all causal (intent) E codes.

The first-listed E code should correspond to the cause of the most serious diagnosis due to an assault, accident, or self-harm, following the order of hierarchy listed above.

9) If the reporting format limits the number of E codes

If the reporting format limits the number of E codes that can be used in reporting clinical data, report the code for the cause/intent most related to the principal diagnosis. If the format permits capture of additional E codes, the cause/intent, including medical misadventures, of the additional events should be reported rather than the codes for place, activity or external status.

b. Place of Occurrence Guideline

Use an additional code from category E849 to indicate the Place of Occurrence for injuries and poisonings. The Place of Occurrence describes the place where the event occurred and not the patient's activity at the time of the event.

Do not use E849.9 if the place of occurrence is not stated.

EXAMPLE

Injury to the left wrist occurred on the playground at the public park. Patient fell off slide, 959.3, E884.0, E849.4, E006.9, E000.8 (S69.92xA, W09.0xxA, Y92.830, Y93.59, Y99.8).

e. Unknown or Suspected Intent Guideline

1) If the intent (accident, self-harm, assault) of the cause of an injury or poisoning is unknown

If the intent (accident, self-harm, assault) of the cause of an injury or poisoning is unknown or unspecified, code the intent as undetermined E980-E989.

EXAMPLE

Laceration of left wrist from sharp glass, intent unknown, 881.02, E986 (S61.512A, Y28.0xxA, Y92.9).

2) If the intent (accident, self-harm, assault) of the cause of an injury or poisoning is questionable

If the intent (accident, self-harm, assault) of the cause of an injury or poisoning is questionable, probable or suspected, code the intent as undetermined E980-E989.

EXAMPLE

Laceration of left wrist from sharp glass, suspected suicide attempt, 881.02, E986 (S61.512A, Y28.0xxA).

f. Undetermined Cause

When the intent of an injury or poisoning is known, but the cause is unknown, use codes: E928.9, Unspecified accident, E958.9, Suicide and self-inflicted injury by unspecified means, and E968.9, Assault by unspecified means.

These E codes should rarely be used, as the documentation in the medical record, in both the inpatient outpatient and other settings, should normally provide sufficient detail to determine the cause of the injury.

g. **Late Effects of External Cause Guidelines**
   1) **Late effect E codes**
      Late effect E codes exist for injuries and poisonings but not for adverse effects of drugs, misadventures and surgical complications.
   2) **Late effect E codes (E929, E959, E969, E977, E989, or E999.1)**
      A late effect E code (E929, E959, E969, E977, E989, or E999.1) should be used with any report of a late effect or sequela resulting from a previous injury or poisoning (905-909).

EXAMPLE | Left wrist with keloid scar due to previous burns from fire (accidental), 701.4, 906.6, E929.4 (L91.0, T23.072S, X08.8xxS).

   3) **Late effect E code with a related current injury**
      A late effect E code should never be used with a related current nature of injury code.
   4) **Use of late effect E codes for subsequent visits**
      Use a late effect E code for subsequent visits when a late effect of the initial injury or poisoning is being treated. There is no late effect E code for adverse effects of drugs. Do not use a late effect E code for subsequent visits for follow-up care (e.g., to assess healing, to receive rehabilitative therapy) of the injury or poisoning when no late effect of the injury has been documented.

EXAMPLE | Subsequent encounter for malunion fracture of right tibia from motor vehicle accident, 733.81, 905.4, E929.0 (S82.201P, V89.2xxS).

i. **Terrorism Guidelines**
   1) **Cause of injury identified by the Federal Government (FBI) as terrorism**
      When the cause of an injury is identified by the Federal Government (FBI) as terrorism, the first-listed E-code should be a code from category E979, Terrorism. The definition of terrorism employed by the FBI is found at the inclusion note at E979. The terrorism E-code is the only E-code that should be assigned. Additional E codes from the assault categories should not be assigned.

EXAMPLE | The patient (civilian) had a head injury due to a terrorist explosion, 959.01, E979.2, E000.8 (S09.90xA, Y38.2x2A, Y99.8).

   2) **Cause of an injury is suspected to be the result of terrorism**
      When the cause of an injury is suspected to be the result of terrorism a code from category E979 should not be assigned. Assign a code in the range of E codes based circumstances on the documentation of intent and mechanism.
   3) **Code E979.9, Terrorism, secondary effects**
      Assign code E979.9, Terrorism, secondary effects, for conditions occurring subsequent to the terrorist event. This code should not be assigned for conditions that are due to the initial terrorist act.

EXAMPLE | The patient (civilian) has chronic posttraumatic stress syndrome following a terrorist attack, subsequent encounter, 309.81, E979.9 (F43.12, Y38.9x2S).

4) Statistical tabulation of terrorism codes

For statistical purposes these codes will be tabulated within the category for assault, expanding the current category from E960-E969 to include E979 and E999.1.

j. Activity Code Guidelines

Assign a code from category E001-E030 to describe the activity that caused or contributed to the injury or other health condition.

Unlike other E codes, activity E codes may be assigned to indicate a health condition (not just injuries) resulted from an activity, or the activity contributed to the condition.

The activity codes are not applicable to poisonings, adverse effects, misadventures or late effects.

Do not assign E030, Unspecified activity, if the activity is not stated.

k. External cause status

A code from category E000, External cause status, should be assigned whenever any other E code is assigned for an encounter, including an Activity E code, except for the events noted below. Assign a code from category E000, External cause status, to indicate the work status of the person at the time the event occurred. The status code indicates whether the event occurred during military activity, whether a non-military person was at work, whether an individual including a student or volunteer was involved in a non-work activity at the time of the causal event.

A code from E000, External cause status, should be assigned, when applicable, with other external cause codes, such as transport accidents and falls. The external cause status codes are not applicable to poisonings, adverse effects, misadventures or late effects.

Do not assign a code from category E000 if no other E codes (cause, activity) are applicable for the encounter.

Do not assign code E000.9, Unspecified external cause status, if the status is not stated.

Remember that E codes identify how an injury occurred and the intent. E codes also identify the place that an injury occurred and describe the activity that caused the injury or other health condition. At the beginning of Chapter 17 in the ICD-9-CM code book, special instructions state, "Use E code(s) to identify the cause and intent of the injury or poisoning (E800-E999)" (Figure 23-1).

Apply the General Coding Guidelines as found in Chapter 5 and the Procedural Guidelines as found in Chapter 6.

17.   INJURY AND POISONING (800–999)

Use E code(s) to identify the cause and intent of the injury or poisoning (E800-E999)

Note:

1. The principle of multiple coding of injuries should be followed wherever possible. Combination categories for multiple injuries are provided for use when there is insufficient detail as to the nature of the individual conditions, or for primary tabulation purposes when it is more convenient to record a single code; otherwise, the component injuries should be coded separately.

Where multiple sites of injury are specified in the titles, the word "with" indicates involvement of both sites, and the word "and" indicates involvement of either or both sites. The word "finger" includes thumb.

2. Categories for "late effect" of injuries are to be found at 905–909.

FIGURE 23-1. Instructional note regarding the use of E code(s) to identify the cause and intent of the injury or poisoning (E800-E999).

ICD-10-CM

Official Guidelines for Coding and Reporting

Please refer to the companion Evolve website for the most current guidelines.

19. Chapter 19: Injury, poisoning, and certain other consequences of external causes (S00-T88)

a. Code Extensions

Most categories in chapter 19 have 7th character extensions that are required for each applicable code. Most categories in this chapter have three extensions (with the exception of fractures): A, initial encounter, D, subsequent encounter and S, sequela.

Extension "A", initial encounter is used while the patient is receiving active treatment for the injury. Examples of active treatment are: surgical treatment, emergency department encounter, and evaluation and treatment by a new physician.

Extension "D" subsequent encounter is used for encounters after the patient has received active treatment of the injury and is receiving routine care for the injury during the healing or recovery phase. Examples of subsequent care are: cast change or removal, removal of external or internal fixation device, medication adjustment, other aftercare and follow up visits following injury treatment.

The aftercare Z codes should not be used for aftercare for injuries. For aftercare of an injury, assign the acute injury code with the 7th character "D" (subsequent encounter).

Extension "S", sequela, is for use for complications or conditions that arise as a direct result of an injury, such as scar formation after a burn. The scars are sequelae of the burn. When using extension "S", it is necessary to use both the injury code that precipitated the sequela and the code for the sequela itself. The "S" is added only to the injury code, not the sequela code. The "S" extension identifies the injury responsible for the sequela. The specific type of sequela (e.g. scar) is sequenced first, followed by the injury code.

b. Coding of Injuries

When coding injuries, assign separate codes for each injury unless a combination code is provided, in which case the combination code is assigned. **Code T07, Unspecified multiple injuries** should not be assigned unless information for a more specific code is not available. **Traumatic** injury codes (S00-T14.9) are not to be used for normal, healing surgical wounds or to identify complications of surgical wounds.

The code for the most serious injury, as determined by the provider and the focus of treatment, is sequenced first.

1) Superficial injuries

Superficial injuries such as abrasions or contusions are not coded when associated with more severe injuries of the same site.

2) Primary injury with damage to nerves/blood vessels

When a primary injury results in minor damage to peripheral nerves or blood vessels, the primary injury is sequenced first with additional code(s) for injuries to nerves and spinal cord (such as category S04), and/or injury to blood vessels (such as category S15). When the primary injury is to the blood vessels or nerves, that injury should be sequenced first.

c. Coding of Traumatic Fractures

The principles of multiple coding of injuries should be followed in coding fractures. Fractures of specified sites are coded individually by site in accordance with both the provisions within categories S02, S12, S22, S32, S42, S49, S52, S59, S62, S72, S79, S82, S89, S92 and the level of detail furnished by medical record content.

A fracture not indicated as open or closed should be coded to closed. A fracture not indicated whether displaced or not displaced should be coded to displaced.

More specific guidelines are as follows:

1) Initial vs. Subsequent Encounter for Fractures

Traumatic fractures are coded using the appropriate 7th character extension for initial encounter (A, B, C) while the patient is receiving active treatment for the fracture. Examples of active treatment are: surgical treatment, emergency department encounter, and evaluation and treatment by a new physician.

The appropriate 7th character for initial encounter should also be assigned for a patient who delayed seeking treatment for the fracture or nonunion.

Fractures are coded using the appropriate 7th character extension for subsequent care for encounters after the patient has completed active treatment of the fracture and is receiving routine care for the fracture during the healing or recovery phase. Examples of fracture aftercare are: cast change or removal, removal of external or internal fixation device, medication adjustment, and follow-up visits following fracture treatment.

Care for complications of surgical treatment for fracture repairs during the healing or recovery phase should be coded with the appropriate complication codes.

Care of complications of fractures, such as malunion and nonunion, should be reported with the appropriate 7th character extensions for subsequent care with nonunion (K, M, N,) or subsequent care with malunion (P, Q, R).

A code from category M80, not a traumatic fracture code, should be used for any patient with known osteoporosis who suffers a fracture, even if the patient had a minor fall or trauma, if that fall or trauma would not usually break a normal, healthy bone.

See Section I.C.13. Osteoporosis.

The aftercare Z codes should not be used for aftercare for **traumatic fractures**. For aftercare of **a traumatic fracture**, assign the acute **fracture** code with the **appropriate** 7th character.

2) Multiple fractures sequencing

Multiple fractures are sequenced in accordance with the severity of the fracture.

20. Chapter 20: External Causes of Morbidity (V01-Y99)

Introduction: These guidelines are provided for the reporting of external causes of morbidity codes in order that there will be standardization in the process. These codes are secondary codes for use in any health care setting.

External cause codes are intended to provide data for injury research and evaluation of injury prevention strategies. These codes capture how the injury or health condition happened (cause), the intent (unintentional or accidental; or intentional, such as suicide or assault), the place where the event occurred the activity of the patient at the time of the event, and the person's status (e.g., civilian, military).

a. General External Cause Coding Guidelines

1) Used with any code in the range of A00.0-T88.9, Z00-Z99

An external cause code may be used with any code in the range of A00.0-T88.9, Z00-Z99, classification that is a health condition due to an external cause. Though they are most applicable to injuries, they are also valid for use with such things as infections or diseases due to an external source, and other health conditions, such as a heart attack that occurs during strenuous physical activity.

2) External cause code used for length of treatment

Assign the external cause code, with the appropriate 7th character (initial encounter, subsequent encounter or sequela) for each encounter for which the injury or condition is being treated.

3) Use the full range of external cause codes

Use the full range of external cause codes to completely describe the cause, the intent, the place of occurrence, and if applicable, the activity of the patient at the time of the event, and the patient's status, for all injuries, and other health conditions due to an external cause.

4) Assign as many external cause codes as necessary

Assign as many external cause codes as necessary to fully explain each cause. If only one external code can be recorded, assign the code most related to the principal diagnosis.

5) The selection of the appropriate external cause code

The selection of the appropriate external cause code is guided by the **Alphabetic Index of** External Causes and by Inclusion and Exclusion notes in the Tabular List.

6) External cause code can never be a principal diagnosis

An external cause code can never be a principal (**first-listed**) diagnosis.

7) Combination external cause codes

Certain of the external cause codes are combination codes that identify sequential events that result in an injury, such as a fall which results in striking against an object. The injury may be due to either event or both. The combination external cause code used should correspond to the sequence of events regardless of which caused the most serious injury.

8) No external cause code needed in certain circumstances

No external cause code from Chapter 20 is needed if the external cause and intent are included in a code from another chapter (e.g. **T36.0x1-** Poisoning by penicillins, accidental (unintentional)).

b. Place of Occurrence Guideline

Codes from category Y92, Place of occurrence of the external cause, are secondary codes for use after other external cause codes to identify the location of the patient at the time of injury or other condition.

A place of occurrence code is used only once, at the initial encounter for treatment. No 7th characters are used for Y92. Only one code from Y92 should be recorded on a medical record. A place of occurrence code should be used in conjunction with an activity code, Y93.

Do not use place of occurrence code Y92.9 if the place is not stated or is not applicable.

c. Activity Code

Assign a code from category Y93, Activity code, to describe the activity of the patient at the time the injury or other health condition occurred.

An activity code is used only once, at the initial encounter for treatment. Only one code from Y93 should be recorded on a medical record. An activity code should be used in conjunction with a place of occurrence code, Y92.

The activity codes are not applicable to poisonings, adverse effects, misadventures or late effects.

Do not assign Y93.9, Unspecified activity, if the activity is not stated.

A code from category Y93 is appropriate for use with external cause and intent codes if identifying the activity provides additional information about the event.

d. Place of Occurrence, Activity, *and Status* Codes Used with other External Cause Code

When applicable, place of occurrence, activity, and external cause status codes are sequenced after the main external cause code(s). Regardless of the number of external cause codes assigned, there should be only one place of occurrence code, one activity code, and one external cause status code assigned to an encounter.

e. If the Reporting Format Limits the Number of External Cause Codes

If the reporting format limits the number of external cause codes that can be used in reporting clinical data, report the code for the cause/intent most related to the principal diagnosis. If the format permits capture of additional external cause codes, the cause/intent, including medical misadventures, of the additional events should be reported rather than the codes for place, activity, or external status.

f. Multiple External Cause Coding Guidelines

More than one external cause code is required to fully describe the external cause of an illness **or** injury. The assignment of external cause codes should be sequenced in the following priority:

If two or more events cause separate injuries, an external cause code should be assigned for each cause. The first listed external cause code will be selected in the following order:

External codes for child and adult abuse take priority over all other external cause codes.

See Section I.C.19., Child and Adult abuse guidelines.

External cause codes for terrorism events take priority over all other external cause codes except child and adult abuse.

External cause codes for cataclysmic events take priority over all other external cause codes except child and adult abuse and terrorism.

External cause codes for transport accidents take priority over all other external cause codes except cataclysmic events, child and adult abuse and terrorism.

Activity and external cause status codes are assigned following all causal (intent) external cause codes.

The first-listed external cause code should correspond to the cause of the most serious diagnosis due to an assault, accident, or self-harm, following the order of hierarchy listed above.

h. Unknown or Undetermined Intent Guideline

If the intent (accident, self-harm, assault) of the cause of an injury or other condition is unknown or unspecified, code the intent as accidental intent. All transport accident categories assume accidental intent.

1) Use of undetermined intent

External cause codes for events of undetermined intent are only for use if the documentation in the record specifies that the intent cannot be **determined.**

i. Late Effects of External Cause Guidelines

1) Late effect external cause codes

Late effects are reported using the external cause code with the 7th character extension "S" for sequela. These codes should be used with any report of a late effect or sequela resulting from a previous injury.

2) Late effect external cause code with a related current injury

A late effect external cause code should never be used with a related current nature of injury code.

3) Use of late effect external cause codes for subsequent visits

Use a late effect external cause code for subsequent visits when a late effect of the initial injury is being treated. Do not use a late effect external cause code for subsequent visits for follow-up care (e.g., to assess healing, to receive rehabilitative therapy) of the injury when no late effect of the injury has been documented.

j. Terrorism Guidelines

1) Cause of injury identified by the Federal Government (FBI) as terrorism

When the cause of an injury is identified by the Federal Government (FBI) as terrorism, the first-listed external cause code should be a code from category Y38, Terrorism. The definition of terrorism employed by the FBI is found at the inclusion note at the beginning of category Y38. Use additional code for place of occurrence (Y92.-). More than one Y38 code may be assigned if the injury is the result of more than one mechanism of terrorism.

2) Cause of an injury is suspected to be the result of terrorism

When the cause of an injury is suspected to be the result of terrorism a code from category Y38 should not be assigned. Suspected cases should be classified as assault.

3) Code Y38.9, Terrorism, secondary effects

Assign code Y38.9, Terrorism, secondary effects, for conditions occurring subsequent to the terrorist event. This code should not be assigned for conditions that are due to the initial terrorist act.

It is acceptable to assign code Y38.9 with another code from Y38 if there is an injury due to the initial terrorist event and an injury that is a subsequent result of the terrorist event.

k. External cause status

A code from category Y99, External cause status, should be assigned whenever any other external cause code is assigned for an encounter, including an Activity code, except for the events noted below. Assign a code from category Y99, External cause status, to indicate the work status of the person at the time the event occurred. The status code indicates whether the event occurred during military activity, whether a non-military person was at work, whether an individual including a student or volunteer was involved in a non-work activity at the time of the causal event.

A code from Y99, External cause status, should be assigned, when applicable, with other external cause codes, such as transport accidents and falls. The external cause status codes are not applicable to poisonings, adverse effects, misadventures or late effects.

Do not assign a code from category Y99 if no other external cause codes (cause, activity) are applicable for the encounter.

An external cause status code is used only once, at the initial encounter for treatment. Only one code from Y99 should be recorded on a medical record.

Do not assign code Y99.9, Unspecified external cause status, if the status is not stated.

Apply the General Coding Guidelines as found in Chapter 5 and the Procedural Guidelines as found in Chapter 7.

GUIDELINE DIFFERENCES BETWEEN ICD-9-CM AND ICD-10-CM

- ICD-10-CM guidelines include instructions regarding the seventh-character extensions used in the injury chapter.
- ICD-10-CM guidelines explain the use of the initial versus subsequent encounter extensions for fractures.
- In ICD-9-CM, the guidelines state that if the intent of the cause of an injury is unknown or questionable, code the intent as undetermined. ICD-10-CM guidelines state that if the cause of an injury or other condition is unkown or unspecified, the intent is coded as accidental. Undetermined intent is only coded if the documentation in the record indicates that the intent cannot be determined.

MAJOR DIFFERENCES BETWEEN ICD-9-CM AND ICD-10-CM

- ICD-10-CM has more notes with instructions to code also any associated injuries.
- Laterality is specified in ICD-10-CM.
- In ICD-9-CM, there is a fourth digit to identify a laceration that is infected or "complicated." In ICD-10-CM, there are instructional notes under the open-wound categories to code also any associated wound infection.
- In ICD-10-CM, fractures are classified as nondisplaced or displaced. If a fracture is not specified, it should be coded to displaced.
- Most of the codes in Chapter 19 utilize the seventh character. Most of the codes use at least the following extensions:
  A Initial encounter
  D Subsequent encounter
  S Sequela
- Complications such as malunion and nonunion of a fracture are reported with the appropriate seventh-character extensions for subsequent care with nonunion (K, M, N) or subsequent care with malunion (P, Q, R).

EXERCISE 23-1

Using the Alphabetic Index for E codes, assign E codes to the following.

1. Bite by spider _____
2. Burn by cigar _____
3. Entanglement in wheel of bike _____
4. Self-inflicted hanging _____
5. Shot by BB gun _____
6. Fall from a ladder in the backyard _____
7. Injury due to lightning _____
8. Patient was bitten by a dog at a public park _____
9. Farmer was injured by a hay mower while mowing hay in the field _____
10. Child was accidentally burned by hot water _____

ANATOMY AND PHYSIOLOGY

The musculoskeletal chapter outlines the anatomy and physiology that is pertinent to injury. Internal organs and the blood vessels may also be involved in an injury. These are outlined in their respective body system chapters.

DISEASE CONDITIONS

Injury and Poisoning (800-999), Chapter 17 in your ICD-9-CM code book, covers a wide range of codes that will be discussed in the next three chapters of this textbook. Categories marked with an asterisk (*) are covered in this chapter. Chapter 24 discusses burns, adverse effects, and poisonings, and Chapter 25 is dedicated to complications associated with surgical and medical care. Injury and poisoning codes are divided into the following categories:

CATEGORY	SECTION TITLES
*800-804	Fracture of Skull
*805-809	Fracture of Neck and Trunk
*810-819	Fracture of Upper Limb
*820-829	Fracture of Lower Limb
*830-839	Dislocation
*840-848	Sprains and Strains of Joints and Adjacent Muscles
*850-854	Intracranial Injury, Excluding Those With Skull Fracture
*860-869	Internal Injury of Thorax, Abdomen, and Pelvis
*870-879	Open Wound of Head, Neck, and Trunk
*880-887	Open Wound of Upper Limb
*890-897	Open Wound of Lower Limb
*900-904	Injury to Blood Vessels
905-909	Late Effects of Injuries, Poisonings, Toxic Effects, and Other External Causes
*910-919	Superficial Injury
*920-924	Contusion With Intact Skin Surface
*925-929	Crushing Injury
*930-939	Effects of Foreign Body Entering Through Orifice
940-949	Burns
*950-957	Injury to Nerves and Spinal Cord
958-959	Certain Traumatic Complications and Unspecified Injuries
960-979	Poisoning by Drugs, Medicinals, and Biological Substances
980-989	Toxic Effects of Substances Chiefly Nonmedicinal as to Source
990-995	Other and Unspecified Effects of External Causes
996-999	Complications of Surgical and Medical Care, Not Elsewhere Classified

The S section is for coding different types of injuries related to single body regions, and the T section is for injuries to unspecified body regions, poisonings, and certain other consequences of external causes. Chapter 19 in the ICD-10-CM code book—Injury, Poisoning, and Certain Other Consequences of External Causes (S00-T88)—is divided into the following categories:

CATEGORY	SECTION TITLES
*S00-S09	Injuries to the Head
*S10-S19	Injuries to the Neck
*S20-S29	Injuries to the Thorax
*S30-S39	Injuries to the Abdomen, Lower Back, Lumbar Spine, Pelvis, and External Genitalia
*S40-S49	Injuries to the Shoulder and Upper Arm
*S50-S59	Injuries to the Elbow and Forearm
*S60-S69	Injuries to the Wrist and Hand
*S70-S79	Injuries to the Hip and Thigh
*S80-S89	Injuries to the Knee and Lower Leg
*S90-S99	Injuries to the Ankle and Foot
*T07	Unspecified Multiple Injuries
*T14	Injury of Unspecified Body Region
*T15-T19	Effects of Foreign Body Entering through Natural Orifice
T20-T32	Burns and Corrosions
T33-T34	Frostbite

CATEGORY	SECTION TITLES
T36-T50	Poisoning by, Adverse Effect of, and Underdosing of Drugs, Medicaments, and Biological Substances
T51-T65	Toxic Effects of Substances Chiefly Nonmedicinal as to Source
T66-T78	Other and Unspecified Effects of External Causes
*T79	Certain Early Complications of Trauma
T80-T88	Complications of Surgical and Medical Care, Not Elsewhere Classified

Fractures

Fractures are divided by the following anatomic sections:

800-804	Fracture of Skull
805-809	Fracture of Spine and Trunk
810-819	Fracture of Upper Limb
820-829	Fracture of Lower Limb

A **fracture** is a break in a bone. Bones are rigid but will bend. However, if the impact or force is too great, the bone will break. There are different types of fractures (Figure 23-2) with varying degrees of complexity. In a minor injury, the bone may just crack and may not break all the way through. In a more severe injury, the bone may shatter, or it may break through the skin. Treatment provided for a fracture depends on the specific bone broken, the severity of the break, and whether it is an "open" or a "closed" fracture.

Fractures fall into two categories:

1. **Closed fracture** or **simple fracture** is diagnosed when the bone is broken, but the skin remains intact. Descriptive words used for a closed fracture include the following:
   * Comminuted—broken, splintered, or crushed into a number of pieces
   * Depressed—portion of the skull that is broken and driven inward
   * Fissured—incomplete fracture that does not split the bone
   * Fracture NOS—not otherwise specified
   * Greenstick—the bone is somewhat bent and is partially broken; occurs in children
   * Impacted—one fractured bone end is wedged into another broken end
   * Linear—straight line fracture
   * Simple—fracture that remains in alignment with little damage to surrounding tissue
   * Slipped epiphysis—separation of the growing end of the bone (epiphysis) from the shaft of the bone; occurs in children and young adults
   * Spiral—occurs when a bone has been twisted apart

2. **Open fracture** or **compound fracture** occurs when the bone exits and is visible through the skin, or a deep wound exposes the bone through the skin. If the wound is superficial and the fracture site is not exposed, the injury is coded as a closed fracture—not an open fracture. Some descriptive words used for an open fracture include the following:
   * Compound—fracture in which the bone is sticking through the skin
   * Infected—condition in which the bone becomes infected by bacteria
   * Missile—penetrating injuries resulting in fractures caused by bullets or stab wounds
   * Puncture—a puncture wound is present. The wound may be related to the injury or to bone fragments
   * Foreign body—presence of a foreign body within the fracture site

If a fracture is not specified as open or closed, it is coded as a closed fracture. If documentation in the record reveals an open wound around the fracture site, it may be necessary to query the physician as to whether this is an open or a closed fracture. In some instances, a fracture is documented as both open and closed. This usually occurs with a severe fracture with fracture fragments, and it should be coded as an open fracture. A **complicated fracture** is a fracture that causes injury to surrounding tissues; it may be open or closed.

FIGURE 23-2. Types of fractures.

Open fractures may be identified by the **Gustilo open fracture classification**, which is based on the mechanism of the injury and the amount of soft tissue and skeletal injury. This classification system is useful in assessing risk of infection and possible amputation.

- Type I: clean wound smaller than 1 cm in diameter, appears clean, simple fracture pattern, minimal soft tissue injury.
- Type II: a laceration greater than 1 cm but with moderate soft tissue injury. Fracture pattern may be more complex.
- Type III: an open segmental fracture or a single fracture with extensive soft tissue injury. Also included are injuries older than 8 hours. Type III injuries are subdivided into three types:
  - Type IIIA: adequate soft tissue coverage of the fracture despite high energy trauma or extensive laceration or skin flaps.
  - Type IIIB: inadequate soft tissue coverage with periosteal stripping and bone exposure. Soft tissue reconstruction is necessary. Wound is contaminated.
  - Type IIIC: any open fracture that is associated with vascular (major arterial) injury that requires repair.

If a physician does not document the exact location of a fracture, *Coding Clinic* (1999:1Q:p5)[1] says it is acceptable to review the entire recording, including the radiology report, to identify the exact location of the fracture. If there is any question as to the appropriate diagnosis, the physician should be queried before assigning a diagnosis code.

EXAMPLE

> The physician documents closed fracture of right tibia. The x-ray report indicates a fracture of the shaft of the right tibia, 823.20, E887 (S82.201A, X58.xxxA).

It is acceptable to use the more specific 823.20 code instead of 823.80 as documented by the physician.

EXAMPLE

> The physician documents closed fracture of right tibia. The x-ray report indicates a fracture through the shaft of the right tibia and fibula.
> In this instance, the physician would need to be queried regarding the fracture of the fibula before code 823.22 (S82.201A, S82.401A, X58.xxxA) is assigned.

Specific coding guidelines assist with sequencing and coding of fractures. The most severe fracture is sequenced first. The fourth digits of fracture codes usually indicate whether a fracture is open or closed; the fifth digits indicate more specific bones or locations within the general site. When a patient presents with multiple fractures, all fractures must be coded. Although multiple fracture categories 819 and 828 are provided, codes from these categories would rarely be used. In the inpatient setting, it may be necessary to query the physician for more specific information.

A **pathologic fracture** is a break in a bone that occurs because of underlying disorders that weaken the bone, including malignancy, benign bone tumor, metabolic disorders, infection, and osteoporosis. A fracture can result from normal stress placed on an abnormal bone. Minor trauma can cause fracture. It is important to determine whether a fracture is pathologic or traumatic, so the appropriate code can be assigned. Coding of pathologic fractures is discussed in Chapter 18. Fractures that are due to a birth injury are classified as perinatal conditions.

Skull Fractures

Skull fracture may be associated with traumatic head injury. Injury to the brain may also occur. In most skull fractures, there is no displacement of broken bones. This is a closed or simple fracture. In severe cases, bone fragments are displaced, resulting in an open and/or depressed skull fracture. Fractures of the skull are frequently encountered after falls, crushing injuries, direct blows to the head, or motor vehicle accidents. A simple skull fracture may have little impact on eventual neurologic outcomes of head trauma. Neurologic outcomes of a skull fracture are determined by the nature of the brain injury. Some trauma patients can have severe neurologic impairment without having a skull fracture. The cranium, which protects the brain, consists of eight bones: occipital, frontal, sphenoidal, ethmoidal, two parietal, and two temporal bones (Figure 23-3). Categories 850 to 854 have fourth- or fifth-digit designations that are specific to the patient's level of consciousness. **Loss of consciousness** (LOC) occurs when a patient is unable to respond to people or to other stimuli. Unconsciousness and other sudden changes in mental status should be treated as a medical emergency.

EXAMPLE

> Fracture of frontal skull bone due to motor vehicle accident involving head-on collision with pick-up truck, unbelted car passenger. The patient did not lose consciousness, 800.01, E812.1, E849.5 (S02.0xxA, V43.63xA, Y92.410).

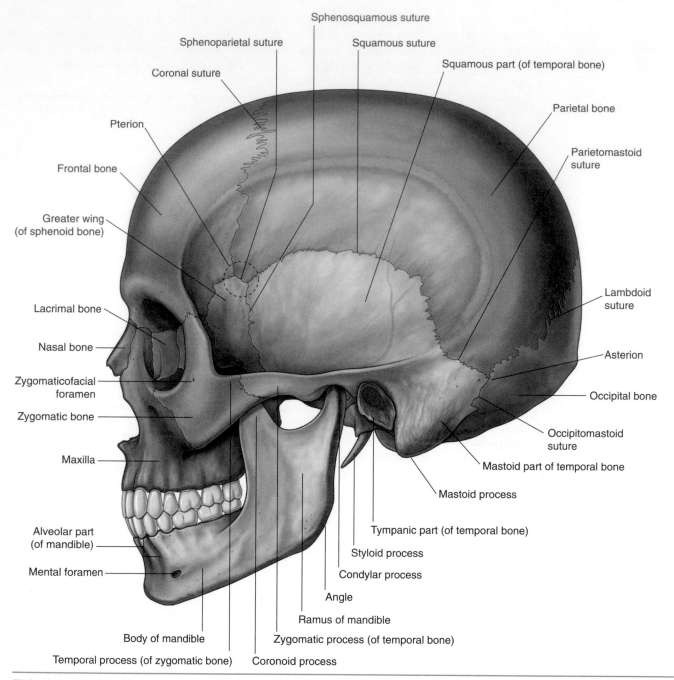

FIGURE 23-3. Lateral view of the skull.

Spine Fractures

As was discussed in Chapter 19, vertebral fractures are often pathologic fractures, particularly in older women with osteoporosis. This chapter focuses on traumatic spinal fractures, which usually occur as the result of motor vehicle accidents, falls, acts of violence, or recreational and sporting activities. Spinal fracture does not necessarily indicate damage to the spinal cord, and a spinal cord injury can occur without a spinal fracture. Injuries to the spinal cord without associated fractures and nerve injuries are assigned to codes 950 to 957. Category 806 includes combination codes for use in cases of spinal fracture with spinal cord injury (Figures 23-4).

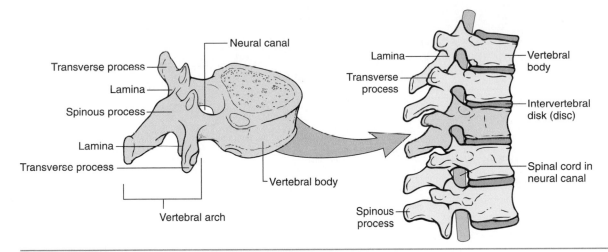

FIGURE 23-4. Lateral view of vertebrae.

Clay shoveler's fracture C7 (nondisplaced) due to strain injury from shoveling while working at construction site, 805.07, E927.8, E849.3, E016.0, E000.0 (S12.601A, Y93.h1, Y92.69, Y99.0).

Upper Limb Fractures

Shoulder and upper arm (Figure 23-5) injuries, including fractures of the clavicle or the upper part of the humerus, are fairly common. Fractures of the scapula are less common. A **Colles' fracture** is a common fracture in adults. In this type of fracture, the lower end of the radius is fractured, and the wrist and the hand are displaced backward. Fractures of the ulna typically occur across the shaft or at the tip of the elbow. Sometimes, the radius is fractured at the same time. Fractures of the radius, which are among the most common of fractures, usually are caused by a fall on an outstretched hand. The disc-shaped head of the bone just below the elbow joint is one of the most common sites of fracture in young adults. Fingers often sustain lacerations, fractures, and tendon ruptures. Fractures are particularly common at the knuckles, usually in the little finger, as the result of a blow.

Right Boxers' fracture (neck of the fifth metacarpal) due to brawl at nightclub. The patient was employed at the nightclub as a bouncer, 815.04, E960.0, E849.6, E000.0 (S62.336A, Y04.0xxA, Y99.0).

Lower Limb Fractures

A fractured hip is usually a fracture of the head or neck of the femur. The nature, symptoms, treatment, and possible complications of a fractured femur depend on whether the bone has been broken across its neck or across the shaft. A fracture in the shaft of the femur usually occurs when the femur is subjected to extreme force, as occurs in a motor vehicle accident.

In most cases, the bone ends are considerably displaced, causing severe pain, tenderness, and swelling. The patella is the triangular bone that protects the knee joint. Fracture is usually caused by a direct blow. The tibia is one of the most commonly fractured bones. It may break across the shaft as the result of a direct blow to the front of the leg, or at the upper end from a blow to the outside of the leg below the knee. The fibula, a very common site of fracture, usually breaks just above the ankle as the result of a harsh twisting motion, such as occurs in severe ankle sprain. Injury to the foot commonly results in fractures of the bones in the toes, caused by stubbing or twisting them or as the result of a falling or crushing injury. The calcaneus may fracture after a fall from a height onto a hard surface (Figures 23-6 and 23-7).

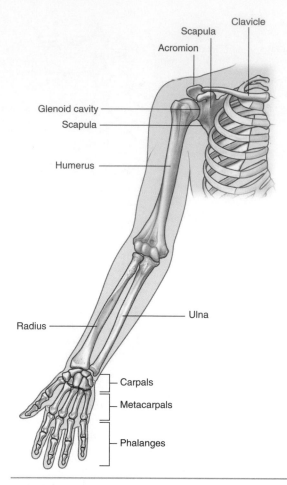

FIGURE 23-5. Bones of the upper limb.

EXAMPLE | Left Dupuytren's fracture due to fall from horse while riding in meadow, 824.4, E828.2, E006.1, E000.8, E849.8 (S82.62xA, V80.010A, Y92.828, Y93.52, Y99.8).

Traumatic Fractures and Fracture Aftercare

Active treatment of a traumatic fracture includes surgery, an Emergency Room encounter, and/or evaluation and treatment by a new physician. According to the guidelines, when a patient is receiving active treatment, the acute fracture code is assigned.

Following the period of active treatment of a traumatic fracture, other encounters may be necessary. These encounters are assigned aftercare V codes. Aftercare may include a cast change or removal, removal of a fixation device, medication adjustments, and other follow-up visits.

EXAMPLE | Patient is admitted for open reduction of right orbital floor fracture. Patient was involved in a fight at a bar last week, and this was the initial encounter for treatment, 802.6, E960.0, E849.6, 76.79 (S02.3xxA, Y04.0xxA, Y92.29, 0NSP0ZZ).

EXAMPLE | Patient had a cast change for traumatic radial shaft fracture, V54.12, 97.11 (S52.309D, 2W0CX2Z).

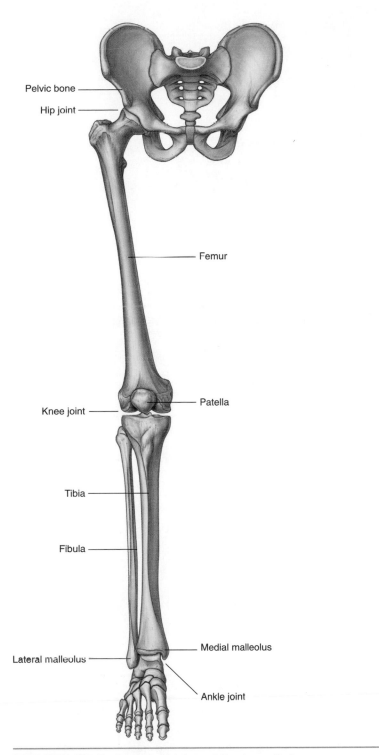

FIGURE 23-6. Bones and joints of the lower limb.

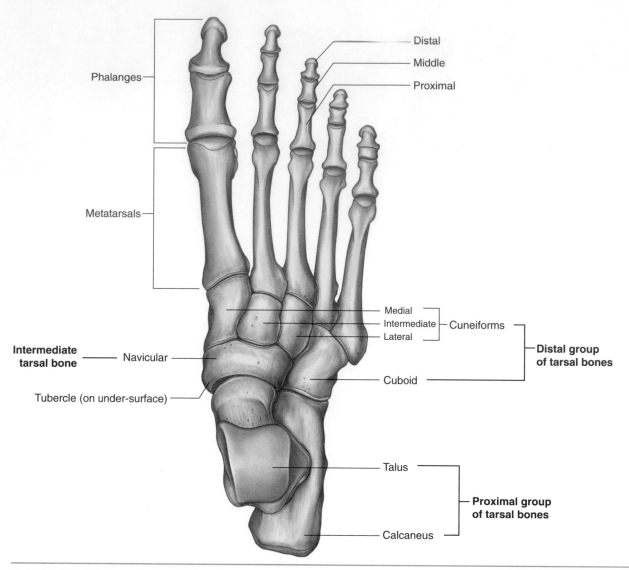

FIGURE 23-7. Dorsal view of right foot.

Assign codes to the following conditions.

1. Type II Salter Harris fracture left fifth proximal phalanx due to fall from scooter   _____

2. Nondisplaced right lateral malleolus fracture due to slipping on gravel while jogging   _____

3. Comminuted left calcaneal fracture due to fall from ladder while doing home repairs   _____

4. Open fracture distal right tibia and fibula due to motorcycle accident involving loss of control on wet highway. Patient was driver of the motorcycle   _____

5. Avulsion fracture of the medial aspect of the left patella as a result of falling on cement at school playground   _____

6. LeFort I fracture due to being hit by baseball during baseball game   _____

7. Fracture cervical spine C1 and C2 due to diving into shallow swimming pool (hitting bottom) at hotel   _____

8. Compound fracture midshaft of right femur due to motorcycle accident with crash into a car   _____

9. Fracture midshaft left clavicle due to tackle during football practice   _____

10. Temporal skull fracture due to self-inflicted gunshot; patient had intracranial hemorrhage   _____

11. Patient was seen for removal of internal fixation device from previous right traumatic tibial fracture   _____

12. Follow-up visit for traumatic pelvic fracture   _____

Dislocations

Dislocation is the displacement of the bones that form a joint. It is the separation of the end of a bone and the joint it meets. A partial or incomplete dislocation is called a **subluxation.** Dislocations may occur as the result of traumatic injury, or they may result from diseases such as rheumatoid arthritis, congenital joint defects, or weakened joints due to previous injury. The shoulder is especially prone to dislocation. The elbow is a common site of dislocation in toddlers. Other sites include fingers, hips, jaws, and spine. Soft tissues such as ligaments, tendons, muscles, and cartilage in and around the joint may stretch or tear as a result of the dislocation. Nerves and blood vessels may also be injured by the dislocated bone.

It is possible for a fracture and dislocation/subluxation to occur at the same anatomic site. In these instances, the Index gives the coder instructions under the main term "Dislocation": It says, "with fracture—*see* Fracture, by site" (Figure 23-8). This means that only the fracture code is assigned for fractures/dislocations at the same site. According to *Coding Clinic* (1990:3Q:p13),[2] it is incorrect to also code the dislocation. Reduction of fracture/

Dislocation (articulation) (closed) (displacement) (simple) (subluxation) 839.8

Note

"Closed" includes simple, complete, partial, uncomplicated, and unspecified dislocation.

"Open" includes dislocation specified as infected or compound and dislocation with foreign body.

"Chronic," "habitual," "old," or "recurrent" dislocations should be coded as indicated under the entry "Dislocation, recurrent"; and "pathological" as indicated under the entry "Dislocation, pathological."

For late effect of dislocation see Late, effect, dislocation.

with fracture - *see* Fracture, by site ◀

FIGURE 23-8. Instruction for dislocation with fracture—see Fracture, by site.

dislocation is coded to reduction of fracture. No additional code is assigned for reduction of a dislocation.

Once a joint has been dislocated, it is not unusual for it to dislocate again; with each recurrence, less force is required to sustain a dislocation. According to *Coding Clinic* (1997:Nov-Dec:p7),[3] only the initial occurrence of the dislocation is coded with an injury code, and all subsequent dislocations of the same joint are coded as recurrent dislocations.

EXAMPLE

> The patient sustained an open dislocation of distal interphalageal joint of right little finger during tackle on school football field during game, 834.12, E886.0, E007.0, E849.4, E000.8 (S63.296A, S61.206A, W03.xxxA, Y92.321, Y93.61, Y99.8).

EXERCISE 23-3

Assign codes to the following conditions.

1. Dislocation right patella due to fall at nursing home _____
2. Dislocation proximal interphalangeal joint left index finger due to jamming finger while playing basketball at gym during high school game _____
3. Recurrent dislocation right shoulder _____
4. Subluxation left elbow due to twisting injury during gymnastics practice at the gym. Patient is 10 years old _____

Sprains and Strains of Joints and Adjacent Muscles

A **sprain** is a stretch and/or tear of a ligament. The severity of the injury depends on whether a tear is partial or complete and on the number of ligaments involved. A **strain** is an injury to a muscle or a tendon. Depending on the severity of the injury, a strain may be the result of an overstretched muscle or tendon, or it can be caused by a partial or complete tear. Often, the patient is unaware of any specific injury. Strains can be acute or chronic. Chronic strains usually result from overuse or prolonged repetitive movement.

EXAMPLE

> The patient has an anterior cruciate ligament sprain due to injury 844.2, E928.9 (S83.519A, X58.xxxA).

EXERCISE 23-4

Assign codes to the following conditions.

1. Sprain left hand due to sliding into third base during baseball game in backyard of private residence _____
2. Strain lumbosacral spine due to overexertion from lifting at factory _____
3. Rupture of left Achilles tendon while playing racquetball due to twisting injury at the gym after work _____
4. SLAP (superior labrum anterior-posterior) lesion on right shoulder while rock climbing and fall from cliff in the mountains _____

INTRACRANIAL INJURY, EXCLUDING THOSE WITH SKULL FRACTURE (850–854)

> **Excludes** *intracranial injury with skull fracture (800–801 and 803–804, except .0 and .5)*
> *open wound of head without intracranial injury (870.0–873.9)*
> *skull fracture alone (800–801 and 803–804 with .0, .5)*

Note: The description "with open intracranial wound," used in the fourth-digit subdivisions, includes those specified as open or with mention of infection or foreign body.

The following fifth-digit subclassification is for use with categories 851–854:

☐ 0 unspecified state of consciousness
1 with no loss of consciousness
2 with brief [less than one hour] loss of consciousness
3 with moderate [1–24 hours] loss of consciousness
4 with prolonged [more than 24 hours] loss of consciousness and return to pre-existing conscious level
5 with prolonged [more than 24 hours] loss of consciousness without return to pre-existing conscious level

> Use fifth-digit 5 to designate when a patient is unconscious and dies before regaining consciousness, regardless of the duration of the loss of consciousness

☐ 6 with loss of consciousness of unspecified duration
☐ 9 with concussion, unspecified

FIGURE 23-9. Fifth digit code assignment for level of consciousness.

Intracranial Injury, Excluding Those With Skull Fracture

Intracranial injuries that are not associated with skull fracture(s) are assigned codes in categories 850-854. A **concussion** is an injury to the brain that results from a significant blow to the head. Length of unconsciousness may relate to severity of the concussion. Most people recover with no ill effects. A patient may have to be admitted to the hospital for observation. The fourth or fifth digit designates the length of time that the patient was unconscious (Figure 23-9). It may be necessary to review the Emergency Room and ambulance records to determine the time that the patient was unconscious.

Traumatic brain injury (TBI) is injury to the brain that may affect the brain's normal functions. Penetrating injuries are injuries in which a foreign object such as a bullet enters the brain. Symptoms vary depending on the areas of the brain that are damaged.

Closed head injury (CHI) results from a blow to the head. Primary brain damage may occur at the time of the injury or accident. Secondary brain damage may result from complications of the injury such as brain swelling, increased intracranial pressure, seizure, infection, fever, hematoma, high or low blood pressure, anemia, and metabolic changes.

EXAMPLE Patient was hospitalized with a concussion due to tripping while jumping rope at school. Unconscious for 5 minutes, 850.11, E885.9, E849.6, E006.5, E000.8 (S06.0x1A, W01.0xxA, Y92.219, Y93.56, Y99.8).

EXERCISE 23-5

Assign codes to the following conditions.

1. Cerebral contusion due to fall on ice in driveway. Positive for loss of consciousness   _____

2. Laceration brain due to impact from motor vehicle accident (MVA). Loss of consciousness lasted longer than 1 hour   _____

3. Subdural hemorrhage due to fall 1 week ago   _____

4. Subarachnoid hemorrhage without regaining consciousness after an all-terrain vehicle (ATV) accident. Patient died after 2 days   _____

Internal Injury of Thorax, Abdomen, and Pelvis

Injury to the internal organs can occur with or without an open wound. Laceration of the spleen may result from blunt trauma without an open wound; injury to the spleen can occur from an open wound due to a gunshot. Types of injuries included in these categories are as follows:

- Blast injuries of internal organs
- Blunt trauma of internal organs
- Bruise of internal organs
- Concussion injuries (except cerebral) of internal organs
- Crushing of internal organs
- Hematoma of internal organs
- Laceration of internal organs
- Puncture of internal organs
- Traumatic rupture of internal organs

The Organ Injury Scaling was developed by the Organ Injury Scaling Committee of the American Association for the Surgery of Trauma. This scale is graded from I through VI for each organ, with I being least severe and V the most severe injury from which the patient may survive. Grade VI injuries are by definition not salvageable. Scales are available for the following organ injuries:

- Thoracic vascular
- Lung
- Heart
- Chest wall
- Diaphragm
- Spleen
- Liver
- Abdominal vascular
- Kidney
- Ureter
- Bladder
- Urethra

Table 23-1 shows the organ injury scale for liver injuries.

These scales can be helpful in coding internal injuries more accurately. They may also be useful for querying the physician about the extent of an internal injury.

Categories 864, Injury to liver (Figure 23-10), 865, Injury to spleen, and 866, Injury to kidney, have fifth-digit subclassifications that may fit into one of the organ injury grade levels.

EXAMPLE | Patient had laceration of right lung due to stab wound (laceration) right chest wall during fight at nightclub, 861.32, E966, E849.6 (S27.331A, S21.311A, X99.9xxA, Y92.29).

TABLE 23-1. ORGAN INJURY SCALING—LIVER[4]

Grade	Injury Description	
I	Hematoma	Subscapular, <10% surface area
	Laceration	Capsular tear, <1 cm parenchymal depth
II	Hematoma	Subscapular, 10%-50% surface area
		Intraparenchymal, <10 cm diameter
	Laceration	1-3 cm parenchymal depth, <10 cm length
III	Hematoma	Subscapular, >50% surface area or expanding. Ruptured subscapular or parenchymal hematoma
		Intraparenchymal hematoma >10 cm or expanding
	Laceration	>3 cm parenchymal depth
IV	Laceration	Parenchymal disruption involving 25%-75% of hepatic lobe, or 1-3 Coinaud's segments in a single lobe
V	Laceration	Parenchymal disruption involving >75% of hepatic lobe or >3 Coinaud's segments within a single lobe
	Vascular	Juxtahepatic venous injuries (i.e., retrohepatic vena cava/ central major hepatic veins)
VI	Vascular	Hepatic avulsion

Advance one grade for multiple injuries to same organ up to grade III.

●864 **Injury to liver**

The following fifth-digit subclassification is for use with category 864:

☐ 0 **unspecified injury**
  1 **hematoma and contusion**
  2 **laceration, minor**
     Laceration involving capsule only, or without significant involvement of hepatic parenchyma [i.e., less than 1 cm deep]
  3 **laceration, moderate**
     Laceration involving parenchyma but without major disruption of parenchyma [i.e., less than 10 cm long and less than 3 cm deep]
  4 **laceration, major**
     Laceration with significant disruption of hepatic parenchyma [i.e., 10 cm long and 3 cm deep]
     Multiple moderate lacerations, with or without hematoma
     Stellate lacerations of liver
☐ 5 **laceration, unspecified**
☐ 9 **other**

FIGURE 23-10. Fifth-digit code assignment for type of liver laceration.

EXERCISE 23-6

Assign codes to the following conditions.

1. Pneumothorax due to stab wound (puncture) of the right chest wall during assault on the street   _____

2. A superficial 5-cm laceration spleen due to blunt trauma from steering wheel of car during head-on collision with another car   _____

3. Grade III laceration liver (involving parenchyma) due to snowmobile accident with collision with a tree in the ditch. Patient was driver   _____

4. Minor contusion of the left kidney due to fall from horse at riding stable   _____

5. Mediastinal hematoma due to MVA, single vehicle with loss of control, passenger   _____

FIGURE 23-11. Laceration of elbow.

Open Wounds

An open wound or **laceration** is an injury that results in a tear in the skin (Figure 23-11). Bruising and swelling can occur around the wound site. Common sites of laceration are body areas with underlying bony support, such as above the eyebrows, on the scalp and face, and over the knees. Categories 870-897 are assigned for traumatic injury; these codes should not be used to identify surgical wounds, nontraumatic wounds or ulcers, decubitus ulcers, and stasis ulcers. Laceration codes are assigned by location and according to whether the wound is complicated. The definition of a **complicated wound** includes delayed healing, delayed treatment, foreign body, and/or infection. An additional code would be assigned to identify the type of infection and any responsible organism. Because a physician says that a wound is complicated or that a complex repair was performed does not necessarily mean that the wound should be coded as complicated. The wound must fit the ICD-9-CM definition of a complicated wound.

EXAMPLE

The patient cut his right eyebrow during fall while downhill skiing; patient fell while skiing at resort, 873.42, E885.3, E003.2, E000.8, E849.4 (S01.111A, V00.321A, Y92.838, Y93.23, Y99.8).

EXAMPLE

Patient presented to the Emergency Room with gravel embedded in laceration of left knee. Patient fell while hiking in the mountains 2 days ago. The wound was cleaned and dressing applied, 891.1, E888.9, E001.0, E000.8, E849.8 (S81.022A, W19.xxxA, Y92.828, Y93.01, Y99.8).

EXERCISE 23-7

Assign codes to the following conditions.

1. Puncture wound left forearm due to dog bite while playing at public park   _____

2. Partial traumatic amputation right little toe due to lawn mower accident   _____

3. Laceration right calf from hatchet injury during camping trip in the mountains. Injury occurred 3 days ago, and no medical attention has been sought until now   _____

4. Wound left foot with glass pieces in wound due to stepping on broken glass at home (single family) while working in the kitchen   _____

Injury to Blood Vessels

Often, injuries to the blood vessels occur in conjunction with other injuries such as fractures, dislocations, open wounds, or lacerations. It is appropriate to assign codes that identify injury to the blood vessels, in addition to fractures and dislocations. Sequencing of codes according to Coding Guidelines depends on which is the primary injury.

EXAMPLE   Injury to the thoracic aorta due to MVA involving collision with train. Patient was the driver of the car, 901.0, E810.0, E849.5 (S25.00xA, V45.5xxA, Y92.410).

EXERCISE 23-8

Assign codes to the following conditions.

1. Crush injury abdomen with minor injury to splenic artery due to being struck and caught between two motor vehicles   _____

2. Injury to abdominal aorta due to accident while passenger on shuttle bus   _____

3. Injury to internal left jugular due to stabbing during assault in parking garage   _____

4. Rupture of right anterior tibial artery due to accidental gunshot (hunting rifle) while hunting in the forest   _____

5. Dislocation of left femoral neck due to injury during game of rugby. Minor damage to the left femoral artery was noted   _____

Superficial Injury

Superficial injuries may manifest in the form of abrasions (Figure 23-12), friction burns, blisters, nonvenomous insect bites, and superficial foreign bodies or splinters (Figure 23-13). The physician may not document the term "superficial," so supporting documentation must be used to determine whether the injury fits into the superficial categories. It is also important to look for documentation about the presence of an infection. As was mentioned previously, it is not necessary to code superficial injuries when a more serious injury has occurred at the same site. The fourth digit identifies whether infection is present. Superficial injury to the eye is coded to category 918 (S05.–).

EXAMPLE   Corneal abrasion due to being struck by tree branch while hiking in the forest, 918.1, E917.9, E001.0, E008.0, E849.8 (S05.00xA, W22.8xxA, Y92.821, Y93.01, Y99.8).

FIGURE 23-12. Abrasion wound of kneecap.

● **910 Superficial injury of face, neck, and scalp except eye**

 Includes: cheek   lip
               ear   nose
               gum   throat

 Excludes *eye and adnexa (918.0–918.9)*

 910.0 Abrasion or friction burn without mention of infection

 910.1 Abrasion or friction burn, infected

 910.2 Blister without mention of infection

 910.3 Blister, infected

 910.4 Insect bite, nonvenomous, without mention of infection

 910.5 Insect bite, nonvenomous, infected

 910.6 Superficial foreign body (splinter) without major open wound and without mention of infection

 910.7 Superficial foreign body (splinter) without major open wound, infected

 ☐ **910.8 Other and unspecified superficial injury of face, neck, and scalp without mention of infection**

 ☐ **910.9 Other and unspecified superficial injury of face, neck, and scalp, infected**

FIGURE 23-13. Fourth-digit classifications for superficial injuries.

EXAMPLE   Laceration and abrasion of right elbow due to fall from scooter at the lake, 881.01, E885.0, E849.8, E000.8 (S51.011A, V00.141A, Y92.828, Y99.8). The abrasion is not coded separately because it occurred at the same site as a more severe injury.

EXAMPLE   Sprain of right ankle and abrasions to left knee due to being knocked down while playing basketball during phys-ed in gym, 845.00, 916.0, E886.0, E007.6, E000.8, E849.4 (S93.401A, S80.212A, W03.xxxA, Y92.310, Y99.8). Abrasions are coded because they occurred at a different site from the sprain.

EXERCISE 23-9

Assign codes to the following conditions.

1. Blister left heel due to rubbing of shoe   _____

2. Infected mosquito bites both legs   _____

3. Abrasions right hand and right knee due to fall from bicycle   _____
   on the driveway at home (single family)

4. Superficial wood splinter right thumb from board on   _____
   construction job site

5. Abrasions and deep laceration of left elbow due to fall while   _____
   playing soccer. Patient was pushed down by opponent during
   high school game

Contusion With Intact Skin Surface

A **contusion** is any injury that results in hemorrhage beneath unbroken skin. Other terms for contusion include "bruise" and "hematoma." Contusions associated with more severe or serious injuries at the same site would not be coded. Occasionally, if a hematoma does not absorb on its own, it may have to be evacuated or aspirated.

| EXAMPLE | Contusion of right quadriceps after tackle in college football game, 924.00, E886.0, E007.0, E000.8, E849.4 (S70.11xA, W03.xxxA, Y92.321, Y93.61). |

| EXAMPLE | Contusion and severe sprain of left ankle after falling into a hole while hiking in the mountains, 845.00, E883.9, E001.0, E849.8, E000.8 (S93.402A, W17.2xxA, Y92.828, Y93.01, Y99.8). |

EXERCISE 23-10

Assign codes to the following conditions.

1. Black eye (right) due to hit by opponent's elbow during   _____
   professional basketball game

2. Subungual hematoma left thumb after hitting with hammer in   _____
   home workshop

3. Bruise left ankle following hit from hockey puck during NHL _____
   practice

4. Hematoma right breast from the seatbelt when involved in   _____
   MVA involving collision with a tree. Patient was alone in the
   vehicle

5. Contusion right shin after tripping on steps leading to the _____
   public high school

Crush Injury

A **crush injury** occurs when a body part is subjected to a high degree of force or pressure, usually after it has been squeezed between two heavy or immobile objects. A crush injury can be more serious than other types of injury such as a fracture or a laceration. In a severe crush, the force of the trauma can damage the underlying tissues, bones, blood vessels, and nerves. Increased pressure from tissue swelling can also damage muscles, blood vessels, and nerves. Instructions say to use additional codes to identify any associated injuries such as the following:

- Fractures
- Internal organs injury
- Intracranial injury

According to *Coding Clinic* (2003:4Q:p76-78),[5] the code for crush injury should be sequenced first.

EXAMPLE | Crush injury of left foot with metatarsal fractures due to dropping car battery on foot at industrial factory, 928.20, 825.25, E916, E849.3, E000.0 (S97.82xA, S92.302A, W20.8xxA, Y92.63, Y99.0).

According to *Coding Clinic* (1993:2Q:p7),[6] assign only the code for the crush injury (925-929.9) when there is also an open wound or a laceration. The Tabular List and the Alphabetic Index do not include any mention of "with open wound" under the section on crush injuries ("Crush, crushing ..." in the Index). However, the note under "Wound, open" in the Index gives direction, "For crush injury, see Crush ..." (Figure 23-14), and the Exclusion note under the section on "Open wound" in the Tabular List clearly excludes "crushing (925-925.9)" (Figure 23-15). Therefore, a code for open wound is not used with a code for crush injury.

EXAMPLE | Employee sustained a crush injury to right pointer finger with 3-cm laceration which happened while fixing combine on the farm, 927.3, E919.0, E849.1, E000.0 (S67.190A, S61.210A, W30.0xxA, Y92.79, Y99.0).

Wound, open (by cutting or piercing instrument) (by firearms) (cut) (dissection) (incised) (laceration) (penetration) (perforating) (puncture) (with initial hemorrhage, not internal) 879.8

Note   For fracture with open wound, see Fracture.

For laceration, traumatic rupture, tear, or penetrating wound of internal organs, such as heart, lung, liver, kidney, pelvic organs, etc., whether or not accompanied by open wound or fracture in the same region, see Injury, internal. For contused wound, see Contusion. For crush injury, see Crush. For abrasion, insect bite (nonvenomous), blister, or scratch, see Injury, superficial.

Complicated includes wounds with:

delayed healing
delayed treatment
foreign body
primary infection

For late effect of open wound, see Late, effect, wound, open, by site.

FIGURE 23-14. Instructional note for coding crush injuries.

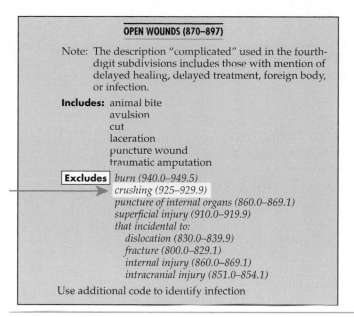

FIGURE 23-15. Crush injuries are excluded from open wound codes.

EXERCISE 23-11

Assign codes to the following conditions.

1. Crush injury left fingers with fractures of distal phalanges due to slamming in car door   _____

2. Crush injury to abdomen with injury to bladder and pelvic fracture   _____

3. Crush injury right foot   _____

4. Crush injury left great toe due to dropping bowling ball on bare foot at the bowling alley during league bowling   _____

5. Crush injury right ankle with 4-cm laceration due to being pinned by farm machinery while working in field   _____

Effects of Foreign Body Entering Through Orifice

A foreign body (FB) can enter the body through natural openings or orifices such as eyes, ears, nose, and mouth. In some cases it may be necessary to seek emergency medical attention for possible removal. One of the most common sites that foreign bodies enter are the eyes. Young children and elderly patients, particularly those with neurologic disorders and/or decreased gag reflexes, are at risk for aspiration and food can become lodged in the esophagus.

EXAMPLE   Small piece of grass from mowing lawn at single family house stuck on right cornea. Grass was removed, 930.0, E914, E016.1, E000.8, E849.0, 98.21 (T15.01xA, Y92.017, 08C8XZZ).

EXERCISE 23-12

Assign codes to the following conditions.

1. Hot dog lodged in distal esophagus of patient with dysphagia. _____
   EGD with removal of hot dog

2. 1-year-old swallowed a penny, and x-rays showed that it was _____
   in the stomach

3. Child put sunflower seed in right nostril; removed with _____
   forceps

4. Patient with cough and hemoptysis was found to have a _____
   chicken bone lodged in right bronchus of the lung;
   bronchoscopy with removal of chicken bone

5. Malodorous vaginal discharge due to retained tampon in _____
   vagina; manually removed

Injury to Nerves and Spinal Cord

Spinal cord injury (SCI) is damage to the spinal cord that causes loss of sensation and motor control. The most common causes of SCI include MVAs, falls, acts of violence, and sporting accidents. SCIs tend to occur where the spine is most flexible, in the regions C5-C7 of the neck and T10-L2 at the base of the rib cage. If SCI is suspected, a computed tomography (CT) scan, magnetic resonance imaging (MRI), or a myelogram may be used as a diagnostic tool. Immediate medical treatment should focus on stabilizing the spine and providing aggressive treatment with corticosteroid drugs to limit damage. Surgery may also be necessary to stabilize the spine or fuse the spine with metal plates or pins. Once the initial injury heals, functional improvements may continue for at least 6 months. After this time, any remaining disability is likely to be permanent. Any nerve damage or injury should be coded, in addition to other injuries.

EXAMPLE
Spinal cord injury at C2 level due to tackle during NFL football game, 952.00, E886.0, E007.0, E000.0, E849.4 (S14.102A, W03.xxxA, Y92.321, Y93.61, Y99.0).

EXERCISE 23-13

Assign codes to the following conditions.

1. Injury to ulnar nerve due to laceration left wrist; accidental _____
   laceration with hunting knife while hunting in woods

2. Radial nerve injury due to fracture of right humerus; injury _____
   occurred when water taxi overturned in rough water

3. Injury to sciatic nerve due to dislocation of left hip; patient _____
   fell on the way to dining room at the nursing home

4. Spinal cord injury T10 due to MVA _____

Certain Traumatic Complications and Unspecified Injuries

A variety of complications may occur as the result of injury. An **air embolism** is formed when air or gas bubbles get into the bloodstream and obstruct the circulation. Trauma to the lungs can cause an air embolism, as may occur in divers from rapid changes of pressure.

A **fat embolism** can occur when fat enters the circulatory system after long bone or pelvic fracture. It usually presents 12 to 48 hours after the injury with symptoms such as tachycardia, tachypnea, elevated temperature, hypoxemia, hypocapnia, thrombocytopenia, and occasionally with mild neurologic symptoms. A petechial rash also appears on the upper portions of the body, including the chest, neck, upper arm, axilla, shoulder, oral mucous membranes, and conjunctivae. Infection, shock, anuria, and subcutaneous emphysema are other examples of complications of trauma.

Category 959 is used for injuries that are unspecified or not otherwise specified. This code is commonly used in the outpatient setting. A patient may have sustained injury to the ankle, but after x-rays and examination, the patient's ankle pain cannot be explained by a more specific code such as fracture, dislocation, or sprain.

EXAMPLE

Patient was hospitalized for treatment of an open traumatic fracture, right femur (shaft), and developed a fat embolism, 821.11, 958.1, E887 (S72.301B, T79.1xxA, X58.xxxA)

EXERCISE 23-14

Assign codes to the following conditions.

1. Pain due to twisting injury to left knee while playing basketball at the gym _____

2. Patient bumped head on kitchen cabinet door at home _____

3. Shoulder injury due to fall on public sidewalk _____

4. Injury to left hip during high school football game due to being pushed down _____

5. Subcutaneous emphysema due to pneumothorax from a stab wound into thorax during a bar fight _____

6. Infection due to second-degree burn on left thigh caused by spilled coffee, subsequent encounter _____

7. Traumatic shock due to blunt intraabdominal injury caused by car pile-up on Interstate highway; patient was the driver of the car _____

FACTORS INFLUENCING HEALTH STATUS AND CONTACT WITH HEALTH SERVICES (V CODES/Z CODES)

In the past, V/Z codes have been considered primarily for use in the outpatient setting. This has changed with the addition of more V/Z codes each year. As was discussed in Chapter 8, it may be difficult to locate V/Z codes in the Index. Coders often say, "I did not know there was a V/Z code for that." Refer to Chapter 8 for a listing of common main terms used to locate V/Z codes.

V/Z codes that may be used with injuries include the following:

V15.51	Personal history of traumatic fracture
V15.59	Personal history of other injury
V15.82	Personal history of traumatic brain injury
V42.4	Organ or tissue replaced by transplant—bone
V43.60	Organ or tissue replaced by other means—unspecified
V43.61	Organ or tissue replaced by other means—shoulder
V43.62	Organ or tissue replaced by other means—elbow
V43.63	Organ or tissue replaced by other means—wrist

V43.64	Organ or tissue replaced by other means—hip
V43.65	Organ or tissue replaced by other means—knee
V43.66	Organ or tissue replaced by other means—ankle
V43.69	Organ or tissue replaced by other means—other
V43.7	Organ or tissue replaced by other means—limb
V48.6	Disfigurements of head
V48.7	Disfigurements of neck and trunk
V49.4	Disfigurements of limbs
V49.60	Upper limb amputation status—unspecified level
V49.61	Upper limb amputation status—thumb
V49.62	Upper limb amputation status—other finger(s)
V49.63	Upper limb amputation status—hand
V49.64	Upper limb amputation status—wrist
V49.65	Upper limb amputation status—below elbow
V49.66	Upper limb amputation status—above elbow
V49.67	Upper limb amputation status—shoulder
V49.70	Lower limb amputation status—unspecified level
V49.71	Lower limb amputation status—great toe
V49.72	Lower limb amputation status—other toe(s)
V49.73	Lower limb amputation status—foot
V49.74	Lower limb amputation status—ankle
V49.75	Lower limb amputation status—below knee (BKA)
V49.76	Lower limb amputation status—above knee (AKA)
V49.77	Lower limb amputation status—hip
V52.0	Fitting and adjustment of prosthetic device and implant—artificial arm
V52.1	Fitting and adjustment of prosthetic device and implant—artificial leg
V53.7	Fitting and adjustment of other device—orthopedic devices
V54.01	Encounter for removal of internal fixation device
V54.09	Other aftercare involving internal fixation device
V54.10	Aftercare for healing traumatic fracture of arm, unspecified
V54.11	Aftercare for healing traumatic fracture of upper arm
V54.12	Aftercare for healing traumatic fracture of lower arm
V54.13	Aftercare for healing traumatic fracture of hip
V54.14	Aftercare for healing traumatic fracture of leg, unspecified
V54.15	Aftercare for healing traumatic fracture of upper leg
V54.16	Aftercare for healing traumatic fracture of lower leg
V54.17	Aftercare for healing traumatic fracture of vertebrae
V54.19	Aftercare for healing traumatic fracture of other bone
V54.81	Aftercare after joint replacement
V54.89	Other orthopedic aftercare
V54.9	Unspecified orthopedic aftercare
V57.1	Other physical therapy
V57.21	Encounter for occupational therapy
V57.22	Encounter for vocational therapy
V57.4	Orthotic training
V57.81	Orthotic training
V58.30	Encounter for change or removal of nonsurgical wound dressing
V58.31	Encounter for change or removal of surgical wound dressing
V58.32	Encounter for removal of sutures
V58.41	Encounter for planned postoperative wound closure
V58.49	Other specified aftercare after surgery

V58.43	Aftercare after surgery for injury and trauma
V59.2	Donor—bone
V64.43	Arthroscopic surgical procedure converted to open procedure
V65.43	Counseling on injury prevention
V66.4	Convalescence and palliative care after treatment of fracture
V67.4	Follow-up examination after treatment of healed fracture
V71.3	Observation after accident at work
V71.4	Observation after other accident
V71.6	Observation after other inflicted injury
V80.01	Special screening for traumatic brain injury

EXAMPLE | Patient was seen for suture removal from the left leg, V58.32, 97.89 (Z48.02, 8EOYXY8).

Admission for Observation Following an Injury

According to *Coding Clinic* (1987:M-A:p1-5),[7] observation codes V71.3, V71.4, and V71.6 should be used when a patient is seen for an injury but after examination and observation no significant physical injury is found. Usually in these cases, patients are admitted to rule out or to be observed for a more serious type of injury. If a patient has minor cuts, bruises, or other superficial injuries, these are coded as secondary diagnoses and the appropriate observation code as the principal.

This V71 (Z04.–) code category is used for patients who are suspected of having an abnormal condition without a sign or a symptom that requires study. After examination and observation, no condition is determined to exist.

EXAMPLE | Patient has a contusion of the forehead and is admitted for observation to rule out a concussion. Patient was the driver of a motor vehicle that lost control while taking a curve on a state road and collided with a tree, V71.4, 920, E815.0, E849.5 (Z04.1, S00.83xA, V47.52xA, Y92.413).

EXERCISE 23-15

Assign codes to the following conditions.

1. Observation following work accident   _____

2. Previous right knee joint replacement   _____

3. Observation after MVA for internal abdominal injuries;   _____
   internal injuries were ruled out, and patient was discharged
   with a diagnosis of contusion abdominal wall

4. Encounter for removal of screw used to stabilize left tibial   _____
   fracture; fracture is well healed, and no complications of the
   fixation device or infections are reported

5. Patient had a previous amputation of the left great toe   _____

6. Patient's x-rays show a healing traumatic fracture of the right   _____
   humerus

COMMON TREATMENTS

Many injuries are diagnosed with the use of imaging procedures such as x-ray, MRI, CT scans, and ultrasound. Treatment depends on the severity of the injury. For very severe injuries, patients may have to be transferred to hospitals that specialize in the care of trauma patients. Surgical intervention may also be required to repair the specific injury or trauma. Pain medications, anti-inflammatories, corticosteroids, and antibiotics may be necessary to alleviate pain and inflammation and to prevent or fight infection.

PROCEDURES

Some of the procedures that may be related to injuries are located in the following chapters of the Procedure Tabular:

Chapter 14, Operations on the Musculoskeletal System (76-84)

Chapter 15, Operations on the Integumentary System (85-86)

Procedures for internal injuries are found within procedural chapters for the respective systems.

Procedures related to injuries in ICD-10-PCS can be located in many tables depending on the procedure performed and the body system involved.

Fracture Treatment

A fracture is classified as "open" or "closed." Treatments for fracture are also classified as "open" or "closed," and the coder should not confuse the type of fracture with the type of procedure. An open fracture may not require open treatment, and a closed fracture may need open reduction. The root operation for reduction of a fracture is reposition. The treatment provided will depend on other injuries and the type and location of the fracture. Reduction or manipulation of bone fragments to their proper anatomic position is necessary for appropriate healing. For fractures that are not displaced, stabilization or immobilization may be all that is necessary to promote healing. Reductions may be performed in the Operating Room or other areas of the hospital, such as the Emergency Room, fracture treatment room, and/or in radiology.

Closed reduction of a fracture occurs when the surgeon manipulates or reduces fractured bones into anatomic alignment without making an incision through the skin and subcutaneous tissue. Closed reduction may include internal fixation. If no incision is made to expose the fracture, it is coded as a closed reduction. Small incision(s) may be made for placement of internal fixation device(s) such as pins, wires, screws, plates, and intramedullary nails. As long as the fracture is not exposed, it is considered a closed fixation. Fixation devices are used to immobilize the fracture, but they do not manipulate or reduce the fracture. Sometimes radiologic guidance is needed for placement of the fixation device(s). It is also possible for a closed reduction to be performed prior to having an open reduction and fixation.

Open reduction of a fracture occurs when the surgeon makes an incision at the fracture site to reduce or manipulate the fracture into anatomic position. Open reduction and internal fixation (ORIF) is a procedure that is very commonly performed for fractures.

External skeletal fixation is another form of fracture treatment (Figure 23-16). This involves insertion of percutaneous pins proximal and distal to the fracture and application of a frame that connects the pins externally. The pins are located internally, except for the portion to which the frame is connected. The frame is located outside the body. These devices can be used to hold a reduced fracture or to assist the surgeon in reducing a fracture. Instructional notes under the "Reduction of fracture and dislocation" category indicate that external skeletal fixation codes may be assigned, in addition to the codes for fracture reduction.

FIGURE 23-16. Example of an external fixation service on the right leg. The left is in a splint.

Repair of Wounds

Suture is a method used to close cutaneous wounds. The root operation for suture of skin and subcutaneous tissue is repair. The risks of bleeding and infection are reduced by approximating skin edges for an aesthetically pleasing and functional result. Routine debridement of wound edges prior to suturing of the wound is considered part of the suturing and should not be coded separately. In ICD-9-CM, suturing of the skin for most sites is coded to 86.59. How deep, how long, or how complex the repair is does not affect ICD-9-CM code assignment. A few body sites require a different code:

- Breast
- Ear
- Eyebrow
- Eyelid
- Nose
- Penis
- Scrotum
- Vulva

No procedure code is assigned for application of adhesive strips or butterfly strips. It is acceptable to assign 86.59 when adhesives such as **Dermabond** are used for wound closure, per *Coding Clinic* (1999:4Q:p23).[8] Sometimes, a combination of adhesives and sutures is used for wound repair.

EXAMPLE | Laceration of left wrist due to suicidal attempt with razor. Laceration was repaired, 881.02, E956, 86.59 (S61.512A, X78.8xxA, 0HQEXZZ). No place of occurrence was given, so no E code is assigned, per guidelines.

EXAMPLE | Laceration of nose due to being hit in nose by surfboard while at beach. Laceration of the skin was repaired, 873.20, E917.0, E002.7, E000.8, E849.8, 21.81 (S01.21xA, W21.89xA, Y92.832, Y99.8, 0HQ1XZZ).

EXERCISE 23-16

Assign codes for all diagnoses and procedures.

1. Laceration to spleen with parenchymal disruption with total splenectomy _____

2. Coco Puff in left ear (auditory canal); removed by physician _____

3. Closed reduction and percutaneous fixation of left supracondylar fracture elbow after fall from monkey bars on elementary school playground _____

4. Manipulation of right shoulder dislocation due to fall while skiing at ski resort _____

5. Suture deep laceration of the right hand due to cut with knife while preparing dinner at home (single family) _____

6. Suture of laceration of the left eyelid that occurred due to falling and hitting edge of coffee table in living room (apartment) _____

7. Open reduction and internal fixation of left hip fracture due to fall _____

8. Open manipulation and internal fixation of left acetabular fracture due to head-on collision (MVA sport utility vehicle) _____

9. Healing traumatic fracture right tibia/fibula with application of short leg cast _____

10. Closed reduction and percutaneous internal fixation of right Bennett's fracture _____

DOCUMENTATION/REIMBURSEMENT/MS-DRGs

Often coding difficulties are due to lack of documentation. Sometimes radiology and other test results are not available at the time of discharge or when the physician is dictating the discharge summary or is reporting the final diagnoses. Documentation may be lacking for how and where an injury happened, so it is difficult to assign appropriate E codes.

Identification and accurate coding of all procedures and diagnoses may be instrumental in MS-DRG assignment. It is also important to code associated chronic conditions that may qualify as comorbid conditions. A thorough review of the record is necessary to identify complications that may occur during the stay. In cases of injury, it is very important to pick up all associated procedures. Often, in trauma cases, surgeons are busy trying to save the life of the patient, and documentation is not their top priority. The record should be reviewed for suturing of arteries or lacerations of internal organs, mechanical ventilation, and debridements. Sometimes, in the repair of fractures resulting from trauma, joint replacement may be necessary.

It is difficult to pinpoint any particular codes that may be frequently missed complications/comorbidities from this chapter. There are numerous injury codes on the CC/MCC listing. It is important to code all injuries with the most serious injury as the principal diagnosis.

Correct Orthopedic Procedure Code

EXAMPLE

An elderly patient falls and fractures right hip (femoral neck) and undergoes ORIF procedure. An error is made in assigning or entering the procedure code in the second case.

DIAGNOSES	CODES	MS-DRG	RW
Fracture hip	820.8, E888.9 (S72.001A, W19.xxxA)	482	1.5372
ORIF	79.35 (0QS604Z)		
Fracture hip	820.8, E888.9 (S72.001A, W19.xxxA)	536	0.7191
Closed reduction without fixation	79.05 (0QS6XZZ)		

Two Diagnoses That Equally Meet the Definition for Principal Diagnosis

EXAMPLE

A patient is admitted with a skull fracture and a right hip fracture. Designation of the principal diagnosis can make a difference in reimbursement. In this case, it may be necessary to query the physician as to which injury is the most serious. If a procedure was performed, that may also help the coder to determine which diagnosis is principal.

DIAGNOSES	CODES	MS-DRG	RW
Fracture hip and skull	820.8, 803.00, E887 (S72.001A, S02.91xA, X58.xxxA)	536	0.7191
Fracture skull and hip	803.00, 820.8, E887 (S02.91xA, S72.001A, X58.xxxA)	085	2.1423

Coding Specificity and MS-DRG With and Without MCC/CC

EXAMPLE

Patient is admitted with fractured ribs. X-ray report reveals fractures of the left third, fourth, fifth, and sixth ribs. No procedures were performed. Patient was also treated for a urinary tract infection.

DIAGNOSES	CODES	MS-DRG	RW
Rib fractures, UTI	807.00, 599.0, E887 (S22.42xA, N39.0, X58.xxxA)	206	0.7575
Rib fracture, 4 ribs, UTI	807.04, 599.0, E887 (S22.42xA, N39.0, X58.xxxA)	184	0.9755

In this example, reimbursement is affected by the more specific ICD-9-CM fracture code, which indicates that four ribs were fractured, and by the assignment of the UTI code (599.0 [N39.0]), which is a CC for MS-DRG 184.

CHAPTER REVIEW EXERCISE

Assign codes for all diagnoses and procedures.

1. Fracture/dislocation right femur due to fall from hospital bed. Contusion right hip _____

2. Closed reduction of recurrent left shoulder dislocation _____

3. Inversion injury right ankle with severe sprain during dismount from gymnastics equipment at local gym (twisting injury) _____

4. Grade III laceration to the bladder due to gunshot wound. Exploratory laparotomy with repair of the bladder laceration. Patient was shot during robbery of gas station _____

5. Crush injury with fracture of the right hand (multiple metacarpals) _____

6. Wound left calf due to dog bite. Wound was cleansed and Steri-Strips applied _____

7. Closed head injury with concussion and brief loss of consciousness (10 minutes) _____

8. Pain caused by anterior dislocation of left shoulder due to tackle during college football game _____

9. Tear of right ulnar collateral ligament of the left thumb–metacarpophalangeal joint due to fall and injury due to ski pole _____

10. Sprain right foot due to fall from trampoline. Trampoline is in neighbor's backyard _____

11. Crush injury with laceration of left foot. Dropped car battery on foot while at work at garage where the patient works _____

12. Hemiarthroplasty due to displaced right femoral neck fracture caused by fall at home (mobile) _____

13. Rib fractures on the left due to child abuse by foster mother _____

14. Open fracture of left tibial shaft with fracture of the fibula. Laceration calf, which exposes the tibia _____

15. Flail chest due to MVA involving collision with train. Patient was driver of pickup truck _____

16. Lacerations of right upper arm with embedded gravel due to fall from bicycle. Repaired with Dermabond and sutures _____

17. Contusions chest and forehead with 2-cm laceration of forehead, which was sutured. Patient was a passenger in a motor vehicle rollover (car) _____

18. Bilateral fractures of the radius. Right upper end and left distal end. Closed reductions bilaterally _____

19. Dislocation of left little finger due to wrestling. This is the third time the patient has dislocated this finger. Closed reduction was performed _____

20. Intertrochanteric fracture left hip with ORIF _____

21. Fracture temporal bone due to fall while skateboarding at park _____

22. Injury to right eye from paintball gun. Injury occurred at paintball recreation site _____

23. Hangman's fracture (C2) due to suicide attempt _____

24. Laceration scalp repaired with staples. Fall from tree in backyard of single family house _____

25. Fracture of L3 requiring fracture repair, posterior spinal fusion L2-L4 using bone grafts from iliac crest, and spinal instrumentation. Pedestrian hit by car _____

26. Closed head injury due to fall from balcony of apartment building. Patient had a brain contusion with LOC _____

27. Subdural hematoma with brief loss of consciousness due to fall from scaffolding at construction site. Hematoma was evacuated in the OR through burr hole _____

28. Peroneal nerve injury due to left fibular fracture (shaft). Patient was kicked while milking cows in the barn at a dairy farm _____

29. Shattered C1-C2 vertebrae with spinal cord injury due to fall from horse _____

Write the correct answer(s) in the space(s) provided.

30. Define open fracture. _____

CHAPTER GLOSSARY

Air embolism: when air or gas bubbles get into the bloodstream and obstruct the circulation.

Closed fracture: injury in which the bone is broken, but the skin remains intact.

Closed head injury: injury that results from a blow to the head.

Closed reduction: the surgeon manipulates or reduces fractured bones into anatomic alignment without making an incision through the skin and subcutaneous tissue.

Colles' fracture: common fracture in adults in which the lower end of the radius is fractured and the wrist and hand are displaced backward.

Complicated fracture: fracture that causes injury to surrounding tissues.

Complicated wound: laceration with delayed healing, delayed treatment, foreign body, and/or infection.

Compound fracture: when the broken bone exits and is visible through the skin, or a deep wound exposes the broken bone through the skin.

Concussion: injury to the brain that results from a significant blow to the head.

Contusion: any mechanical injury that results in hemorrhage beneath unbroken skin.

Crush injury: when a body part is subjected to a high degree of force or pressure, usually after it has been squeezed between two heavy or immobile objects.

Dermabond: liquid skin adhesive used to close skin lacerations.

Dislocation: displacement of the bones that form a joint; separation of the end of a bone from the joint it meets.

External skeletal fixation: form of fracture treatment that involves insertion of percutaneous pins proximal and distal to the fracture and application of a frame that connects the pins externally.

Fat embolism: when fat enters the circulatory system after long bone or pelvic fracture.

Fracture: break in a bone.

Gustilo open fracture classification: classification based on the mechanism of the injury and the amount of soft tissue and skeletal injury that is useful in assessing risk of infection and possible amputation.

Laceration: an injury that results in a tear in the skin.

Loss of consciousness: when a patient is unable to respond to people or other stimuli.

Open fracture: when the broken bone exits and is visible through the skin, or a deep wound exposes the broken bone through the skin.

Open reduction: when the surgeon makes an incision at the fracture site to reduce or manipulate the fracture into anatomic position.

Pathologic fracture: break in a bone that occurs because of underlying disorders that weaken the bone, including malignancy, benign bone tumor, metabolic disorder, infection, and osteoporosis.

Simple fracture: injury in which the bone is broken, but the skin remains intact.

Spinal cord injury: damage to the spinal cord that causes loss of sensation and motor control.

Sprain: stretch and/or tear of a ligament.

Strain: injury to a muscle or a tendon.

Subluxation: partial or incomplete dislocation.

Suture: method for closing cutaneous wounds.

Traumatic brain injury: injury to the brain that may result in interference with the brain's normal functions.

REFERENCES

1. American Hospital Association. *Coding Clinic for ICD-9-CM* 1999:1Q:p5. Fracture site specified in radiology report.
2. American Hospital Association. *Coding Clinic for ICD-9-CM* 1990:3Q:p13. Fracture with dislocation.
3. American Hospital Association. *Coding Clinic for ICD-9-CM* 1997:Nov-Dec:p7. Recurrent shoulder dislocation.
4. From American Association for the Surgery of Trauma, Chicago, Illinois.
5. American Hospital Association. *Coding Clinic for ICD-9-CM* 2003:4Q:p76-78. Crushing injury.
6. American Hospital Association. *Coding Clinic for ICD-9-CM* 1993:2Q:p7. Crush injury with open wound.
7. American Hospital Association. *Coding Clinic for ICD-9-CM* 1987:M-A:p1-5. Observation and evaluation for suspected conditions—Guidelines.
8. American Hospital Association. *Coding Clinic for ICD-9-CM* 1999:4Q:p23. Dermabond application—correction.

24

Burns, Adverse Effects, and Poisonings

(ICD-9-CM Chapter 17, Codes 800-995, ICD-10-CM Chapters 19 and 20, Codes S00-Y99)

LEARNING OBJECTIVES

1. Apply and assign the correct ICD-9-CM and ICD-10-CM codes in accordance with Official Guidelines for Coding and Reporting
2. Identify major differences between ICD-9-CM and ICD-10-CM related to burns, adverse effects, and poisonings
3. Identify the various types of burns
4. Differentiate between an adverse effect and a poisoning
5. Assign the correct V/Z codes, E codes, and procedure codes related to burns, adverse effects, and poisonings
6. Identify common treatments
7. Explain the importance of documentation in relation to MS-DRGs for reimbursement

ABBREVIATIONS/ ACRONYMS

AKA above-knee amputation

CC complication/comorbidity

HBOT hyperbaric oxygen therapy

ICD-9-CM *International Classification of Diseases, 9th Revision, Clinical Modification*

ICD-10-CM *International Classification of Diseases, 10th Revision, Clinical Modification*

ICD-10-PCS *International Classification of Diseases, 10th Revision, Procedure Coding System*

MS-DRG Medicare Severity diagnosis-related group

MVA motor vehicle accident

OR Operating Room

SIRS systemic inflammatory response syndrome

UTI urinary tract infection

ICD-9-CM

Official Guidelines for Coding and Reporting

Please refer to the companion Evolve website for the most current guidelines.

17. Chapter 17: Injury and Poisoning (800-999)

Only guidelines applicable to this chapter are included; therefore the numbers or letters are not sequential.

c. Coding of Burns

Current burns (940-948) are classified by depth, extent and by agent (E code). Burns are classified by depth as first degree (erythema), second degree (blistering), and third degree (full-thickness involvement).

1) Sequencing of burn and related condition codes

Sequence first the code that reflects the highest degree of burn when more than one burn is present.

a. When the reason for the admission or encounter is for treatment of external multiple burns, sequence first the code that reflects the burn of the highest degree.

EXAMPLE

Second-degree burns of the left hand and first-degree burns of the left forearm, 944.20, 943.11, E988.1 (T23.202A, T22.112A).

b. When a patient has both internal and external burns, the circumstances of admission govern the selection of the principal diagnosis or first-listed diagnosis.

c. When a patient is admitted for burn injuries and other related conditions such as smoke inhalation and/or respiratory failure, the circumstances of admission govern the selection of the principal or first-listed diagnosis.

2) Burns of the same local site

Classify burns of the same local site (three-digit category level, 940-947) but of different degrees to the subcategory identifying the highest degree recorded in the diagnosis.

EXAMPLE

Second- and third-degree burns of the right thigh, 945.36, E988.1 (T24.311A).

3) Non-healing burns

Non-healing burns are coded as acute burns.
Necrosis of burned skin should be coded as a non-healed burn.

EXAMPLE

Necrosis of third-degree burn on the buttock, subsequent visit, 942.34 (T21.35xD).

4) Code 958.3, Posttraumatic wound infection

Assign code 958.3, Posttraumatic wound infection, not elsewhere classified, as an additional code for any documented infected burn site.

EXAMPLE | Infected burn right foot, subsequent visit, 945.02, 958.3, T79.8xxD (T25.021D, L08.9).

5) Assign separate codes for each burn site

When coding burns, assign separate codes for each burn site. Category 946 Burns of Multiple specified sites, should only be used if the location of the burns are not documented.

Category 949, Burn, unspecified, is extremely vague and should rarely be used.

EXAMPLE | Multiple burns over the entire body. The patient expired before he could be admitted, 949.0 (T30.0).

6) Assign codes from category 948, Burns

Burns classified according to extent of body surface involved, when the site of the burn is not specified or when there is a need for additional data. It is advisable to use category 948 as additional coding when needed to provide data for evaluating burn mortality, such as that needed by burn units. It is also advisable to use category 948 as an additional code for reporting purposes when there is mention of a third-degree burn involving 20% or more of the body surface.

In assigning a code from category 948:

Fourth-digit codes are used to identify the percentage of total body surface involved in a burn (all degree).

Fifth-digits are assigned to identify the percentage of body surface involved in third-degree burn.

Fifth-digit zero (0) is assigned when less than 10% or when no body surface is involved in a third-degree burn.

Category 948 is based on the classic "rule of nines" in estimating body surface involved: head and neck are assigned 9%, each arm 9%, each leg 18%, the anterior trunk 18%, posterior trunk 18%, and genitalia 1%. Providers may change these percentage assignments where necessary to accommodate infants and children who have proportionately larger heads than adults and patients who have large buttocks, thighs, or abdomen that involve burns.

EXAMPLE | The patient has second-degree (3%) and third-degree (5%) burns of the trunk and first-degree burns (2%) of the right arm, 942.30, 943.10, 948.10, E988.1 (T21.30xA, T22.10xA, T31.10).

7) Encounters for treatment of late effects of burns

Encounters for the treatment of the late effects of burns (i.e., scars or joint contractures) should be coded to the residual condition (sequelae) followed by the appropriate late effect code (906.5-906.9). A late effect E code may also be used, if desired.

EXAMPLE | Contracture of the skin of the right index finger due to burn from fire injury 6 months ago, 709.2, 906.6, E929.4 (L90.5, T23.021S, X08.8xxS).

8) Sequelae with a late effect code and current burn

When appropriate, both a sequelae with a late effect code, and a current burn code may be assigned on the same record (when both a current burn and sequelae of an old burn exist).

d. Coding of Debridement of Wound, Infection, or Burn

Excisional debridement involves surgical removal or cutting away, as opposed to a mechanical (brushing, scrubbing, washing) debridement.

For coding purposes, excisional debridement is assigned to code 86.22.

Nonexcisional debridement is assigned to code 86.28.

EXAMPLE Surgical debridement of infected burn on right foot performed by physical therapist, subsequent visit, 945.02, 958.3, 86.22 (T25.021D, T79.8xxD, L08.9, 0HBMXZZ).

e. Adverse Effects, Poisoning and Toxic Effects

The properties of certain drugs, medicinal and biological substances or combinations of such substances, may cause toxic reactions. The occurrence of drug toxicity is classified in ICD-9-CM as follows:

1) Adverse Effect

When the drug was correctly prescribed and properly administered, code the reaction plus the appropriate code from the E930-E949 series. Codes from the E930-E949 series must be used to identify the causative substance for an adverse effect of drug, medicinal and biological substances, correctly prescribed and properly administered. The effect, such as tachycardia, delirium, gastrointestinal hemorrhaging, vomiting, hypokalemia, hepatitis, renal failure, or respiratory failure, is coded and followed by the appropriate code from the E930-E949 series.

Adverse effects of therapeutic substances correctly prescribed and properly administered (toxicity, synergistic reaction, side effect, and idiosyncratic reaction) may be due to (1) differences among patients, such as age, sex, disease, and genetic factors, and (2) drug-related factors, such as type of drug, route of administration, duration of therapy, dosage, and bioavailability.

2) Poisoning

(a) Error was made in drug prescription

Errors made in drug prescription or in the administration of the drug by provider, nurse, patient, or other person, use the appropriate poisoning code from the 960-979 series.

EXAMPLE While in the hospital, the nurse accidentally gave the patient 40 mg of Lasix instead of the ordered 20-mg dosage. The patient suffered no ill effects, 974.4, E858.5, E849.7 (T50.1x1A, Y92.230).

(b) Overdose of a drug intentionally taken

If an overdose of a drug was intentionally taken or administered and resulted in drug toxicity, it would be coded as a poisoning (960-979 series).

EXAMPLE The patient intentionally overdosed with 20 Valium tablets. The patient is in a coma, 969.4, 780.01, E950.3 (T42.4x2A, R40.20).

(c) Nonprescribed drug taken with correctly prescribed and properly administered drug

If a nonprescribed drug or medicinal agent was taken in combination with a correctly prescribed and properly administered drug, any drug toxicity or other reaction resulting from the interaction of the two drugs would be classified as a poisoning.

(d) Interaction of drug(s) and alcohol

When a reaction results from the interaction of a drug(s) and alcohol, this would be classified as poisoning.

(e) Sequencing of poisoning

When coding a poisoning or reaction to the improper use of a medication (e.g., wrong dose, wrong substance, wrong route of administration) the poisoning code is sequenced first, followed by a code for the manifestation. If there is also a diagnosis of drug abuse or dependence to the substance, the abuse or dependence is coded as an additional code.

See Section I.C.3.a.6.b. if poisoning is the result of insulin pump malfunctions and Section I.C.19 for general use of E-codes.

EXAMPLE Chest pain due to accidental poisoning from cocaine. The patient uses cocaine on a daily basis, 970.81, 786.50, 305.61, E854.3 (T40.5x1A, R07.9, F14.10).

3) Toxic Effects

(a) Toxic effect codes

When a harmful substance is ingested or comes in contact with a person, this is classified as a toxic effect. The toxic effect codes are in categories 980-989.

(b) Sequencing toxic effect codes

A toxic effect code should be sequenced first, followed by the code(s) that identify the result of the toxic effect.

(c) External cause codes for toxic effects

An external cause code from categories E860-E869 for accidental exposure, codes E950.6 or E950.7 for intentional self-harm, category E962 for assault, or categories E980-E982, for undetermined, should also be assigned to indicate intent.

EXAMPLE A 2-year-old accidentally drank lye, causing burns to the mouth and throat, 983.2, 947.0, E864.2 (T54.3x1A, T28.5xxA).

g. SIRS due to Non-infectious Process

The systemic inflammatory response syndrome (SIRS) can develop as a result of certain non-infectious disease processes, such as trauma, malignant neoplasm, or pancreatitis. When SIRS is documented with a noninfectious condition, and no subsequent infection is documented, the code for the underlying condition, such as an injury, should be assigned, followed by code 995.93, Systemic inflammatory response syndrome due to noninfectious process without acute organ dysfunction, or 995.94, Systemic inflammatory response syndrome due to noninfectious process with acute organ dysfunction. If an acute organ dysfunction is documented, the appropriate code(s) for the associated acute organ dysfunction(s) should be assigned in addition to code 995.94. If acute organ dysfunction is documented, but it cannot be determined if the acute organ dysfunction is associated with SIRS or due to another condition (e.g., directly due to the trauma), the provider should be queried.

When the noninfectious condition has led to an infection that results in SIRS, *see Section I.C.1.b.11 for the guideline for sepsis and severe sepsis associated with a noninfectious process.*

EXAMPLE Patient has SIRS due to accidental burns in a street car fire. Patient has second- (3%) and third-degree (5%) burns of the trunk and first-degree burns of the right arm, 942.30, 943.10, 948.00, 995.93, E829.4, E849.5 (T21.30xA, T22.10xA, T31.10, R65.10, V82.9xxA, Y92.818).

a. **General E Coding Guidelines**
   7) **External cause code(s) with systemic inflammatory response syndrome (SIRS)**
      An external cause code is not appropriate with a code from subcategory 995.9, unless the patient also has another condition for which an E code would be appropriate (such as an injury, poisoning, or adverse effect of drugs).
b. **Place of Occurrence Guideline**
   Use an additional code from category E849 to indicate the Place of Occurrence for injuries and poisonings. The Place of Occurrence describes the place where the event occurred and not the patient's activity at the time of the event.
      Do not use E849.9 if the place of occurrence is not stated.
c. **Adverse Effects of Drugs, Medicinal and Biological Substances Guidelines**
   1) **Do not code directly from the Table of Drugs**
      Do not code directly from the Table of Drugs and Chemicals. Always refer back to the Tabular List.
   2) **Use as many codes as necessary to describe**
      Use as many codes as necessary to describe completely all drugs, medicinal or biological substances.
         If the reporting format limits the number of E codes, and there are different fourth digit codes in the same three digit category, use the code for "Other specified" of that category of drugs, medicinal or biological substances. If there is no "Other specified" code in that category, use the appropriate "Unspecified" code in that category.
         If the reporting format limits the number of E codes, and the codes are in different three digit categories, assign the appropriate E code for other multiple drugs and medicinal substances.

EXAMPLE   Patient was treated for epistaxis, which is likely due to the patient's long-term use of Coumadin for atrial fibrillation. Patient was taking the Coumadin as prescribed, 784.7, 427.31, V58.61, E934.2 (T45.515A, R04.0, I48.0, Z79.01).

   3) **If the same E code would describe the causative agent**
      If the same E code would describe the causative agent for more than one adverse reaction, assign the code only once.
   4) **If two or more drugs, medicinal or biological substances**
      If two or more drugs, medicinal or biological substances are reported, code each individually unless the combination code is listed in the Table of Drugs and Chemicals. In that case, assign the E code for the combination.
   5) **When a reaction results from the interaction of a drug(s)**
      When a reaction results from the interaction of a drug(s) and alcohol, use poisoning codes and E codes for both.

EXAMPLE   A patient combined Percodan with beer and was stuporous and drowsy, 965.09, 980.0, 780.09, E980.0, E980.9 (T40.2x1A, T51.0x1A, R40.1, R40.0).

   6) **Codes from the E930-E949 series**
      Codes from the E930-E949 series must be used to identify the causative substance for an adverse effect of drug, medicinal and biological substances, correctly prescribed and properly administered. The effect, such as tachycardia, delirium, gastrointestinal hemorrhaging, vomiting, hypokalemia, hepatitis, renal failure, or respiratory failure, is coded and followed by the appropriate code from the E930-E949 series.

EXAMPLE

> Hypokalemia due to Lasix therapy for congestive heart failure, 276.8, 428.0, E944.4 (T50.1x5A, E87.6, I50.9).

d. Child and Adult Abuse Guideline

1) Intentional injury

When the cause of an injury or neglect is intentional child or adult abuse, the first listed E code should be assigned from categories E960-E968, Homicide and injury purposely inflicted by other persons, (except category E967). An E code from category E967, Child and adult battering and other maltreatment, should be added as an additional code to identify the perpetrator, if known.

EXAMPLE

> A wife was seen with head and face injuries due to spousal abuse. The patient had been struck repeatedly in the face and head, 995.81, 959.01, 959.09, E968.9, E967.3 (T74.11xA, S09.93xA, S09.90xA, Y04.2xxA, Y07.01).

2) Accidental intent

In cases of neglect when the intent is determined to be accidental E code E904.0, Abandonment or neglect of infant and helpless person, should be the first listed E code.

Apply the General Coding Guidelines as found in Chapter 5 and the Procedural Guidelines as found in chapter 6.

At the beginning of Chapter 17 in the ICD-9-CM code book, special instructions say, "Use E code(s) to identify the cause and intent of the injury or poisoning (E800-E999)" (Figure 24-1).

17. INJURY AND POISONING (800–999)

Use E code(s) to identify the cause and intent of the injury or poisoning (E800-E999)

Note:

1. The principle of multiple coding of injuries should be followed wherever possible. Combination categories for multiple injuries are provided for use when there is insufficient detail as to the nature of the individual conditions, or for primary tabulation purposes when it is more convenient to record a single code; otherwise, the component injuries should be coded separately.

   Where multiple sites of injury are specified in the titles, the word "with" indicates involvement of both sites, and the word "and" indicates involvement of either or both sites. The word "finger" includes thumb.

2. Categories for "late effect" of injuries are to be found at 905–909.

FIGURE 24-1. Instructional note regarding the use of E code(s) to identify the cause and intent of injury or poisoning (E800-E999).

ICD-10-CM

**Official
Guidelines for
Coding and
Reporting**

Please refer to the companion Evolve website for the most current guidelines.

19. Chapter 19: Injury, poisoning, and certain other consequences of external causes (S00-T88)

d. Coding of Burns and Corrosions

The ICD-10-CM **makes a distinction** between burns and corrosions. The burn codes are for thermal burns, except sunburns, that come from a heat source, such as a fire or hot appliance. The burn codes are also for burns resulting from electricity and radiation. Corrosions are burns due to chemicals. The guidelines are the same for burns and corrosions.

Current burns (T20-T25) are classified by depth, extent and by agent (X code). Burns are classified by depth as first degree (erythema), second degree (blistering), and third degree (full-thickness involvement). Burns of the eye and internal organs (T26-T28) are classified by site, but not by degree.

1) Sequencing of burn and related condition codes

Sequence first the code that reflects the highest degree of burn when more than one burn is present.

a. When the reason for the admission or encounter is for treatment of external multiple burns, sequence first the code that reflects the burn of the highest degree.

b. When a patient has both internal and external burns, the circumstances of admission govern the selection of the principal diagnosis or first-listed diagnosis.

c. When a patient is admitted for burn injuries and other related conditions such as smoke inhalation and/or respiratory failure, the circumstances of admission govern the selection of the principal or first-listed diagnosis.

2) Burns of the same local site

Classify burns of the same local site (three-**character** category level, T20-T28) but of different degrees to the subcategory identifying the highest degree recorded in the diagnosis.

3) Non-healing burns

Non-healing burns are coded as acute burns.

Necrosis of burned skin should be coded as a non-healed burn.

4) Infected Burn

For any documented infected burn site, use an additional code for the infection.

5) Assign separate codes for each burn site

When coding burns, assign separate codes for each burn site. Category T30, Burn and corrosion, body region unspecified is extremely vague and should rarely be used.

6) Burns and Corrosions Classified According to Extent of Body Surface Involved

Assign codes from category T31, Burns classified according to extent of body surface involved, or T32, Corrosions classified according to extent of body surface involved, when the site of the burn is not specified or when there is a need for additional data. It is advisable to use category T31 as additional coding when needed to provide data for evaluating burn mortality, such as that needed by burn units. It is also advisable to use category T31 as an additional code for reporting purposes when there is mention of a third-degree burn involving 20 percent or more of the body surface.

Categories T31 and T32 are based on the classic "rule of nines" in estimating body surface involved: head and neck are assigned nine percent, each arm nine percent, each leg 18 percent, the anterior trunk 18 percent, posterior trunk 18 percent, and genitalia one percent. Providers may change these percentage assignments where necessary to accommodate infants and children who have proportionately larger heads than adults, and patients who have large buttocks, thighs, or abdomen that involve burns.

7) Encounters for treatment of late effects of burns

Encounters for the treatment of the late effects of burns or corrosions (i.e., scars or joint contractures) should be coded with a burn or corrosion code with the 7th character "S" **for** sequela.

8) Sequelae with a late effect code and current burn

When appropriate, both a code for a current burn or corrosion with 7th character extension "A" or "D" and a burn or corrosion code with extension "S" may be assigned on the same record (when both a current burn and sequelae of an old burn exist). Burns and corrosions do not heal at the same rate and a current healing wound may still exist with sequela of a healed burn or corrosion.

9) Use of an external cause code with burns and corrosions

An external cause code should be used with burns and corrosions to identify the source and intent of the burn, as well as the place where it occurred.

e. Adverse Effects, Poisoning, Underdosing and Toxic Effects

Codes in categories T36-T65 are combination codes that include the substances related to adverse effects, poisonings, toxic effects and underdosing, as well as the external cause. No additional external cause code is required for poisonings, toxic effects, adverse effects and underdosing codes.

A code from categories T36-T65 is sequenced first, followed by the code(s) that specify the nature of the adverse effect, poisoning, or toxic effect. Note: This sequencing instruction does not apply to underdosing codes (fifth or sixth character "6", for example T36.0x6-).

1) Do not code directly from the Table of Drugs

Do not code directly from the Table of Drugs and Chemicals. Always refer back to the Tabular List.

2) Use as many codes as necessary to describe

Use as many codes as necessary to describe completely all drugs, medicinal or biological substances.

3) If the same code would describe the causative agent

If the same code would describe the causative agent for more than one adverse reaction, poisoning, toxic effect or underdosing, assign the code only once.

4) If two or more drugs, medicinal or biological substances

If two or more drugs, medicinal or biological substances are reported, code each individually unless **a** combination code is listed in the Table of Drugs and Chemicals.

5) The occurrence of drug toxicity is classified in ICD-10-CM as follows:

(a) Adverse Effect

Assign the appropriate code for adverse effect (for example, T36.0x5-) when the drug was correctly prescribed and properly administered. Use additional code(s) for all manifestations of adverse effects. Examples of manifestations are tachycardia, delirium, gastrointestinal hemorrhaging, vomiting, hypokalemia, hepatitis, renal failure, or respiratory failure.

(b) Poisoning

When coding a poisoning or reaction to the improper use of a medication (e.g., overdose, wrong substance given or taken in error, wrong route of administration), assign the appropriate code from categories T36-T50. Poisoning codes have an associated intent: accidental, intentional self-harm, assault and undetermined. Use additional code(s) for all manifestations of poisonings.

If there is also a diagnosis of abuse or dependence on the substance, the abuse or dependence is coded as an additional code.

Examples of poisoning include:

(i) Error was made in drug prescription

Errors made in drug prescription or in the administration of the drug by provider, nurse, patient, or other person.

(ii) Overdose of a drug intentionally taken

If an overdose of a drug was intentionally taken or administered and resulted in drug toxicity, it would be coded as a poisoning.

(iii) Nonprescribed drug taken with correctly prescribed and properly administered drug

If a nonprescribed drug or medicinal agent was taken in combination with a correctly prescribed and properly administered drug, any drug toxicity or other reaction resulting from the interaction of the two drugs would be classified as a poisoning.

(iv) Interaction of drug(s) and alcohol

When a reaction results from the interaction of a drug(s) and alcohol, this would be classified as poisoning.

See Section I.C.4. if poisoning is the result of insulin pump malfunctions.

(c) Underdosing

Underdosing refers to taking less of a medication than is prescribed by a provider or a manufacturer's instruction. For underdosing, assign the code from categories T36-T50 (fifth or sixth character "6").

Codes for underdosing should never be assigned as principal or first-listed codes. If a patient has a relapse or exacerbation of the medical condition for which the drug is prescribed because of the reduction in dose, then the medical condition itself should be coded.

Noncompliance (Z91.12-, Z91.13-) or complication of care (Y63.61, Y63.8-Y63.9) codes are to be used with an underdosing code to indicate intent, if known.

(d) Toxic Effects

When a harmful substance is ingested or comes in contact with a person, this is classified as a toxic effect. The toxic effect codes are in categories T51-T65.

Toxic effect codes have an associated intent: accidental, intentional self-harm, assault and undetermined.

f. Adult and child abuse, neglect and other maltreatment

Sequence first the appropriate code from categories T74.- **(Adult and child abuse, neglect and other maltreatment, confirmed)** or T76.- **(Adult and child abuse, neglect and other maltreatment, suspected)** for abuse, neglect and other maltreatment, followed by any accompanying mental health or injury code(s).

If the documentation in the medical record states abuse or neglect it is coded as confirmed **(T74.-)**. It is coded as suspected if it is documented as suspected **(T76.-)**.

For cases of confirmed abuse or neglect an external cause code from the assault section (X92-Y08) should be added to identify the cause of any physical injuries. A perpetrator code (Y07) should be added when the perpetrator of the abuse is known. For suspected cases of abuse or neglect, do not report external cause or perpetrator code.

If a suspected case of abuse, neglect or mistreatment is ruled out during an encounter code Z04.71, Suspected adult physical and sexual abuse, ruled out, or code Z04.72, Suspected child physical and sexual abuse, ruled out, should be used, not a code from T76.

See Section I.C.15.r Abuse in a pregnant patient.

20. Chapter 20: External Causes of Morbidity (VO1- Y99)

g. Child and Adult Abuse Guideline

Adult and child abuse, neglect and maltreatment are classified as assault. Any of the assault codes may be used to indicate the external cause of any injury resulting from the confirmed abuse.

For confirmed cases of abuse, neglect and maltreatment, when the perpetrator is known, a code from Y07, Perpetrator of maltreatment and neglect, should accompany any other assault codes.

See Section I.C.19. Adult and child abuse, neglect and other maltreatment

Apply the General Coding Guidelines as found in Chapter 5 and the Procedural Guidelines as found in Chapter 7.

GUIDELINE DIFFERENCES BETWEEN ICD-9-CM AND ICD-10-CM

- ICD-10-CM does not have a code to identify posttraumatic wound infection. An infected burn site is coded with an additional code for the infection.
- Late effects for burns are coded differently in ICD-10-CM. The burn code is assigned with the seventh character *S,* for *sequela.* A code to identify the sequela is also assigned (e.g., contracture, scar, etc.).
- In ICD-10-CM, adverse effects, poisoning, underdosing, and toxic effects are combination codes that identify the substance and the external cause.
- Underdosing codes are new in ICD-10-CM. To identify the medication that has been underdosed, a T code is assigned. According to the ICD-10-CM guidelines, the T code should not be assigned as the principal or first-listed code. The medical

condition that is exacerbated because of the lower dose should be sequenced before the T code.

MAJOR DIFFERENCES BETWEEN ICD-9-CM AND ICD-10-CM

- In ICD-10-CM, there are specific codes for **corrosive burns**, which are burns due to a chemical. A code to identify the chemical and intent is sequenced before the corrosive burn code.
- The coding of adverse effects and poisonings is different in ICD-10-CM. In ICD-9-CM, an adverse effect is coded with whatever manifestation(s) describe the effect and the appropriate E code to identify the drug. In ICD-9-CM, a poisoning is coded with the appropriating poisoning code, followed by any manifestation codes and the appropriate E codes to identify the intent of the poisoning. In ICD-10-CM, the same code is used for adverse effects and poisonings to identify the substance. The fifth and sixth digits identify the circumstances, and the seventh digit identifies the encounter as initial, subsequent, or for treatment of sequelae.
- ICD-10-CM codes can be used to identify underdosing, taking less of a medication than is prescribed or less than the manufacturer's instructions, with a negative effect on health. A code for noncompliance or failure in dosage during surgical or medical care should also be assigned.
- In ICD-10-CM a dummy placeholder or letter *x* is used in some codes in this chapter along with seventh-character extensions.

ANATOMY AND PHYSIOLOGY

All areas of the body may be involved in an injury. These are outlined in their respective body system chapters.

DISEASE CONDITIONS

This chapter discusses the following categories from Chapter 17 in your ICD-9-CM code book:

CATEGORY	SECTION TITLES
905-909	Late Effects of Injuries, Poisonings, Toxic Effects, and Other External Causes
940-949	Burns
958-959	Certain Traumatic Complications and Unspecified Injuries
960-979	Poisoning by Drugs, Medicinals, and Biologic Substances
980-989	Toxic Effects of Substances Chiefly Nonmedicinal to Source
990-995	Other and Unspecified Effect of External Causes

Chapter 25 is dedicated to complications of surgical and medical care.

Injury, Poisoning, and Certain Other Consequences of External Causes (S00-T88), Chapter 19 in the ICD-10-CM code book, is divided into the following categories:

CATEGORY	SECTION TITLES
T20-T32	Burns and Corrosions
T33-T34	Frostbite
T36-T50	Poisoning by, Adverse Effect of, and Underdosing of Drugs, Medicaments, and Biologic Substances
T51-T65	Toxic Effects of Substances Chiefly Nonmedicinal as to Source
T66-T78	Other and Unspecified Effects of External Causes

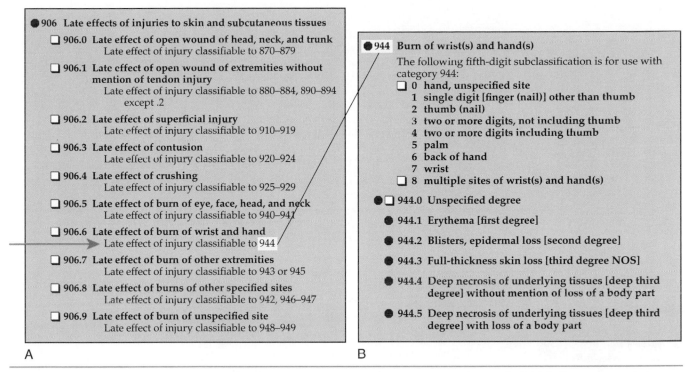

FIGURE 24-2. A, Categories for late effects of injuries to skin and subcutaneous tissues. **B,** 944 is the category that would have been assigned for the acute injury.

Late Effects of Injuries, Poisonings, Toxic Effects, and Other External Causes

Once the acute nature of an injury, poisoning, or adverse effect has resolved, some residual effects that have remained may require medical treatment. The residual effect is sequenced first, followed by the appropriate late effect code. In Chapter 5, the coding and sequencing of late effects were discussed. In this chapter, late effects due to traumatic injury, poisoning, and adverse effects are covered. Remember, a late effect may occur at any time after the acute injury, poisoning, or adverse effect has resolved. No specific time frames are required.

Late effect categories are as follows:

905	Late effects of musculoskeletal and connective tissue injuries
906	Late effects of injuries to skin and subcutaneous tissues (Figure 24-2, A)
907	Late effects of injuries to the nervous system
908	Late effects of other and unspecified injuries
909	Late effects of other and unspecified external causes (includes poisoning and adverse effects)

To locate the late effect code, look under the main term "Late" and then verify in the Tabular. The Tabular indicates which conditions from categories 800 to 999 are the cause of the residual condition.

EXAMPLE   Scar of left wrist due to previous burn by fire, 709.2, 906.6, E929.4 (L90.5, T23.072S, X08.8xxS).
     Late effect of injury classifiable to 944 (see Figure 24-2, *B*).

It may be necessary to assign the appropriate E code to indicate the late effects of accidental injury from category E929. Code assignment for E codes may depend on facility policy. Often, documentation is insufficient to reveal how the accident happened.

E929.0	Late effects of motor vehicle accident
E929.1	Late effects of other transport accident
E929.2	Late effects of accidental poisoning
E929.3	Late effects of accidental fall
E929.4	Late effects of accident caused by fire
E929.5	Late effects of accident due to natural and environmental factors
E929.8	Late effects of other accidents
E929.9	Late effects of unspecified accident
E989	Late effects of injury, undetermined whether accidental or purposely inflicted

There are also late effect E codes for late effects of accidental poisonings, suicide attempts, and complications of medical care.

EXAMPLE Patient has a cicatrix of left hand due to accidental burn that occurred 1 year ago from a bonfire, 709.2, 906.6, E929.4 (L90.5, T23.002S, X03.0xxS).

EXAMPLE Patient is being treated for avascular necrosis following previous left scaphoid fracture due to old sports injury with fall, 733.49, 905.2, E929.3 (M87.242, S62.002S).

EXERCISE 24-1

Assign codes to the following conditions.

1. Nonunion of left lateral humeral condylar fracture; patient fell 2 months ago (accidental injury) _____

2. Traumatic arthritis due to severe sprain of right ankle 3 years ago (accidental injury) _____

3. Phantom limb pain due to traumatic AKA (above-knee amputation); patient was in a motorcycle accident 6 months ago _____

4. Spastic quadriplegia due to complete C3 spinal cord injury from diving accident 5 years ago _____

5. Hypoxic brain injury due to suicide attempt by strangulation 1 year ago _____

Burns

It may be necessary to transport burn victims to a hospital that has a specialized unit for care of the burn patient. Plastic surgeons, anesthesiologists, nurses, dietitians, and physical and occupational therapists assist the burn patient through the acute and recovery phases of their injury. As a result, many facilities only stabilize the burn patient in the Emergency Room and then transport to a burn unit, or only less critical burn patients are admitted for care.

The Coding Guidelines offer advice on the coding and sequencing of burn injury codes. As with other injuries, it is necessary to assign separate codes for each burn site. Codes are available for multiple sites, but these should be used only if the documentation is insufficient to allow assignment of more specific burn codes.

Burn severity is classified by degrees (Figure 24-3):

- First-degree burn: **erythema** or redness of the skin
- Second-degree burn: formation of blisters with epidermal loss
- Third-degree burn: full-thickness skin loss
- Fourth-degree burn: deep **necrosis** of underlying tissues or deep third-degree burn

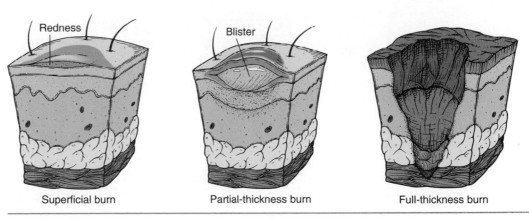

Redness

Blister

Superficial burn

Partial-thickness burn

Full-thickness burn

FIGURE 24-3. Depths of burns.

The guidelines instruct the coder to sequence the code that reflects the highest degree of burn first.

EXAMPLE   Patient was seen in the ER for second-degree burns of the left calf and first-degree burns of the right foot due to uncontrolled grass fire in woods, 945.24, 945.12, E892, E849.8 (T24.232A, T25.121A, X01.0xxA, Y92.828).

Often, a burn will be described as having different degrees at the same site. It is only necessary to assign the code that identifies the highest degree of burn.

EXAMPLE   Examination of the patient shows erythema and blisters to the right wrist due to burn from an iron. The accident occurred at the patient's house, 944.27, E924.8, E849.0, E013.3, E000.8 (T23.271A, X15.8xxA, Y92.019, Y93.e4, Y99.8).

Although the physician did not state first- or second-degree burn, by the description, this burn is a first- (erythema) and second-degree (blister) burn, so it would be coded to the most severe burn, which is second-degree.

For a variety of reasons, a burn may not heal quickly, or it may become infected. A nonhealing burn is coded as an acute burn. It is possible to have burns that occurred at the same time, and some may have healed completely while others have not yet healed. If the burn contains necrotic tissue, it is coded as an acute burn. It is possible to have late effects (e.g., scar, contracture) of a burn along with a nonhealing burn. Sometimes, late effects remain after the burn has healed, and these still require treatment. Residual conditions are late effects; therefore, these should be coded with the residual condition sequenced first followed by the appropriate late effect code. A late effect E code may also be assigned.

Sunburns or burns due to friction are excluded from the burn codes; this is noted in the Excludes note at the beginning of the burn section (Figure 24-4).

EXAMPLE   Patient has third-degree burn on chest wall due to house fire, 942.32, E890.3, E849.0 (T21.31xA, X00.0xxA, Y92.019).

EXAMPLE   Patient has a nonhealing third-degree burn of abdominal wall with keloid scar forming on right shoulder burn, subsequent visit. Burns due to accidental injury in house fire, 942.33, 701.4, 906.7, E890.3, E929.4 (T21.32xD, L91.0, T22.051S, X00.0xxD, X00.0xxS, Y92.019).

FIGURE 24-4. Friction burns and sunburn are excluded from the burn section.

FIGURE 24-5. Invasive pseudomonal burn wound infection, stage 2C.

Code 958.3, Posttraumatic wound infection, can be used as an additional code to indicate that the burn has become infected. The acute burn code would be sequenced first (Figure 24-5).

EXAMPLE | Patient is being treated for an infected burn right palm from a hot light bulb, subsequent visit, 944.05, 958.3, E924.8 (T23.051D, T79.8xxD, L08.9, X15.8xxD).

Category 948 is provided to identify the extent of body surface that is involved by burns and to indicate the percentage of body surface that has third-degree burns. According to the classic "rule of nines," in estimating involved body surface, head and neck are assigned 9%, each arm 9%, each leg 18%, anterior trunk 18%, posterior trunk 18%, and genitalia 1%. These percentage assignments may change as necessary to accommodate infants and children who have proportionately larger heads than adults and patients who have large buttocks, thighs, or abdomens that involve burns (Figure 24-6). The percentages of body surface involvement must be documented by a healthcare professional for code assignment. Percentages should not be calculated by the coder.

Categories 948 (T30) and/or 949 can be used when the site of the burn is not specified. Category 948 can be used with categories 940-947 when the site is specified. In some instances, the burns may be so extensive that detailed documentation is not provided. A specialized burn assessment form to document burn location, type, and body percentage is often used in burn centers.

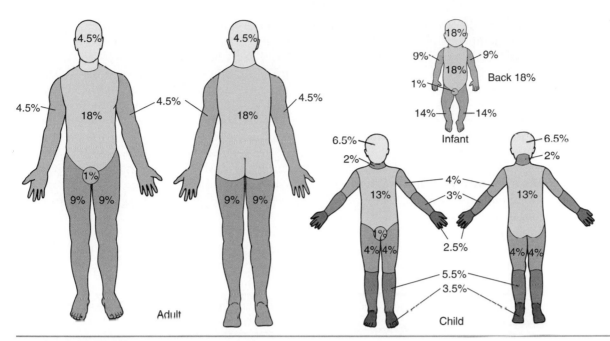

FIGURE 24-6. Rule of nines.

EXAMPLE	Patient has second- (3%) and third-degree (5%) burns of the trunk and first-degree burns (2%) of the right arm due to fire on a street car, 942.30, 943.10, 948.10, E803.1, E849.5 (T21.30xA, T22.10xA, T31.10, V82.9xxA, Y92.818).

EXERCISE 24-2

Assign codes to the following conditions. (If percentage of the body burned is not documented, do not assign a code from category 948.)

1. Nonhealing second-degree burn left thigh due to hot coffee spill, subsequent encounter _____

2. Second- and third-degree burns trunk, and second- and third-degree burns both legs due to fire at night club; in all, 35% of the body was burned, 25% third-degree _____

3. First-degree burn wrist and second-degree burns fingers and hand due to firework explosion while playing in backyard _____

4. Infected second-degree burn buttock, subsequent encounter _____

5. Alkaline burn left cornea due to caustic soda while working in a paper manufacturing factory _____

6. Hypertrophic scar of burn to right cheek _____

7. Friction burn left elbow due to accidental fall on carpeted stairs at patient's home _____

8. Patient in house fire with multiple burns over 60% of body, 30% third-degree; patient was stabilized and prepared for transport to burn unit; fire was due to accidental causes _____

Adverse Effects of Drugs and Medicinals

An **adverse effect** can occur due to ingestion or exposure to drugs or other medicinal and biologic substances. It is a reaction to a drug that has been taken according to the prescription or instructions on the label of over-the-counter drugs. To code an adverse effect, at least two codes are required: one code for the adverse effect (e.g., rash, nausea, headache) and a therapeutic-use E code (E930-E949) for the drug responsible for the adverse effect. These E codes are located in the Table of Drugs and Chemicals.

The Table of Drugs and Chemicals (Figure 24-7), which is also known as the Alphabetic Index to Poisoning and External Causes of Adverse Effects of Drugs and Other Chemical Substances, is located after the Alphabetic Index. This Table is used to identify external causes of adverse effects that are due to drugs or chemicals. The drug responsible for the adverse effect must first be identified and then located in the Index under the therapeutic column. If a specific drug cannot be located, the generic name should be determined or the category of the drug identified (e.g., antihypertensive, antianginal, antineoplastic). Once the drug or drug category has been located in the Index, the E code from the therapeutic-use column is assigned. The adverse effect code(s) are sequenced before the therapeutic E code(s).

Because drugs have generic and brand names, and these are used interchangeably, it may be difficult to locate the drug in the Index. A drug reference book or an Internet search can be used to determine the generic name or category of the drug.

EXAMPLE	Hematuria due to Coumadin, which is taken for atrial fibrillation, 599.70, E934.2, 427.31, V58.61 (T45.515A, R31.9, I48.0, Z79.01). Hematuria in this case is the adverse effect of medication that was properly prescribed and properly taken. An E code for the therapeutic use of Coumadin is also assigned.

EXAMPLE	Patient presented with hypokalemia due to long-term use of diuretics, 276.8, V58.69, E944.4 (T50.2x5A, E87.6, Z79.899). Hypokalemia is the adverse effect of the diuretic.

EXAMPLE	Dizziness caused by Claritin, which was taken per instructions on the label, 780.4, E933.0 (T45.0x5A, R42). Claritin is not listed in the Table of Drugs and Chemicals, but an Internet search reveals that loratadine is the generic name, and this is not listed either. Claritin is classified as an antihistamine that can be located in the table.

EXERCISE 24-3

Using a drug reference book or the Internet, specify drug category or generic name for the following drugs.

1. Lunesta   _____
2. Cardizem   _____
3. Bactrim   _____
4. Zoloft   _____
5. Ditropan   _____

It is possible that an adverse effect to some drugs may be based on an abnormal laboratory result. Sometimes a physician will document "toxicity" based on these laboratory results. According to *Coding Clinic* (1997:1Q:p16),[1] for a drug toxicity with no documented adverse reaction, assign code 796.0 (R89.2). If the patient has any symptoms, then the symptom codes are assigned along with the appropriate E code for therapeutic use.

EXAMPLE	Dilantin toxicity per laboratory report. Patient is asymptomatic. The Dilantin dosage will be adjusted and Dilantin levels monitored. Patient takes Dilantin for seizure disorder, 796.0, 345.90, E936.1 (T42.0x5A, R56.9, G40.909).

| | External Cause (E-Code) | | | | | |
Substance	Poisoning	Accident	Therapeutic Use	Suicide Attempt	Assault	Undetermined
1-propanol	980.3	E860.4	—	E950.9	E962.1	E980.9
2-propanol	980.2	E860.3	—	E950.9	E962.1	E980.9
2,4-D (dichlorophenoxyacetic acid)	989.4	E863.5	—	E950.6	E962.1	E980.7
2,4-toluene diisocyanate	983.0	E864.0	—	E950.7	E962.1	E980.6
2,4,5-T (trichlorophenoxyacetic acid)	989.2	E863.5	—	E950.6	E962.1	E980.7
14-hydroxydihydromorphinone	965.09	E850.2	E935.2	E950.0	E962.0	E980.0
ABOB	961.7	E857	E931.7	E950.4	E962.0	E980.4
Abrus (seed)	988.2	E865.3	—	E950.9	E962.1	E980.9
Absinthe	980.0	E860.1	—	E950.9	E962.1	E980.9
beverage	980.0	E860.0	—	E950.9	E962.1	E980.9
Acenocoumarin, acenocoumarol	964.2	E858.2	E934.2	E950.4	E962.0	E980.4
Acepromazine	969.1	E853.0	E939.1	E950.3	E962.0	E980.3
Acetal	982.8	E862.4	—	E950.9	E962.1	E980.9
Acetaldehyde (vapor)	987.8	E869.8	—	E952.8	E962.2	E982.8
liquid	989.89	E866.8	—	E950.9	E962.1	E980.9
Acetaminophen	965.4	E850.4	E935.4	E950.0	E962.0	E980.0
Acetaminosalol	965.1	E850.3	E935.3	E950.0	E962.0	E980.0
Acetanilid(e)	965.4	E850.4	E935.4	E950.0	E962.0	E980.0
Acetarsol, acetarsone	961.1	E857	E931.1	E950.4	E962.0	E980.4
Acetazolamide	974.2	E858.5	E944.2	E950.4	E962.0	E980.4
Acetic	—	—	—	—	—	—
acid	983.1	E864.1	—	E950.7	E962.1	E980.6
with sodium acetate (ointment)	976.3	E858.7	E946.3	E950.4	E962.0	E980.4
irrigating solution	974.5	E858.5	E944.5	E950.4	E962.0	E980.4
lotion	976.2	E858.7	E946.2	E950.4	E962.0	E980.4
anhydride	983.1	E864.1	—	E950.7	E962.1	E980.6
ether (vapor)	982.8	E862.4	—	E950.9	E962.1	E980.9
Acetohexamide	962.3	E858.0	E932.3	E950.4	E962.0	E980.4
Acetomenaphthone	964.3	E858.2	E934.3	E950.4	E962.0	E980.4
Acetomorphine	965.01	E850.0	E935.0	E950.0	E962.0	E980.0
Acetone (oils) (vapor)	982.8	E862.4	—	E950.9	E962.1	E980.9
Acetophenazine (maleate)	969.1	E853.0	E939.1	E950.3	E962.0	E980.3
Acetophenetidin	965.4	E850.4	E935.4	E950.0	E962.0	E980.0
Acetophenone	982.0	E862.4	—	E950.9	E962.1	E980.9
Acetorphine	965.09	E850.2	E935.2	E950.0	E962.0	E980.0
Acetosulfone (sodium)	961.8	E857	E931.8	E950.4	E962.0	E980.4
Acetrizoate (sodium)	977.8	E858.8	E947.8	E950.4	E962.0	E980.4
Acetylcarbromal	967.3	E852.2	E937.3	E950.2	E962.0	E980.2
Acetylcholine (chloride)	971.0	E855.3	E941.0	E950.4	E962.0	E980.4
Acetylcysteine	975.5	E858.6	E945.5	E950.4	E962.0	E980.4
Acetyldigitoxin	972.1	E858.3	E942.1	E950.4	E962.0	E980.4
Acetyldihydrocodeine	965.09	E850.2	E935.2	E950.0	E962.0	E980.0
Acetyldihydrocodeinone	965.09	E850.2	E935.2	E950.0	E962.0	E980.0
Acetylene (gas) (industrial)	987.1	E868.1	—	E951.8	E962.2	E981.8
incomplete combustion of - see Carbon monoxide, fuel, utility	—	—	—	—	—	—
tetrachloride (vapor)	982.3	E862.4	—	E950.9	E962.1	E980.9
Acetyliodosalicylic acid	965.1	E850.3	E935.3	E950.0	E962.0	E980.0
Acetylphenylhydrazine	965.8	E850.8	E935.8	E950.0	E962.0	E980.0
Acetylsalicylic acid	965.1	E850.3	E935.3	E950.0	E962.0	E980.0
Achromycin	960.4	E856	E930.4	E950.4	E962.0	E980.4
ophthalmic preparation	976.5	E858.7	E946.5	E950.4	E962.0	E980.4
topical NEC	976.0	E858.7	E946.0	E950.4	E962.1	E980.4
Acidifying agents	963.2	E858.1	E933.2	E950.4	E962.0	E980.4
Acids (corrosive) NEC	983.1	E864.1	—	E950.7	E962.1	E980.6
Aconite (wild)	988.2	E865.4	—	E950.9	E962.1	E980.9
Aconitine (liniment)	976.8	E858.7	E946.8	E950.4	E962.0	E980.4
Aconitum ferox	988.2	E865.4	—	E950.9	E962.1	E980.9
Acridine	983.0	E864.0	—	E950.7	E962.1	E980.6
vapor	987.8	E869.8	—	E952.8	E962.2	E982.8
Acriflavine	961.9	E857	E931.9	E950.4	E962.0	E980.4
Acrisorcin	976.0	E858.7	E946.0	E950.4	E962.0	E980.4

FIGURE 24-7. Excerpt from the Table of Drugs and Chemicals.

Assign codes to the following conditions.

1. Hives due to Bactrim taken to treat UTI (urinary tract
    infection) _____

2. Diarrhea due to erythromycin used to treat acute bronchitis _____

3. Headache due to Nitrostat taken for angina _____

4. Constipation due to narcotics used after surgery _____

5. Decreased sex drive due to treatment with Zoloft for
    depression _____

6. Digoxin toxicity from Digoxin taken for congestive heart
    failure; drug was taken as prescribed _____

7. Dizziness and irregular heartbeat due to Inderal, which was
    taken for hypertension _____

8. Tachycardia due to albuterol, which was administered for
    asthma _____

Poisonings

It is sometimes confusing to determine the difference between an adverse effect and
a poisoning. Poisoning from medication(s) occurs when:

■ The wrong medication is taken—patient took a medication that is not currently
prescribed for them

■ The wrong dose is taken—patient took two tablets instead of one (double the dosage)

■ Intentional overdose—patient took large amount of medication or other drug or
chemical

■ Nonprescribed drug (including illegal drugs and alcohol) interacts with a
prescription medication—patient took an over-the-counter medication that causes
some reaction with prescribed medication

The poisoning code is always sequenced first and is found in the Table of Drugs and
Chemicals under the heading "poisoning." It is possible to assign more than one poisoning
code along with corresponding E codes, to describe a poisoning if more than one substance
or drug is responsible. A poisoning requires at least two codes: one code for the poisoning
and an E code to describe the circumstances of the poisoning. These E codes are located
in the Table of Drugs and Chemicals. Remember, E codes can never be sequenced as a
principal diagnosis.

The selection of the appropriate E code for poisonings can be confusing. Unlike
adverse effects where the only option for E code assignment is an E code from the "therapeutic" column, poisoning E codes are assigned according to circumstances surrounding
this poisoning. The circumstances (intent) include the following:

■ Accidental
■ Suicide attempt
■ Assault
■ Undetermined

According to the guidelines:

■ If the intent (accident, self-harm, assault) of the cause of an injury or poisoning is
unknown, code the intent as undetermined, E980-E989.

■ If the intent (accident, self-harm, assault) is questionable, probable, or suspected,
code the intent as undetermined, E980-E989.

If the manifestation(s) of the poisoning is documented, it should be coded as a secondary diagnosis. Manifestations could include chest pain, vomiting, lethargy, coma, and so
forth.

According to *Coding Clinic* (1993:1Q:p25),[2] when a patient is admitted for chest pain due to cocaine intoxication, this is considered a poisoning, and the code for the cocaine poisoning (970.81) is the principal diagnosis. An additional code for the manifestation of chest pain is assigned, along with a code for the drug abuse.

EXAMPLE   Patient admitted for a suicide attempt with multiple medications, including Naproxen, Keppra, and acetaminophen mixed with beer. Patient was somnolent on arrival in the ER, 965.61, 966.3, 965.4, 980.0, 780.09, E950.0, E950.4, E950.9 (T39.312A, T42.6x2A, T39.1x2A, T51.0x2A, R40.0).
(Both Naproxen and acetaminophen are coded to E950.0, so this E code needs to be assigned only once.)

EXAMPLE   Patient became weak, had labored breathing, and had altered mental status caused by an accidental overdose of codeine, 965.09, 780.79, 786.09, 780.97, E850.2 (T40.2x1A, R53.1, R06.4, R41.82).
The manifestations of the overdose are the weakness, breathing problems, and alteration in mental status.

EXERCISE 24-5

Assign codes to the following conditions.

1. Patient took ampicillin that belonged to his wife; patient developed hives caused by the ampicillin   _____

2. Patient became stuporous and lethargic after taking Valium according to prescription, then drinking a couple of beers; accidental intent   _____

3. The patient accidentally received the higher dosage of potassium while in hospital; no effects were noted   _____

4. Cocaine-induced chest pain; patient is a known cocaine abuser with a daily habit; accidental intent   _____

5. Suicide attempt with acetaminophen; patient has nausea and vomiting with abdominal pain   _____

6. Toddler accidentally drank bottle of Visine; the toddler was having labored breathing and was very irritable   _____

7. Patient was taking extra doses of Lasix to reduce swelling of lower extremities; patient is hypokalemic and takes Lasix for congestive heart failure   _____

8. Patient became dizzy and very drowsy after taking one of spouse's Vicodin tablets and drinking a couple of alcoholic beverages and smoking marijuana   _____

Toxic Effects of Substances Chiefly Nonmedicinal to Source

Numerous toxic substances can cause ill effects. Categories 980 to 989 identify these types of reactions. Reactions range from mild events such as headache to life-threatening conditions such as anaphylactic shock. At the beginning of this section, instructions are provided on the use of additional codes to specify the nature of the toxic effect.

EXAMPLE   Patient admitted with alcohol poisoning due to intake of vodka, 980.0, E980.9 (T51.0x1A).

EXERCISE 24-6

Assign codes to the following conditions.

1. Angioedema due to penicillin taken as prescribed   _____

2. Accidental lead poisoning from paint with anemia and muscle weakness   _____

3. Unconscious due to carbon monoxide poisoning caused by motor vehicle fumes, suicide attempt   _____

4. Tremors, low-grade fever, weight loss, and extreme fatigue due to mercury toxicity caused by exposure while working with dental fillings   _____

Other and Unspecified Effect of External Causes

Categories 990 to 995 are used to identify the effects that external causes such as radiation, temperature, heat, light, and air pressure may have on the human body. According to *Coding Clinic* (1997:2Q:p12),[3] it is unacceptable to use 995.20, Unspecified adverse effect of a drug, medicinal or biologic substance in the inpatient setting. This code should be assigned only in the outpatient setting and only in rare circumstances. The record should be reviewed to find further documentation of any specific adverse effect.

EXAMPLE   Patient developed an adverse reaction to codeine, 995.29, E935.2 (T40.2x5A, T88.7xxA).

Adult/Child Abuse

Domestic violence, elder abuse, and child abuse occur more often than one might think. Healthcare providers are required to report to the proper authorities any suspicions of abuse and/or neglect. Four major types of abuse have been identified:
1. Physical abuse
2. Sexual abuse
3. Emotional abuse
4. Neglect

The codes for child abuse range from 995.50 to 995.59. These codes must be assigned as the principal diagnosis according to *Coding Clinic* (1996:4Q:p40-41).[4] The code book gives instructions on the use of additional code(s), if applicable, to identify any associated injuries (Figure 24-8) and the appropriate E code to identify the perpetrator. The codes for adult abuse are from 995.80 to 995.85 and there are similar instructions to code any associated injuries as an additional code with an E code to identify the perpetrator. The adult abuse codes must be assigned as the principal diagnosis according to *Coding Clinic* (1996:4Q:p41-42).[5]

EXAMPLE   The child was admitted for moderate malnutrition because of neglect by the mother, 995.52, 263.0, E904.0, E967.2 (T74.02xA, E44.0, Y07.12).

Systemic Inflammatory Response Syndrome (SIRS)

Systemic inflammatory response syndrome (SIRS) is a serious medical condition that can occur in response to an infection or to noninfectious causes such as severe trauma, burns, and complications of surgery. It may also occur in diseases such as pancreatitis and AIDS.

SIRS may be diagnosed when two or more of the following criteria are present:
- Heart rate >90 beats per minute
- Body temperature <36° or >38°C
- Tachypnea (high respiratory rate) >20 breaths per minute or, on blood gas, a $PaCo_2$ <4.3 kPa (32 mm Hg)

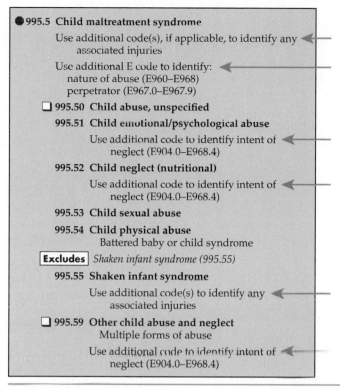

FIGURE 24-8. Instructions to use additional code(s) to identify any associated injuries caused by child maltreatment.

- White blood cell count <4000 cells/mm^3 or >12,000 cells/mm^3 (<4 × 10^9 or >12 × 10^9 cells/L), or the presence of greater than 10% immature neutrophils.

  Because of instructional notes in the code book to "code first underlying infection or condition," the SIRS codes will generally not be the principal diagnosis. In patients with trauma, the most severe injury would be the principal diagnosis and the SIRS code would be assigned as a secondary code. It is possible for organ dysfunction to occur as a result of trauma, and this would be coded to SIRS due to noninfectious process with organ dysfunction.

EXAMPLE

Patient has SIRS due to accidental burns in a street car fire. Patient has second- (3%) and third-degree (5%) burns of the trunk and first-degree burns of the right arm, 942.30, 943.10, 948.00, 995.93, E803.1, E849.5 (T21.30xA, T22.10xA, T31.0, R65.0, V82.9xxA, Y92.818).

EXERCISE 24-7

Assign codes to the following conditions.

1. Frostbite toes and fingers due to spending night outdoors in blizzard   _____

2. Heatstroke due to high temperature while at beach   _____

3. Anaphylactic shock due to peanut butter   _____

4. Seasickness while on cruise   _____

5. Shaken baby syndrome with subdural hematoma and retinal hemorrhages. The baby was shaken by the babysitter   _____

6. Headache, confusion, and seizure caused by arsenic poisoning. Wife was trying to harm the patient   _____

FACTORS INFLUENCING HEALTH STATUS AND CONTACT WITH HEALTH SERVICES (V CODES/Z CODES)

In the past, V/Z codes have been considered primarily for use in the outpatient setting. This has changed with the addition of more V/Z codes each year. As was discussed in Chapter 8, it may be difficult to locate V/Z codes in the Index. Coders often say, "I did not know there was a V/Z code for that." It is important for the coder to be familiar with different types and uses of V/Z codes. Refer to Chapter 8 for a listing of common main terms used to locate V/Z codes. See Chapter 23 for V codes used for injuries.

V14.0	Personal history of allergy to medicinal agents—penicillin
V14.1	Personal history of allergy to medicinal agents—other antibiotic agent
V14.2	Personal history of allergy to medicinal agents—sulfonamides
V14.2	Personal history of allergy to medicinal agents—other anti-infective agents
V14.4	Personal history of allergy to medicinal agents—anesthetic agent
V14.5	Personal history of allergy to medicinal agents—narcotic agent
V14.6	Personal history of allergy to medicinal agents—analgesic agent
V14.7	Personal history of allergy to medicinal agents—serum or vaccine
V14.8	Personal history of allergy to medicinal agents—other specified medicinal agents
V14.9	Personal history of allergy to medicinal agents—unspecified medicinal agent
V15.07	Allergy other than to medicinal agents—latex
V15.08	Allergy other than to medicinal agents—radiographic dye
V15.41	History of physical abuse
V15.52	History of emotional abuse
V15.49	Other psychological trauma
V15.59	Personal history of other injury
V15.6	History of poisoning
V15.84	Exposure to asbestos
V15.86	Personal history of contact with and (suspected) exposure to lead
V61.11	Counseling for victim of spousal and partner abuse
V61.21	Counseling for victim of child abuse
V61.22	Counseling for perpetrator of parental child abuse
V62.83	Counseling for perpetrator of physical/sexual abuse
V71.5	Observation after alleged rape or seduction
V71.6	Observation after other inflicted injury
V71.81	Observation and evaluation for other specified suspected conditions—abuse and neglect
V87.01	Contact with and (suspected) exposure to arsenic
V87.02	Contact with and (suspected) exposure to uranium
V87.09	Contact with and (suspected) exposure to other hazardous metals
V87.11	Contact with and (suspected) exposure to aromatic amines
V87.12	Contact with and (suspected) exposure to benzene
V87.19	Contact with and (suspected) exposure to other hazardous aromatic compounds
V87.2	Contact with and (suspected) exposure to other potentially hazardous chemicals
V87.39	Contact with and (suspected) exposure to other potentially hazardous substances

EXAMPLE Patient was exposed to asbestos while working in a shipyard years ago, V15.84 (Z77.090).

EXAMPLE Patient wears a bracelet because of allergy to penicillin, V14.0 (Z88.0).

EXERCISE 24-8

Assign codes to the following conditions.

1. History of allergy to latex _____
2. History of allergy to Bactrim _____
3. Patient has a history of anaphylactic shock due to bee sting _____
4. History of rape _____
5. History of hives due to contrast media or radiologic dye _____
6. Observation for suspected physical abuse (adult) _____

COMMON TREATMENTS

Treatment will depend on the type and severity of the injury. Pain medications, anti-inflammatories, corticosteroids, and antibiotics may be necessary to alleviate pain and inflammation and to prevent or fight infection.

PROCEDURES

Debridement

Debridement of burns is probably the most common procedure that will be assigned in this chapter. The root operation for debridement is excision. There are very specific guidelines regarding the use of debridement codes. If any question arises as to whether a debridement was **excisional** or **nonexcisional**, a query may be necessary. Debridements can be performed in many settings in the hospital including at the bedside, so documentation may be difficult to locate. Debridements do not have to be performed in the Operating Room. Debridements may also be performed by physical therapists, wound care nurses, and other healthcare professionals in addition to physicians.

According to *Coding Clinic* (1999:1Q:p8-9),[6] when an extensive debridement goes beyond the skin and subcutaneous tissue into the muscle, tendon, and/or bone it is appropriate to "assign only a code for the deepest layer of debridement when multiple layers of the same site are debrided." If a patient had a debridement of skin, subcutaneous tissue, muscle, and bone, the bone is the deepest layer and debridement of the bone 77.67 is the only procedure code assigned.

EXAMPLE | Excisional debridement of infected burn right palm performed by physical therapist, subsequent visit. Patient was burned by hot light bulb, 944.05, 958.3, E924.8, 86.22 (T23.051D, L08.9, X15.8xxD, 0HBFXZZ).

EXAMPLE | Excisional debridement of fourth-degree burn lower back by physician. Accidentally burned in house fire, 942.44, E890.3, E849.0, 86.22 (T21.34xA, X00.0xxA, Y92.019, 0HB6XZZ).

Hyperbaric Oxygen Therapy

Hyperbaric oxygen therapy (HBOT) is a treatment in which the patient's entire body is placed in a transparent, airtight chamber at increased atmospheric pressure. The patient breathes in 100% pure oxygen. This increased oxygen flow in the body helps to improve healing within the tissues and helps to get rid of toxic gases in the case of a poisoning. The ICD-10-PCS codes for HBOT can be found in the extracorporeal assistance and performance section.

HBOT is helpful in treating medical conditions such as the following:

- Air or gas embolism (in divers or following bypass surgery)
- Decompensation sickness in divers (bends)
- Burns and other wounds
- Carbon monoxide poisoning
- Smoke inhalation
- Near drowning, near electrocution or near hanging
- Diabetic ulcers/skin ulcers

EXAMPLE

Patient is being treated with HBOT for decompression sickness while surfacing while scuba diving in the ocean, 993.3, E902.2, E849.8, E002.4, 93.95 (T70.3xxA, W94.21xA, Y92.832, Y93.15, 6A150ZZ).

EXERCISE 24-9

Assign codes for all diagnoses and procedures.

1. Z-plasty to release scar contracture forearm _____

2. Nonexcisional debridement of second-degree burn right knee by wound care nurse _____

3. Excisional debridement of second- and third-degree burns back performed at the patient's bedside _____

4. Debridement to the soft tissue of deep burns left thigh _____

5. Full-thickness skin graft to deep third-degree burn area of the right hand. Graft from patient (subsequent encounter) _____

DOCUMENTATION/REIMBURSEMENT/MS-DRGs

Often, coding challenges are due to lack of documentation. Sometimes radiology and other test results are not available at the time of discharge or when the physician is dictating the discharge summary or is reporting the final diagnoses.

Documentation of how, when, and where an injury occurred, along with good descriptions of the injury, is often lacking. It may not be important to the physician that the accident occurred on the school playground instead of the backyard of the patient's home. Surgical procedures such as skin grafting, excisional debridement, or mechanical ventilation can make a difference in reimbursement.

Burns have their own major diagnostic category, or MDC—22. The following Medicare Severity diagnosis-related groups (MS-DRGs) fall into the burn MDC:

- 927 Extensive burns or full-thickness burns with mechanical ventilation 96 hours with skin graft
- 928 Full-thickness burn with skin graft or inhalation injury with CC/MCC
- 929 Full-thickness burn with skin graft or inhalation injury without CC/MCC
- 933 Extensive burns or full-thickness burns with mechanical ventilation 96 hours without skin graft
- 934 Full-thickness burn without skin graft of inhalation injury
- 935 Nonextensive burns

By the titles of these MS-DRGs, it is evident that the type of burn, mechanical ventilation, skin graft procedure, presence of an inhalation injury, and/or CC/MCC determines the MS-DRG assignment.

Frequently missed complications/comorbidities from this chapter are difficult to pinpoint. The CC/MCC listing contains numerous injury codes. It is important to code all injuries with the most serious injury as the principal diagnosis. Codes for complications related to trauma are also important.

Correct Procedure Code

EXAMPLE   A patient was admitted with third-degree burns to the abdomen and second-degree burns to the face with burn injury to the lungs. The patient was on a mechanical ventilator for 5 days. Documentation of mechanical ventilation may be difficult to find within the health record. The calculation of ventilation hours can also affect the MS-DRG assignment.

DIAGNOSES	CODES	MS-DRG	RW
Burns abdomen, face, and lungs	947.1, 942.33, 941.20, (T27.1xxA, T21.32xA, T20.20xA)	207	5.2068
Ventilation 96+ hours	96.72 (5A1955Z)		
Burns abdomen, face, and lungs	947.1, 942.33, 941.20 (T27.1xxA, T21.32xA, T20.20xA)	208	2.2630
Ventilation less than 96 hours (30 hours)	96.71 (5A1945Z)		
Burns abdomen and face	942.33, 941.20 (T21.32xA, T20.20xA)	934	1.3556
No ventilation			

The MS-DRG assignment is affected by the burn injury to the lung and the use of mechanical ventilation.

Adverse Effect Versus Poisoning

If an adverse effect is incorrectly coded as a poisoning, or if a poisoning is incorrectly coded as an adverse effect, reimbursement can be affected.

EXAMPLE   The patient's physician recently adjusted the dosage of the patient's digitalis, which the patient takes for congestive heart failure. The patient took the medication as directed by the physician but became severely nauseated. This is an adverse effect associated with digitalis because the patient took the medication as prescribed by the physician.

DIAGNOSES	CODES	MS-DRG	RW
Coded as Adverse Effect			
Nausea due to digitalis toxicity with congestive heart failure	787.02, 428.0, E942.1 (T46.0x5A, R11.0, I50.9)	392	0.7173
Coded as Poisoning			
Nausea due to digitalis toxicity with congestive heart failure	972.1, 787.02, 428.0, E980.4 (T46.0x1A, R11.0, I50.9)	918	0.6269

The term "toxicity" does not necessarily indicate a poisoning. This case should be coded as an adverse effect. If this case had been coded as a poisoning, the facility would have received a lower reimbursement than was supported by the documentation in the health record.

CHAPTER REVIEW EXERCISE

Assign codes for all diagnoses and procedures. Explain why it is an adverse effect or a poisoning.

1. Alcoholic drank rubbing alcohol, undetermined circumstances _____

2. Anaphylactic shock due to bee sting _____

3. Gastrointestinal bleeding due to excessive use of aspirin for chronic low back pain (accidental) _____

4. Orthostatic hypotension due to Nitro-Bid taken for stable angina _____

_____

5. Depression due to Keppra, which was taken for a seizure disorder _____

_____

6. Accidental ingestion of Drano with burns mouth and esophagus _____

_____

7. Drug-induced dementia due to Lithium. Lithium is taken for bipolar disorder_____

_____

8. Coma due to accidental alcohol poisoning with blood alcohol of 0.3_____

_____

9. Abnormal level of mercury in blood indicating poisoning. No symptoms_____

_____

10. Accidental injury with chemical burns to eyelids from Roundup chemical used on the job doing farm work_____

_____

11. Weakness and tremor due to Lithium toxicity. Patient has bipolar affective disease and is currently depressed. Lithium taken as prescribed_____

_____

12. Drug-induced hepatitis due to isoniazid, which is being taken because of exposure to tuberculosis_____

_____

13. Bite by poisonous rattlesnake _____

_____

14. Steroid-induced hyperglycemia _____

_____

15. Paralytic ileus due to interaction of anticholinergics and codeine _____

_____

Assign codes for all diagnoses and procedures.

16. Sunburn neck, back, and back of legs after spending day at water park_____

17. Chemical burn on right knee due to leaking ice pack that was used for knee injury. The skin is reddened with no blister formation_____

18. History of exposure to lead. No apparent symptoms _____

19. Malunion of radial shaft fracture. Previous accidental injury _____

20. Firefighter suffers smoke inhalation after fighting warehouse fire _____

21. Hypothermia due to cold weather. Patient is homeless and lives in alley _____

22. Second-degree burns to left foot due to accidental scald injury with hot water from bathroom sink at home _____

23. Toddler with third- and fourth-degree burns buttocks, lower legs, and feet. Patient was put into boiling water by the mother's boyfriend. Twenty percent of his body was affected _____

24. Extensive burns 50% of body with 18% third-degree. Patient was in a motor vehicle accident (MVA) _____

25. SIRS due to crush injury to chest. Patient was driver of MV that hit deer on roadway _____

26. Second-degree burns right hand and third-degree burns left hand due to grease fire at restaurant. Excisional debridement of left hand done in the Operating Room _____

Write the correct answer(s) in the space(s) provided.

27. Name two things that can make a difference in the assignment of a burn MS-DRG.

_____

_____

28. Describe the difference between excisional and nonexcisional debridement.

_____

29. What degree of burn results in full-thickness skin loss?

_____

30. Define adverse effect of a drug.

_____

31. Second-degree burns right hand and third-degree burns left hand due to grease fire at restaurant. Excisional debridement of left hand done in the Operating Room

_____

CHAPTER GLOSSARY

Adverse effect: pathologic manifestation due to ingestion or exposure to drugs or other chemical substances.

Corrosive burn: burn due to a chemical.

Erythema: redness of the skin.

Excisional debridement: surgical removal or cutting away of devitalized tissue, necrosis, or slough.

Hyperbaric oxygen therapy (HBOT): treatment in which the patient's entire body is placed in a transparent, airtight chamber at increased atmospheric pressure.

Necrosis: death of cells.

Nonexcisional debridement: removal of devitalized tissue by brushing, irrigating, scrubbing, or washing.

Residual condition or effect: when the acute phase of an illness or injury has passed, but a residual condition or health problem remains.

Systemic inflammatory response syndrome: a serious medical condition that can occur in response to infectious or noninfectious causes, such as severe trauma, burns, or complications of surgery.

REFERENCES

1. American Hospital Association. *Coding Clinic for ICD-9-CM* 1997:1Q:p16. Correction—Dilantin toxicity.
2. American Hospital Association. *Coding Clinic for ICD-9-CM* 1993:1Q:p25. Cocaine intoxication with chest pain.
3. American Hospital Association. *Coding Clinic for ICD-9-CM* 1997:2Q:p12. Clarification—Unspecified adverse effect of drug.
4. American Hospital Association. *Coding Clinic for ICD-9-CM* 1996:4Q:p40-41. Sequencing of child abuse codes.
5. American Hospital Association. *Coding Clinic for ICD-9-CM* 1996:4Q:p41-42. Adult abuse coding.
6. American Hospital Association. *Coding Clinic for ICD-9-CM* 1999:1Q:p8-9. Extensive wound debridement.

25

Complications of Surgical and Medical Care

LEARNING OBJECTIVES

1. Apply and assign the correct ICD-9-CM and ICD-10-CM codes in accordance with Official Guidelines for Coding and Reporting

2. Identify major differences between ICD-9-CM and ICD-10-CM related to complications of surgical and medical care

3. Identify complications of surgical and medical care

4. Assign the correct V/Z codes, E codes, and procedure codes related to complications of surgical and medical care

5. Explain the importance of documentation in relation to MS-DRGs for reimbursement

ABBREVIATIONS/ ACRONYMS

CKD chronic kidney disease

DVT deep vein thrombosis

ECT electroconvulsive therapy

ESRD end-stage renal disease

ICD-9-CM *International Classification of Diseases, 9th Revision, Clinical Modification*

ICD-10-CM *International Classification of Diseases, 10th Revision, Clinical Modification*

ICD-10-PCS *International Classification of Diseases, 10th Revision, Procedure Coding System*

IUD intrauterine device

MS-DRG Medicare Severity diagnosis-related group

PE pulmonary embolism

THR total hip replacement

TPN total parenteral nutrition

TURP transurethral resection of the prostate

UTI urinary tract infection

VAP ventilator-assisted pneumonia

VSD ventricular septal defect

ICD-9-CM

Official Guidelines for Coding and Reporting

Please refer to the companion Evolve website for the most current guidelines.

Section II. Selection of a Principal Diagnosis

G. Complications of surgery and other medical care

When the admission is for treatment of a complication resulting from surgery or other medical care, the complication code is sequenced as the principal diagnosis. If the complication is classified to the 996-999 series and the code lacks the necessary specificity in describing the complication, an additional code for the specific complication should be assigned.

Section I. Conventions, general coding guidelines and chapter specific guidelines

C. Chapter-Specific Guidelines

1. **Chapter 1: Infectious and Parasitic Diseases (001-139)**

   b. **Septicemia, Systemic Inflammatory Response Syndrome (SIRS), Sepsis, Severe Sepsis, and Septic Shock**

      10) **Sepsis due to a Postprocedural Infection**

         (a) **Documentation of causal relationship**

            As with all postprocedural complications, code assignment is based on the provider's documentation of the relationship between the infection and the procedure.

         (b) **Sepsis due to postprocedural infection**

            In cases of postprocedural sepsis, the complication code, such as code 998.59, Other postoperative infection, or 674.3x, Other complications of obstetrical surgical wounds should be coded first, followed by the appropriate sepsis codes (systemic infection code and either code 995.91 or 995.92). An additional code(s) for any acute organ dysfunction should also be assigned for cases of severe sepsis.

EXAMPLE

The patient was readmitted after undergoing surgery last week; the patient is being treated for postoperative sepsis, 998.59, 038.9, 995.91, E879.9 (T81.4xxA, A41.9, Y83.9).

---

2. **Chapter 2: Neoplasms (140-239)**

   c. **Coding and sequencing of complications**

      4) **Treatment of a complication resulting from a surgical procedure**

         When the admission/encounter is for treatment of a complication resulting from a surgical procedure, designate the complication as the principal or first-listed diagnosis if treatment is directed at resolving the complication.

   i. **Malignant neoplasm associated with transplanted organ**

      A malignant neoplasm of a transplanted organ should be coded as a transplant complication. Assign first the appropriate code from subcategory 996.8, Complications of transplanted organ, followed by code 199.2, Malignant neoplasm associated with transplanted organ. Use an additional code for the specific malignancy.

EXAMPLE | Hernia of colostomy with repair of parastomal hernia. The colostomy was performed 1 year ago during colon cancer resection. The patient is no longer receiving treatment, and the cancer was completely resected, 569.69, V10.05, E878.3, 46.42 (K94.09, Z85.038, Y83.3, 0WQFXZ2).

3. Chapter 3: Endocrine, Nutritional, and Metabolic Diseases and Immunity Disorders (240-279)
   a. Diabetes mellitus
   6) **Insulin pump malfunction**
      (a) **Underdose of insulin due insulin pump failure**
          An underdose of insulin due to an insulin pump failure should be assigned 996.57, Mechanical complication due to insulin pump, as the principal or first listed code, followed by the appropriate diabetes mellitus code based on documentation.
      (b) **Overdose of insulin due to insulin pump failure**
          The principal or first listed code for an encounter due to an insulin pump malfunction resulting in an overdose of insulin, should also be 996.57, Mechanical complication due to insulin pump, followed by code 962.3, Poisoning by insulins and antidiabetic agents, and the appropriate diabetes mellitus code based on documentation.
   7) **Secondary Diabetes Mellitus**
      (i) **Secondary diabetes mellitus due to pancreatectomy**
          For postpancreatectomy diabetes mellitus (lack of insulin due to the surgical removal of all or part of the pancreas), assign code 251.3, Postsurgical hypoinsulinemia. Assign a code from subcategory 249, **Secondary diabetes mellitus and a code from subcategory V88.1, Acquired absence of pancreas** as additional codes. Code also any diabetic manifestations (e.g., diabetic nephrosis 581.81).

EXAMPLE | Patient presents with a kink in the tubing of the insulin pump. This has resulted in diabetic ketoacidosis, 996.57, 250.13, E879.8 (T85.694A, E10.10, Y84.8).

6. Chapter 6: Diseases of Nervous System and Sense Organs (320-389)
   a. Pain—Category 338
   2) **Pain due to devices, implants and grafts**
      Pain associated with devices, implants or grafts left in a surgical site (for example painful hip prosthesis) is assigned to the appropriate code(s) found in Chapter 17, Injury and Poisoning. Use additional code(s) from category 338 to identify acute or chronic pain due to presence of the device, implant or graft (338.18-338.19 or 338.28-338.29).

EXAMPLE | Patient presents with acute pain secondary to a displaced nail in the right femur, 996.49, 338.19, 729.5, E878.1 (T84.124A, G89.18, M79.604, Y83.1).

   3) **Postoperative Pain**
      Post-thoracotomy pain and other postoperative pain are classified to subcategories 338.1 and 338.2, depending on whether the pain is acute or chronic. The default for post-thoracotomy and other postoperative pain not specified as acute or chronic is the code for the acute form.

      Routine or expected postoperative pain immediately after surgery should not be coded.
   (a) **Postoperative pain not associated with specific postoperative complication**
      Postoperative pain not associated with a specific postoperative complication is assigned to the appropriate postoperative pain code in category 338.

     (b) **Postoperative pain associated with specific postoperative complication**

Postoperative pain associated with a specific postoperative complication (such as painful wire sutures) is assigned to the appropriate code(s) found in Chapter 17, Injury and Poisoning. If appropriate, use additional code(s) from category 338 to identify acute or chronic pain (338.18 or 338.28). If pain control/management is the reason for the encounter, a code from category 338 should be assigned as the principal or first-listed diagnosis in accordance with *Section I.C.6.a.1.a above.*

     (c) **Postoperative pain as principal or first-listed diagnosis**

Postoperative pain may be reported as the principal or first-listed diagnosis when the stated reason for the admission/encounter is documented as postoperative pain control/management.

     (d) **Postoperative pain as secondary diagnosis**

Postoperative pain may be reported as a secondary diagnosis code when a patient presents for outpatient surgery and develops an unusual or inordinate amount of postoperative pain.

The provider's documentation should be used to guide the coding of postoperative pain, as well as *Section III. Reporting Additional Diagnoses* and *Section IV. Diagnostic Coding and Reporting in the Outpatient Setting.*

See Section II.I.2 for information on sequencing of diagnoses for patients admitted to hospital inpatient care following post-operative observation.

See Section II.J for information on sequencing of diagnoses for patients admitted to hospital inpatient care from outpatient surgery.

See Section IV.A.2 for information on sequencing of diagnoses for patients admitted for observation.

7. Chapter 7: Disease and Circulatory System (390-459)
  c. Postoperative cerebrovascular accident

A cerebrovascular hemorrhage or infarction that occurs as a result of medical intervention is coded to 997.02, Iatrogenic cerebrovascular infarction or hemorrhage. Medical record documentation should clearly specify the cause-and-effect relationship between the medical intervention and the cerebrovascular accident in order to assign this code. A secondary code from the code range 430-432 or from a code from subcategories 433 or 434 with a fifth digit of "1" should also be used to identify the type of hemorrhage or infarct.

This guideline conforms to the use additional code note instruction at category 997. Code 436, Acute, but ill-defined, cerebrovascular disease, should not be used as a secondary code with code 997.02.

EXAMPLE The patient had a postoperative cerebrovascular accident, which was embolic in nature. The patient initially had been admitted for treatment of coronary artery arteriosclerosis with CABG (left internal mammary artery and two saphenous vein grafts were used). Cardiopulmonary bypass was used during the surgery, 414.01, 997.02, 434.11, 36.12, 36.15, 39.61, E878.2, E849.7 (I25.10, I97.820, I63.40, 021109W, 02100A9, 5A1221Z).

17. Chapter 17: Injury and Poisoning (800-999)
  f. Complications of care
    1) Complications of care
      (a) **Documentation of complications of care**

As with all procedural or postprocedural complications, code assignment is based on the provider's documentation of the relationship between the condition and the procedure.

    2) Transplant complications
      (a) **Transplant complications other than kidney**

Codes under subcategory 996.8, Complications of transplanted organ, are for use for both complications and rejection of transplanted organs. A transplant complication code is only assigned if the complication affects the function of the transplanted organ. Two codes are required to fully describe a transplant complication, the appropriate code from subcategory 996.8 and a secondary code that identifies the complication.

Pre-existing conditions or conditions that develop after the transplant are not coded as complications unless they affect the function of the transplanted organs.

See I.C.18.d.3) for transplant organ removal status.

See I.C.2.i for malignant neoplasm associated with transplanted organ.

EXAMPLE   A patient with a previous intestinal transplant presents with diarrhea, which has been diagnosed as acute graft-versus-host disease, 996.87, 279.51, 787.91, E878.0 (T86.858, D89.810, R19.7, Y83.0).

(b) Chronic kidney disease and kidney transplant complications
Patients who have undergone kidney transplant may still have some form of chronic kidney disease (CKD) because the kidney transplant may not fully restore kidney function. Code 996.81 should be assigned for documented complications of a kidney transplant, such as transplant failure or rejection or other transplant complication. Code 996.81 should not be assigned for post kidney transplant patients who have chronic kidney (CKD) unless a transplant complication such as transplant failure or rejection is documented. If the documentation is unclear as to whether the patient has a complication of the transplant, query the provider.

For patients with CKD following a kidney transplant, but who do not have a complication such as failure or rejection, *see section I.C.10.a.2, Chronic kidney disease and kidney transplant status.*

EXAMPLE   Patient with history of kidney transplant presents to the ER with gastroenteritis. His review of systems documents CKD and hypertension, 558.9, 403.90, 585.9, V42.0 (K52.9, I12.9, N18.9, Z94.0).

EXAMPLE   Patient with history of kidney transplant presents to hospital in acute renal failure due to rejection, 996.81, 584.9, E878.0 (T86.11, N17.9, Y83.0).

3) Ventilator associated pneumonia
(a) Documentation of Ventilator associated Pneumonia
As with all procedural or postprocedural complications, code assignment is based on the provider's documentation of the relationship between the condition and the procedure.

Code 997.31, Ventilator associated pneumonia, should be assigned only when the provider has documented ventilator associated pneumonia (VAP). An additional code to identify the organism (e.g., *Pseudomonas aeruginosa*, code 041.7) should also be assigned. Do not assign an additional code from categories 480-484 to identify the type of pneumonia.

Code 997.31 should not be assigned for cases where the patient has pneumonia and is on a mechanical ventilator but the provider has not specifically stated that the pneumonia is ventilator-associated pneumonia.

If the documentation is unclear as to whether the patient has a pneumonia that is a complication attributable to the mechanical ventilator, query the provider.

EXAMPLE	Patient was hospitalized last month and was on a ventilator for exacerbation of COPD. She presents to the hospital today with pneumonia, 486, 496 (J18.9, J44.9).

EXAMPLE	Patient was recently admitted for an acute exacerbation of CHF for which she was placed on a ventilator. She presents to the hospital today with ventilator associated pneumonia. Sputum cultures were taken and this pneumonia was found to be due to MRSA, 997.31, 041.12, 428.0, E879.8, E849.7 (J95.851, I50.9, Z16, Y84.8, Y92.23).

> **(b) Patient admitted with pneumonia and develops VAP**
> A patient may be admitted with one type of pneumonia (e.g., code 481, Pneumococcal pneumonia) and subsequently develop VAP. In this instance, the principal diagnosis would be the appropriate code from categories 480-484 for the pneumonia diagnosed at the time of admission. Code 997.31, Ventilator associated pneumonia, would be assigned as an additional diagnosis when the provider has also documented the presence of ventilator associated pneumonia.

EXAMPLE	Patient was admitted to the hospital in acute respiratory failure due to pneumonia. She is placed in the ICU intubated and on a vent for 48 hours. She is transferred to the floor after 3 days where she develops a high fever. The physician documents ventilator associated pneumonia due to pseudomonas aeruginosa, 518.81, 486, 997.31, 041.7, 96.71, 96.04, E849.7, E879.8 (J96.00, J18.9, J95.851, B96.5, Y84.8, Y92.230, 0BH17EZ, 5A1945Z).

> **19. Chapter 19: Supplemental Classification of External Causes of Injury and Poisoning (E-codes, E800-E999)**
> **h. Misadventures and Complications of Care Guidelines**
> **1) Code range E870-E876**
> Assign a code in the range of E870-E876 if misadventures are stated by the provider.
> **2) Code range E878-E879**
> Assign a code in the range of E878-E879 if the provider attributes an abnormal reaction or later complication to a surgical or medical procedure, but does not mention misadventure at the time of the procedure as the cause of the reaction.

EXAMPLE	The colon was accidentally perforated during routine screening colonoscopy in the ambulatory surgical suite. The colon was sutured, V76.51, 998.2, 46.75, 45.23, E870.8, E849.7 (Z12.11, K91.71, Y83.0, 0DJD8ZZ, 0DQE8ZZ).

Apply the General Coding Guidelines as found in Chapter 5 and the Procedural Guidelines as found in Chapter 6.

ICD-10-CM

Official
Guidelines for
Coding and
Reporting

Please refer to the companion Evolve website for the most current guidelines.

Section II. Selection of a Principal Diagnosis

G. Complications of surgery and other medical care

When the admission is for treatment of a complication resulting from surgery or other medical care, the complication code is sequenced as the principal diagnosis. If the complication is classified to the T80-T88 series and the code lacks the necessary specificity in describing the complication, an additional code for the specific complication should be assigned.

C. Chapter Specific Guidelines

  1. Chapter 1: Certain Infectious and Parasitic Diseases (A00-B99)

   d. Sepsis, Severe Sepsis, and Septic Shock

    5) Sepsis due to a postprocedural infection

      Sepsis resulting from a postprocedural infection is a complication of medical care. For such cases, the postprocedural infection code, such as, T80.2, Infections following infusion, transfusion, and therapeutic injection, T81.4, Infection following a procedure, T88.0, Infection following immunization, or O86.0, Infection of obstetric surgical wound, should be coded first, followed by the code for the specific infection. If the patient has severe sepsis the appropriate code from subcategory R65.2 should also be assigned with the additional code(s) for any acute organ dysfunction.

  2. Chapter 2: Neoplasms (C00-D49)

   c. Coding and sequencing of complications

    4) Treatment of a complication resulting from a surgical procedure

      When the admission/encounter is for treatment of a complication resulting from a surgical procedure, designate the complication as the principal or first-listed diagnosis if treatment is directed at resolving the complication.

   l. Sequencing of neoplasm codes

    5) Complication from surgical procedure for treatment of a neoplasm

      When an encounter is for treatment of a complication resulting from a surgical procedure performed for the treatment of the neoplasm, designate the complication as the principal/**first-listed** diagnosis. See guideline regarding the coding of a current malignancy versus personal history to determine if the code for the neoplasm should also be assigned.

   r. Malignant neoplasm associated with transplanted organ

      A malignant neoplasm of a transplanted organ should be coded as a transplant complication. Assign first the appropriate code from category T86.-, Complications of transplanted **organs and tissue**, followed by code C80.2, Malignant neoplasm associated with transplanted organ. Use an additional code for the specific malignancy.

  4. Chapter 4: Endocrine, Nutritional, and Metabolic Diseases (E00-*E89*)

   a. Diabetes mellitus

    5) Complications due to insulin pump malfunction

     (a) Underdose of insulin due *to* insulin pump failure

      An underdose of insulin due to an insulin pump failure should be assigned to a code from subcategory T85.6, Mechanical complication of other specified internal and external prosthetic devices, implants and grafts, that specifies the type of pump malfunction, as the principal or **first-listed** code, followed by code T38.3x6-, Underdosing of insulin and oral hypoglycemic [antidiabetic] drugs. Additional codes for the type of diabetes mellitus and any associated complications due to the underdosing should also be assigned.

     (b) Overdose of insulin due to insulin pump failure

      The principal or **first-listed** code for an encounter due to an insulin pump malfunction resulting in an overdose of insulin, should also be T85.6-, Mechanical complication of other specified internal and external prosthetic devices, implants and grafts, followed by code T38.3x1-, Poisoning by insulin and oral hypoglycemic [antidiabetic] drugs, accidental (unintentional).

6) **Secondary Diabetes Mellitus**
(b) **Assigning and Sequencing secondary diabetes codes and its causes**
(i) **Secondary diabetes mellitus due to pancreatectomy**
For postpancreatectomy diabetes mellitus (lack of insulin due to the surgical removal of all or part of the pancreas), assign code E89.1, **Postprocedural** hypoinsulinemia. Assign a code from category **E13** and a code from **subcategory Z90.41-, Acquired absence of pancreas**, as additional codes.
6. **Chapter 6: Diseases of Nervous System and Sense Organs (G00-G99)**
b. **Pain—Category G89**
2) **Pain due to devices, implants and grafts**
See Section I.C.19. Pain due to medical devices
3) **Postoperative Pain**
The provider's documentation should be used to guide the coding of postoperative pain, as well as *Section III. Reporting Additional Diagnoses* and *Section IV. Diagnostic Coding and Reporting in the Outpatient Setting.*
The default for post-thoracotomy and other postoperative pain not specified as acute or chronic is the code for the acute form.
Routine or expected postoperative pain immediately after surgery should not be coded.
(a) **Postoperative pain not associated with specific postoperative complication**
Postoperative pain not associated with a specific postoperative complication is assigned to the appropriate postoperative pain code in category G89.
(b) **Postoperative pain associated with specific postoperative complication**
Postoperative pain associated with a specific postoperative complication (such as painful wire sutures) is assigned to the appropriate code(s) found in Chapter 19, Injury, poisoning, and certain other consequences of external causes. If appropriate, use additional code(s) from category G89 to identify acute or chronic pain (G89.18 or G89.28).
9. **Chapter 9: Diseases of Circulatory System (I00-I99)**
c. **Intraoperative and Postprocedural *Cerebrovascular Accident***
Medical record documentation should clearly specify the cause- and-effect relationship between the medical intervention and the cerebrovascular accident in order to assign a code for intraoperative or postprocedural cerebrovascular accident. Proper code assignment depends on whether it was an infarction or hemorrhage and whether it occurred intraoperatively or postoperatively. If it was a cerebral hemorrhage, code assignment depends on the type of procedure performed.
19. **Chapter 19: Injury, poisoning, and certain other consequences of external causes (S00-T88)**
g. **Complications of care**
1) **Complications of care**
(a) **Documentation of complications of care**
As with all procedural or postprocedural complications, code assignment is based on the provider's documentation of the relationship between the condition and the procedure.
2) **Pain due to medical devices**
Pain associated with devices, implants or grafts left in a surgical site (for example painful hip prosthesis) is assigned to the appropriate code(s) found in Chapter 19, Injury, poisoning, and certain other consequences of external causes. Specific codes for pain due to medical devices are found in the T code section of the ICD-10-CM. Use additional code(s) from category G89 to identify acute or chronic pain due to presence of the device, implant or graft (G89.18 or G89.28).
3) **Transplant complications**
(a) **Transplant complications other than kidney**
Codes under category T86, Complications of transplanted organs and tissues, are for use for both complications and rejection of transplanted organs. A transplant complication code is only assigned if the complication affects the function of the transplanted organ. Two codes are required to fully describe a transplant complication: the appropriate code from category T86 and a secondary code that identifies the complication.

Pre-existing conditions or conditions that develop after the transplant are not coded as complications unless they affect the function of the transplanted organs.

See I.C.21.c.3 for transplant organ removal status

See I.C.2.r for malignant neoplasm associated with transplanted organ.

(b) Chronic kidney disease and kidney transplant complications

Patients who have undergone kidney transplant may still have some form of chronic kidney disease (CKD) because the kidney transplant may not fully restore kidney function. Code T86.1- should be assigned for documented complications of a kidney transplant, such as transplant failure or rejection or other transplant complication. Code T86.1- should not be assigned for post kidney transplant patients who have chronic kidney (CKD) unless a transplant complication such as transplant failure or rejection is documented. If the documentation is unclear as to whether the patient has a complication of the transplant, query the provider.

For patients with CKD following a kidney transplant, but who do not have a complication such as failure or rejection, see section I.C.14. Chronic kidney disease and kidney transplant status.

4) Complication codes that include the external cause

As with certain other T codes, some of the complications of care codes have the external cause included in the code. The code includes the nature of the complication as well as the type of procedure that caused the complication. No external cause code indicating the type of procedure is necessary for these codes.

5) Complications of care codes within the body system chapters

Intraoperative and postprocedural complication codes are found within the body system chapters with codes specific to the organs and structures of that body system. These codes should be sequenced first, followed by a code(s) for the specific complication, if applicable.

Apply the General Coding Guidelines as found in Chapter 5 and the Procedural Guidelines as found in Chapter 7.

GUIDELINE DIFFERENCES BETWEEN ICD-9-CM AND ICD-10-CM

- Many ICD-10-CM complications of care include the external cause within the code.
- Many complication-of-care codes are found within the body system chapters.
- Pain due to a medical device is assigned codes found in the T-code section.

MAJOR DIFFERENCES BETWEEN ICD-9-CM AND ICD-10-CM

- The section on foreign bodies left behind during a procedure has been expanded to include the type of procedure.
- Many more complications of care are located in specific body system chapters.
- The coding for complications of kidney transplants has been expanded to include specific types of complications.

ANATOMY AND PHYSIOLOGY

Complications of surgical or medical care can affect any of the body systems. The anatomy and physiology of these body systems are outlined in their respective chapters. Find below some general guidelines that apply to complications.

CODING COMPLICATIONS

Several general guidelines should be kept in mind when coding complications.

- No time limit: can occur after medical care or surgery, either immediately or years later.
- Complications after surgery or medical care should be documented as such. Routine events such as fever in the immediate postoperative period are not considered postoperative complications.
- Coding of complications does not imply that poor care or improper care has been delivered.
- Codes for complications may be located in the chapter for specified body sites or under abortion and pregnancy.
- Codes for complications that affect multiple sites or body systems are usually located in codes 996 through 999.
- "**Iatrogenic**" is a term that is used to signify that a condition is a result or complication of treatment.
- When in doubt as to whether the condition occurred as the result of a procedure or medical care, it is best practice to query the physician.
- Complications of surgical and medical care require an E code in the range of E878-E879 for abnormal reactions or later complications, or E870-E879 if misadventure is stated.
- When the admission is for treatment of a complication resulting from surgery or other medical care, the complication code is sequenced as the principal diagnosis.
- If the complication is classified to 996-999 and the code lacks necessary specificity to describe the complication, an additional code should be assigned for the specific complication.
- Codes in the complication chapter are early postprocedural complications, and those found in other chapters may be described as late functional disorders, i.e. postmastectomy lymphedema, postsurgical ovarian failure.

Locating Complication Codes in the Alphabetic Index

When looking for a complication code in the Index, the condition for which the patient is admitted should be located first (Figures 25-1 and 25-2).

EXAMPLE

Patient was readmitted for treatment of postoperative ileus following appendectomy, 997.4, 560.1, E878.6 (K91.89, K56.7, Y83.6).

EXAMPLE

Anemia due to acute blood loss following a right total knee replacement using metal and plastic components for osteoarthritis, 715.36, 285.1, E878.1, E849.7, 81.54 (M17.9, D62, Y83.1, Y92.239, OSRC0JZ).

Ileus (adynamic) (bowel) (colon) (inhibitory) (intestine) (neurogenic) (paralytic) 560.1
  arteriomesenteric duodenal 537.2
  due to gallstone (in intestine) 560.31
  duodenal, chronic 537.2
  following gastrointestinal surgery 997.49
  gallstone 560.31
  mechanical (*see also* Obstruction, intestine) 560.9
  meconium 777.1
    due to cystic fibrosis 277.01
  myxedema 564.89
  postoperative 997.49 ◄
  transitory, newborn 777.4

FIGURE 25-1. Postoperative ileus.

Anemia *(Continued)*
    pernicious (combined system disease)
        (congenital) (dorsolateral spinal de-
        generation) (juvenile) (myelopathy)
        (neuropathy) (posterior sclerosis)
        (primary) (progressive) (spleen)
        281.0
    of or complicating pregnancy 648.2
    pleochromic 285.9
        of sprue 281.8
    portal 285.8
    posthemorrhagic (chronic) 280.0
        acute 285.1
        newborn 776.5
    postoperative
        due to (acute) blood loss 285.1 ◄──────
            chronic blood loss 280.0
        other 285.9

FIGURE 25-2. Postoperative blood loss anemia.

Complications *(Continued)*
    surgical procedures *(Continued)*
        stitch abscess 998.59
        transplant - *see* Complications, graft
        ureterostomy malfunction 997.5
        urethrostomy malfunction 997.5
        urinary NEC 997.5
        vascular
            mesenteric artery 997.71
            other vessels 997.79
            peripheral vessels 997.2
            renal artery 997.72
        wound infection 998.59
    therapeutic misadventure NEC 999.9
        surgical treatment 998.9
    tracheostomy 519.00 ◄──────

FIGURE 25-3. Tracheostomy complication.

When no entry is found under the main term for the condition, the term "complication" should be referenced (Figures 25-3 and 25-4).

EXAMPLE   Patient is admitted with tracheal stenosis of tracheostomy site, 519.02, E878.3 (J95.03, Y83.3).
    Note that this complication code is located in the respiratory chapter.

EXAMPLE   Patient admitted with cystitis due to indwelling urinary catheter, 996.64, 595.9, E879.6 (T83.51xA, N30.90, Y84.6).

Locating External Causes of Injury and Poisoning to Correspond with Complication Coding

To locate the corresponding external cause code for complications, begin by locating the Alphabetic Index to External Causes. This Index follows the Alphabetic Index to Diseases. Locate the term *complication* to see the cross-references to other index entries (Figure 25-5).
    For further detail on external cause codes, refer to Chapter 23 of this textbook.

EXAMPLE   During spinal surgery, the surgeon accidentally nicks the dura due to the amount of adhesions present, 349.31, E870.0 (G97.42, Y83.8) (Figure 25-6).

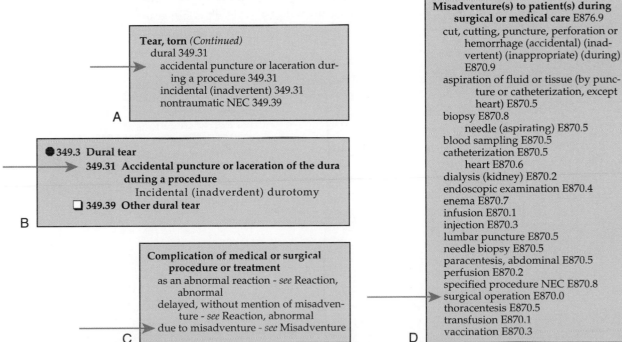

Complications (Continued)
  due to (presence of) any device, implant, or graft classified to 996.0–996.5 NEC 996.70
    with infection or inflammation - see Complications, infection or inflammation, due to (presence of) any device, implant, or graft classified to 996.0–996.5 NEC
  arterial NEC 996.74
    coronary NEC 996.03
      atherosclerosis - see Arteriosclerosis, coronary
    embolism 996.72
    occlusion NEC 996.72
    specified type NEC 996.72
    thrombus 996.72
    renal dialysis 996.73
  arteriovenous fistula or shunt NEC 996.74
  bone growth stimulator 996.78
  breast NEC 996.79
  cardiac NEC 996.72
    defibrillator 996.72
    pacemaker 996.72
    valve prosthesis 996.71
  catheter NEC 996.79
    spinal 996.75
    urinary, indwelling 996.76

FIGURE 25-4. Urinary catheter complications.

Complication of medical or surgical procedure or treatment
  as an abnormal reaction – see Reaction, abnormal
  delayed, without mention of misadventure – see Reaction, abnormal
  due to misadventure – see Misadventure

FIGURE 25-5. Cross-references to other index entries under "complication".

Tear, torn (Continued)
  dural 349.31
    accidental puncture or laceration during a procedure 349.31
    incidental (inadvertent) 349.31
    nontraumatic NEC 349.39

A

●349.3 Dural tear
  349.31 Accidental puncture or laceration of the dura during a procedure
        Incidental (inadverdent) durotomy
  ☐ 349.39 Other dural tear

B

Complication of medical or surgical procedure or treatment
  as an abnormal reaction - see Reaction, abnormal
  delayed, without mention of misadventure - see Reaction, abnormal
  due to misadventure - see Misadventure

C

Misadventure(s) to patient(s) during surgical or medical care E876.9
  cut, cutting, puncture, perforation or hemorrhage (accidental) (inadvertent) (inappropriate) (during) E870.9
  aspiration of fluid or tissue (by puncture or catheterization, except heart) E870.5
  biopsy E870.8
    needle (aspirating) E870.5
  blood sampling E870.5
  catheterization E870.5
    heart E870.6
  dialysis (kidney) E870.2
  endoscopic examination E870.4
  enema E870.7
  infusion E870.1
  injection E870.3
  lumbar puncture E870.5
  needle biopsy E870.5
  paracentesis, abdominal E870.5
  perfusion E870.2
  specified procedure NEC E870.8
  surgical operation E870.0
  thoracentesis E870.5
  transfusion E870.1
  vaccination E870.3

D

FIGURE 25-6. ICD-9-CM excerpts showing correct code assignment for the previous example. **A** and **B,** Code 349.31 in the Alphabetic Index and the Tabular List. **C** and **D,** Code E870.0 in the Alphabetic Index and the Tabular List.

CHAPTER-SPECIFIC COMPLICATIONS

Complications of the Digestive System

Patients who have had some or part of their stomachs removed or who have undergone gastric bypass surgery may be susceptible to a condition known as "**dumping syndrome**." This condition occurs when undigested contents of the stomach are transported to the small intestine too quickly. The symptoms of this condition may include abdominal cramping, nausea, and diarrhea, to name a few. Dumping syndrome may in turn result in weight loss or malnutrition. This syndrome may be treated with dietary changes, as well as with medications.

EXAMPLE | Patient presents with abdominal pain following a gastric bypass performed for obesity. It is determined that she suffers from dumping syndrome, and dietary changes are suggested, 564.2, E878.2 (K91.1, Y83.2).

Complications of Gastrostomy, Colostomy, Enterostomy

Ostomies are surgically created openings into the body (Figure 25-7). Enterostomies and colostomies are created to discharge waste products from the body; gastrostomies are typically used for feeding or aspirating the contents of the stomach. Often, these surgically created openings result in complications. Complications associated with these openings are caused by a variety of problems such as infection, blockage of the opening, drainage or leakage around the opening, breakage of the device, and granulation of tissue.

If a patient presents to the hospital with a chief complaint of a percutaneous endoscopic gastrostomy (PEG) tube falling out, the principal diagnosis would be V55.1 (Z43.1), or attention to gastrostomy, because no complications resulted from the gastrostomy itself. This is described in detail in *Coding Clinic* (1997:3Q:p8).[1]

EXAMPLE | Patient is admitted for a clogged gastrostomy tube, V55.1 (Z43.1).

EXAMPLE | Patient is being treated for an enterocutaneous fistula in the colostomy, 569.69, E878.3 (K94.09, Y83.3).

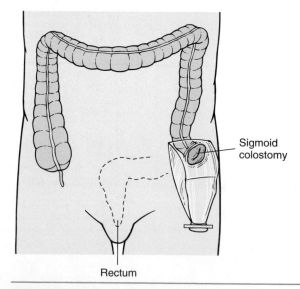

Sigmoid colostomy

Rectum

FIGURE 25-7. Colostomy. The opening in the colon is brought to the surface of the skin to divert feces into an external pouch worn by the patient.

| EXAMPLE | Patient presents with cellulitis of the abdomen due to an infected colostomy site. The organism responsible for the cellulitis is *Staph aureus,* 569.61, 682.2, 041.11, E878.3 (K94.02, L03.311, B95.6, Y83.3). |

Complications of the Genitourinary System

Occasionally, hematuria occurs as the result of a traumatic injury due to forceful removal of a urinary catheter. According to *Coding Clinic* (1985:Nov-Dec:p15),[2] this is coded as injury of the urethra, with hematuria assigned as an additional code. In some cases, it may be appropriate to assign an E code to indicate the cause and intent of the injury.

| EXAMPLE | Hematuria due to patient pulling out indwelling urinary catheter, 867.0, 599.70, E928.9 (S37.30xA, R31.9, X58.xxxA). |

Hematuria is expected after many urinary procedures and should not be coded unless it is excessive and has been documented as such by the physician.

Complications of Dialysis

Several complications may result from dialysis treatment. Many of these conditions are included in other chapters of the ICD-9-CM book. **Dialysis disequilibrium syndrome**, which is characterized by weakness, dizziness, headache, and, in severe cases, mental status changes, is a complication of dialysis. Electrolyte imbalances such as hyperkalemia, hyponatremia, hypocalcemia, hypermagnesemia and acidosis may also occur. Hypotension and fluid overload can complicate the care of the patient on dialysis. Occasionally, some of these conditions occur because the patient has been noncompliant with dialysis treatment and/or medications and diet. Complications associated with dialysis catheters may be due to infection or mechanical malfunction. If an infection is present, an additional code may be needed to identify specified infections and causative organisms.

| EXAMPLE | Patient with ESRD was admitted to the hospital with noncardiogenic fluid overload due to noncompliance with dialysis treatment. Patient has a history of CHF and is on Lasix, 276.69, 428.0, 585.6, V45.12 (E87.79, I50.9, N18.6, Z91.15). |

| EXAMPLE | Patient has dialysis disequilibrium syndrome due to hemodialysis for end-stage renal failure, 276.9, 585.6, V45.12, E879.1 (E87.8, N18.6, Z99.2, Y84). |

| EXAMPLE | Leakage of peritoneal dialysis catheter. Patient is on dialysis for end-stage renal disease. Peritoneal catheter was removed, 996.56, 585.6, V45.11, E879.1, 97.82 (T85.631A, N18.6, Z99.2, Y84.1, 0WPGX0Z). |

Complications of the Musculoskeletal System

Common complications of joint replacement include infection, blood clot, nerve injury, loosening, dislocation, wear and tear, and breakage of the prosthesis. It may be necessary to remove the prosthesis and insert a new prosthesis. According to *Coding Clinic* (1997:3Q:p13),[3] "any time the joint is replaced or revised after the initial replacement this would be considered a revision."

| EXAMPLE | Patient presents with dislocation of a right hip replacement. A revision must be performed, 996.42, 81.53, E878.1, V43.64 (T84.020A, Y83.1, 0SW90JZ) (Figure 25-8). |

Complications *(Continued)*
  mechanical *(Continued)*
    device NEC *(Continued)*
      cardiac 996.00
        automatic implantable defibril-
          lator 996.04
        long-term effect 429.4
        specified NEC 996.09
      contraceptive, intrauterine 996.32
      counterpulsation, intra-aortic 996.1
      fixation, external, with internal
          components 996.49
      fixation, internal (nail, rod, plate)
          996.40
      genitourinary 996.30
        specified NEC 996.39
      insulin pump 996.57
      nervous system 996.2
      orthopedic, internal 996.40
        prosthetic joint *(see also* Compli-
            cations, mechanical, device,
            orthopedic, prosthetic, joint)
            996.47
      prosthetic NEC 996.59
        joint *(see also* Complications,
            prosthetic joint) 996.47
          articular bearing surface wear
            996.46
          aseptic loosening 996.41
          breakage 996.43
          dislocation 996.42 ◄

FIGURE 25-8. Complication of hip replacement.

FIGURE 25-9. Surgical correction of malunion ankle fracture.

Malunion/Nonunion of Fractures

Malunion of a fracture occurs when the fracture fragments have united but are not properly aligned. Incorrectly positioned bones may demonstrate angulation, rotation, and shortening. The degree and severity of the malunion will determine the selection of treatment, which may include surgery (Figure 25-9).

Nonunion of a fracture occurs when bony healing is not achieved at the fracture site. A fracture site that fails to heal within approximately 6 to 9 months of the injury represents a nonunion (Figure 25-10).

Malunion or nonunion may occur as the result of insufficient or improper reduction and immobilization, infection, metabolic bone disease, poor nutrition, and/or inadequate blood supply. Improper healing may be noted in cases of traumatic fracture and pathologic fracture and is considered a "late effect" of a fracture.

FIGURE 25-10. Nonunion of the lateral humeral condyle.

EXAMPLE | Patient's x-rays showed nonunion of left tibial shaft fracture, which is a late effect of a fall, 733.82, 905.4, E929.3 (S82.202K, W19xxxS).

EXAMPLE | Patient presents with pain and swelling in the ankle status postcasting 3 weeks ago. Patient suffered a closed fracture of the left ankle. It is determined that the patient has a malunion of the fracture, and the patient is scheduled next week for surgery to correct the malunion, 733.81 (S82.892P).

Complications of the Nervous System and Sense Organs

One of the most common complications discussed in this chapter is a spinal headache. A spinal headache, which is also known as a postdural puncture headache, may occur following a spinal tap (lumbar puncture) or spinal anesthesia. These headaches are caused by spinal fluid that is leaking from the puncture site of the procedure. The patient may experience nausea, vomiting, dizziness, ringing in the ears, and/or sensitivity to light. Treatment for the headache consists of lying flat and drinking fluids, particularly those that include caffeine. If these conservative treatments do not help, an epidural blood patch to seal the puncture hole may be required.

EXAMPLE	Patient develops a severe headache 1 day postlumbar puncture performed because of high fever and stiff neck to rule out meningitis, 349.0, 780.60, 723.5, 03.31, E879.8, E849.7 (G97.1, R50.9, M43.6, Y83.4, 00903ZX).

Complications of the Respiratory System

A **pulmonary embolism** (PE) is a blockage in an artery of the lung that can be life threatening. This blockage commonly is caused by a blood clot that started in the leg and then traveled to the lung. A pulmonary embolism may occur as a result of a surgical procedure. If a patient has recently had surgery and presents with sudden shortness of breath, chest pain, or cough, a pulmonary embolism may be suspected. To determine whether a patient has a PE, scans or angiograms may be performed. Treatment consists of anticoagulant drugs such as heparin. When a condition is the result of treatment, it is referred to as iatrogenic.

EXAMPLE	Patient presents with shortness of breath and chest pain. Two weeks before presentation, the patient had a right total hip replacement. A pulmonary angiogram is performed, as is a Doppler ultrasound of the legs. The attending documents that the patient is positive for both a pulmonary embolism and a lower right leg deep vein thrombosis secondary to recent surgery, 415.11, 997.2, 453.40, V43.64, E878.1 (T81.72xA, I26.99, I82.401, Z96.649, Y83.1).

A pneumothorax is another condition that can result from medical treatment. A **pneumothorax** is air in the space around the lung. Procedures such as central venous lines, chest tubes, and mechanical ventilation may inadvertently cause a traumatic pneumothorax. A patient may have symptoms of chest pain or shortness of breath. A chest x-ray or CT scan can be used to diagnose this condition.

EXAMPLE	Patient with a chronic cough undergoes a left transbronchial right lung biopsy. A chest x-ray is performed following this procedure, and a pneumothorax is noted. Attending physician decides that because the pneumothorax is small, the condition will be monitored by chest x-ray, 786.2, 512.1, 33.27, E878.8, E849.7, R05 (J95.81, Y83.8, Y92.234, 0BBK8ZX).

Patients with tracheostomies often develop complications related to the tracheostomy site. A patient can have infection or bleeding or mechanical complications at the site.

EXAMPLE	Patient presents with cellulitis of the neck secondary to an infected tracheostomy site, 519.01, 682.1, E878.3 (J95.02, L03.221, Y83.3).

COMPLICATIONS NOT ELSEWHERE CLASSIFIED

Complications of Surgical and Medical Care, codes 996-999 in ICD-9-CM and codes T80-T88 in ICD-10-CM, are found in Chapter 17 in the ICD-9-CM code book and in Chapter 19 in the ICD-10-CM code book.

Mechanical Complications

It is important to pay particular attention to the many Excludes notes in this chapter. **Mechanical complications** involve equipment malfunctions. Some types of mechanical malfunctions are breakdown, displacement, leakage, obstruction, perforation, and protrusion.

Complications *(Continued)*
  mechanical *(Continued)*
    prosthesis NEC 996.59
      bile duct 996.59
      breast 996.54
      chin 996.59
      ocular lens 996.53
      reconstruction, vas deferens 996.39
    reimplant NEC 996.59
      extremity *(see also* Complications,
        reattached, extremity) 996.90
      organ *(see also* Complications, trans-
        plant, organ, by site) 996.80
    repair - *see* Complications, mechani-
      cal, graft
    respirator [ventilator] V46.14
    shunt NEC 996.59
      arteriovenous, surgically created
        996.1
      ventricular (communicating) 996.2
    stent NEC 996.59 ◄

FIGURE 25-11. Complications of devices.

| EXAMPLE | Patient has ascending cholangitis related to clogged biliary stent, 996.59, 576.1, E878.8 (T85.590A, K83.0, Y83.8) (Figure 25-11). |

| EXAMPLE | Patient has a leaking breast implant, 996.54, E878.1 (T85.43xA, Y83.1). |

Infections Due to Prosthetic Device, Implants, and Grafts

The presence of a device, implant, or graft carries a risk of infection. It is important to note that the codes in this section may give instruction to use an additional code to identify specified infections.

| EXAMPLE | Patient has sepsis due to a dialysis catheter, 999.31, 038.9, 995.91, E879.1 (T80.21xA, A41.9, Y84.1). |

| EXAMPLE | Patient has acute osteomyelitis of femur secondary to infected right hip replacement, 996.66, 730.05, V43.64, E878.1 (T84.51xA, M86.151, Z96.641, Y83.1). |

Other Complications of Internal Prosthetic Devices, Implants, and Grafts

When problems result from the use of a device, implant, or graft that are **NOT** due to infection or mechanical problems, category 996.7X should be selected. Often, devices that have been implanted become stenosed or occluded by thrombus or embolism. *Coding Clinic* (2008:3Q:p11)[4] describes the difference between "end stent" and "in stent" stenosis of a patient who had previous coronary artery stenting. In stent stenosis occurs when there is an obstruction within the stent, and code 996.72 is assigned. End stent stenosis could refer to the tip of the stent or could also refer to the vessel closest to the stent. If an adjacent coronary vessel to the stent is obstructed, then code 414.01 would be assigned, whereas if the stent itself is clogged or obstructed, then code 996.72 would be assigned.

| EXAMPLE | Patient is admitted to remove prosthetic right hip because of severe hip pain, 996.77, V43.64, E878.1, 80.05 (T84.84xA, Y83.1, 0SP90JZ). |

EXAMPLE | Patient with a right arm dialysis graft in place is admitted because of an embolism in the graft. Patient has ESRD. An upper vein thrombectomy was performed, 996.73, 453.9, 585.6, E878.2, 39.49 (T82.818A, I82.89, N18.6, Y84.1, 05CY0ZZ).

EXAMPLE | Patient with CAD is admitted because of coronary artery stent restenosis and to insert new drug-eluting stent, 996.72, 414.01, 00.66, 36.07, 00.40, 00.45, E878.1 (T82.857A, I25.10, Y83.8, 027034Z).

Complications of Transplanted Organ

Coding Clinic (1998:3Q:p3)[5] advises the coder to examine the documentation when a postorgan transplant patient presents for medical care to determine whether there are complications of the transplanted organ.

Complications of a transplanted organ include rejection or any posttransplant illnesses that affect the function of a transplanted organ. If illness affects the transplanted organ, two codes are required. The exceptions per guidelines are those patients with a kidney transplant and chronic kidney disease (CKD). In those cases 996.81 should be used only for complications such as rejection or failure or a medical condition such as infection affecting the transplanted organ.

EXAMPLE | Acute pyelonephritis postkidney transplant, 996.81, 590.10, E878.0 (T86.13, N10, Y83.0).

Posttransplant surgical complications that do not affect the function of the transplanted organ are coded to the specific surgical complications.

EXAMPLE | Patient presents for heart transplant due to primary cardiomyopathy and postoperatively develops renal failure, 425.4, 997.5 586, E878.0, E849.7, 37.51 (I42.9, N99.0, N19, Y83.0, Y92.239, 02YA0Z0).
In this case, the complication is affecting the urinary system, not the heart, which is the transplanted organ.

Preexisting conditions or medical conditions that develop after transplant are not coded as complications unless they affect the transplanted organ. Code V42.X (Z94.-) is used as an additional code to identify transplant status when no complications are associated with the transplanted organ. Codes V42.X (V94.-) and 996.8X (T86) are **NEVER** used together.

EXAMPLE | Patient is admitted for treatment of primary liver cancer. Patient had a liver transplant 2 years ago, 996.82, 199.2, 155.0, E878.0 (T86.49, C80.2, C22.8, Y83.0).

Ventilator-Associated Pneumonia (VAP)

As with any postprocedural complication, code assignment must be based on provider documentation of the relationship between the procedure and condition. In the case of ventilator-associated pneumonia, the provider must document the association of the use of a ventilator with the pneumonia. If the documentation is unclear about the association, the provider may be queried. The only codes assigned for ventilator-associated pneumonia are 997.31 (J95.851) and the causative organism if known. A specific code for pneumonia (480-484) is not assigned.

It is possible for a patient to be admitted with pneumonia and later develop ventilator-associated pneumonia. In this case, the code for pneumonia would be assigned as the principal diagnosis with the complication code for the VAP assigned as a secondary diagnosis.

Ventilation pneumonitis is not the same as ventilator-associated pneumonia. Ventilation pneumonitis is the result of inhalation of organisms growing in air conditioning systems.

EXAMPLE

Patient is admitted to the hospital with pneumonia. After reviewing the records from an outside hospital, the physician documents that it appears this pneumonia is due to the use of a ventilator on the previous admission, 997.31, E879.8, E849.7 (J95.851, Y84.3, Y92.239).

EXERCISE 25-1

Assign codes to the following conditions.

1. Displacement of a pacemaker electrode, initial encounter _____
2. Obstruction secondary to a stenosis of an atrioventricular dialysis shunt, initial encounter; patient has ESRD _____
3. Protrusion of a nail from a right femur fixation, subsequent encounter _____
4. Failure of artificial skin graft, initial encounter _____
5. Patient with indwelling urinary catheter presents with sepsis due to catheter, initial encounter _____
6. Patient with peritoneal dialysis catheter presents with inflammation of the skin around the catheter; patient had ESRD, initial encounter _____
7. Patient with pelvic inflammatory disease attributed to an intrauterine device (IUD), subsequent encounter _____
8. Patient is admitted for removal of her intramedullary rod because of acute leg pain, subsequent encounter _____
9. Cellulitis of the skin of the right knee due to right knee replacement, initial encounter _____
10. Patient with a transplanted lung presents with pneumonia _____
11. Patient is rejecting transplanted kidney _____
12. Patient has graft-versus-host disease; status postbone marrow transplant _____
13. Patient with an intestine transplant presents with dehydration _____
14. Patient with a ventricular shunt presents with severe headache due to stenosis of the shunt; patient has hydrocephalus _____
15. Patient with an abscess of a gastrostomy tube site due to *Staph aureus* _____
16. Patient with left pleural effusion develops iatrogenic pneumothorax following insertion of a chest tube _____

Complications Affecting Specified Body Systems, Not Elsewhere Classified

This category is to be used if the patient's complication is not better classified in another category, such as mechanical complication or infection of a device. It is important to note that the instructional note under category 997 advises the use of an additional code to identify the specific complication.

EXAMPLE	Patient develops postoperative congestive heart failure after endoscopic transurethral resection of the prostate (TURP) for BPH, 600.00, 997.1, 428.0, E878.4, E849.7, 60.29 (N40.0, I97.131, I50.9, Y83.6, Y92.239, 0VB08ZZ).

EXAMPLE	Patient received a total hip replacement (THR) 3 weeks ago and now presents with a postoperative deep vein thrombosis (DVT) in the lower extremity, 997.2, 453.40, E878.1, V43.64 (T81.72xA, I97.89, I82.409, Y83.1).

EXAMPLE	Patient is status post-TURP for BPH, which was performed as an outpatient 2 days ago. Patient is now admitted with postoperative acute renal failure, 997.5, 584.9, E878.6 (N99.0, Y83.6).

The amputation stump complication, per *Coding Clinic* (1995:4Q:p82),[6] is used to describe complications as current or as late effects. Phantom limb pain (353.6) is excluded from these codes.

EXAMPLE	Patient was admitted with a neuroma of amputation stump of the right leg, 997.61, E878.5 (T87.33, Y83.5).

Other Complications of Procedures, Not Elsewhere Classified

This category describes complications that may occur as the result of procedures but are not described by other specific codes. A second code to identify the exact type of complication may be required with category 998.

A relatively common complication of surgery is wound **dehiscence**. Wound dehiscence is the opening of layers of a surgical wound. The symptoms of this condition can be pain, fever, and/or inflammation. It can be caused by any of the following and is most common in abdominal surgeries.

- Sutures too tight
- Infection at the wound site
- Vitamin C deficiency
- Tension of the wound caused by lifting or straining

EXAMPLE	Patient is admitted for treatment of a postoperative wound infection. The patient has developed cellulitis of the abdominal wound, 998.59, 682.2, E878.9 (T81.4xxA, L03.311, Y83.8).

EXAMPLE	Dehiscence of an external abdominal wound following cholecystectomy, 998.32, E878.6 (T81.31xA, Y83.6).

Complications of Medical Care, Not Elsewhere Classified

Sometimes, complications occur that are not the result of surgical procedures but of medical care. Examples of medical care might include infusions, transfusions, total parenteral nutrition (TPN), dialysis, and vaccinations.

EXAMPLE	After transfusion, patient presents with thrombophlebitis of right arm, 999.2, E879.8, 451.84 (T80.1xxA, I80.8, Y84.8).

EXAMPLE	Sepsis due to central line, 999.32, 038.9, 995.91, E879.8 (T80.21xA, A41.9, Y84.8).

EXERCISE 25-2

Assign codes to the following conditions.

1. During a surgical procedure, patient goes into cardiac arrest _____

2. After a surgical procedure, patient develops aspiration pneumonia _____

3. Patient has a hemicolectomy and is readmitted to the hospital for intractable postoperative vomiting _____

4. After spine surgery, patient becomes oliguric _____

5. Patient is admitted for a *Staphylococcus aureus* infection of a right amputation stump of the lower extremity _____

6. Patient is admitted for removal of a sponge left in during a hysterectomy, initial encounter _____

7. Patient develops a seroma of the operative wound, initial encounter _____

8. Patient develops anaphylactic shock after a blood transfusion, initial encounter _____

9. Patient develops seizures after electroconvulsive therapy (ECT) _____

DOCUMENTATION/REIMBURSEMENT/MS-DRGs

Often, coding difficulties are due to lack of documentation. Sometimes pathology and other test results are not available at the time of discharge or when the physician is dictating the discharge summary or reporting the final diagnoses. Significant MS-DRG differences may result should the wrong principal diagnosis be selected.

UTI as a Principal Diagnosis Versus UTI as a Postoperative Complication

EXAMPLE A patient presents with UTI and the physician states status post-prostatectomy 2 days prior to this admit.

DIAGNOSES	CODES	MS-DRG	RW
UTI	599.0 (N39.0)	690	0.7864
UTI as a postop infection	997.5 (N99.89)	699	0.9999
	599.0 (N39.0)		
	E879.6 (Y83.6)		

When patients have central lines, dialysis catheters, ports, or indwelling urinary catheters, to name a few and they present with bacteremia/sepsis, it is important for the coder to verify whether the bacteremia/sepsis is due to the presence of these devices.

It is also important to realize that physicians do not often use the term "complication." If it is stated as UTI following appendectomy, it may be necessary to query the physician as to whether this is a postop complication.

Pneumonia as a Principal Diagnosis Versus Pneumonia as a Transplant Complication

EXAMPLE

Patient with a transplanted lung presents with pneumonia.

DIAGNOSES	CODES	MS-DRG	RW
Pneumonia h/o kidney transplant	486 (J18.9)	194	
	V42.0 (Z94.0)		1.0152
Pneumonia in transplanted lung	996.84 (T86.812)	205	1.2972
	486 (J18.9)		

In this case, if the transplant guideline was not applied, "a transplant code is only assigned if the complication affects the function of the transplant organ," a significant difference in payment would occur.

CHAPTER REVIEW EXERCISE

Where applicable, assign codes for diagnoses, procedures, and V/Z codes and external cause codes.

1. Postoperative septicemia, initial encounter _____

2. Internal wound dehiscence, initial encounter _____

3. Patient with abdominal adhesions due to surgical instrument left in body cavity, initial encounter _____

4. Perforation of coronary artery due to coronary artery stent insertion _____

5. During hemicolectomy, doctor inadvertently makes a rent in the intestine _____

6. Inflammation of the external stoma of the urinary tract _____

7. Rejection of a skin graft _____

8. Failure of an insulin pump; patient has type I diabetes, initial encounter _____

9. Thrombophlebitis of the right lower extremity as the result of saphenous vein graft harvest, initial encounter _____

10. Stroke after surgery, encounter _____

11. Acute renal failure after surgery _____

12. Shock due to surgery, initial encounter _____

13. Severe hypertension after surgery _____

14. Hematoma of surgical site _____

15. After a blood transfusion, patient develops high fever _____

16. Cytomegalovirus infection in transplanted kidney _____

17. Patient had a traumatic amputation of the right upper extremity 1 year ago after a farm accident; he presents with a neuroma of the amputation stump _____

CHAPTER GLOSSARY

Dehiscence: opening of a surgical wound.

Dialysis disequilibrium syndrome: characterized by weakness, dizziness, headache, and, in severe cases, mental status changes.

Dumping syndrome: when undigested contents of the stomach are transported to the small intestine too quickly.

Iatrogenic: caused by medical treatment.

Malunion: when the fracture fragments have united but are not properly aligned. Incorrectly positioned bones may demonstrate angulation, rotation, and shortening.

Mechanical complication: when a device or equipment malfunctions.

Nonunion: when bony healing is not achieved at the fracture site. A fracture site that fails to heal within approximately 6 to 9 months of the injury represents a nonunion.

Ostomies: surgically created openings in the body.

Pneumothorax: air in space around the lung.

Pulmonary embolism: blood clot(s) in the pulmonary artery that causes blockage in the artery.

REFERENCES

1. American Hospital Association. *Coding Clinic for ICD-9-CM* 1997:3Q:p8. Dislodged gastrostomy tube.
2. American Hospital Association. *Coding Clinic for ICD-9-CM* 1985:Nov-Dec:p15. Trauma resulting from patient pulling out urinary catheter.
3. American Hospital Association. *Coding Clinic for ICD-9-CM* 1997:3Q:p13. Hip prosthesis removal with total hip replacement.
4. American Hospital Association. *Coding Clinic for ICD-9-CM* 2008:3Q:p11. End stent restenosis.
5. American Hospital Association. *Coding Clinic for ICD-9-CM* 1998:3Q:p3. Complication of transplanted organs.
6. American Hospital Association. *Coding Clinic for ICD-9-CM* 1995:4Q:p82. Amputation stump complication.

Reimbursement Methodologies

LEARNING OBJECTIVES

1. Describe the complexities of MS-DRGs and hospital reimbursement
2. Explain the difference between optimization and maximization
3. Identify key elements of a UB-04
4. Describe the elements and purpose of the charge description master (CDM)
5. Explain medical necessity
6. Calculate case-mix index (CMI)
7. Explain the role of Quality Improvement Organizations (QIOs)
8. Explain the purpose of PEPPER
9. Explain the purpose of Recovery Audit Contract (RAC)
10. Describe the purpose of a clinical documentation improvement program

ABBREVIATIONS/ ACRONYMS

AHIMA American Health Information Management Association
ALOS average length of stay
CC complication/comorbidity
CDIP Clinical Documentation Improvement Program

CDM charge description master
CHF congestive heart failure
CMI case-mix index
CMS Centers for Medicare and Medicaid Services
COPD chronic obstructive pulmonary disease

CPT *Current Procedural Terminology*
DHHS U.S. Department of Health and Human Services
GMLOS geometric length of stay
HCPCS Healthcare Common Procedure Coding System

HH Home Health

HMO Health Maintenance Organization

HPR hospital payment rate

ICD-9-CM *International Classification of Diseases, 9th Revision, Clinical Modification*

ICD-10-CM *International Classification of Diseases, 10th Revision, Clinical Modification*

ICD-10-PCS *International Classification of Diseases, 10th Revision, Procedure Coding System*

IPPS Inpatient Prospective Payment System

LCDs local coverage determinations

LMRP local medical review policies

LOS length of stay

LTC long-term care

MAC Medicare Administrative Contractor

MDC major diagnostic category

MI myocardial infarction

MIC Medicaid Integrity Contractor

MS-DRG Medicare Severity diagnosis-related group

NCDs national coverage determinations

NPI National Provider Identifier

PEPPER Program for Evaluating Payment Patterns Electronic Report

PPO Preferred Provider Organization

PPS Prospective Payment System

QIO Quality Improvement Organization

RAC Recovery Audit Contract

RPS retrospective payment system

RW relative weight

SNF skilled nursing facility

SOW scope of work

TEFRA Tax Equity and Fiscal Responsibility Act

UB-04 Uniform Bill-04

ZPIC Zone Program Integrity Contractor

INTRODUCTION TO REIMBURSEMENT

Reimbursement or payment for healthcare services has evolved over time into a complicated system with many rules and guidelines that must be followed if proper payment is to be received from third party payers. Rules and guidelines vary, depending on which healthcare setting or third party payer is involved. A **third party payer** makes payments on behalf of the patient for health services. Third party payers may include government programs, insurance companies, and managed care plans.

Private Plans

A variety of private plans (commercial payer) are provided by companies such as Blue Cross/Blue Shield, Aetna, Cigna, and Travelers. These plans are available in different formats, including the following:

- **Self-insured plans**—self-insurance fund set up by an employer to provide health claim benefits for employees.
- **Health Maintenance Organization (HMO)**—type of managed care in which hospitals, physicians, and other providers contract to provide health care for patients, usually at a discounted rate.
- **Preferred Provider Organization (PPO)**—type of managed care in which hospitals, physicians, and other providers have an arrangement with a third party payer to provide health care at discounted rates to third party payer clients.

Because Medicare is the predominant payer for healthcare services, this text focuses on Medicare's reimbursement system. Of note, many private and commercial payers have adopted the Medicare reimbursement system.

Government Plans

Medicare is a federal entitlement program administered by the Centers for Medicare and Medicaid Services (CMS) for patients over 65 years of age, certain disabled individuals, and those with end-stage renal disease.

Medicaid is a federal and state insurance plan, administered by the states and managed by the Social Security Administration of the federal government for patients whose income and resources are insufficient to pay for health care.

TRICARE, previously known as CHAMPUS (Civilian Health and Medical Program for the Uniformed Services), is a medical program for active duty military members, qualified family members, non–Medicare-eligible retirees, and their family members.

Workers' Compensation is a requirement of the federal government for employers to cover employees who are injured or become sick on the job. It is managed by various plans chosen by the employer or by state governments.

Medicare

After many years of debate in Congress, in July 1965, the House and Senate passed the bill that established Medicare, an insurance program designed to provide all older adults with comprehensive healthcare coverage at an affordable cost. In 1972, Medicare eligibility was extended to people with disabilities and those with end-stage renal disease.

The Social Security Act was responsible for the establishment of the Medicare program. As a result of this, the government became more involved in the delivery of health care. The government wanted to ensure that Medicare participants received both quality health care and medically necessary services.

Medicare is a federal health insurance program that is divided into parts according to the type of coverage.

Part A: Hospital Insurance. To be eligible for Part A hospital insurance, one must have worked or must have had a spouse who worked a minimum of 40 quarters of Medicare-covered employment. Part A of Medicare pays for inpatient hospital, skilled nursing facility, and some home health care. Medicare pays all costs for each benefit period (60 days), except for the deductible (which changes each year).

Part B: Medical Insurance. To be eligible for Part B insurance, one must meet the same requirements as for Part A. A premium (which changes each year) is deducted from a person's social security check for Part B coverage. Part B Medicare covers Medicare-eligible physician services, outpatient hospital services, certain home health services, and durable medical equipment. A yearly deductible (that changes each year) and a 20% co-payment amount are applied to these services.

Part C: Medicare Advantage Plans. Medicare Advantage Plans are run by private companies and are similar to HMOs and PPOs. They provide more choices and sometimes additional benefits. They offer all the benefits provided by Part A and Part B, but some also may provide prescription drug coverage (Part D). Patients may be required to use certain hospitals and physicians in the service area.

Part D: Prescription Drug Coverage. This is an optional program for prescription drug coverage. Medicare prescription drug coverage is available to anyone who is covered by Medicare.

DIAGNOSIS-RELATED GROUPS/MEDICARE SEVERITY DIAGNOSIS-RELATED GROUPS

DRGs were developed at Yale University in the late 1960s to monitor quality of care and utilization of services. DRGs were not intended to be a means of determining hospital reimbursement. In 1982, the Tax Equity and Fiscal Responsibility Act (TEFRA) mandated limits on Medicare payments to hospitals. The government decided to use the DRG classification system, a prospective payment system (PPS), to pay for services rendered to Medicare inpatients. A **prospective payment system** is a method of reimbursement in which payment is made according to a predetermined, fixed amount rather than on the basis of billed charges.

The government implemented a PPS in an effort to control the costs of inpatient hospital stays. The DRG system had some inequities in that a patient with multiple complication(s) or comorbid condition(s) is assigned that same DRG and receives the same payment as the patient who has just one complication or comorbid condition. Larger hospitals and tertiary care centers may present greater financial risks because they routinely care for patients who

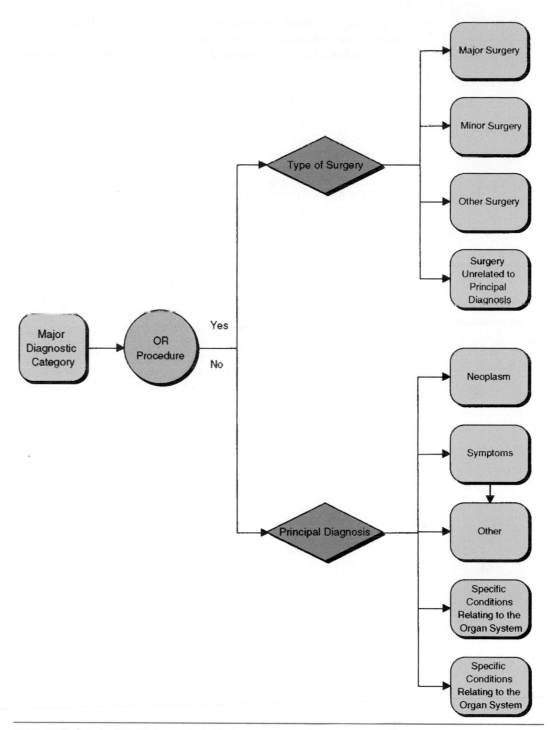

FIGURE 26-1. MS-DRG structure for a major diagnostic category (MDC).

are severely ill. As a result, CMS implemented the Medicare Severity diagnosis-related groups (MS-DRGs), which became effective on October 1, 2007.

ICD-9-CM codes are used to determine the MS-DRG. First, a patient is assigned to an MDC (Figure 26-1) on the basis of the principal diagnosis code; next, it is determined whether the case is a "medical" or a "surgical" case. If no procedures are identified, a medical MS-DRG is assigned. Patients who undergo a valid operating room procedure or another non–operating room procedure that affects MS-DRG assignment are assigned a surgical MS-DRG. It is logical that a patient who has undergone a surgical procedure would use more resources because of costs associated with anesthesia, operating and recovery rooms, and additional nursing care.

The MS-DRG classification system is divided into 25 major diagnostic categories (MDCs), which are based on all possible principal diagnoses that often correspond with an organ system.

MDC 1	Diseases and Disorders of the Nervous System
MDC 2	Diseases and Disorders of the Eye
MDC 3	Diseases and Disorders of the Ear, Nose, Mouth, and Throat
MDC 4	Diseases and Disorders of the Respiratory System
MDC 5	Diseases and Disorders of the Circulatory System
MDC 6	Diseases and Disorders of the Digestive System
MDC 7	Diseases and Disorders of the Hepatobiliary System and Pancreas
MDC 8	Diseases and Disorders of the Musculoskeletal System and Connective Tissue
MDC 9	Diseases and Disorders of the Skin, Subcutaneous Tissue, and Breast
MDC 10	Endocrine, Nutritional, and Metabolic Diseases and Disorders
MDC 11	Diseases and Disorders of the Kidney and Urinary Tract
MDC 12	Diseases and Disorders of the Male Reproductive System
MDC 13	Diseases and Disorders of the Female Reproductive System
MDC 14	Pregnancy, Childbirth, and the Puerperium
MDC 15	Newborns and Other Neonates with Conditions Originating in the Perinatal Period
MDC 16	Diseases and Disorders of the Blood and Blood-Forming Organs and Immunologic Disorders
MDC 17	Myeloproliferative Diseases and Disorders, and Poorly Differentiated Neoplasms
MDC 18	Infectious and Parasitic Diseases (Systemic or unspecified sites)
MDC 19	Mental Diseases and Disorders
MDC 20	Alcohol/Drug Use and Alcohol/Drug-Induced Organic Mental Disorders
MDC 21	Injuries, Poisonings, and Toxic Effects of Drugs
MDC 22	Burns
MDC 23	Factors Influencing Health Status and Other Contacts with Health Services
MDC 24	Multiple Significant Trauma
MDC 25	Human Immunodeficiency Virus Infections
PreMDC	Heart Transplant or Implant of Heart Assist System — MS-DRG 001/002
	ECMO or Trach with Mechanical Ventilation 96+ Hr or PDX Except Face, Mouth, and Neck with Major OR — MS-DRG 003
	Trach with Mechanical Ventilation 96+ Hr or PDX Except Face, Mouth, and Neck without Major OR — MS-DRG 004
	Liver Transplant — MS-DRG 005/006
	Lung Transplant — MS-DRG 007
	Simultaneous Pancreas/Kidney Transplant — MS-DRG 008
	Pancreas Transplant — MS-DRG 010
	Tracheostomy for Face, Mouth, and Neck Diagnoses — MS-DRG 011/012/013
	Allogeneic Bone Marrow Transplant — MS-DRG 014
	Autologous Bone Marrow Transplant — MS-DRG 015

Other factors influencing MS-DRG assignment include:

- Patient's sex
- Patient's discharge disposition or status
- Secondary diagnoses and the presence or absence of complications or comorbidities (CC) or major complication or comorbidities (MCC)
- Birth weight for neonates
- Procedures used as proxy for CC/MCC

There are 745 MS-DRGs that group patients who have similar diagnoses, lengths of stay, and need for resources into a particular MS-DRG with a set payment rate. Specialized software called a **grouper** is used to assign the appropriate MS-DRG. Groupers are often included in the **encoder** or coding software that is used to assign diagnosis and procedure codes.

After completing a thorough review of the health record, the coder must determine the principal diagnosis on the basis of the UHDDS definition. The **principal diagnosis** is "the condition established after study to be chiefly responsible for occasioning the admission of the patient to the hospital for care." Then, codes for all secondary diagnoses and procedures can be assigned. Grouper software is used to determine the appropriate MS-DRG.

Changes may be made to ICD-9-CM codes on April 1 and/or October 1 each year. The government also makes changes to the MS-DRG system annually on October 1. These changes are published in the *Federal Register,* which is the official daily publication for rules, proposed rules, and notices of U.S. federal agencies and organizations, as well as for executive orders and other presidential documents. MS-DRG changes are first published as a proposed rule, and a comment period is generally provided for the public prior to publishing of the final rule. The conversion of the MS-DRGs to ICD-10-CM/PCS was completed, and the *ICD-10 Definitions Manual* was posted in October of 2009. A team of researchers, physicians, clinical coding experts, MS-DRG analysts, and software programmers were involved in this conversion project.

MS-DRG OPTIMIZATION

Optimization is the process of striving to obtain optimal reimbursement or the highest possible payment to which the facility is legally entitled on the basis of coded data supported by documentation in the health record. It is often said that "If it is not documented, it was not done." If services were performed and not documented, payment for these services may be denied. On the other hand, **maximization** is the manipulation of codes to receive maximum reimbursement without supporting documentation in the health record or with disregard for coding conventions, guidelines, and UHDDS definitions. Maximization is unethical and is addressed in the American Health Information Management Association (AHIMA) Standards of Ethical Coding, which can be found in Chapter 1.

Not all MS-DRGs are affected by the presence of a secondary diagnosis. It can be determined by the MS-DRG title whether the MS-DRG is affected by the absence or presence of a CC or MCC. A **complication** is a condition that arises during a patient's hospitalization that may lead to increased resource use. A **comorbidity** is a preexisting condition (i.e., is present on admission) that may lead to increased resource use. The fact that a physician documents that a diagnosis is a complication during a patient's stay does not necessarily mean that diagnosis will fit the definition of a complication in the MS-DRG assignment. A physician may also document that the patient had no complications during hospital stay, and an assigned secondary diagnosis may qualify as a CC or MCC for that particular MS-DRG.

EXAMPLE

MS-DRG 193, Simple pneumonia and pleurisy with MCC, 1.4796.
MS-DRG 194, Simple pneumonia and pleurisy with CC, 1.0152.
MS-DRG 195, Simple pneumonia and pleurisy without MCC/CC, 0.7096.

In the above example, one way to optimize MS-DRG 195 would be to review the record further for documentation of a secondary diagnosis that would qualify as CC or MCC.

Other ways to optimize in the above case would be to review the record for the following:
- An organism that is responsible for the pneumonia
- Respiratory neoplasm
- Septicemia
- Mechanical ventilation
- Opportunistic lung infection in a patient with HIV
- Tracheostomy with mechanical ventilation over 96 hours

Remember to optimize; supporting documentation must be included in the health record and the definition for principal diagnosis must be met.

Some of the most commonly missed CCs or MCCs include the following:
- Atrial flutter
- Atelectasis

- Cachexia
- Cardiogenic shock
- Cardiomyopathy
- Cellulitis
- Chronic kidney disease, stages IV-V, including end-stage
- Chronic obstructive pulmonary disease (COPD)—exacerbation
- Diabetes mellitus with complications
- Hematemesis
- Hyponatremia
- Malnutrition
- Melena
- Pleural effusion
- Pneumothorax
- Respiratory failure
- Urinary tract infection

MS-DRG REIMBURSEMENT

Each MS-DRG payment is determined by two basic factors:
1. Relative weight of assigned MS-DRG
2. Individual hospital payment rate or base rate

Each of the more than 745 MS-DRGs is assigned a relative weight. The average relative weight factor is 1.0000. If a particular MS-DRG used twice as many resources as the average, it would be assigned a relative weight of 2.0000. If a particular MS-DRG used half as many resources as the average, it would be assigned a relative weight of 0.5000. Each year, MS-DRG relative weights are updated to reflect the following:

- Changes in treatment patterns
- Technology
- Any other factors that may change the use of hospital resources

Each hospital is assigned a base dollar amount as the hospital payment rate for a relative weight of 1.0000. Larger facilities that have more complicated cases and provide additional services may have higher hospital payment rates than smaller rural facilities. The individual hospital payment rate or base dollar amount is determined by the following:

- A regional or national adjusted standardized amount that considers the type of hospital
- Designation of large urban, urban, or rural hospital
- Wage index for the geographic area where the hospital is located

A hospital payment rate can change from time to time. It usually changes once a year, effective on October 1.

Relative weight (RW) is multiplied by the hospital's payment rate (HPR) to equal that hospital's MS-DRG reimbursement.

$$RW \times HPR = \text{MS-DRG payment}$$

EXAMPLE

A patient who is admitted with pneumonia and is being treated for a urinary tract infection, which is a CC, is assigned to MS-DRG 194.

Simple pneumonia and pleurisy with CC are assigned. If this hospital's payment rate is $4000.00, the MS-DRG payment would be calculated as follows. MS-DRG 194 has a relative weight of 1.0152.

$$1.0152(RW) \times \$4000.00(HPR) = \$4060.80(\text{MS-DRG payment})$$

The MS-DRG payment is not based on actual charges for that patient during the hospital stay. If the patient had actual charges that totaled more than $10,000.00, the hospital would be paid only the MS-DRG payment. The hospital would not be able to bill the patient for any additional charges other than the deductible and/or coinsurance amounts. If the patient had a hospital bill that totaled $3500.00, the hospital would still be paid the MS-DRG payment. The hospital would lose reimbursement in the first scenario but would gain reimbursement in the second case scenario.

The intent with a PPS system is that hospitals would know what they are going to be reimbursed for a particular type of patient before they render any services. The old payment method, or a retrospective payment system (RPS), was based on actual charges or a percentage of charges; this did not promote best practices and quality care because the hospital was paid on the basis of charges, and the higher the charges, the higher the payment. The amount of the payment is determined after the patient has been cared for and the charges assessed. If a patient experienced complications and the hospital bill went higher, the hospital was still paid. PPS provides incentive to decrease patient complications. Hospitals must provide quality care in an efficient manner to maintain a healthy bottom line.

Each hospital stay will fit into one and only one MS-DRG category. For example, if a patient was admitted because of osteoarthritis for a hip replacement and had a myocardial infarction (MI) 2 days after the procedure, the hip replacement MS-DRG is the one that will be assigned. No additional MS-DRG is assigned to pay for the costs associated with the MI. However, the MI is an MCC, and increased reimbursement would be received because of the assignment of an MS-DRG with MCC.

If more than one procedure is performed, the procedure in the highest surgical group will determine the MS-DRG assignment. For example, if the patient had a breast biopsy and a mastectomy during the same hospital stay, the mastectomy would determine the surgical MS-DRG.

UB-04

Uniform Bill-04, or UB-04, or CMS-1450 is the paper claim form (Figure 26-2) that is used to submit bills to Medicare and other third party payers. The first uniform bill was introduced in 1982 and was called the UB-82. Prior to that time, each and every insurance or third party payer had its own forms. The uniform bill made it much easier for patients and hospital billing offices to submit claims to all insurance companies in a timely manner. Some different completion requirements may apply for an individual payer.

The UB-04 consists of fields for 12 diagnosis codes (nine diagnosis codes and three E codes) and six procedure codes. Codes affecting reimbursement need to be sequenced in the top nine codes in order for codes to be submitted on the UB-04. The same applies to the top six procedure codes. A code for the admitting diagnosis is also required. The admitting diagnosis does not have to be the same as the principal diagnosis.

When errors in coding occur, the hospital may resubmit the billing data with revised codes on the claim or UB-04. For Medicare patients, the hospital has 60 days from the date of the MS-DRG payment to request a review of the original MS-DRG assignment. After 60 days, no resubmissions for higher payment can be made. If an error was found that meant a lower payment for the hospital, the adjustment should be made as soon as possible. For the most part, hospital billing or claim forms are submitted electronically. There are specific formats that are required by HIPAA (Health Insurance Portability and Accountability Act). Most healthcare organizations use the HIPPA-approved ANSI (American National Standards Institute) ASC (Accredited Standards Committee) X12 standards as the format for various electronic documents. Because of ICD-10 and other industry changes, the current 4010 X12 standards need to be upgraded. All providers, payers, and clearinghouses will need to comply with the version 5010 X12 standards for electronic claims processing by January 1, 2012.

CHARGE DESCRIPTION MASTER

The **chargemaster** or **charge description master (CDM)** is a listing of the services, procedures, drugs, and supplies that can be applied to a patient's bill. A chargemaster often contains many data items to properly identify a particular charge. Some of those data items include:

FIGURE 26-2. UB-04—Form used to submit inpatient claims.

- **Department number**—Ancillary departments such as radiology, laboratory, and emergency room will have a specific hospital departmental number.
- **Charge description number**—This is a number that designates a particular service or procedure; it is used to generate a charge on a patient bill.
- Description of service, procedure, drug, or supply—This is a brief description of the procedure or service. If there is a corresponding HCPCS code, the description should match the code description.
- HCPCS code (includes CPT codes)—Codes will be assigned to all applicable CDM items. Not all items will have an HCPCS code.
- **Revenue code**—This four-digit code is utilized on the UB-04 to indicate a particular type of service. Revenue code 0351 would be used when billing a CT scan of the head, and code 0352 would be used for a CT scan of the body.
- Price or charge of the service, procedure, drug, or supply—The charge for the item is also shown.

MEDICAL NECESSITY

Medicare and other third-party payers only want to pay for items and services that are reasonable and necessary. Medicare may only pay for services that are "reasonable and necessary for the diagnosis or treatment of illness or injury or to improve the functioning of a malformed body member." There are policies that outline the criteria for what is determined to be reasonable and necessary and what meets **medical necessity** guidelines. These policies include **national coverage determinations** (**NCDs**; Figure 26-3) and **local coverage determinations** (**LCDs**), previously known as local medical review policies (LMRPs). These may include certain time frames for testing, certain age requirements, and that a particular diagnosis or condition must be present for a procedure or treatment to be considered medically necessary.

POST–ACUTE CARE TRANSFER POLICY

The U.S. Congress, through the Balanced Budget Act of 1997, required CMS to begin applying a slightly different payment methodology when transferring from acute care to a post–acute care setting. This payment methodology was already in place for transfers from an acute facility to another short-term acute care facility. Complicated formulas are used to determine the transfer-adjusted payment.

It was found that shortly after admission, many patients were transferred to other post–acute care settings, so CMS figured it was overpaying the hospitals for these patients. CMS created special rules for certain MS-DRGs when patients were discharged immediately after their hospitalization to a rehabilitation hospital, a skilled nursing facility (SNF), a long-term care (LTC) hospital, or home health care. These MS-DRGs are called "transfer MS-DRGs." This started in 1999 with 10 transfer MS-DRGs. It has expanded to 273 transfer MS-DRGs. Although a patient may be grouped in a transfer MS-DRG, a payment reduction occurs only if all of the following conditions are met:
- The patient is in a transfer MS-DRG.
- The patient was a "short-stay" or early discharge (LOS+1 < GMLOS).
- The patient was transferred to a SNF, home health care, a rehab hospital, or a long-term care hospital.

CASE-MIX INDEX

MS-DRGs provide a means of defining and measuring a hospital's **case-mix index** (CMI), in other words, how sick its patients are. Following are interrelated parts of case-mix:
- Severity of illness
- Prognosis

220.4 - Mammograms
(Rev. 1, 10-03-03)
CIM 50-21

A diagnostic mammography is a radiologic procedure furnished to a man or woman with signs and symptoms of breast disease, or a personal history of breast cancer, or a personal history of biopsy – proven benign breast disease, and includes a physician's interpretation of the results of the procedure. A diagnostic mammography is a covered service if it is ordered by a doctor of medicine or osteopathy as defined in §1861 (r) (1) of the Act. A screening mammography is a radiologic procedure furnished to a woman without signs or symptoms of breast disease, for the purpose of early detection of breast cancer, and includes a physician's interpretation of the results of the procedure. A screening mammography has limitations as it must be, at a minimum a two-view exposure (cranio-caudal and a medial lateral oblique view) of each breast. Payment may not be made for a screening mammography performed on a woman under age 35. Payment may be made for only one screening mammography performed on a woman over age 34, but under age 40. For an asymptomatic woman over age 39, payment may be made for a screening mammography performed after at least 11 months have passed following the month in which the last screening mammography was performed.

A radiological mammogram is a covered diagnostic test under the following conditions:

• A patient has distinct signs and symptoms for which a mammogram is indicated;

• A patient has a history of breast cancer; or

• A patient is asymptomatic but, on the basis of the patient's history and other factors the physician considers significant, the physician's judgment is that a mammogram is appropriate.

Use of mammograms in routine screening of: (1) asymptomatic women aged 50 and over, and (2) asymptomatic women aged 40 or over whose mothers or sisters have had the disease, is considered medically appropriate, but would not be covered for Medicare purposes.

Cross-reference:

The Medicare Benefit Policy Manual, Chapter 15, "Covered Medical and Other Health Services," §80.

The Medicare Benefit Policy Manual, Chapter 1, "Inpatient Hospital Services," §50

FIGURE 26-3. An example of National Coverage Determinations.

- Treatment difficulty
- Need for intervention
- Resource intensity

To calculate case-mix, add the relative weight of the MS-DRG assigned to each patient discharged during a specific time period. Then divide the total relative weight by the number of patients in that time period. The resultant value represents the case-mix index. Some facilities may calculate their Medicare case-mix along with overall case-mix, which includes all patients. This value may be calculated each month, quarterly, and/or at the end of each fiscal year. If great variations in the case-mix are seen from month to month, hospital administration may want an explanation. For example, if the hospital was undergoing renovations in the surgery department and the number of surgeries for the month was significantly lower than usual, this change may cause a facility's case-mix to drop.

EXAMPLE

During the month of June, the following Medicare patients were discharged from Hospital A:

2 patients	MS-DRG 194	RW 1.0152
2 patients	MS-DRG 292	RW 1.0302
1 patient	MS-DRG 192	RW 0.7220
3 patients	MS-DRG 302	RW 0.9755
2 patients	MS-DRG 065	RW 1.1667

A total of 10 patients are included. To perform a manual calculation, add the following:

1.0152
1.0152
1.0302
1.0302
0.7220
0.9755
0.9755
0.9755
1.1667
1.1667
TOTAL   10.0727 is the total of the relative weights of the 10 patients listed above.

The next step is to divide the total relative weight by the number of patients. 10.0727 divided by 10 = 1.0073. This is the CMI for this group of patients.

Usually, these figures are calculated with the use of software programs and can be calculated using certain parameters such as specific third party payer, by date, by physician, or by clinical service. If significant coding errors and/or errors in MS-DRG assignment occur, the CMI may not be accurate.

QUALITY IMPROVEMENT ORGANIZATION

Quality improvement organizations (QIOs) work for consumers, healthcare providers, and hospitals to make sure that patients are getting the "right care at the right time in the appropriate setting." A total of 53 QIOs have been created, one for each state and territory and for the District of Columbia. This network acts under the direction of CMS and is contracted to monitor the quality of health care and to make sure that Medicare pays only for services that are reasonable and necessary. QIO functions under three-year contract cycles called *scopes of work* (SOWs).

PEPPER

The Program for Evaluating Payment Patterns Electronic Report (PEPPER) is an electronic report that is sent to a hospital that contains hospital-specific information for 13 target areas. These target areas are specific MS-DRGs that have been identified as being at risk for payment errors. PEPPER was developed to assist QIOs with their Hospital Payment Monitoring Programs (HPMPs) to identify and prevent payment errors due to billing, MS-DRG assignment, coding, and/or admission necessity issues. CMS announced at the beginning of 2009 that it will continue to require the QIOs to provide hospitals with these reports.

RECOVERY AUDIT CONTRACT

The Recovery Audit Contract (RAC) Initiative was implemented as a result of section 306 of the Medicare Prescription Drug, Improvement, and Modernization Act of 2003 (MMA). Congress directed the Department of Health and Human Services (DHHS) to conduct a three-year demonstration project using Recovery Audit Contractors (RACs) to detect and correct improper Medicare payments—both overpayments and underpayments. Under the demonstration project, RACs reviewed claims for hospital inpatient and outpatient, skilled nursing facility, physician, ambulance, laboratory, and durable medical equipment in California, Florida, New York, Massachusetts, South Carolina, and Arizona. At the conclusion of the project in March of 2008, more than $900 million in overpayments was returned to the Medicare Trust Fund, and almost $38 million in underpayments was paid to healthcare providers/facilities. RACs are paid on a contingency fee basis, receiving a percentage of the improper payments collected from providers/facilities.

CMS is using lessons learned from the RAC demonstration project to improve its permanent program. A permanent RAC program is now in place for all 50 states.

Currently, four recovery audit contractors (RACs) are available:

- Region A: Diversified Collection Services, Inc., of Livermore, California
- Region B: CGI Technologies and Solutions, Inc., of Fairfax, Virginia
- Region C: Connolly Consulting Associates, Inc., of Wilton, Connecticut
- Region D: HealthDataInsights, Inc., of Las Vegas, Nevada

Other groups that are contracting with state and federal agencies to identify improper billing and overpayments include:

- Medicare Administrative Contractors (MACs) are the companies that process Part A and Part B Medicare claims. They are responsible for overseeing the accuracy of claims completion and the determination of correct payments for services. Because they review both Part A and Part B claims, they are able to review for discrepancies between the two sets of claims.
- Zone Program Integrity Contractors (ZPICs), who serve the same jurisdictions as the MACs and are authorized to conduct investigations, provide support to law enforcement and audit the Medicare advantage plans. They may also focus on Medicare billing targets.
- Medicaid Integrity Contractors (MICs) are in charge of reviewing and auditing Medicaid claims for inappropriate payments or fraud. They use a data-driven approach to identify some of the following target areas:
  - Services after the death of a beneficiary
  - Duplicate claims
  - Unbundling of services
  - Outpatient claims with service dates that overlap an inpatient stay

MICs also conduct medical record reviews to ensure that payment was made for medically necessary services, services that are covered, that payment was made correctly, and that the services were billed properly with the correct diagnosis and procedure codes.

DATA QUALITY

In Chapter 1, it was mentioned that coded data have many purposes.[1] In November 2007, AHIMA published a position statement on the "Consistency of Healthcare Diagnostic and Procedural Coding." It states that accurate and complete coded data are critical for:

- Healthcare delivery
- Research
- Public reporting
- Reimbursement
- Policy making

All users must consistently apply the same official coding rules, conventions, guidelines, and definitions. AHIMA promotes the idea that coding professionals are educated and certified to assign and validate codes and to assist with policy development related to coding accuracy.

As reimbursement and coding systems evolve, it is important to remember that the codes that are assigned today will have a role in the reimbursement system(s) of tomorrow, so it is imperative that each health record be coded accurately and completely.

CLINICAL DOCUMENTATION IMPROVEMENT PROGRAM

Incomplete, inaccurate, and illegible documentation has been a problem in health care for years. With the evolution of reimbursement systems that are based on documentation and coded data, it is imperative that hospitals make improvements in their clinical documentation. A clinical documentation improvement program (CDIP) will depend on the facility's needs and must work within the culture and framework of the organization. The success of any improvement type of program is dependent on the participation of the "right" team players. It is extremely important to get physician support and buy-in because physicians are responsible for much of the documentation within the health record.

One of the goals of a CDIP is to improve the facility's CMI. Case-mix data can be used for comparison with other facilities and for monitoring trends within the facility. Better documentation, along with accurate and complete coding of the health record, should lead to better reimbursement and increased CMI.

The manner in which documentation is collected should be analyzed so improvements can be made to capture complete and accurate clinical documentation. As hospitals convert from paper to electronic records, the time is ideal for assessing all forms of documentation.

Many facilities are employing Clinical Documentation Specialists who concurrently review patient records and query the attending physician about documentation that may be missing or incomplete within the patient's record. Most documentation issues can be resolved before the patient is discharged, and the record will have more complete and accurate documentation for assigning codes. This should reduce the number of physician queries asked by the coder. Because greater specificity is required for ICD-10-CM and ICD-10-PCS, good documentation will be even more important.

CHAPTER REVIEW EXERCISE

Choose the best answer to the followings questions.

1. A preexisting condition that is present on admission and may lead to increased resource use
   A. Complication
   B. Comorbidity
   C. Morbidity
   D. Other diagnosis

2. The condition that, after study, is established as chiefly responsible for occasioning the admission of the patient to the hospital is called the
   A. Primary diagnosis
   B. Provisional diagnosis
   C. Principal diagnosis
   D. Major diagnosis

3. DRG stands for
   A. Drug-related gastritis
   B. Diagnostic related groups
   C. Diagnosis-related group
   D. Diagnostic regulation by government

4. The billing form that is currently in use in hospitals is
   A. UB-87
   B. UB-04
   C. UB-82
   D. UB-92

5. Calculate the case-mix for the following patients using the weights from the MS-DRG Table on the Evolve website:

2 patients	MS-DRG 690
3 patients	MS-DRG 292
1 patient	MS-DRG 069
2 patients	MS-DRG 378

Complete the following questions.

6. Identify four MS-DRGs that appear on the post-transfer policy listing.

_____

_____

7. List four commonly missed CCs or MCCs.

_____

_____

8. What organization is the QIO in your state?

_____

9. Explain the purpose of a recovery audit contractor.

_____

_____

10. What date has been set to the full implementation of a permanent RAC program?

_____

CHAPTER GLOSSARY

Case-mix index: a measurement used by hospitals to define how sick their patients are.

Charge description number: a number that designates a particular service or procedure, used to generate a charge on a patient bill.

Chargemaster or **charge description master (CDM):** a listing of the services, procedures, drugs, and supplies that can be applied to a patient's bill.

Comorbidity: a preexisting condition (i.e., it is present on admission) that may lead to increased resource use.

Complication: a condition that arises during a patient's hospitalization that may lead to increased resource use.

Department number: ancillary departments such as radiology, laboratory, and Emergency Room will have a specific hospital departmental number.

Encoder: coding software that is used to assign diagnosis and procedure codes.

Grouper: specialized software used to assign the appropriate MS-DRG.

Health Maintenance Organization (HMO): type of managed care in which hospitals, physicians, and other providers contract to provide health care for patients, usually at a discounted rate.

Local coverage determinations (LCDs): local policy that may include certain time frames for testing, certain age requirements, and that a particular diagnosis or condition must be present for a procedure or treatment to be considered medically necessary.

Maximization: the manipulation of codes to result in maximum reimbursement without supporting documentation in the health record or with disregard for coding conventions, guidelines, and UHDDS definitions.

Medical necessity: criteria or guidelines for what is determined to be reasonable and necessary for a particular medical service.

National coverage determinations (NCDs): national policy that may include certain time frames for testing, certain age requirements, and that a particular diagnosis or condition be present for a procedure to be considered medically necessary.

Optimization: the process of striving to obtain optimal reimbursement or the highest possible payment to which a facility is legally entitled on the basis of documentation in the health record.

Preferred Provider Organization (PPO): type of managed care in which hospitals, physicians, and other providers have an arrangement with a third party payer to provide health care at discounted rates to third party payer clients.

Principal diagnosis: condition established after study to be chiefly responsible for occasioning the admission of the patient to the hospital for care.

Prospective payment system: method of reimbursement in which payment is made on the basis of a predetermined, fixed amount rather than for billed charges.

Reimbursement: payment for healthcare services.

Revenue code: a four-digit code that is utilized on the UB-04 to indicate a particular type of service.

Self-insured plans: self-insurance fund is set up by an employer to provide health claim benefits for employees.

Third party payer: makes payments for health services on behalf of the patients; may be a government program, insurance company, or managed care plan.

REFERENCE

1. American Health Information Management Association (AHIMA). Statement on consistency of health care diagnostic and procedural coding (AHIMA Position Statement, December 2007).

Outpatient Coding

CHAPTER OUTLINE

Outpatient Terminology
ICD-9-CM Official Guidelines for Coding and Reporting
ICD-10-CM Official Guidelines for Coding and Reporting
Guideline Differences Between ICD-9-CM and ICD-10-CM
Procedure Coding in the Outpatient Setting
APCs as Reimbursement
Chapter Review Exercise
Chapter Glossary
References

LEARNING OBJECTIVES

1. Explain terminology as related to the outpatient setting
2. Identify major differences between ICD-9-CM and ICD-10-CM related to outpatient conditions
3. Describe the difference between inpatient coding guidelines and outpatient coding guidelines
4. Describe what CPT coding is, when it is used, and the official guideline source
5. Apply Diagnostic Coding and Reporting Guidelines for Outpatient Services
6. Assign ICD-9-CM codes for outpatient services
7. Explain the purpose and use of APCs

ABBREVIATIONS/ ACRONYMS

AICD automatic implantable cardioverter-defibrillator

AMA American Medical Association

APC Ambulatory Payment Classification

COPD chronic obstructive pulmonary disease

CPT Current Procedural Terminology

CVA cerebrovascular accident

DEXA dual-energy x-ray absorptiometry

ER Emergency Room

HCPCS Healthcare Common Procedure Coding System

ICD-9-CM *International Classification of Diseases, 9th Revision, Clinical Modification*

ICD-10-CM *International Classification of Diseases, 10th Revision, Clinical Modification*

ICD-10-PCS *International Classification of Diseases, 10th Revision, Procedure Coding System*

MRI magnetic resonance imaging

MS-DRG Medicare Severity diagnosis-related group

OPPS Outpatient Prospective Payment System

PCP primary care provider

UTI urinary tract infection

OUTPATIENT TERMINOLOGY

Terminology in the outpatient setting is often confusing. Outpatient services may be provided in a variety of settings:

■ Doctor's office
■ Clinic
■ Ambulatory surgery, which may also be called outpatient surgery, "in and out" surgery, same day surgery, or same day care

- Emergency Room (ER)
- **Observation unit,** a unit to which unstable patients are admitted for a stay of less than 48 hours
- **Ancillary service** visits/clinic visits (i.e., radiology, laboratory, chemotherapy, radiation therapy)

These outpatient services are called visits or **encounters.** Encounters may require hospital services and/or **professional services** (services rendered by a physician or a nonphysician practitioner). For example, a patient receiving a chest x-ray in a hospital setting will have a hospital bill for the chest x-ray and a professional service bill from the radiologist for the reading of the x-ray.

The term "principal diagnosis" as used in the inpatient setting does not apply in the outpatient setting. The outpatient term that is synonymous with "principal diagnosis" is "first-listed diagnosis" or "primary diagnosis."

ICD-9-CM

Official Guidelines for Coding and Reporting

Please refer to the companion Evolve website for the most current guidelines.

Section IV. Diagnostic Coding and Reporting Guidelines for Outpatient Services

These coding guidelines for outpatient diagnoses have been approved for use by hospitals/providers in coding and reporting hospital-based outpatient services and provider-based office visits.

Information about the use of certain abbreviations, punctuation, symbols, and other conventions used in the ICD-9-CM Tabular List (code numbers and titles), can be found in Section IA of these guidelines, under "Conventions Used in the Tabular List." Information about the correct sequence to use in finding a code is also described in Section I.

The terms encounter and visit are often used interchangeably in describing outpatient service contacts and, therefore, appear together in these guidelines without distinguishing one from the other.

Though the conventions and general guidelines apply to all settings, coding guidelines for outpatient and provider reporting of diagnoses will vary in a number of instances from those for inpatient diagnoses, recognizing that:

The Uniform Hospital Discharge Data Set (UHDDS) definition of principal diagnosis applies only to inpatients in acute, short-term, long-term care and psychiatric hospitals.

Coding guidelines for inconclusive diagnoses (probable, suspected, rule out, etc.) were developed for inpatient reporting and do not apply to outpatients.

A. Selection of first-listed condition

In the outpatient setting, the term first-listed diagnosis is used in lieu of principal diagnosis.

In determining the first-listed diagnosis the coding conventions of ICD-9-CM, as well as the general and disease specific guidelines take precedence over the outpatient guidelines.

In the outpatient setting, the first-listed diagnosis is the reason for the encounter. The first-listed diagnosis may often be a symptom.

EXAMPLE

Patient presents to physician's office with complaints of headache and slurred speech. Physician suspects that this patient is experiencing a transient ischemic attack (TIA) or a cerebrovascular accident (CVA). The patient is sent directly to the hospital. The first-listed diagnosis for the physician office visit is 784.59 (R51), headache, with a secondary diagnosis of 784.5 (R47.81), slurred speech.

> Diagnoses often are not established at the time of the initial encounter/visit. It may take two or more visits before the diagnosis is confirmed.
>
> The most critical rule involves beginning the search for the correct code assignment through the Alphabetic Index. Never begin searching initially in the Tabular List as this will lead to coding errors.

It is common in the outpatient setting for a patient to present to a physician's office with symptoms, for administrative reasons, for follow-up on conditions that no longer exist, or with abnormal findings. A code from the Supplementary Classification of Factors Influencing Health Status and Contact with Health Services (V codes) may often be the most appropriate code. Refer to Chapter 8 for greater detail on assigning V codes.

EXAMPLE

A child presents to his physician's office for a required camp physical, V70.3 (Z02.89).
　　To locate this code in the Alphabetic Index, look under the main term "Admission for, exam."

EXAMPLE

A healthcare worker is stuck by a needle used on a patient with acquired immunodeficiency syndrome (AIDS), V01.79 (Z20.6).
　　To locate this code in the Alphabetic Index, look under the main term "Exposure to."

EXAMPLE

A patient is visiting her oncologist's office for her yearly visit 5 years status post left mastectomy for breast cancer, V67.09, V10.3, V45.71 (Z08, Z90.12, Z85.3).
　　This code is located in the Alphabetic Index under "Admission for follow-up exam—surgery" and "History, malignant neoplasms, breast." *Coding Clinic* (1984 M-J:p10)[1] instructs coding of follow-up visits for cancer patients treated with surgery, who currently have no evidence of cancer, to code V67.09, follow-up exam following other surgery.

EXAMPLE

A patient presents to her physician's office with a strong family history of breast cancer. She is interested in prophylactic removal of both breasts, V16.3 (Z80.3).
　　This code is located in the Alphabetic Index under "History, family, malignant neoplasm."

1. Outpatient Surgery
When a patient presents for outpatient surgery, code the reason for the surgery as the first-listed diagnosis (reason for the encounter), even if the surgery is not performed due to a contraindication.

EXAMPLE

A patient reports to the outpatient surgery department for an arthroscopic meniscectomy for a torn meniscus on the right knee. The patient injured her meniscus when she tripped over the cat. The patient is administered anesthesia and is found to be in atrial fibrillation. The surgeon decides that it is best not to proceed with the procedure but wishes to consult with a cardiologist and reschedule. The primary diagnosis is the torn meniscus; atrial fibrillation is coded secondarily along with canceled surgery and the E code for the accident, 836.2, 427.31, V64.1, E885.9 (S83.206A, I48.0, Z53.09, W01.0xxA).

2. Observation Stay
When a patient is admitted for observation for a medical condition, assign a code for the medical condition as the first-listed diagnosis.

When a patient presents for outpatient surgery and develops complications requiring admission to observation, code the reason for the surgery as the first reported diagnosis (reason for encounter), followed by codes for the complications as secondary diagnoses.

EXAMPLE

A patient is admitted to outpatient surgery with cholelithiasis and is scheduled for a laparoscopic cholecystectomy. The surgery proceeds uneventfully. In the recovery room, the patient is found to have hypotension. The surgeon decides to admit the patient for observation, 574.20, 458.9 (K80.20, I95.9).

B. Codes from 001.0 through V89

The appropriate code or codes from 001.0 through V89 must be used to identify diagnoses, symptoms, conditions, problems, complaints, or other reason(s) for the encounter/visit.

EXAMPLE

When presenting to a doctor's office, a patient often presents with symptoms such as cough or leg pain. At the end of the visit, the physician may not know the cause of the leg pain and therefore may make the assessment that leg pain is probably the result of muscle strain. Therefore, in this case, the code would be 729.5 (M79.606) for leg pain.

C. Accurate reporting of ICD-9-CM diagnosis codes

For accurate reporting of ICD-9-CM diagnosis codes, the documentation should describe the patient's condition, using terminology which includes specific diagnoses as well as symptoms, problems, or reasons for the encounter. There are ICD-9-CM codes to describe all of these.

EXAMPLE

A patient is scheduled for cataract surgery and has congestive heart failure. The surgeon asks the patient's cardiologist for a preoperative consult, V72.81, 428.0, 366.9 (Z01.810, I50.9, H26.9).

D. Selection of codes 001.0 through 999.9

The selection of codes 001.0 through 999.9 will frequently be used to describe the reason for the encounter. These codes are from the section of ICD-9-CM for the classification of diseases and injuries (e.g., infectious and parasitic diseases; neoplasms; symptoms, signs, and ill-defined conditions, etc.).

E. Codes that describe symptoms and signs

Codes that describe symptoms and signs, as opposed to diagnoses, are acceptable for reporting purposes when a diagnosis has not been established (confirmed) by the provider. Chapter 16 of ICD-9-CM, Symptoms, Signs, and Ill-defined conditions (codes 780.0-799.9) contain many, but not all codes for symptoms.

EXAMPLE

When a patient is seen in a physician's office for a problem-oriented visit, it is often a symptom that will be reported as the first-listed diagnosis. A patient may come to the office with abdominal pain, and the physician suspects it is due to diverticulitis. The patient is sent for testing. The first-listed diagnosis for this encounter is 789.00 (R10.9).

On the return visit, test results reveal that the patient does indeed have diverticulitis; therefore, the follow-up visit code would be 562.11 (K57.92).

F. Encounters for circumstances other than a disease or injury
ICD-9-CM provides codes to deal with encounters for circumstances other than a disease or injury. The Supplementary Classification of factors Influencing Health Status and Contact with Health Services (V01.0-**V91.99**) is provided to deal with occasions when circumstances other than a disease or injury are recorded as diagnosis or problems. *See Section I.C.18 for information on V-codes.*

EXAMPLE

A patient is planning on donating an organ and is seen by his family physician. The patient must be examined so it can be determined whether he can qualify as a donor, V70.8 (Z00.5).

EXAMPLE

A patient who is on Coumadin therapy for history of DVT is required to visit a Coumadin clinic weekly until the levels of medication are adjusted, V58.83, V58.61, V12.51 (Z51.81, Z79.01, Z86.71).

G. Level of Detail in Coding
1. ICD-9-CM codes with 3, 4, or 5 digits
ICD-9-CM is composed of codes with either 3, 4, or 5 digits. Codes with three digits are included in ICD-9-CM as the heading of a category of codes that may be further subdivided by the use of fourth and/or fifth digits, which provide greater specificity.
2. Use of full number of digits required for a code
A three-digit code is to be used only if it is not further subdivided. Where fourth-digit subcategories and/or fifth-digit subclassifications are provided, they must be assigned. A code is invalid if it has not been coded to the full number of digits required for that code.
See also discussion under Section I.B.3., General Coding Guidelines, Level of Detail in Coding.
H. ICD-9-CM code for the diagnosis, condition, problem, or other reason for encounter/visit
List first the ICD-9-CM code for the diagnosis, condition, problem, or other reason for encounter/visit shown in the medical record to be chiefly responsible for the services provided. List additional codes that describe any coexisting conditions. In some cases the first-listed diagnosis may be a symptom when a diagnosis has not been established (confirmed) by the physician.

It is important when coding outpatient services that codes for all coexisting conditions are also assigned.

EXAMPLE

A patient presents to his primary care provider (PCP) with a cough and a fever and a long history of chronic obstructive pulmonary disease (COPD). After reviewing the chest x-ray, the physician determines that the patient has pneumonia, 486, 496 (J18.9, J44.9).

I. Uncertain diagnosis
Do not code diagnoses documented as "probable," "suspected," "questionable," "rule out," or "working diagnosis" or other similar terms indicating uncertainty. Rather, code the condition(s) to the highest degree of certainty for that encounter/visit, such as symptoms, signs, abnormal test results, or other reason for the visit. **Please note:** This differs from the coding practices used by short-term, acute care, long-term care and psychiatric hospitals.

Coding Clinic (2005:3Q:p21-22)[2] has also identified the term "compatible" to fall into the same category as possible and probable and a diagnosis described as "compatible with" is not coded in the outpatient setting. The condition should only be coded to the highest degree of certainty for that encounter.

EXAMPLE

A patient presents to her doctor with complaints of weight gain, decreased libido, and cold intolerance. The physician sends her to the laboratory for blood work with a diagnosis of probable hypothyroidism. She is to return in 2 weeks for results of the blood work, which comes back positive for hypothyroidism.
> First visit: 783.1, 799.81, 780.99 (R63.5, R68.82, R68.89)
> Second visit: 244.9 (E03.9)

J. Chronic diseases
Chronic diseases treated on an ongoing basis may be coded and reported as many times as the patient receives treatment and care for the condition(s).

EXAMPLE

A patient is scheduled for a return visit every 6 months for hypercholesterolemia, 272.0 (E78.0).

K. Code all documented conditions that coexist
Code all documented conditions that coexist at the time of the encounter/visit, and require or affect patient care treatment or management. Do not code conditions that were previously treated and no longer exist. However, history codes (V10-V19) may be used as secondary codes if the historical condition or family history has an impact on current care or influences treatment.

EXAMPLE

A patient presents to a physician's office with a complaint of low back pain and is on medications for hypertension and hypercholesterolemia. During the visit the patient's blood pressure is checked and blood was drawn to check cholesterol levels, 724.2, 401.9, 272.0 (M54.5, I10, E78.0).

This case follows the rule of coding coexisting conditions that affect the management of the patient. The physician must take into account the patient's other history and medications before prescribing medication for the back pain.

L. Patients receiving diagnostic services only
For patients receiving diagnostic services only during an encounter/visit, sequence first the diagnosis, condition, problem, or other reason for encounter/visit shown in the medical record to be chiefly responsible for the outpatient services provided during the encounter/visit. Codes for other diagnoses (e.g., chronic conditions) may be sequenced as additional diagnoses.

For encounters for routine laboratory/radiology testing in the absence of any signs, symptoms, or associated diagnosis, assign V72.5 and/**or** a code from subcategory V72.6. If routine testing is performed during the same encounter as a test to evaluate a sign, symptom, or diagnosis, it is appropriate to assign both the V code and the code describing the reason for the non-routine test.

EXAMPLE

A patient who presents to radiology for a chest x-ray may have a working diagnosis such as cough/rule out pneumonia. The ordering physician documents that the patient also has a history of asthma for which he takes albuterol, prn. On reading the x-ray the radiologist documents COPD with no evidence of pneumonia, 786.2, 493.20 (R05, J44.9).

Per *Coding Clinic* (2000:1Q:p4),[3] in the outpatient setting it is permissible to assign codes based on radiology and pathology documentation. This differs from the inpatient setting where diagnoses documented by radiologists and/or pathologists must be confirmed by attending physicians.

For outpatient encounters for diagnostic tests that have been interpreted by a physician, and the final report is available at the time of coding, code any confirmed or definitive diagnosis(es) documented in the interpretation. Do not code related signs and symptoms as additional diagnoses.

Please note: This differs from the coding practice in the hospital inpatient setting regarding abnormal findings on test results.

EXAMPLE

As in the previous example, a patient presents to radiology for a cough/rule out pneumonia and history of asthma, and after the chest x-ray is performed, the radiologist interprets the x-ray as pneumonia and COPD, 486, 493.20 (J18.9, J44.9).

The code for the symptom would not be assigned.

M. Patients receiving therapeutic services only

For patients receiving therapeutic services only during an encounter/visit, sequence first the diagnosis, condition, problem, or other reason for encounter/ visit shown in the medical record to be chiefly responsible for the outpatient services provided during the encounter/visit. Codes for other diagnoses (e.g., chronic conditions) may be sequenced as additional diagnoses.

EXAMPLE

Patient presents to the physician's office monthly for a vitamin B_{12} shot for pernicious anemia, 281.0 (D51.0).

The only exception to this rule is that when the primary reason for the admission/encounter is chemotherapy, radiation therapy, or rehabilitation, the appropriate V code for the service is listed first, and the diagnosis or problem for which the service is being performed listed second.

EXAMPLE

A patient presents to a physician's office for chemotherapy for pancreatic cancer, V58.11, 157.9, 99.25 (Z51.11, C25.9).

N. Patients receiving preoperative evaluations only

For patients receiving preoperative evaluations only, sequence first a code from category V72.8, Other specified examinations, to describe the pre-op consultations. Assign a code for the condition to describe the reason for the surgery as an additional diagnosis. Code also any findings related to the pre-op evaluation.

EXAMPLE   Patient is planning surgery for an abdominal aortic aneurysm (AAA). The surgeon requests that the patient see her primary care provider for a preoperative evaluation. This patient is well known to her primary care provider and has additional chronic diagnoses of hypertension, hypercholesterolemia, and history of breast cancer, V72.84, 401.9, 272.0, V10.3, 441.4 (Z01.818, I10, E78.0, Z85.3, I71.4).

O. Ambulatory surgery

For ambulatory surgery, code the diagnosis for which the surgery was performed. If the postoperative diagnosis is known to be different from the preoperative diagnosis at the time the diagnosis is confirmed, select the postoperative diagnosis for coding, since it is the most definitive.

EXAMPLE   A patient undergoes surgery to remove a left breast mass. The mass is sent to the pathology department, where a diagnosis of breast cancer is confirmed, 174.9 (C50.912).

However, if the pathology report was unequivocal and was sent for a second opinion, the breast mass would be the primary diagnosis, 611.72 (N63).

P. Routine outpatient prenatal visits

For routine outpatient prenatal visits when no complications are present, codes V22.0, Supervision of normal first pregnancy, or V22.1, Supervision of other normal pregnancy, should be used as the principal diagnosis. These codes should not be used in conjunction with chapter 11 codes.

EXAMPLE   Patient was seen at 22 weeks for prenatal visit. There are no problems noted. Patient has a 3-year-old daughter, V22.1 (Z34.82).

ICD-10-CM
 	
Official Guidelines for Coding and Reporting
	Please refer to the companion Evolve website for the most current guidelines.
	Section IV. Diagnostic Coding and Reporting Guidelines for Outpatient Services
	These coding guidelines for outpatient diagnoses have been approved for use by hospitals/ providers in coding and reporting hospital-based outpatient services and provider-based office visits.
	    Information about the use of certain abbreviations, punctuation, symbols, and other conventions used in the ICD-10-CM Tabular List (code numbers and titles), can be found in Section IA of these guidelines, under "Conventions Used in the Tabular List." Information about the correct sequence to use in finding a code is also described in Section I.
	    The terms encounter and visit are often used interchangeably in describing outpatient service contacts and, therefore, appear together in these guidelines without distinguishing one from the other.
	    Though the conventions and general guidelines apply to all settings, coding guidelines for outpatient and provider reporting of diagnoses will vary in a number of instances from those for inpatient diagnoses, recognizing that:
	    The Uniform Hospital Discharge Data Set (UHDDS) definition of principal diagnosis applies only to inpatients in acute, short-term, long-term care and psychiatric hospitals.
	    Coding guidelines for inconclusive diagnoses (probable, suspected, rule out, etc.) were developed for inpatient reporting and do not apply to outpatients.

A. Selection of first-listed condition

In the outpatient setting, the term first-listed diagnosis is used in lieu of principal diagnosis.

In determining the first-listed diagnosis the coding conventions of ICD-10-CM, as well as the general and disease specific guidelines take precedence over the outpatient guidelines.

Diagnoses often are not established at the time of the initial encounter/visit. It may take two or more visits before the diagnosis is confirmed.

The most critical rule involves beginning the search for the correct code assignment through the Alphabetic Index. Never begin searching initially in the Tabular List as this will lead to coding errors.

1. Outpatient Surgery

When a patient presents for outpatient surgery (same day surgery), code the reason for the surgery as the first-listed diagnosis (reason for the encounter), even if the surgery is not performed due to a contraindication.

2. Observation Stay

When a patient is admitted for observation for a medical condition, assign a code for the medical condition as the first-listed diagnosis.

When a patient presents for outpatient surgery and develops complications requiring admission to observation, code the reason for the surgery as the first reported diagnosis (reason for the encounter), followed by codes for the complications as secondary diagnoses.

B. Codes from A00.0 through T88.9, Z00-Z99

The appropriate code(s) from A00.0 through T88.9, Z00-Z99 must be used to identify diagnoses, symptoms, conditions, problems, complaints, or other reason(s) for the encounter/visit.

C. Accurate reporting of ICD-10-CM diagnosis codes

For accurate reporting of ICD-10-CM diagnosis codes, the documentation should describe the patient's condition, using terminology which includes specific diagnoses as well as symptoms, problems, or reasons for the encounter. There are ICD-10-CM codes to describe all of these.

D. Codes that describe symptoms and signs

Codes that describe symptoms and signs, as opposed to diagnoses, are acceptable for reporting purposes when a diagnosis has not been established (confirmed) by the provider. Chapter 18 of ICD-10-CM, Symptoms, Signs, and Abnormal Clinical and Laboratory Findings Not Elsewhere Classified (codes R00-R99) contain many, but not all codes for symptoms.

E. Encounters for circumstances other than a disease or injury

ICD-10-CM provides codes to deal with encounters for circumstances other than a disease or injury. The Factors Influencing Health Status and Contact with Health Services codes (Z00-99) **are** provided to deal with occasions when circumstances other than a disease or injury are recorded as diagnosis or problems.

See Section I.C.21. Factors influencing health status and contact with health services.

F. Level of Detail in Coding

1. ICD-10-CM codes with 3, 4, 5, *6 or 7 characters*

ICD-10-CM is composed of codes with 3, 4, 5, 6 or 7 **characters**. Codes with three **characters** are included in ICD-10-CM as the heading of a category of codes that may be further subdivided by the use of **fourth,** fifth, sixth or seventh **characters to** provide greater specificity.

2. Use of full number of *characters* required for a code

A three-**characters** code is to be used only if it is not further subdivided. A code is invalid if it has not been coded to the full number of characters required for that code, including the 7th character extension, if applicable.

G. **ICD-10-CM code for the diagnosis, condition, problem, or other reason for encounter/visit**

List first the ICD-10-CM code for the diagnosis, condition, problem, or other reason for encounter/visit shown in the medical record to be chiefly responsible for the services provided. List additional codes that describe any coexisting conditions. In some cases the first-listed diagnosis may be a symptom when a diagnosis has not been established (confirmed) by the physician.

H. **Uncertain diagnosis**

Do not code diagnoses documented as "probable", "suspected," "questionable," "rule out," or "working diagnosis" or other similar terms indicating uncertainty. Rather, code the condition(s) to the highest degree of certainty for that encounter/visit, such as symptoms, signs, abnormal test results, or other reason for the visit.

Please note: This differs from the coding practices used by short-term, acute care, long-term care and psychiatric hospitals.

I. **Chronic diseases**

Chronic diseases treated on an ongoing basis may be coded and reported as many times as the patient receives treatment and care for the condition(s)

J. **Code all documented conditions that coexist**

Code all documented conditions that coexist at the time of the encounter/visit, and require or affect patient care treatment or management. Do not code conditions that were previously treated and no longer exist. However, history codes (categories Z80-Z87) may be used as secondary codes if the historical condition or family history has an impact on current care or influences treatment.

K. **Patients receiving diagnostic services only**

For patients receiving diagnostic services only during an encounter/visit, sequence first the diagnosis, condition, problem, or other reason for encounter/visit shown in the medical record to be chiefly responsible for the outpatient services provided during the encounter/visit. Codes for other diagnoses (e.g., chronic conditions) may be sequenced as additional diagnoses.

For encounters for routine laboratory/radiology testing in the absence of any signs, symptoms, or associated diagnosis, assign Z01.89, Encounter for other specified special examinations. If routine testing is performed during the same encounter as a test to evaluate a sign, symptom, or diagnosis, it is appropriate to assign both the V code and the code describing the reason for the non-routine test.

For outpatient encounters for diagnostic tests that have been interpreted by a physician, and the final report is available at the time of coding, code any confirmed or definitive diagnosis(es) documented in the interpretation. Do not code related signs and symptoms as additional diagnoses.

Please note: This differs from the coding practice in the hospital inpatient setting regarding abnormal findings on test results.

L. **Patients receiving therapeutic services only**

For patients receiving therapeutic services only during an encounter/visit, sequence first the diagnosis, condition, problem, or other reason for encounter/visit shown in the medical record to be chiefly responsible for the outpatient services provided during the encounter/visit. Codes for other diagnoses (e.g., chronic conditions) may be sequenced as additional diagnoses.

The only exception to this rule is that when the primary reason for the admission/encounter is chemotherapy or radiation therapy, the appropriate Z code for the service is listed first, and the diagnosis or problem for which the service is being performed listed second.

M. **Patients receiving preoperative evaluations only**

For patients receiving preoperative evaluations only, sequence first a code from subcategory Z01.81, Encounter for pre-procedural examinations, to describe the pre-op consultations. Assign a code for the condition to describe the reason for the surgery as an additional diagnosis. Code also any findings related to the pre-op evaluation.

N. Ambulatory surgery
For ambulatory surgery, code the diagnosis for which the surgery was performed. If the postoperative diagnosis is known to be different from the preoperative diagnosis at the time the diagnosis is confirmed, select the postoperative diagnosis for coding, since it is the most definitive.

O. Routine outpatient prenatal visits
See Section I.C.15. Routine outpatient prenatal visits.

P. Encounters for general medical examinations with abnormal findings
The subcategories for encounters for general medical examinations, Z00.0-, provide codes for with and without abnormal findings. Should a general medical examination result in an abnormal finding, the code for general medical examination with abnormal finding should be assigned as the first listed diagnosis. A secondary code for the abnormal finding should also be coded.

Q. Encounters for routine health screenings
See Section I.C.21. Factors influencing health status and contact with health services, Screening

Apply the General Coding Guidelines as found in Chapter 5.

GUIDELINE DIFFERENCES BETWEEN ICD-9-CM AND ICD-10-CM

The guidelines for coding outpatient conditions in ICD-9-CM and ICD-10-CM are nearly identical. The only differences appear in ICD-10-CM where guidelines have been added for encounters for general medical exams with abnormal findings. There is now a code in ICD-10-CM for general medical exams with and without abnormal findings. There is also a cross reference in the guidelines directing the user to go to the Section on Factors influencing health status and contact with health services, Screening, to code encounters for routine health screenings.

PROCEDURE CODING IN THE OUTPATIENT SETTING

When procedures are reported for inpatient coding, ICD-9-CM Volume 3 is used. In ICD-10, procedures are coded from ICD-10-PCS for inpatient coding. In the outpatient setting, procedure codes are assigned from the **Current Procedural Terminology (CPT)** published by the American Medical Association (AMA). Per *Coding Clinic* (2008:1Q:p15),[4] ICD-9-CM procedure codes are not to be reported for claim submission on outpatient encounters. According to the Health Insurance Portability and Accountability Act (HIPAA), "The use of ICD-9-CM procedure codes is restricted to the reporting of inpatient procedures by the hospital." Hospitals may still elect to code outpatient visits with ICD-9-CM procedure codes for non–claim-related purposes. CPT is a coding system for reporting medical services and procedures performed by healthcare providers. Physicians report office visits using CPT codes (Figure 27-1) to describe the service provided, along with diagnostic codes from ICD-9-CM to describe why the service was performed.

CPT is Level I of the Healthcare Common Procedure Coding System (HCPCS). CPT is published yearly by the AMA. Revisions are effective for dates of service after January 1 of each year. CPT codes are five-digit numeric codes.

Level II of HCPCS consists of alphanumeric codes (Figure 27-2). These codes, which are used to identify drugs, medical supplies, and durable medical equipment, are maintained by the HCPCS National Panel, which is composed of Blue Cross/Blue Shield, the Health Insurance Association of America, and Centers for Medicare and Medicaid Services (CMS).

Mastectomy Procedures

19300   Mastectomy for gynecomastia

19301   Mastectomy, partial (eg, lumpectomy, tylectomy, quadrantectomy, segmentectomy);

19302   with axillary lymphadenectomy

(For placement of radiotherapy afterloading balloon/brachytherapy catheters, see 19296-19298)

19303   Mastectomy, simple, complete

FIGURE 27-1. Example of CPT codes (Level I HCPCS).

Chemotherapy Drugs *J9000-J9999*

J9000   **Doxorubicin HCl, 10 mg**
Use this code for Adriamycin PFS, Adriamycin RDF, Rubex.
MED: 100-2, 15, 50

J9001   **Doxorubicin HCl, all lipid formulations, 10 mg**
Use this code for Doxil.
MED: 100-2, 15, 50

J9010   **Alemtuzumab, 10 mg**
Use this code for Campath.

J9015   **Aldesleukin, per single use vial**
Use this code for Proleukin, IL-2, Interleukin.
MED: 100-2, 15, 50

FIGURE 27-2. Example of HCPCS Level II codes.

EXAMPLE   Patient with acute appendicitis had laparoscopic appendectomy, 540.9 (K35.80), 44970 (CPT code).

EXAMPLE   Patient with right carpal tunnel syndrome had an endoscopic carpal tunnel release, 354.0 (G56.01) 29848-RT (CPT code).

APCs AS REIMBURSEMENT

Ambulatory Payment Classifications (APCs) became effective on August 1, 2000. APCs constitute a reimbursement system that is similar to Medicare Severity diagnosis-related groups (MS-DRGs), which are used in the inpatient setting. APCs categorize outpatient procedures into similar groups for payment purposes (Figure 27-3). This is Medicare's Outpatient Prospective Payment System (OPPS). Assignment to an APC is based primarily on CPT codes. One of the big differences between MS-DRGs and APCs is that more than one APC may be assigned per claim.

APC	Group Title	SI	Relative Weight	Payment Rate	National Unadjusted Copayment	Minimum Unadjusted Copayment	* Indicates a Change
	Addendum A.-OPPS APCs for CY 2010						
0001	Level I Photochemotherapy	S	0.5302	$35.74	.	$7.15	
0002	Fine Needle Biopsy/Aspiration	T	1.5111	$101.86	.	$20.38	
0003	Bone Marrow Biopsy/Aspiration	T	3.0998	$208.95	.	$41.79	
0004	Level I Needle Biopsy/Aspiration Except Bone Marrow	T	4.5991	$310.01	.	$62.01	
0005	Level II Needle Biopsy/Aspiration Except Bone Marrow	T	7.8145	$526.74	.	$105.35	
0006	Level I Incision & Drainage	T	1.4557	$98.12	.	$19.63	
0007	Level II Incision & Drainage	T	12.6217	$850.78	.	$170.16	
0008	Level III Incision & Drainage	T	19.4063	$1,308.10	.	$261.62	
0012	Level I Debridement & Destruction	T	0.4436	$29.90	.	$5.98	
0013	Level II Debridement & Destruction	T	0.8789	$59.24	.	$11.85	
0015	Level III Debridement & Destruction	T	1.5412	$103.89	.	$20.78	
0016	Level IV Debridement & Destruction	T	2.7982	$188.62	.	$37.73	
0017	Level VI Debridement & Destruction	T	21.2653	$1,433.41	.	$286.69	
0019	Level I Excision/Biopsy	T	4.3625	$294.06	$64.51	$58.82	
0020	Level II Excision/Biopsy	T	8.2028	$552.92			
0021	Level III Excision/Biopsy	T	17.4975	$1,179.44			
0022	Level IV Excision/Biopsy	T	23.3880	$1,576.49			

FIGURE 27-3. Example of APCs.

CHAPTER REVIEW EXERCISE

Answer questions or assign ICD-9-CM codes for all diagnoses and procedures.

1. Outpatient visits are only visits to physicians' offices.
   A. True
   B. False

2. The same coding guidelines apply to inpatient and outpatient settings.
   A. True
   B. False

3. What is another name for "in and out" surgery?
   _____

4. What is the term in the outpatient setting for principal diagnosis?
   _____

5. Is an encounter the same as a visit?
   _____

6. A coder should always begin the search for the correct code in the Tabular List.
   A. True
   B. False

7. Patient presents to office with burning on urination. Physician performs a urinalysis, which is sent out to the laboratory. Physician prescribes antibiotics for presumed urinary tract infection (UTI).   _____

8. Patient presents to ER stating that she has been raped. A rape kit is used to determine whether the rape actually occurred. Results were negative.   _____

9. Patient presents to the gynecologist's office for a routine Pap and pelvic examination.   _____

10. Postmenopausal patient is sent for dual-energy x-ray absorptiometry (DEXA) scan to evaluate status of bone loss. _____

11. Diabetic patient is sent to nutritionist for dietary counseling. _____

12. Child presents to physician's office for routine vaccination. The physician decides not to administer because the child has a cold. _____

13. Patient and husband present to clinical social worker for marriage counseling. _____

14. Patient had a malignant neoplasm of the lung removed. She presents to the surgeon for routine aftercare. _____

15. Patient presents to physician's office for reprogramming of an automatic implantable cardioverter-defibrillator (AICD). _____

16. Patient presents to physician's office complaining of dizziness. _____

17. Patient presents to physician's office complaining of testicular pain. Physician prescribes antibiotics and says the symptoms are compatible with epididymitis. _____

18. Patient presents to physician's office as a possible bone marrow donor for her sister. _____

19. Patient presents to physician's office with severe headache. Physician sends patient for magnetic resonance imaging (MRI) and notes to rule out cerebrovascular accident (CVA) in a patient with a history of hypertension and coronary artery disease. _____

20. Patient is seen in doctor's office for abdominal pain. After examination, the physician states that this is probably due to diverticulitis in that the patient has known diverticulum. He also notes that this patient has a history of alcohol abuse and is currently drinking on a daily basis. _____

21. Patient presents to doctor's office with fever, cough, and muscle aches and pains. Physician is uncertain as to whether these symptoms are an exacerbation of her COPD or whether she has viral pneumonia. Laboratory work is ordered. _____

CHAPTER GLOSSARY

Ambulatory Payment Classifications (APCs): used for outpatient prospective payment.

Ancillary services: services provided by a hospital that are additional to a professional service, such as laboratory work and radiology and pathology services.

Current Procedural Terminology (CPT): a coding system for reporting medical services and procedures.

Encounters: face-to-face visits with a healthcare provider.

Level II of HCPCS: codes used to identify drugs, medical supplies, and durable medical equipment.

Observation unit: area outside the emergency department where unstable patients are admitted for a stay of less than 48 hours. The patient is observed for admission to the hospital or discharge to home.

Professional service: service rendered by a physician or a nonphysician practitioner.

REFERENCES

1. American Hospital Association. *Coding Clinic for ICD-9-CM* 1984:M-J:p10. Follow-up for malignancy—Sequencing.
2. American Hospital Association. *Coding Clinic for ICD-9-CM* 2005:3Q:p21-22. Consistent with and compatible with.
3. American Hospital Association. *Coding Clinic for ICD-9-CM* 2000:1Q:p4. Radiologist diagnosis.
4. American Hospital Association. *Coding Clinic for ICD-9-CM* 2008:1Q:p15. Reporting ICD-9-CM procedure codes for outpatient procedures.

Glossary

Ablation Correction of abnormal heart rhythm by burning of abnormal heart tissue through radiofrequency or other methods such as laser, microwave, or freezing.

Abortion Termination of a pregnancy by natural causes or by medical intervention.

Abscess A localized collection of pus that causes swelling.

Abstracting Extracting data from the health record.

Acromegaly Condition that results when hypersecretion of human growth hormone (hGH) occurs after puberty, along with overgrowth of the face, hands, feet, and soft tissues.

Acute A short and relatively severe course.

Acute renal failure Sudden and severe impairment of renal function characterized by oliguria, increased serum urea, and acidosis.

Addison's disease Adrenocortical insufficiency that may be caused by neoplasms, surgical removal of the adrenal gland, autoimmune processes, tuberculosis, hemorrhage, and/or infection.

Adenocarcinomas Malignancies of epithelial glandular tissue such as those found in the breast, prostate, and colon.

Adhesion Scar tissue that forms an abnormal connection between body parts.

Adjunct codes Add-on codes to a primary procedure to provide additional information about the primary procedure that was performed.

Admission diagnosis Diagnosis that brings the patient to the hospital. This will often be a symptom.

Admitting diagnosis The condition that requires the patient to be hospitalized.

Adverse effect Pathologic manifestation due to ingestion or exposure to drugs or other chemical substances.

Affective disorders A category of mental health problems that includes major depressive disorders and bipolar disorders.

AIDS Acquired immunodeficiency syndrome, an incurable disease of the immune system caused by a virus.

Air embolism When air or gas bubbles get into the bloodstream and obstruct the circulation.

Alimentary canal Comprises the mouth, pharynx, esophagus, stomach, small intestine, and large intestine.

Allograft Graft of tissue between individuals of the same species.

Alphabetic Index The index found in the ICD-9-CM book for both disease conditions and procedures.

Alteration Modifying the natural anatomic structure of a body part without affecting the function of the body part (e.g., breast augmentation).

Alzheimer's disease Disorder of the brain that causes a progressive decline in mental and physical function.

Ambulatory Payment Classifications (APCs) Used for outpatient prospective payment.

Amnioinfusion The insertion of normal saline or lactated Ringer's solution into the amniotic sac.

Ancillary services Services provided by a hospital that are additional to a professional service, such as laboratory work and radiology and pathology services.

Anemia Occurs when hemoglobin drops, which interrupts the transport of oxygen throughout the body.

Aneurysm Bulging or ballooning out of a vessel.

Angiodysplasia Type of AVM characterized by dilated or fragile blood vessels.

Angioplasty A procedure performed to treat coronary artery disease. An inflated balloon compresses plaque against artery walls.

Anomaly A deviation from normal standards (e.g., as in congenital defects).

Anorexia Loss of appetite.

Antepartum Time from conception until delivery or childbirth with regard to the mother.

Anterior Front of the body or an organ.

Anthrax A bacterial infection usually found in wild or domestic animals.

Anticoagulant medications Medications that are used to prevent venous thrombi.

Antiplatelet medications Medications that are used to prevent clumping of platelets or formation of an arterial thrombus.

Apgar Test used to measure the condition of a newborn at birth.

Aphasia Impairment of speech expression and/or word understanding.

Apheresis Procedure that separates different components of blood and removes a certain part of the blood, such as occurs in leukapheresis, plateletpheresis, and plasmapheresis.

Aplastic anemia Reduction in new blood cells due to impairment or failure of bone marrow function.

Appendectomy Removal of the appendix.

Appendicitis Inflammation of the appendix.

Arteriovenous malformation Defect that arises during fetal development.

Arthropathy Disease that affects the joints.

Arthroscopic Minimally invasive surgery that involves the use of highly specialized instruments to perform surgery through very small incisions on joints.

Arthroscopic approach An arthroscope is used to examine and perform closed procedures within a joint.

Asbestosis Lung disease due to inhalation of asbestos.

Aspiration pneumonia Inflammation of the lungs and bronchial tubes due to aspiration of foreign material into the lung.

Assistance Taking over a portion of a physiological function by extracorporeal means.

Asthma Chronic disease that affects the airways that carry air into and out of the lungs.

Asthmatic bronchitis Underlying asthmatic problem in patients in whom asthma has become so persistent that clinically significant chronic airflow obstruction is present despite antiasthmatic therapy.

Asymptomatic Without any symptoms.

Atherosclerosis Type of arteriosclerosis wherein fatty substances such as plaque block or clog the arteries.

Atmospheric control Extracorporeal control of atmospheric pressure and composition.

Atrophy When a gland becomes smaller.

Attention deficit disorder A common childhood disorder characterized by inattention and impulsivity.

Attention deficit hyperactivity disorder A common childhood disorder characterized by inattention, hyperactivity, and impulsivity.

Autograft Graft of tissue from another site on the same individual.

Autoimmune disorder Disorder that occurs when the immune system attacks itself inappropriately.

Autologous Originating from the recipient, rather than from a donor; tissue transferred from the same individual's body (e.g., a skin graft taken from one part of the body and transferred to another part of the body on the same individual).

Autologous transfusion Transfusion of a patient's own blood. Blood may have been donated before an elective procedure.

Autonomic nervous system Consists of both sensory and motor functions that involve the central nervous system and internal organs.

Bacteremia Bacteria in blood, which is a laboratory finding.

Bariatrics Branch of medicine that is concerned with the management (prevention or control) of obesity and allied diseases.

Baritosis Lung disease due to inhalation of barium.

Barrett's esophagus Precancerous condition that usually occurs in people with chronic GERD.

Benign Neoplasm or tumor; means that it is not malignant.

Benign prostatic hyperplasia Condition resulting in enlargement of the prostate gland; usually occurs in men older than 50 years of age.

Benign prostatic hypertrophy Condition resulting in enlargement of the prostate gland; usually occurs in men older than 50 years of age.

Bilateral procedure Operative procedure performed on paired anatomic organs or tissues during the same operative session.

Biological response modifier (BRM) Immunotherapy that can destroy cancer cells, stimulate the immune system to destroy cancer cells, or change cancer cells to normal cells.

Biopsy Removal of a representative sample for pathologic examination and diagnosis.

Bipolar disorder Brain disorder that causes unusual shifts in a person's mood, energy, and ability to function. Different from the normal ups and downs that everyone goes through; symptoms of bipolar disorder; can be severe.

Black lung Lung disease due to inhalation of coal dust.

Blalock-Taussig procedure Procedure used to treat patients with tetralogy of Fallot who have insufficient pulmonary arterial flow.

Blood Viscous fluid that circulates through the vessels of the circulatory system as a result of the pumping action of the heart.

Blood pressure The force that blood puts on the arterial walls when the heart beats.

BNP (Brain natriuretic peptide) A hormone that is produced by the heart; a BNP test measures the amount of BNP that is found in the heart.

Body mass index Uses weight and height to estimate body fat.

Bone marrow biopsy Diagnostic procedure that is used to identify types of anemia and cell deficiencies and to detect leukemia.

Bowel resection Removal of a portion of the bowel.

Brachytherapy Placement of radioactive material directly into or near the cancer.

Bradycardia Slow heart rate, generally fewer than 60 beats per minute.

Bronchi The two air tubes that branch off the trachea and deliver air to both lungs.

Bronchitis Lower respiratory tract or bronchial tree infection characterized by cough, sputum production, and wheezing.

Bronchopulmonary dysplasia Chronic lung disease that develops in babies during the first 4 weeks after birth.

Bronchoscopy Diagnostic endoscopic procedure in which a tube with a tiny camera on the end is inserted through the nose or mouth into the lungs.

Bursitis Inflammation of a bursa, which is a tiny, fluid-filled sac that is found between muscles, tendons, and bones that reduces friction and facilitates movement.

Bypass Altering the route of passage of the contents of a tubular body part (CABG).

Calculus A stone. Calculi, which vary in size, can develop anywhere in the urinary tract.

Candidiasis A fungal infection also known as a *yeast infection*.

Capillaries Smallest blood vessel through which material passes to and from the bloodstream.

Carbuncle Cluster of boils.

Carcinoma in situ Malignant cells that remain within the original site with no spread or invasion into neighboring tissue.

Carcinomas Malignant tumors originating from epithelial tissue (e.g., in the skin, bronchi, and stomach).

Cardiac arrest Sudden loss of heart function.

Cardiomyopathy A disorder of the muscles of the heart chambers that impedes heart function.

Carryover line Used when an entry will not fit on a single line.

Case-mix index A measurement used by hospitals to define how sick their patients are.

Cataract Clouding of the lens of the eye causing obstructed vision.

Category A single three-digit code that describes a disease or a similarly related group of conditions.

Caudal Toward the tail.

Cellulitis Inflammation of the tissue with possible abscess.

Cervical dysplasia Abnormal growth of cells on the surface of the cervix.

Cervical intraepithelial neoplasia (CIN) Dysplasia that is seen on a biopsy of the cervix.

Cervix The neck of the uterus that serves as an outlet from the uterus.

Chancre An ulcer that forms during the first stage of syphilis.

Change To take out or off a device from a body part and put back an identical or similar device, in or on the same body part, without cutting or puncturing the skin or a mucous membrane (e.g., change gastrostomy tube).

Charge description number A number that designates a particular service or procedure, used to generate a charge on a patient bill.

Chargemaster or Charge description master (CDM) A listing of the services, procedures, drugs, and supplies that can be applied to a patient's bill.

Chemoembolization Intra-arterial administration of chemotherapy with collagen particles to enhance the delivery of chemotherapy to the targeted area.

Chemotherapy The use of drugs or medications to treat disease.

Chief complaint The reason, in the patient's own words, for presenting to the hospital.

Choledocholithiasis Stone lodged in the bile duct.

Cholelithiasis An abnormal condition of stones in the gallbladder.

Cholesteatoma Growth in the middle ear that usually results from repeated ear infections.

Chronic Persistent over a long period.

Chronic bronchitis Condition defined by a mucus-producing cough most days of the month, 3 months out of a year for 2 successive years with no other underlying disease to explain the cough.

Chronic obstructive pulmonary disease General term used to describe a lung disease in which the airways become obstructed, making it difficult for air to get into and out of the lungs.

Chylothorax Milky fluid consisting of lymph and fat (chyle) that accumulates in the pleural space.

Cirrhosis Liver disease wherein scar tissue replaces healthy tissue and blocks blood flow.

Classification Grouping together of items as for storage and retrieval.

Cleft lip/palate Opening in the lip or palate of an infant that occurs in utero.

Closed fracture Injury in which the bone is broken, but the skin remains intact.

Closed head injuries Injuries that result from a blow to the head.

Closed reduction The surgeon manipulates or reduces fractured bones into anatomic alignment without making an incision through the skin and subcutaneous tissue.

Clostridium difficile Microorganisms that are a leading cause of pseudomembranous colitis; also known as *C. diff*.

Coagulation defect Breakdown in the clotting process of the blood.

Coal workers' pneumoconiosis Lung disease due to inhalation of coal dust.

Cognitive deficit Disorder in thinking, learning, awareness, or judgment.

Cognitive impairment A decline in mental activities associated with thinking, learning, and memory.

Colles' fracture Common fracture in adults in which the lower end of the radius is fractured, and the wrist and the hand are displaced backward.

Colostomy A procedure that uses the colon to create an artificial opening.

Combination code A single code used to classify two diagnoses; or a diagnosis with an associated secondary process (manifestation); or a diagnosis with an associated complication.

Communicable Easily spread from one person to another.

Community-acquired pneumonia Broad term used to define pneumonias that are contracted outside of the hospital or nursing home setting.

Comorbidity A preexisting condition (i.e., it is present on admission) that may lead to increased resource use.

Complete abortion Abortion in which all the products of conception are expelled.

Complete remission There are no signs or symptoms of the cancer.

Compliance Adherence to accepted standards.

Complicated fracture Fracture that causes injury to surrounding tissues.

Complicated wound Laceration with delayed healing, delayed treatment, foreign body and/or infection.

Complication A condition that arises during a patient's hospitalization that may lead to increased resource use.

Compound fracture When the broken bone exits and is visible through the skin, or a deep wound exposes the broken bone through the skin.

Compression Putting pressure on a body region.

Computer assisted surgery (CAS) Adjunctive procedure that allows increased visualization and more precise navigation while remaining minimally invasive.

Concussion Injury to the brain that results from a significant blow to the head.

Conduction disorder Abnormalities of cardiac impulses.

Condyloma Wart-type growth found usually in the genital or anal area.

Congenital anomaly An abnormal condition present at birth.

Connecting words Subterms that denote a relationship between a main term or a subterm and an associated condition or etiology.

Consultant Healthcare provider who is asked to see the patient to provide expert opinion outside the expertise of the requester.

Contaminant A cultured organism that a physician does not believe is responsible for causing a particular infection.

Continuous ambulatory peritoneal dialysis Type of peritoneal dialysis that takes about 15 minutes and is performed 3 to 4 times per day and once at night.

Continuous cycling peritoneal dialysis Type of peritoneal dialysis that uses a cycling machine and is performed while the patient sleeps.

Control Stopping, or attempting to stop, postprocedural bleeding (e.g., control of post-tonsillectomy hemorrhage).

Contusion Any mechanical injury that results in hemorrhage beneath unbroken skin.

Conventions General rules for use in classification that must be followed for accurate coding.

Core biopsy Procedure in which a large needle is used to extract a core sample.

Coronary artery bypass graft Surgery performed to bypass an occluded coronary artery.

Corrosive burn Burn due to a chemical.

Cranial Toward the head.

Creation Making a new structure that does not take the place of a body part (creation of vagina in males for sex reassignment).

Credential Degree, certificate, or award that recognizes a course of study taken in a specific field and that acknowledges the competency required.

Crohn's disease Inflammation of the GI tract, especially the small and large intestine.

Crush injury When a body part is subjected to a high degree of force or pressure, usually after it has been squeezed between two heavy or immobile objects.

Current Procedural Terminology (CPT) A coding system for reporting medical services and procedures.

Cushing's syndrome Condition that results in excessive circulating cortisol levels caused by chronic hypersecretion of the adrenal cortex.

Cystic fibrosis Genetic (inherited) condition that affects the cells that produce mucus, sweat, saliva, and digestive juices. Instead of being thin and slippery, these secretions are thick and sticky, plugging up tubes, ducts, and passageways, especially in the pancreas and lungs.

Cystitis Lower tract infection that affects the bladder.

Cystocele When the bladder descends and presses into the wall of the vagina.

Cystoscopy Approach used for many procedures of the urinary tract.

Cystourethrocele A urethrocele in conjunction with a cystocele.

Debridement Removal of devitalized tissue, necrosis, or slough.

Debulking Procedures performed when it is impossible to remove the tumor entirely.

Decompression Extracorporeal elimination of undissolved gas from body fluids.

Decubitus ulcer Skin ulcer also known as a bed sore.

Deep brain stimulator A device implanted to control tremors.

Deep vein thrombosis A blood clot that forms in a deep vein.

Deficit Reduction Act (DRA) Mandates all acute-care facilities reimbursed under MS-DRGs to identify and report diagnoses that are present at the time of a patient's admission.

Dehiscence Opening of a surgical wound.

Dehydration Occurs when the body does not have enough water or fluids as it should.

Delirium tremens Life-threatening condition that may involve severe mental or neurologic changes, such as delirium and/or hallucinations.

Delivery Assisting the passage of the products of conception from the genital canal.

Dementia Progressive deterioration of mental faculties characterized by impairment of memory and one or more cognitive impairments such as language, reasoning and judgment, or calculation and problem-solving abilities.

Department number Ancillary departments such as, radiology, laboratory, and Emergency Room will have a specific hospital departmental number.

Depression Affective disorder that is characterized by sadness, lack of interest in everyday activities and events, and a sense of worthlessness.

Dermabond Liquid skin adhesive used to close skin lacerations.

Dermatitis Inflammation of the skin.

Dermis Layer of skin below the epidermis.

Destruction Physical eradication of all or a portion of a body part by the direct use of energy, force, or a destructive agent (e.g., ablation of endometriosis).

Detachment Cutting off all or a portion of the upper or lower extremities (e.g., above-knee amputation).

Detoxification Active management of withdrawal symptoms in a patient who is physically dependent on alcohol or drugs.

Diabetes insipidus Deficiency in the release of vasopressin by the posterior pituitary gland.

Diabetes mellitus Chronic syndrome of impaired carbohydrate, protein, and fat metabolism caused by insufficient production of insulin by the pancreas or faulty utilization of insulin by the cells.

Diagnosis Identification of a disease through signs, symptoms, and tests.

Dialysis disequilibrium syndrome Characterized by weakness, dizziness, headache, and, in severe cases, mental status changes.

Diaphragm Dome-shaped muscles at the bottom of the lungs that assist in the process of breathing and in the exchange of oxygen/carbon dioxide.

Differential diagnosis When a symptom may represent a variety of diagnoses.

Dilation Expanding an orifice or the lumen of a tubular body part (e.g., PTCA).

Discharge summary A review of the patient's hospital course. This summary details the reason for admission or tests or procedures performed and how the patient responded.

Dislocation Displacement of the bones that form a joint; separation of the end of a bone from the joint it meets.

Dissection A tear in wall of a vessel.

Disseminated intravascular coagulation Disorder that results in depletion of clotting factors in the blood.

Distal Farther from the median plane; term is often used to describe a location in the limbs.

Diverticula Small pouches in the lining of the mucous membranes of an organ.

Division Cutting into a body part, without draining fluids and/or gases from it in order to separate or transect the part (e.g., osteotomy).

Dorsal Back of the body or an organ.

Dorsopathies Conditions or diseases that affect the back or spine.

Drainage Taking or letting out fluids and/or gases from a body part (e.g., paracentesis).

Dressing Putting material on a body region for protection.

Dumping syndrome When undigested contents of the stomach are transported to the small intestine too quickly.

Dyscalculia Learning disability that affects a child's ability to do mathematical calculations.

Dysgraphia Learning disability that affects a child's ability to coordinate movements such as writing.

Dyslexia Learning disability that affects a child's ability to understand or use spoken or written language.

Dysmetabolic Syndrome X Characterized by abdominal obesity, insulin resistance, dyslipidemia, and elevated blood pressure or hypertension.

Ectopic Type of pregnancy that occurs when the egg is implanted outside the cavity of the uterus.

Eczema Type of dermatitis characterized by itching.

Edentulism The complete loss of teeth.

Effaced Cervical thinning.

Elderly obstetric patient 35 years or older at date of delivery.

Elective abortion Elective termination of pregnancy.

Electroconvulsive therapy Psychiatric treatment in which electricity is used to induce seizures.

Electromagnetic therapy Extracorporeal treatment by electromagnetic rays.

Electromyelogram A test that measures electrical activity in muscles and nerves.

Electrophysiologist Physician trained in electrical disorders of the heart.

Embolus Clot that travels to another part of the body.

Emphysema Chronic lung disease of gradual onset that can be attributed to chronic infection and inflammation or irritation from cigarette smoke.

Empiric Initiation of treatment prior to making a definite diagnosis.

Empyema Pus that accumulates in the pleural space.

Encoder Coding software that is used to assign diagnosis and procedure codes.

Encounters Face-to-face visits with a healthcare provider.

Endocarditis Inflammation of the lining of the heart chambers and valves.

Endocrine system Body system composed of many glands that secrete hormones that regulate bodily functions; it works with the nervous system to maintain body activities and homeostasis and to respond to stress.

Endogenous Type of dermatitis caused by something taken internally, such as medication.

Endometriosis A chronic condition in which endometrial material, the tissue that lines the inside of the uterus, grows outside the uterus and attaches to other organs in the pelvic cavity.

Endometritis Inflammation of the uterus.

Endoscopic Examinations and procedures performed with an instrument that examines any cavity of the body with a rigid or a flexible scope.

Endoscopic biopsy Biopsy that is performed during endoscopic examination.

Epidermis Outermost layer of skin.

Epilepsy Disorder of the brain that is characterized by abnormal electrical discharges from the brain cells.

Eponym Term for a disease, structure, procedure, or syndrome that has been named for a person.

Erythema Redness of the skin.

Erythrocytes Another name for red blood cells that are made in the marrow of bones; their main responsibility is to carry oxygen around the body and remove carbon dioxide. These are the cells that give blood its red color.

Ethics Moral standard.

Etiology Cause or origin of a disease or condition.

Euvolemia State of normal body fluid volume.

Excision Cutting out or off, without replacement, a a portion of a body part (e.g., partial nephrectomy).

Excisional Removal by surgical cutting.

Excisional biopsy Total removal of local small masses or growths.

Excisional debridement Surgical removal or cutting away of devitalized tissue, necrosis, or slough.

Exhibitionism Recurrent intense sexual urges and fantasies of exposing the genitals to an unsuspecting stranger.

Exogenous Type of dermatitis caused by contact with a substance.

Exophthalmos Bulging of the eyes.

External Procedures performed directly on the skin or mucous membrane, and procedures performed indirectly by the application of external force through the skin or mucous membrane (e.g., tonsillectomy).

External skeletal fixation Form of fracture treatment that involves insertion of percutaneous pins proximal and distal to the fracture and application of a frame that connects the pins externally.

Extirpation Taking or cutting out solid matter from a body part (e.g., thrombectomy).

Extracorporeal shock wave lithotripsy Used to break up kidney stones into small particles that can then pass through the urinary tract into the urine.

Extraction Pulling or stripping out or off all or a portion of a body part by force (e.g., bone marrow biopsy).

Facet joints Small, stabilizing joints located between and behind adjacent vertebrae.

Fallopian tube Delivers the mature egg to the uterus for fertilization.

Fascia Tissue just below the skin that covers and separates the underlying layers of muscle.

Fat embolism When fat enters the circulatory system after long bone or pelvic fracture.

Federal Register The official daily publication for rules, proposed rules, and notices of U.S. federal agencies and organizations.

Fetishism Recurrent intense sexual urges and fantasies of using inanimate objects for sexual arousal or orgasm. Objects commonly used include female clothing such as shoes, earrings, or undergarments.

Fibromas Neoplasms of fibrous connective tissue.

Fibromyalgia One of the most common diseases affecting the muscles; it is characterized by widespread muscle pain associated with chronic fatigue.

Fine needle aspiration Procedure in which a very small needle is used; works best for masses that are superficial or easily accessible.

Fistula Abnormal passage or communication between two internal organs, or leading from an organ to the surface of the body. It can also be an abnormal passage between an artery and a vein.

Fluid overload Occurs when there is too much fluid in the body.

Foregut Bronchi and stomach (sites of carcinoid neoplasm).

Fracture Break in a bone.

Fragmentation Breaking solid matter in a body part into pieces (e.g., extracorporeal shock wave lithotripsy).

Free flap Involves the cutting of skin, fat, blood vessels, and muscle free from its location and moving it to the chest area.

Fundoplication Surgery in which the fundus of the stomach is wrapped around the esophagus.

Furuncle A boil.

Fusion Joining together portions of an articular body part, rendering the articular body part immobile (e.g., spinal fusion).

Gastroenteritis Inflammation of the stomach and intestines.

Generalized anxiety disorder Chronic, exaggerated worry, tension, and irritability that may be without cause or may be more intense than the situation warrants.

Genetic Inherited.

Genital prolapse When pelvic organs such as the uterus, bladder, and rectum shift from their normal anatomic positions and protrude into the vagina or press against the wall of the vagina.

Gigantism Condition that occurs when hypersecretion of hGH occurs before puberty, along with proportionate overgrowth of all bodily tissues, especially the long bones.

Glaucoma Disorder of the optic nerve that may result in vision loss.

Glomerulonephritis Inflammation of the glomeruli of the kidneys.

Goiter Enlargement of the thyroid gland.

Gonorrhea Disease caused by a bacterium and transmitted by sexual contact.

Grading Pathologic examination of tumor cells. Degree of cell abnormality determines the grade of cancer.

Graft-versus-host disease (GVHD) Common complication that can occur after a stem cell or bone marrow transplant in which the newly transplanted material attacks the transplant recipient's body.

Graves' disease The most common form of hyperthyroidism; it occurs through an autoimmune response that attacks the thyroid gland, resulting in overproduction of the thyroid hormone thyroxine.

Gravid Pregnant.

Grouper Specialized software used to assign the appropriate MS-DRG.

Gustilo open fracture classification Based on the mechanism of the injury and the amount of soft tissue and skeletal injury and is useful in assessing risk of infection and possible amputation.

HAART Highly active antiretroviral therapy, a group of drugs given to AIDS patients for prophylaxis.

Habitual aborter A woman who miscarries at least three consecutive times.

Hashimoto's disease Inflammation of the thyroid gland that often results in hypothyroidism.

Health Maintenance Organizations (HMOs) Type of managed care in which hospitals, physicians, and other providers contract to provide health care for patients, usually at a discounted rate.

Healthcare provider Person who provides care to a patient.

Heart failure Impaired function of the heart's pumping ability.

Hematemesis Vomiting of blood.

Hematochezia Bright red blood in stool.

Hematopoiesis Development of blood cells that occurs in the bone marrow and lymphatic tissue of normal adults.

Hematuria The presence of blood in the urine.

Hemiplegia Paralysis of half of the body.

Hemodialysis Process that uses a machine called a hemodialyzer to remove wastes from the blood.

Hemolysis The breaking down of red blood cells.

Hemolytic anemias Result from abnormal or excessive destruction of red blood cells.

Hemophilia A Most common type of hemophilia; deficiency or abnormality in clotting factor VIII.

Hemophilia B Another name for Christmas disease, which results from a deficiency of factor IX.

Hemophilia C Mild form of hemophilia with decreased factor XI.

Hemothorax Blood that accumulates in the pleural space.

Hepatitis An inflammation of the liver.

Hernia Protrusion of an organ or tissue through an abnormal opening in the body.

Herniorrhaphy Repair of a hernia.

Herpes simplex A virus also known as a *cold sore* or *fever blister*.

Herpes zoster A disease caused by the same virus that causes chickenpox.

Heterograft Graft of skin from another species, such as a graft from a pig to a human.

Hindgut Colon and rectum (sites of carcinoid neoplasms).

Histologic type Type of tissue or cell in which the neoplasm occurs.

HIV Human immunodeficiency virus, the virus that affects the immune system and can progress to AIDS.

Hives Skin condition also known as urticaria, wherein the skin reacts with welts; characterized by itching.

Homeostasis The ability of an organism or cell to maintain internal equilibrium by adjusting its physiologic processes.

Homograft Graft from one individual to another of the same species; also known as an allograft.

Hormones Substances secreted by glands that can regulate bodily functions, such as urinary output, cellular metabolic rate, and growth and development.

Hybrid A combination of formats producing similar results (i.e., paper and electronic records).

Hydrocephalus Cerebrospinal fluid collection in the skull.

Hydronephrosis Abnormal dilatation of the renal pelvis caused by pressure from urine that cannot flow past an obstruction in the urinary tract.

Hydroureter Accumulation of urine in the ureters.

Hyperbaric oxygen therapy (HBOT) Treatment in which the patient's entire body is placed in a transparent, airtight chamber at increased atmospheric pressure.

Hyperemesis gravidarum Excessive vomiting in pregnancy.

Hyperglycemia Condition that results when glucose or blood sugar becomes abnormally high. This is a relatively common event in patients with diabetes.

Hyperparathyroidism Condition that results when an overactive parathyroid gland secretes excessive parathyroid hormone, causing increased levels of circulating calcium associated with loss of calcium in the bone.

Hyperpituitarism Increased production of the pituitary hormones, particularly the human growth hormone (hGH).

Hyperplasia Enlargement of a gland.

Hypersomnia Excessive sleep.

Hyperthermia Extracorporeal raising of body temperature.

Hyperthyroidism Abnormality of the thyroid gland in which secretion of thyroid hormone is usually increased and is no longer under the regulatory control of hypothalamic-pituitary centers.

Hypertrophy Enlargement of a gland.

Hypervitaminosis Toxicity resulting from an excess of any vitamin, especially fat-soluble vitamins such as A, D, and K.

Hypervolemia Occurs when there is too much fluid in the body.

Hypoglycemia Condition that results when glucose or blood sugar becomes abnormally low.

Hypomania Milder form of mania, but this "feel good" mood can change to depression or mania.

Hypoparathyroidism Underactive parathyroid gland that results in decreased levels of circulating calcium.

Hypopituitarism Condition caused by low levels of pituitary hormones. Hormones secreted by the pituitary gland can affect the functions of other glands.

Hypoplasia Atrophy; condition that results when a gland becomes smaller.

Hypothermia Extracorporeal lowering of body temperature.

Hypothyroidism Condition caused by low levels of pituitary hormones. Hormones secreted by the pituitary gland can affect the functions of other glands.

Hypovolemia Occurs due to decreased plasma volume.

Hypoxia Insufficient oxygen in the blood.

Iatrogenic Caused by medical treatment.

ICD-10-CM *International Classification of Diseases, 10th Revision, Clinical Modification.*

ICD-10-PCS *International Classification of Diseases, 10th Revision, Procedure Coding System.*

Idiopathic Causative factor is unknown.

Ileostomy End of small intestine brought out through the abdominal wall.

Ileus Absence of normal movement within the intestine.

Immobilization Limiting or preventing motion of a body region.

Immune system The body's major defense mechanism that responds to invasion of the body by foreign substances.

Immunotherapy Administration of agents that stimulate the immune system's response against tumors.

Impaction Condition that occurs when stool in the rectum becomes so hard that it cannot be passed normally.

Incidental appendectomy Appendectomy performed at the time of another procedure with no known disease process in the appendix.

Incisional biopsy Procedure in which a representative sample of a tumor mass is removed to permit pathologic examination.

Incompetent cervix Cervix begins to open before baby is ready to be born.

Incomplete abortion Abortion in which not all of the products of conception are expelled.

Inevitable abortion Abortion that occurs when symptoms are present and a miscarriage will happen.

Infection Invasion of the body with organisms that have the potential to cause disease.

Inferior Position of the body or an organ relative to the vertical axis of the body.

Influenza Contagious viral infection of the respiratory tract that causes coughing, difficulty breathing, headache, muscle aches, and weakness.

Insertion Putting in a nonbiological appliance that monitors, assists, performs, or prevents a physiological function but does not physically take the place of a body part (e.g., insertion of pacemaker lead).

Insomnia Difficulty falling asleep, wakefulness, and early morning awakening.

Inspection Visually and/or manually exploring a body part (e.g., diagnostic arthroscopy).

Integral Essential part of a disease process.

Integumentary Another name for skin.

Intertrigo Dermatitis in areas where friction may occur.

Intractable Not manageable.

Introduction Putting in or on a therapeutic, diagnostic, nutritional, physiological, or prophylactic substance except blood or blood products.

Intussusception Bowel becomes obstructed when a portion of the intestine telescopes into another portion.

Irrigation Putting in or on a cleansing substance.

Joints Means of joining two bones together.

Juvenile rheumatoid arthritis Type of arthritis that affects children, usually between the ages of 2 and 5 years.

Klinefelter's syndrome A sex chromosome disorder that occurs in males and is caused by an extra X chromosome.

Kyphoplasty Procedure performed to treat and stabilize fractures of the spine.

Kyphosis Excessive posterior curvature of the thoracic spine that may not be detected until a hump in the upper back is noticeable.

Labia Surrounds the vaginal opening.

Labor Process by which the products of conception are expelled from the uterus.

Laceration An injury that results in a tear in the skin.

Lactation Process of milk production from mammary glands.

Laparoscopic approach Uses a laparoscope to examine and perform closed procedures within the abdomen.

Late effect code Used when the acute phase of an illness or injury has passed, but a residual condition or health problem remains.

Lateral Position of a structure that is to the side of the body.

Legal blindness Severe or profound impairment in both eyes.

Leiomyoma Tumor or growth within the walls of the uterus. Also called *uterine fibroid.*

Leukemia Cancer of the white blood cells that begins in the blood-forming cells of the bone marrow.

Leukocytes White blood cells increase in number to battle infection, inflammation, and other diseases.

Leukocytosis Increase in the number of white cells in the blood; it may be a sign of infection or may indicate stress on the body.

Level II HCPCS Codes used to identify drugs, medical supplies, and durable medical equipment.

Ligaments Dense, fibrous bands of connective tissue that provide stability for the joint.

Limited coverage Procedures that are identified by the Medicare Code Editor as procedures covered under limited circumstances.

Lipoma Growth of fat cells within a capsule that usually is found just below the skin.

Lobar pneumonia Synonym for pneumococcal pneumonia or pneumonia due to *Streptococcus pneumoniae* pneumonia.

Local coverage determinations (LCDs) Local policy that may include certain time frames for testing, certain age requirements, and that a particular diagnosis or condition must be present for a procedure or treatment to be considered medically necessary.

Lordosis Exaggerated inward curvature of the spine that may be caused by increased abdominal girth due to obesity, pregnancy, or abdominal tumor.

Loss of consciousness When a patient is unable to respond to people or other stimuli.

Lyme disease An inflammatory disease caused by bacteria carried by ticks.

Lymphadenitis Inflammation of a lymph node that usually is caused by a bacterial infection.

Lymphoma Cancer of the lymphatic system.

Lysis Destruction of adhesions.

Macular degeneration Vision loss in the central portion of the eye, leaving the patient with peripheral vision or low vision.

Main term Term that identifies disease conditions or injuries, it is identified in bold print and set flush with the left margin of each column in the Alphabetic Index.

Major depressive disorder Characterized by one or more major depressive episodes with a history of mania, hypomania, or mixed episodes.

Malignancy Neoplasm that has the ability to invade adjacent structures and spread to distant sites.

Malignant ascites Excess fluid which contains malignant cells accumulates in the abdomen or peritoneum.

Malignant hypertension Rapidly rising blood pressure, usually in excess of 140 mm Hg diastolic with findings of visual impairment and symptoms or signs of progressive cardiac failure.

Malignant pleural effusion Fluid accumulates in the pleural space and contains malignant cells.

Mallory-Weiss Bleeding laceration of the esophagogastric junction.

Malnutrition Nutrition disorder caused by primary deprivation of protein energy caused by poverty or self-imposed starvation, or associated with deficiency diseases such as cancer.

Malunion When the fracture fragments have united but are not properly aligned. Incorrectly positioned bones may demonstrate angulation, rotation, and shortening.

Mammographic localization Procedure that may be necessary to assist the surgeon in identifying the area of breast tissue that must be biopsied or excised.

Mania The other side of depression, in which a person feels so good it is like a "high"; may do risky things.

Manifestation Symptom or condition that is the result of a disease.

Manipulation Manual procedure that involves a directed thrust to move a joint past the physiological range of motion without exceeding the anatomical limit.

Map Locating the route of passage of electrical impulses and/or locating functional areas in a body part (e.g., cardiac mapping).

Marfan's syndrome An inherited condition that affects connective tissue and is caused by gene mutation.

Masochism The act or sense of gaining pleasure from experiencing physical or psychological pain.

Mastication Chewing of food.

Mastitis Inflammation or infection of the breast.

Mastoiditis Infection of the mastoid bone of the skull.

Maximization The manipulation of codes to result in maximum reimbursement without supporting documentation in the health record or with disregard for coding conventions, guidelines, and UHDDS definitions.

McBurney's point Area of the abdomen that, when touched, causes pain that may be indicative of appendicitis.

Measurement Determining the level of a physiological or physical function at a point in time.

Mechanical complication When a device or equipment malfunctions.

Mechanical ventilation Use of a machine to induce alternating inflation and deflation of the lungs; to regulate the exchange rate of gases in the blood.

Meconium Material in the intestine of a fetus.

Medial Position of a structure closer to the median plane than is another structure in the body.

Medical necessity Criteria or guidelines for what is determined to be reasonable and necessary for a particular medical service.

Medicare Code Editor Software that detects errors in coding on Medicare claims.

Melanomas Malignant changes of melanin cells.

Melena Dark blood in stool.

Meningitis Infection in the fluid of a person's spinal cord and brain.

Mental retardation Disorder in which a person's overall intellectual functioning is well below average, with an intelligence quotient (IQ) around 70 or less.

Metastasis Spread of a cancer from one part of the body to another, as in the appearance of neoplasms in parts of the body separate from the site of the primary tumor.

Midgut Small intestine and appendix (sites of carcinoid neoplasms).

Miscarriage Spontaneous termination of pregnancy before the fetus has reached 20 weeks.

Missed abortion Pregnancy with fetal demise before 20 weeks; products of conception are not expelled.

Mixed incontinence Combination of stress and urge incontinence.

Mixed mood Ternating between mania and depression very quickly.

Molar pregnancy Fertilized ovum is converted to a mole.

Monitoring Determining the level of a physiological or physical function repetitively over a period of time.

Mood disorder Condition that occurs with a change in mood over a prolonged period.

Morbid obesity Applies to patients who are 50% to 100% or 100 pounds above their ideal body weight. A BMI of 40 or higher defines morbid obesity.

Morphology The study of neoplasms.

Morphology codes (M codes) Codes that identify the type of cell that has become neoplastic and its biological activity or behavior.

MS-DRG grouper Software that assigns MS-DRG using diagnosis and procedure codes.

Mucositis An inflammation/ulceration of the digestive tract commonly occurring in the oral cavity.

Multigravida A woman with two or more pregnancies.

Multiparity A woman with two or more pregnancies.

Muscular dystrophy Type of myopathy.

Myasthenia gravis Chronic autoimmune disorder that manifests as muscle weakness of varying degrees.

Mycobacterium avium-intercellulare A mycobacteria found in soil and water.

Myeloma Malignancy that originates in the bone marrow.

Myelopathy Compression of the spinal cord.

Myocardial infarction Heart attack.

Myopathy Disorder that affects muscles, usually resulting in weakness or atrophy.

Myxedema Skin and tissue disorder that is usually due to severe prolonged hypothyroidism.

Nadir The lowest level.

National coverage determinations (NCDs) National policy that may include certain time frames for testing, certain age requirements, and that a particular diagnosis or condition be present for a procedure to be considered medically necessary.

NEC Abbreviation for "not elsewhere classifiable" that means "other specified."

Necrosis Death of cells.

Necrotic Dead tissue that lacks a blood supply.

Necrotizing fasciitis (or "flesh-eating disease") A rare but serious condition in which an infection occurs in the tissues below the skin.

Neoplasm Abnormal growth.

Nephrolithiasis Kidney stone.

Nephrotic syndrome Condition marked by proteinuria (protein in the urine), low levels of protein in the blood, hypercholesterolemia, and swelling of the eyes, feet, and hands.

Neutropenia Abnormal decrease in granular leukocytes in the blood.

Nomenclature System of names that are used as the preferred terminology.

Non-OR procedure affecting DRG assignment Procedure code recognized by the MS-DRG Grouper as a non–operating room procedure that may affect MS-DRG assignment.

Noncovered OR procedure A procedure code categorized by the Medicare Code Editor as a noncovered operating room procedure, for which Medicare does not provide reimbursement.

Nonessential modifier Term that is enclosed in parentheses; its presence or absence does not affect code assignment.

Nonexcisional debridement Removal of devitalized tissue by brushing, irrigating, scrubbing, or washing.

Noninvasive ventilation Ventilation without an invasive artificial airway (i.e., endotracheal tube or tracheostomy).

Nonunion When bony healing is not achieved at the fracture site. A fracture site that fails to heal within approximately 6 to 9 months of the injury represents a nonunion.

NOS Abbreviation for "not otherwise specified" that means "unspecified."

Nosocomial Hospital-acquired infection.

Nosocomial pneumonia Pneumonia that is acquired while the patient is residing in a hospital-type setting.

NSTEMI Non–ST elevation myocardial infarction.

Nursing home-acquired pneumonia Pneumonia that is acquired in a nursing home or extended care facility.

Obesity Condition defined as an increase in body weight beyond the limitation of skeletal and physical requirements, caused by excessive accumulation of fat in the body.

Observation unit Area outside the emergency department where unstable patients are admitted for a stay of less than 48 hours. The patient is observed for admission to the hospital or is discharged to home.

Occlusion Completely closing an orifice or lumen of a tubular body part (e.g., tubal ligation).

Occult blood Blood found only by laboratory inspection.

Omit code An instructional note found in Volume 3 that denotes that no code is to be assigned; it generally is used for coding approaches and closures that are integral to an operative procedure.

Oophoritis Inflammation of the ovaries.

Open Cutting through the skin, mucous membrane, and any other body layers necessary to expose the site of the procedure (e.g., abdominal hysterectomy).

Open fracture When the broken bone exits and is visible through the skin, or a deep wound exposes the broken bone through the skin.

Open reduction When the surgeon makes an incision at the fracture site to reduce or manipulate the fracture into anatomic position.

Open with percutaneous endoscopic assistance Cutting through the skin, mucous membrane, and any other body layers necessary to expose the site of the procedure; and entry of instrumentation, by puncture or minor incision, through the skin, mucous membrane, and any other body layers necessary to aid in the performance of the procedure (e.g., laparoscopic-assisted vaginal hysterectomy).

Oppositional defiant disorder Pattern of uncooperative, defiant, and hostile behavior toward authority figures that does not involve major antisocial violations, is not accounted for by the child's developmental stage, and results in significant functional impairment.

Optimization The process of striving to obtain optimal reimbursement or the highest possible payment to which a facility is legally entitled on the basis of documentation in the health record.

Organic brain syndrome General term used to describe the decrease in mental function due to other physical disease(s).

Osteoarthritis Type of arthritis that develops as the result of wear and tear on the joints.

Osteomyelitis Infection of the bone that often starts in another part of the body and spreads to the bone via the blood.

Osteoporosis Metabolic bone disorder that results in decreased bone mass and density.

Ostomies Surgically created openings into the body.

Other procedures Methodologies that attempt to remediate or cure a disorder or disease.

Otitis media Middle ear infection.

Ovaries Produce female hormones and eggs.

Overflow incontinence The constant dribbling of urine.

Packing Putting material in a body region or orifice.

Palliative Procedure performed to correct a condition that is causing problems for the patient.

Pancytopenia Decrease in production of erythrocytes (red blood cells), leukocytes (white blood cells), and thrombocytes (platelets).

Panic disorder Terrifying experience that occurs suddenly without warning. Physical symptoms include pounding heart, chest pains, dizziness, nausea, shortness of breath, trembling, choking, fear of dying, sweating, feelings of unreality, numbness, hot flashes or chills, and a feeling of going out of control or "crazy."

Parasitic Organism that lives on or takes nourishment from another organism.

Parenteral When medications are administered other than through the digestive tract, such as by intravenous or intramuscular injection.

Parkinson's disease Progressive and chronic motor system disorder.

Partial remission There are still a few signs and symptoms of the cancer, and the cancer cells have significantly decreased.

Pathologic fracture Break in a bone that occurs because of underlying disorders that weaken the bone, including malignancy, benign bone tumor, metabolic disorder, infection, and osteoporosis.

Pedicle graft or flap Involves identifying a flap that remains attached to its original blood supply and tunneling it under the skin to a particular area such as the breast.

Pelvic inflammatory disease When vaginal or cervical infections spread and involve the uterus, fallopian tubes, ovaries, and surrounding tissues.

Percutaneous Entry of instrumentation, by puncture or minor incision, through the skin, mucous membrane, and any other body layers necessary to reach the site of the procedure (e.g., needle biopsy liver).

Percutaneous endoscopic Entry of instrumentation, by puncture or minor incision, through the skin, mucous membrane, and any other body layers necessary to reach and visualize the site of the procedure (e.g., laparoscopic cholecystectomy).

Percutaneous endoscopic gastrostomy A tube put through the abdominal wall into the stomach with the use of a scope.

Percutaneous nephrolithotomy Procedure in which the surgeon uses a nephroscope to remove a stone. At times, an ultrasonic or electrohydraulic probe is used to break up the stone, and the fragments are then removed.

Percutaneous vertebroplasty Technique in which x-ray guidance is used to inject an acrylic cement through a needle into a collapsed or weakened vertebra; procedure is performed to treat pain caused by compression fractures of the vertebrae.

Performance Completely taking over a physiological function by extracorporeal means.

Pericarditis Inflammation of the covering of the heart.

Perinatal period Before birth through the first 28 days of life.

Peristalsis Rhythmic muscle contractions that move food down the digestive tract.

Peritoneal dialysis When the peritoneal membrane in the patient's own body is used with a dialysate solution to filter out the wastes and excess fluids.

Personality disorder A pattern of behavior that can disrupt many aspects of a person's life.

Phacoemulsification Incision is made on the side of the cornea and the lens material is softened, broken, and suctioned out.

Pheresis Extracorporeal separation of blood products.

Phlebitis Inflammation of a vein.

Phobia Irrational anxiety or fear that can interfere with one's everyday life or daily routine.

Phototherapy Extracorporeal treatment by light rays.

Physician Licensed medical doctor.

Platelets Another name for thrombocytes. Platelets circulate in the blood and assist in the clotting process.

Pleural effusion Fluid that accumulates in the pleural space because of trauma or disease.

Pneumoconioses Lung diseases due to chronic inhalation of inorganic (mineral) dust that are often due to occupational exposure.

Pneumonia Infection of the lungs that may be caused by a variety of organisms, including viruses, bacteria, and parasites.

Pneumothorax Air in space around the lung.

Poliomyelitis A viral disease that affects the nerves.

Polymyalgia rheumatica Syndrome classified as a rheumatic disease that is characterized by severe aching and stiffness in the neck, shoulder girdle, and pelvic girdle.

Posterior Back of the body or an organ.

Postlaminectomy syndrome Term used to describe patients who have undergone spine surgery and have some degree of recurrent spinal and/or leg pain due to the build up of scar tissue.

Postpartum After delivery or childbirth.

Postterm pregnancy Pregnancy longer than 40 weeks up to 42 weeks.

Posttraumatic stress disorder Anxiety disorder that is triggered by memories of a traumatic event.

Precipitate labor Rapid labor and delivery.

Preeclampsia Pregnancy complication characterized by hypertension, edema, and/or proteinuria.

Preferred Provider Organization (PPO) Type of managed care in which hospitals, physicians, and other providers have an arrangement with a third party payer to provide health care at discounted rates to third party payer clients.

Pregestational Condition present prior to pregnancy.

Premature labor Labor that occurs before the 37th week of pregnancy.

Prenatal Before birth.

Present on admission (POA) An indicator to differentiate between conditions, that develop during a particular hospital encounter or if a condition was present at the time of admission.

Preventive or prophylactic surgery Procedure performed to remove tissue that has the potential to become cancerous.

Primary osteoarthritis Idiopathic degenerative condition that occurs in previously intact joints, with no apparent initiating factor.

Primary site Site at which the neoplasm begins or originates.

Primigravida First pregnancy.

Principal diagnosis Condition established after study to be chiefly responsible for occasioning the admission of the patient to the hospital for care.

Principal procedure Procedure performed for definitive treatment, rather than for diagnostic or exploratory purposes, or one that was necessary to take care of a complication.

Procedure A diagnostic or therapeutic process performed on a patient.

Professional service Service rendered by a physician or a nonphysician practitioner.

Progress notes Daily recordings by healthcare providers of patient progress.

Prolonged pregnancy Beyond 42 weeks of pregnancy.

Prone Lying on the stomach, face down.

Prophylactic Medication or treatment used to prevent a disease from occurring.

Prospective payment system Method of reimbursement in which payment is made on the basis of a predetermined, fixed amount rather than for billed charges.

Prostate-specific antigen (PSA) Protein produced by the prostate gland.

Prostatitis Inflammation of the prostate that can be acute and/or chronic in nature and is due to a bacterium or inflammation that is not caused by a bacterial infection.

Proteinuria Protein in urine.

Proximal Closer to the median plane.

Pruritus Itching.

Psoriasis Inflammation of skin caused by a fault in the immune system.

Psychosis Impairment in mental state in which the perception of reality has become distorted.

Puerperium Time from delivery through the first 6 weeks postpartum.

Pulmonary edema Condition in which fluid accumulates in the lungs.

Pulmonary embolism A blood clot(s) in the pulmonary artery that causes blockage in the artery.

Pulmonary hypertension High blood pressure in the arteries that supply blood to the lungs.

Purpura Ecchymoses or small hemorrhages in the skin, mucous membranes, or serosal surfaces due to blood disorders, vascular abnormalities, or trauma.

Pyelonephritis Upper tract infection that involves the kidneys.

Radiation Use of high-energy radiation to treat cancer.

Radiculopathy Compression of a nerve root.

Reattachment Putting back in or on all or a portion of a separated body part to its normal location or other suitable location.

Rectocele Descent of the rectum and pressing of the rectum against the vaginal wall.

Rectovesical fistula A communication between the bladder and the rectum.

Rehabilitation Structured program with the goal of stopping and recovering from the use of alcohol and/or drugs.

Reimbursement Payment for healthcare services.

Release Freeing a body part from an abnormal physical constraint (e.g., lysis of adhesions) or location to a more suitable location (e.g., reattachment of finger).

Removal Taking out or off a device from a body part (e.g., removal of a chest tube).

Renal colic Intense pain associated with the body's efforts to try to force the stone through the ureters.

Repair Restoring, to the extent possible, a body part to its normal anatomic structure and function (herniorrhaphy).

Replacement Putting in or on biological or synthetic material that physically takes the place and/or performs the function of all or a portion of a body part (total knee replacement).

Reposition Moving to its normal location or other suitable location all or a portion of a body part (e.g., fracture reduction).

Resection Cutting out or off, without replacement, all of a body part (e.g., total lobectomy of lung).

Residual condition or effect When the acute phase of an illness or injury has passed, but a residual condition or health problem remains.

Respiratory failure General term that describes ineffective gas exchange across the lungs by the respiratory system.

Respiratory system System that supplies the body with oxygen (O_2).

Restoration Returning, or attempting to return, a physiological function to its original state by extracorporeal means.

Restorative or reconstructive Surgery performed to restore function and enhance aesthetic appearance after surgery.

Restriction Partially closing an orifice or lumen of a tubular body part (e.g., Nissen fundoplication).

Revenue code A four-digit code that is utilized on the UB-04 to indicate a particular type of service.

Review of systems Question-and-answer period that occurs between a patient and a healthcare provider during which any healthcare issues are reviewed.

Revision Correcting, to the extent possible, a malfunctioning or displaced device (e.g., adjustment of knee prosthesis).

Rhabdomyolysis Breakdown of muscle fibers resulting in the release of muscle fiber contents into the circulation.

Rheumatoid arthritis Chronic, inflammatory systemic disease that affects the joints, often causing deformity.

Robotic-assisted surgery Minimally invasive technique that utilizes robotic arms to manipulate the surgical equipment and tools.

Sadism The act or sense of gaining pleasure from inflicting physical or psychological pain on another.

Salpingitis Inflammation of the fallopian tubes, which are the most common site of pelvic inflammation.

Sarcomas Malignant growths of connective tissue (e.g., muscle, cartilage, lymph tissue, and bone).

Schizophrenia Disorder of the brain characterized by trouble differentiating between real and unreal experiences, along with problems with logical thinking, normal emotional responses to others, and appropriate behavior in social situations.

Scleroderma Chronic, progressive disease characterized by hardening of the skin and scarring of internal organs.

Scoliosis Deviation of the vertical line of the spine.

Screening examination One that occurs in the absence of any signs or symptoms. It involves examination of an asymptomatic individual to detect a given disease, typically by means of an inexpensive diagnostic test.

Sebum Substance secreted from the sebaceous gland.

Secondary diabetes mellitus Form of the disease that develops as a result of another disease or condition.

Secondary osteoarthritis Degenerative disease of the joints that results from some predisposing condition such as trauma or disease.

Secondary thrombocytopenia Decrease in the number of platelets due to specific diseases or external causes, such as drugs, blood transfusions, and overhydration.

Section Consists of a group of three-digit categories that represent diseases or conditions that are similar.

See A mandatory cross-reference that advises the coder to go to another main term.

See also Cross-reference that instructs the coder about the possibility that there may be a better main term elsewhere in the Alphabetic Index.

Self-insured plans Self-insurance fund is set up by an employer to provide health claim benefits for employees.

Sepsis SIRS due to infection.

Septic shock A condition caused by infection and sepsis. It can cause multiple organ failure and death.

Septicemia The presence in the blood of pathologic microorganisms that cause systemic illness.

Sequelae Late or residual effect of an acute disease.

Shock wave therapy Extracorporeal treatment by shock waves.

Shunting Procedure to drain fluid from brain to relieve pressure.

Sialolithiasis Stones in the salivary glands.

Sickle cell anemia One of the most common hemolytic anemias, in which the shape of the red blood cell changes from a disc to a crescent or "sickle," causing obstruction of small blood vessels and eventual damage throughout the body.

Siderosis Lung disease due to inhalation of iron oxide.

Sign Objective evidence of a disease or of a patient's condition as perceived by the patient's examining physician.

Significant procedure A procedure is considered significant if it is surgical in nature, carries a procedural risk, carries an anesthetic risk, and/or requires specialized training.

Simple fracture Injury in which the bone is broken, but the skin remains intact.

Sinusitis A condition in which the linings of one or more sinuses become infected, usually because of viruses or bacteria.

SIRS Systemic inflammatory response syndrome, which can be caused by infection or trauma.

Sleep apnea Disorder characterized by breathing interruption during sleep.

Somatic nervous system Sends sensory (taste, hearing, smell) information to the central nervous system.

Somnolence Sleepiness.

Spinal bifida A disorder that involves incomplete development of the brain, spinal cord, and/or their protective coverings.

Spinal cord injury Damage to the spinal cord that causes loss of sensation and motor control.

Spinal decompression Surgical procedure that frees space for the nerves in the spinal canal.

Spinal fusion The creation of a solid bone bridge between two or more adjacent vertebrae to enhance stability between levels of the spine.

Spinal stenosis Narrowing of the central spinal canal or the areas of the spine where the nerve roots exit (neuroforamina).

Splenomegaly Enlarged spleen.

Spondylolisthesis Condition in which one vertebra slips on another.

Spondylosis (or spinal osteoarthritis) Degenerative disorder that may cause loss of normal spinal structure and function.

Spontaneous abortion Loss of a fetus due to natural causes; also known as *miscarriage*.

Spontaneous pneumothorax Pneumothorax that is not caused by trauma.

Sprain Stretch and/or tear of a ligament.

Squamous intraepithelial lesion (SIL) Dysplasia of the cervix that is identified on a Pap smear.

Staging Means of categorizing a particular cancer that assists in determination of a patient's treatment plan and the need for further therapy.

Staging surgeries Procedures performed to help the clinician determine the extent of disease; these generally are more accurate than laboratory and imaging tests.

Stannosis Lung disease due to inhalation of tin particles.

Stasis dermatitis Skin condition due to poor circulation (venous insufficiency) that is characterized by swelling, skin discoloration, weeping, itching, and scaly skin.

Stasis ulcer Ulcer associated with varicose veins.

STEMI ST elevation myocardial infarction.

Stenosis Abnormal narrowing.

Steroid-induced diabetes Diabetes that is caused by the use of steroids.

Stillbirth Born dead.

Stoma An artificial opening.

Strain Injury to a muscle or a tendon.

Stress incontinence Involuntary loss of small amounts of urine due to increased pressure resulting from coughing, sneezing, or laughing.

Stroke Cerebrovascular accident or brain infarction.

Subacute Somewhat acute; between chronic and acute.

Subcategory A fourth-digit code that provides additional information or specificity.

Subclassification A fifth-digit code that provides even greater specificity.

Subcutaneous Inner layer of the skin that contains fat and sweat glands.

Subluxation Partial or incomplete dislocation.

Subterm Gives more specific information about a main term. Subterms identify site, type, or etiology of a disease condition or injury. Also, modifiers that are indented to the right of the main term.

Superior Position of the body or an organ relative to the vertical axis of the body.

Supine Lying on the back, face up.

Supplement Putting in or on biological or synthetic material that physically reinforces and/or augments the function of a portion of a body part (e.g., herniorrhaphy with mesh).

Suture Method for closing cutaneous wounds.

Symptom Subjective evidence of a disease or of a patient's condition as perceived by the patient.

Syphilis A sexually transmitted disease (STD) that is caused by bacteria.

Systemic inflammatory response syndrome A serious medical condition that can occur in response to infectious or noninfectious causes, such as severe trauma, burns, or complications of surgery.

Systemic lupus erythematosus Chronic, inflammatory autoimmune disease that can damage connective tissue anywhere in the body.

Tabular List Section of the ICD-9-CM book that contains the code listing, along with exclusion or inclusion notes.

Tachycardia Fast heart rate, generally greater than 100 beats per minute.

Tendons Connective tissue that attaches muscle to bone.

Terminology Words and phrases that apply to a particular field.

Tetany A continuous muscle spasm.

Thalassemia Hereditary disease that is similar to sickle cell anemia and occurs in varying degrees.

Therapeutic abortion Abortion performed when the pregnancy is endangering the mother's health, or when the fetus has a condition that is incompatible with life.

Third party payer Makes payments for health services on behalf of the patients; may be a government program, insurance company, or managed care plan.

Thoracentesis Puncture of the chest wall to remove fluid (pleural effusion) from the space between the lining of the outside of the lungs (pleura) and the wall of the chest.

Thoracoscopic approach A thoracoscope is used to examine and perform closed procedures within the thorax.

Threatened abortion Abortion that occurs when symptoms are present that indicate the possibility of a miscarriage.

Thrombocytes Another name for platelets. Thrombocytes circulate in the blood and assist in the clotting process.

Thrombus A blood clot that forms and remains in a vein.

Thyrotoxic crisis/storm Complication of hyperthyroidism associated with a sudden intensification of symptoms combined with fever, rapid pulse, and delirium.

TIPS (transjugular intrahepatic portosystemic shunt) A procedure in which the portal vein is connected to one of the hepatic veins and a stent is inserted.

Topography Location.

Trachea (windpipe) Body part responsible for filtering the air that we breathe.

Tracheostomy Procedure in which an artificial opening is made in the front of the windpipe (trachea) through the skin of the neck.

Traction Exerting a pulling force on a body region in a distal direction.

Transfer Moving, without taking out, all or a portion of a body part to another location to take over the function of all or a portion of a body part (e.g., pedicle skin flap).

Transfusion Putting in blood or blood products.

Transient ischemic attack A stroke that lasts for only a few minutes.

Transplantation Putting in or on all or a portion of a living body part taken from another individual or animal to physically take the place and/or function of all or a portion of a similar body part (kidney transplant).

Transurethral resection of the prostate Endoscopic removal of prostate tissue.

Transvestism Assuming the appearance, manner, or roles traditionally associated with members of the opposite sex (cross-dressing).

Traumatic brain injury Injury to the brain that may result in interference with the brain's normal functions.

Treatment Manual treatment to eliminate or alleviate somatic dysfunction and related disorders.

Trisomy Extra chromosome.

Tube thoracostomy Insertion of chest tube(s) to drain blood, fluid, or air and allow full expansion of the lungs.

Tuberculosis (TB) An infection caused by *Mycobacterium tuberculosis*.

Tumor lysis syndrome (TLS) Development of electrolyte and metabolic disturbances that can occur after treatment of cancer, usually lymphoma and leukemia, and sometimes even without treatment.

Ulcer Open sore of the skin.

Ulcerative colitis An inflammatory bowel disease.

Ultrasound therapy Extracorporeal treatment by ultrasound.

Ultraviolet light therapy Extracorporeal treatment by ultraviolet light.

Undifferentiated Tumor cells that are highly abnormal (e.g., immature, primitive).

Ureterolithiasis Ureter stone.

Urethritis Infection of the urethra.

Urethrocele When the urethra presses into the vagina.

Urethrovaginal fistula Abnormal passage between the urethra and the vagina.

Urge incontinence Sudden and involuntary loss of large amounts of urine.

Urinary tract infection General term used to describe infection in any area of the urinary tract.

Urolithiasis A stone in the urinary tract.

Urosepsis Infection of urinary site.

Urticaria Another name for hives.

Uterine prolapse Descent of the uterus and the cervix into the vaginal canal.

Uterus A muscular organ that serves as an incubator for the developing fetus.

Vagal nerve stimulator A device to control seizures.

Vagina A muscular tube that extends from the vaginal opening to the uterus.

Vaginal vault prolapse Condition that may occur following a hysterectomy, when the top of the vagina descends.

Valid OR procedure A procedure that may affect MSG-DRG assignment.

Varicose veins Enlarged, twisted veins that usually occur in the legs.

Ventral Front of the body or an organ.

Vesicouterine fistula Communication between the bladder and the uterus.

Vesicovaginal fistula Communication between the bladder and the vagina.

Via natural or artificial opening Entry of instrumentation through a natural or artificial external opening to reach the site of the procedure (e.g., endotracheal intubation).

Via natural or artificial opening endoscopic Entry of instrumentation through a natural or artificial external opening to reach and visualize the site of the procedure (e.g., colonoscopy).

Viral meningitis A viral infection of the fluid in the spinal cord and around the brain.

Vitamin deficiency Condition caused by many different factors, such as poor nutrient absorption, digestive tract disorders, lifestyle issues (e.g., alcohol, smoking, medication, overexercising), chronic illness, age, and many other factors.

Volume depletion May be the result of either dehydration or hypovolemia.

Volvulus An abnormal twisting of the intestine that may impair blood flow to the intestine.

Voyeurism Recurrent intense sexual urges and fantasies involving observing unsuspecting people who are naked, disrobing, or engaging in sexual activity.

Vulva The external covering to the vagina.

Vulvar intraepithelial neoplasia (VIN) Certain changes that can occur in the skin that covers the vulva.

Well-differentiated Tumor cells that closely resemble mature, specialized cells.

West Nile A viral disease that is spread to individuals by a mosquito bite.

Whipple procedure A procedure that generally involves removal of the gallbladder, common bile duct, part of the duodenum, and head of the pancreas.

Young obstetric patient Younger than 16 years at date of delivery.

Xenograft Graft to an individual from another species; also known as a *heterograft*.

Abbreviations/ Acronyms

AAPC American Academy of Professional Coders

ABG arterial blood gas

ACS acute coronary syndrome

ADD attention deficit disorder

ADHD attention deficit hyperactivity disorder

AF atrial fibrillation

AGA appropriate for gestational age

AHA American Hospital Association

AHFS American Hospital Formulary Service

AHIMA American Health Information Management Association

AHQA American Health Quality Association

AICD automatic implantable cardioverter-defibrillator

AIDS acquired immunodeficiency syndrome

AKA above-knee amputation

ALL acute lymphocytic leukemia

ALOS average length of stay

AMA American Medical Association

AMI acute myocardial infarction

AML acute myeloid leukemia

APC Ambulatory Payment Classification

ARF acute renal failure

ARI acute renal insufficiency

AROM artificial rupture of membranes

ASA aspirin

ASCUS atypical squamous cells of undetermined significance

ATV all-terrain vehicle

AV arteriovenous

AV atrioventricular

AVM arteriovenous malformation

AVR aortic valve replacement

BAL bronchoalveolar lavage

BIPAP bilevel positive airway pressure

BMI body mass index

BMT bone marrow transplant

BNP brain natriuretic peptide

BP blood pressure

BPD biliopancreatic diversion

BPD bronchopulmonary dysplasia

BPH benign prostatic hypertrophy

BRM biological response modifier

BUN blood urea nitrogen

C. DIFF *Clostridium difficile*

CAB coronary artery bypass

CABG coronary artery bypass graft

CAD coronary artery disease

CAP community-acquired pneumonia

CAPD continuous ambulatory peritoneal dialysis

CAS computer assisted surgery

CAT computerized axial tomography

CBC complete blood count

CC chief complaint

CC complication/comorbidity

CCA Certified Coding Associate

CCPD continuous cycling peritoneal dialysis

CCS Certified Coding Specialist

CCS-P Certified Coding Specialist—Physician Based

CCU coronary care unit

CD4 Cluster of differentiation 4

CDC Centers for Disease Control and Prevention

CDIP Clinical Documentation Improvement Program

CDM charge description master

CEA cultured epidermal autograft

CEUs continuing education units

CF cystic fibrosis

CHB complete heart block

CHD congenital heart disease

CHF congestive heart failure

CHI closed head injury

CIN cervical intraepithelial neoplasia

CKD chronic kidney disease

CLL chronic lymphocytic leukemia

CMI case-mix index

CML chronic myelogenous leukemia

CMS Centers for Medicare and Medicaid Services

CNS central nervous system

COPD chronic obstructive pulmonary disease

CPAP continuous positive airway pressure

CPC Certified Professional Coder

CPC-H Certified Professional Coder—Hospital Based

CPD cephalopelvic disproportion

CPK creatine phosphokinase

CPK-MB creatine phosphokinase, isoenzyme MB

CPT *Current Procedural Terminology*

CRF chronic renal failure

CRI chronic renal insufficiency

CRT cardiac resynchronization therapy

CRT-D cardiac resynchronization treatment defibrillator

CRT-P cardiac resynchronization treatment pacemaker

CSF cerebrospinal fluid

CT computerized tomography

CVA cerebrovascular accident

CVL central venous line

CXR chest x-ray

D&C dilatation and curettage

DBS deep brain stimulation

DCIS ductal carcinoma in situ

DES drug-eluting stent

DEXA dual-energy x-ray absorptiometry (bone density)

DHHS U.S. Department of Health and Human Services

DI diabetes insipidus

DIC disseminated intravascular coagulation

DIEP deep inferior epigastric perforator

DJD degenerative joint disease

DOE dyspnea on exertion

DM diabetes mellitus

DMAC disseminated *Mycobacterium avium-intracellulare* complex

DOB date of birth

DRA Deficit Reduction Act

DRGs diagnosis-related groups

DS discharge summary

DSM-IV *Diagnostic and Statistical Manual of Mental Disorders, Fourth Edition*

DSM-IV-TR *Diagnostic and Statistical Manual of Mental Disorders, Fourth Edition, Text Revision*

DTs delirium tremens

DVT deep vein thrombosis

E. coli *Escherichia coli*

ECMO extracorporeal membrane oxygenation

ECT electroconvulsive therapy

ED emergency department

EDC estimated date of confinement

EEG electroencephalogram

EGD esophogastroduodenoscopy

EKG/ECG electrocardiogram

EMG electromyelogram

EMS emergency medical services

EP electrophysiologic

ER Emergency Room

ERCP endoscopic retrograde cholangiopancreatography

ESRD end-stage renal disease

ESWL extracorporeal shock wave lithotripsy

FB foreign body

FNA fine needle aspiration

FSG focal segmental glomerulosclerosis

FTSG full-thickness skin graft

FUO fever of unknown origin

GAP gluteal artery perforator

GEMs General Equivalence Mappings

GERD gastroesophageal reflux disease

GFR glomerular filtration rate

GI gastrointestinal

GMLOS geometric length of stay

GN glomerulonephritis

GPO Government Printing Office

GVHD graft-versus-host disease

H. flu *Haemophilus influenzae*

H&P history and physical

HAC hospital acquired conditions

HAART highly active antiretroviral therapy

HBOT hyperbaric oxygen therapy

HCC hepatocellular carcinoma

hCG human chorionic gonadotropin

HCPCS Healthcare Common Procedure Coding System

Hct hematocrit

HCVD hypertensive cardiovascular disease

Hgb hemoglobin

hGH human growth hormone

HGSIL high-grade squamous intraepithelial lesion

HH home health

HIPAA Health Insurance Portability and Accountability Act

HIV human immunodeficiency virus

HIVAN HIV-associated nephropathy

HMO Health Maintenance Organization

HPI history of present illness

HPR hospital's payment rate

HPV human papillomavirus

HSIL high-grade intraepithelial lesion

HSV herpes simplex virus

HTN hypertension

I&D incision and drainage

ICD internal cardiac defibrillator

ICD-9-CM *International Classification of Diseases, 9th Revision, Clinical Modification*

ICD-10-CM *International Classification of Diseases, 10th Revision, Clinical Modification*

ICD-10-PCS *International Classification of Diseases, 10th Revision, Procedure Coding System*

ICD-O *International Classification of Diseases for Oncology*

ICU intensive care unit

ICV implantable cardioverter

IDDM insulin-dependent diabetes mellitus

Ig immunoglobulin

IOL induction of labor

IOL intraocular lens

IOP intraocular pressure

IPPS Inpatient Prospective Payment System

IPPV intermittent positive pressure ventilation

IQ intelligence quotient

ITP idiopathic thrombocytopenic purpura

IUD intrauterine device

IUGR intrauterine growth retardation

IV intravenous

IVDU intravenous drug use

JRA juvenile rheumatoid arthritis

LAD left anterior descending

LAVH laparoscopically assisted vaginal hysterectomy

LCA left coronary artery

LCDs local coverage determinations

LD learning disability/difficulty

LDMF latissimus dorsi musculocutaneous flap

LGA large for gestational age

LGIB lower gastrointestinal bleed

LH luteinizing hormone

LLL lower left lobe

LMRP local medical review policies

LOC loss of consciousness

LOS length of stay

LP lumbar puncture

LSIL low-grade intraepithelial lesion

LTC long-term care

LTCS low transverse cesarean section

LUTS lower urinary tract symptoms

MAC Medicaid Administrative Contractor

MAC *Mycobacterium avium-intracellulare* complex

MAI *Mycobacterium avium-intracellulare*

MAO monoamine oxidase

MAR medication administration record

MCE Medicare Code Editor

MDC major diagnostic category

MEN multiple endocrine neoplasia

MI myocardial infarction

MIC Medicaid Integrity Contractor

MR mental retardation

MRA magnetic resonance angiography

MRCP mental retardation, cerebral palsy

MRI magnetic resonance imaging

MRSA methicillin-resistant *Staphylococcus aureus*

MSAFP maternal serum alpha-fetoprotein

MS-DRG Medicare Severity diagnosis–related group

MSSA methicillin-susceptible *Staphylococcus aureus*

MUGA multiple-gated acquisition

MVA motor vehicle accident

MVP mitral valve prolapse

MVR mitral valve replacement

NCDs national coverage determinations

NCHS National Center for Health Statistics

NEC not elsewhere classifiable

NHL non-Hodgkins' lymphoma

NICU neonatal intensive care unit

NIDDM non–insulin-dependent diabetes mellitus

NKF National Kidney Foundation

NOS not otherwise specified

NPH normal pressure hydrocephalus

NPI National Provider Identifier

NPPV noninvasive positive pressure ventilation

NPRM Notice of Proposed Rule Making

NQMI non–Q wave myocardial infarction

NSAID nonsteroidal antiinflammatory drug

NSCLC non–small cell lung cancer

NST nonstress test

NSTEMI non–ST elevation myocardial infarction

O_2 oxygen

OA osteoarthritis

OB obstetrics

OBS organic brain syndrome

OIG Office of the Inspector General

OM obtuse marginal

OM otitis media

OP note operative note

OPPS Outpatient Prospective Payment System

OR Operating Room

ORIF open reduction with internal fixation

OSA obstructive sleep apnea

$Paco_2$ partial pressure of carbon dioxide in arterial blood

Pao_2 partial pressure of oxygen in arterial blood

PCI percutaneous coronary intervention

PCP *Pneumocystis carinii* pneumonia

PCP primary care provider

PDA patent ductus arteriosus

PDA posterior descending artery

PDT photodynamic therapy

PE pulmonary embolism

PEG percutaneous endoscopic gastrostomy

PEPPER Program for Evaluating Payment Patterns Electronic Report

PHT pulmonary hypertension

PICC peripherally inserted central catheter

PID pelvic inflammatory disease

PIH pregnancy-induced hypertension

PKU phenylketonuria

PMR polymyalgia rheumatica

POA present on admission

POCs products of conception

PPH primary pulmonary hypertension

PPO Preferred Provider Organization

PPS Prospective Payment System

PROM premature rupture of membranes

PSA prostate-specific antigen

PT prothrombin time

PTA prior to admission

PTCA percutaneous transluminal coronary angioplasty

PTL preterm labor

PTSD posttraumatic stress disorder

PTT partial thromboplastin time

PUD peptic ulcer disease

PV percutaneous vertebroplasty

QIO Quality Improvement Organization

RA rheumatoid arthritis

RA right atrium

RAC Recovery Audit Contract

RAD reactive airway disease

RBBB right bundle branch block

RCA right coronary artery

RCC renal cell carcinoma

RDS respiratory distress syndrome

RFA radiofrequency ablation

RHD rheumatic heart disease

RHIA Registered Health Information Administrator

RHIT Registered Health Information Technician

RPGN rapidly progressive glomerulonephritis

RPR rapid plasma reagin

RPS retrospective payment system

RSV respiratory syncytial virus

RUL right upper lobe

RW relative weight

SARS severe acute respiratory syndrome

SCI spinal cord injury

SCID severe combined immunodeficiency

SCLC small cell lung cancer

SGA small for gestational age

SIADH syndrome of inappropriate antidiuretic hormone secretion

SIDS sudden infant death syndrome

SIEA superficial inferior epigastric artery

SIL squamous intraepithelial lesion

SIRS systemic inflammatory response syndrome

SLAP superior labrum anterior–posterior

SLE systemic lupus erythematosus

SNF skilled nursing facility

SNOMED Systematized Nomenclature of Medicine

SOAP Subjective/Objective Assessment Plan

SOB shortness of breath

SOM serous otitis media

SOW scope of work

SSS sick sinus syndrome

STAPH aureus *Staphylococcus aureus*

STD sexually transmitted disease

STEMI ST elevation myocardial infarction

STSG split-thickness skin graft

SVD spontaneous vaginal delivery

SVT supraventricular tachycardia

SZ seizure

TB tuberculosis

TBI traumatic brain injury

TEFRA Tax Equity and Fiscal Responsibility Act

THR total hip replacement

TIA transient ischemic attack

TIPS transjugular intrahepatic portosystemic shunt

TJC The Joint Commission

TLS tumor lysis syndrome

TOF tetralogy of Fallot

TPA tissue plasminogen activator

TPN total parenteral nutrition

TPR temperature, pulse, and respiration

TRALI transfusion-related acute lung injury

TRAM transverse rectus abdominis musculocutaneous

TSH thyroid-stimulating hormone

TTN transitory tachypnea of the newborn

TULIP transurethral ultrasound-guided laser-induced prostatectomy

TUMT transurethral microwave thermotherapy

TUNA transurethral needle ablation of the prostate

TURP transurethral resection of the prostate

UB-04 Uniform Bill-04

UGIB upper gastrointestinal bleed

UHDDS Uniform Hospital Discharge Data Set
UPIN Unique Physician Identification Number
USA unstable angina
UTI urinary tract infection
VAD vascular access device
VAP ventilator-assisted preumonia
VATS video-assisted thoracic surgery
VBAC vaginal birth after cesarean section
VBG vertical banded gastroplasty

VDRL Venereal Disease Research Laboratory
VIN vulvar intraepithelial neoplasia
VLAP visual laser ablation of the prostate
VPS ventriculoperitoneal shunt
VRE vancomycin-resistant *enterococcus*
VSD ventricular septal defect
WBC white blood cell
WHO World Health Organization
ZPIC Zone Program Integrity Contractor

Illustration Credits

Chapter 1
Figure 1-1: Courtesy American Health Information Management Association. 1-2: Courtesy American Academy of Professional Coders.

Chapter 2
Figures 2-1, 2-9, 2-11, 2-12: From Abdelhak M, Grostick S, Hanken MA, Jacobs EB (eds). Health Information: Management of a Strategic Resource, 2nd ed. St. Louis, Saunders, 2001.

Chapter 9
Figures 9-2: From Kumar V, Cotran RS, Robbins SJ. Robbins Basic Pathology, 7th ed. Philadelphia, Saunders, 2003. 9-3: Courtesy Dr. John J. Kepers, Kansas City, Kansas. 9-4: From Behrman RE, Kleigman RM, Arvin AM. Slide set for Nelson Textbook of Pediatrics, 15th ed. Philadelphia, Saunders, 1996. 9-5: From Frazier MS, Drzymkowski JW. Essentials of Human Diseases and Conditions, 4th ed. St. Louis, Saunders, 2009.

Chapter 10
Figure 10-1: From Chabner D. The Language of Medicine, 8th ed. St. Louis, Saunders, 2007. 10-5: From Odom RB, James WD, Berger TG. Andrews' Diseases of the Skin, 9th ed. Philadelphia, Saunders, 2000. 10-6: From Doughty DB, Jackson DB. Gastrointestinal Disorders—Mosby's Clinical Nursing Series, 5th ed. St. Louis, Mosby, 1993. 10-7: From Cotran RS, Kumar V, Collins T. Robbins Pathologic Basis for Disease, 6th ed. Philadelphia, Saunders, 1999. 10-8: From Kumar V, Abbas AK, Fausto N. Robbins & Cotran Pathologic Basis of Disease, 7th ed. Philadelphia, Saunders, 2005. 10-9, 10-10, 10-11, 10-13: From Damjanov I. Pathology for the Health Professions, 3rd ed. St. Louis, Saunders, 2006. 10-12: From Huether SE, McCance KL. Understanding Pathophysiology, 3rd ed. St. Louis, Mosby, 2004. 10-14: From Gould BE. Pathophysiology for the Health Professions, 3rd ed. St. Louis, Saunders, 2006. 10-15: Burkitt HG, Quick RG. Essential Surgery, 3rd ed. London, Churchill Livingstone, 2002.

Chapter 11
Figures 11-5, 11-9: From Chabner D. The Language of Medicine, 8th ed. St. Louis, Saunders, 2007. 11-8: From Lookingbill DP, Marks JG. Principles of Dermatology, 3rd ed. Philadelphia, Saunders, 2000.

Chapter 12
Figures 12-2, 12-7: From Chabner D. The Language of Medicine, 8th ed. St. Louis, Saunders, 2007. 12-3: From Swartz M. Textbook of Physical Diagnosis, 4th ed. Philadelphia, Saunders, 2002. 12-4: Courtesy Paul W. Ladenson, MD, The Johns Hopkins University and Hospital, Baltimore, Maryland. 12-5, 12-16, 12-17, 12-21: From Damjanov I. Pathology for the Health Professions, 3rd ed. St. Louis, Saunders, 2006. 12-6: From Seidel HM, Ball JW, Dains JE, Benedict GW. Mosby's Guide to Physical Examination, 4th ed. St. Louis, Mosby, 1998. 12-14A: From Thibodeau GA. Anatomy and Physiology. 4th ed. St. Louis, Times Mirror/Mosby College Publishing, 1987. 12-13:

Courtesy Dr. Edmund Beard, Cleveland, Ohio. 12-14B: From Beuschlein F, Strasburger CJ, Siegerstetter V, et al. Acromegaly caused by secretion of growth hormone by a non-Hodgkins lymphoma. N Engl J Med 2000;342:1871-1876. Copyright 2000, Massachusetts Medical Society. All rights reserved. 12-14C: From Little JW, Falace D, Miller C, Rhodus NL. Dental Management of the Medically Compromised Patient, 7th ed. St. Louis, Mosby, 2008. 12-18: From Zitelli BJ, Davis HW. Atlas of Pediatric Physical Diagnosis, 4th ed. St. Louis, Mosby, 2002. 12-18: From Kumar V, Abbas AK, Fausto N. Robbins & Cotran Pathologic Basis of Disease, 7th ed. Philadelphia, Saunders, 2005. 12-22: Courtesy MiniMed Technologies, Sylmar, California; from Mosby's Medical, Nursing, and Allied Health Dictionary, 6th ed. St. Louis, Mosby, 2002.

Chapter 14
Figures 14-1, 14-2, 14-3, 14-4, 14-5, 14-14: From Chabner D. The Language of Medicine, 8th ed. St. Louis, Saunders, 2007. 14-7: From Damjanov I. Pathology for the Health Professions, 3rd ed. St. Louis, Saunders, 2006. 14-8, 14-9, 14-10, 14-11, 14-12, 14-17: From Frazier MS, Drzymkowski JW. Essentials of Human Diseases and Conditions, 4th ed. St. Louis, Saunders, 2009. 14-15: Courtesy Ophthalmic Photography at the University of Michigan, WK Kellogg Eye Center, Ann Arbor, Michigan. 14-18: From Lewis SM, Heitkemper MM, Dirksen SR. Medical-Surgical Nursing: Assessment and Management of Clinical Problems, 5th ed. St. Louis, Mosby, 2000.

Chapter 15
Figure 15-3: From Patton KT, Thibodeau GA. Mosby's Handbook of Anatomy and Physiology. St. Louis, Mosby, 2000. 15-4: From Applegate EJ. The Anatomy and Physiology Learning System, 2nd ed. Philadelphia, Saunders, 2000. 15-5, 15-9, 15-11, 15-12, 15-16: From Frazier MS, Drzymkowski JW. Essentials of Human Diseases and Conditions, 4th ed. St. Louis, Saunders, 2009. 15-6: ©2008, Bayer Schering Pharma AG. www.thrombosisadviser.com. 15-7: From Gould BE. Pathophysiology for the Health Professions, 3rd ed. Philadelphia, Saunders, 2000. 15-8, 15-13: From Damjanov I. Pathology for the Health Professions, 2nd ed. St. Louis, Saunders, 2006. 15-10: Modified from Ignatavicius DD, Workman ML. Medical-Surgical Nursing: Critical Thinking for Collaborative Care, 4th ed. Philadelphia, Saunders, 2002. 15-14, 15-15, 15-17, 15-18: From Chabner D. The Language of Medicine, 8th ed. St. Louis, Saunders, 2007. 15-19: From Drake RL, Vogl W, Mitchell AWM. Gray's Anatomy for Students. Philadelphia, Churchill Livingstone, 2005. 15-20: From Lewis SM, Heitkemper MM, Dirksen SR. Medical-Surgical Nursing: Assessment and Management of Clinical Problems, 5th ed. St. Louis, Mosby, 2000.

Chapter 16
Figure 16-2: From Gould BE. Pathophysiology for the Health Professions, 3rd ed. St. Louis, Saunders, 2006. 16-6A, B: From Kumar V, Abbas AK, Fausto N. Robbins & Cotran Pathologic Basis of Disease, 7th ed. Philadelphia, Saunders, 2005. 16-6C: Courtesy Paul Emmerson and Seneca College of Applied Arts and Technology, Toronto, Ontario, Canada. 16-7: Courtesy Dr.

W. Thurlback, Vancouver, BC, Canada. 16-10, 16-11, 16-12A, 16-13: From Chabner D. The Language of Medicine, 8th ed. St. Louis, Saunders, 2007. 16-12B: From Black JM, Hawks JH, Keene AM. Medical-Surgical Nursing: Clinical Management for Positive Outcomes, 6th ed. Philadelphia, Saunders, 2001.

Chapter 17
Figure 17-1: Redrawn from Miller M. Pathophysiology: Principles of Disease. Philadelphia, Saunders, 1983. 17-2: From Buck CJ. Saunders 2010 ICD-9-CM, Volumes 1, 2, and 3. St. Louis, Saunders, 2010. 17-3: From Damjanov I. Pathology for the Health-Related Professions, 2nd ed. Philadelphia, Saunders, 2000. 17-6: From Damjanov I. Pathology for the Health Professions, 3rd ed. St. Louis, Saunders, 2006. 17-7, 17-9A, 17-14, 17-15: From Chabner D. The Language of Medicine, 8th ed. St. Louis, Saunders, 2007. 17-8: From Cotran RS, Kumar V, Collins T. Robbins Pathologic Basis for Disease, 6th ed. Philadelphia, Saunders, 1999. 17-9B: From Kumar V, Abbas AK, Fausto N. Robbins & Cotran Pathologic Basis of Disease, 7th ed. Philadelphia, Saunders, 2005. 17-10: From Patton KT, Thibodeau GA. Anatomy and Physiology, 7th ed. St. Louis, Mosby, 2010. 17-11: From Dorland's Illustrated Medical Dictionary, 31st ed. Philadelphia, Saunders, 2007. 17-12, 17-13: From Frazier MS, Drzymkowski JW. Essentials of Human Diseases and Conditions, 4th ed. St. Louis, Saunders, 2009.

Chapter 18
Figure 18-1: From Chabner D. The Language of Medicine, 8th ed. St. Louis, Saunders, 2007. 18-2A: From Lookingbill D, Marks J. Principles of Dermatology, 2nd ed. Philadelphia, Saunders, 1993. 18-2B: From Lawrence CM, Cox NH. Physical Signs in Dermatology: Color Atlas and Text. London, Mosby Europe, 1993. 18-3: From Murphy GF, Herzberg AJ. Atlas of Dermatopathology. Philadelphia, Saunders, 1996. 18-4: From Dorland's Illustrated Medical Dictionary, 31st ed. Philadelphia, Saunders, 2007. 18-5: From Callen J, Greer K, Hood A, et al. Color Atlas of Dermatology. Philadelphia, Saunders, 1993. 18-7: From McCarthy JG, et al (eds): Plastic Surgery, vol 7, Philadelphia, WB Saunders, 1990.

Chapter 19
Figure 19-1, 19-12: From Dorland's Illustrated Medical Dictionary, 31st ed. Philadelphia, Saunders, 2007. 19-2, 19-14A, B: From Frazier MS, Drzymkowski JW. Essentials of Human Diseases and Conditions, 4th ed. St. Louis, Saunders, 2009. 19-3: Thibodeau GA, Patton KT: The Human Body in Health and Disease, 4th ed. St. Louis, Mosby, 2005. 19-5: From Chabner D. The Language of Medicine, 8th ed. St. Louis, Saunders, 2007. 19-6, 19-8, 19-12, 19-13: From Damjanov I. Pathology for the Health Professions, 3rd ed. St. Louis, Saunders, 2006. 19-11: From Mettler FA, Jr. Essentials of Radiology, 2nd ed. Philadelphia, Saunders, 2004. 19-15: From Zitelli BJ, Davis HW. Atlas of Pediatric Physical Diagnosis, 4th ed. St. Louis, Mosby, 2002. 19-16: From Buck CJ. Step-by-Step Medical Coding, 2010 edition. St. Louis, Saunders, 2010. 19-17: From Duthie EH Jr, Katz PR, Malone M. Practice of Geriatrics, 4th ed. Philadelphia, Saunders, 2007.

Chapter 20
Figures 20-1, 20-6, 20-16, 20-17, 20-20: From Gould BE. Pathophysiology for the Health Professions, 3rd ed. St. Louis, Saunders, 2006. 20-2, 20-3: From Frazier MS, Drzymkowski JW. Essentials of Human Diseases and Conditions, 4th ed. St. Louis, Saunders, 2009. 20-4, 20-11, 20-19, 20-22, 20-23: From Chabner D. The Language of Medicine, 8th ed. St. Louis, Saunders, 2007. 20-5, 20-7, 20-8, 20-10, 20-12, 20-15: From Damjanov I. Pathology for the Health Professions, 3rd ed. St. Louis, Saunders, 2006. 20-18: From Dorland's Illustrated Medical Dictionary, 31st ed. Philadelphia, Saunders, 2007.

Chapter 21
Figures 21-1, 21-2, 21-4A, 21-9: From Frazier MS, Drzymkowski JW. Essentials of Human Diseases and Conditions, 4th ed. St. Louis, Saunders, 2009. 21-3, 21-10: From Dorland's Illustrated Medical Dictionary, 31st ed. Philadelphia, Saunders, 2007. 21-4B: From Damjanov I, Linder J. Pathology: A Color Atlas. St. Louis, Mosby, 1999. 21-5, 21-11: From Chabner D. The Language of Medicine, 8th ed. St. Louis, Saunders, 2007.

Chapter 22
Figures 22-1, 22-3: From Frazier MS, Drzymkowski JW. Essentials of Human Diseases and Conditions, 4th ed. St. Louis, Saunders, 2009. 22-2: From Gould BE. Pathophysiology for the Health Professions, 3rd ed. St. Louis, Saunders, 2006. 22-4: From Dorland's Illustrated Medical Dictionary, 31st ed. Philadelphia, Saunders, 2007. 22-5: From Behrman RE, Kleigman RM, Arvin AM. Slide set for Nelson Textbook of Pediatrics, 15th ed. Philadelphia, Saunders, 1996. 22-6: From Baralos M, Baramki TA. Medical Cytogenics. Baltimore, Lippincott Williams and Wilkins, 1967. 22-7: From Damjanov I. Pathology for the Health Professions, 3rd ed. St. Louis, Saunders, 2006. 22-8: Modified from O'Toole M (ed). Miller-Keane Encyclopedia of Medicine, Nursing, and Allied Health, 6th ed. Philadelphia, Saunders, 1997.

Chapter 23
Figure 23-2: From Gould BE. Pathophysiology for the Health Professions, 3rd ed. St. Louis, Saunders, 2006. 23-3, 23-5, 23-6, 23-7: From Drake RL, Vogl W, Mitchell AWM. Gray's Anatomy for Students. Philadelphia, Churchill Livingstone, 2005. 23-4: From Chabner D. The Language of Medicine, 8th ed. St. Louis, Saunders, 2007. 23-11, 23-12: From Henry MC, Stapleton ER. EMT Prehospital Care, 3rd ed. Philadelphia, Saunders, 2004. 23-16: Buck CJ. Step-by-Step Medical Coding, 2008. Philadelphia, Saunders, 2008.

Chapter 24
Figures 24-3, 24-6: From Frazier MS, Drzymkowski JW. Essentials of Human Diseases and Conditions, 4th ed. St. Louis, Saunders, 2009. 24-5: From Cohen J, Powderly WG: Infectious Diseases, 2nd ed. Philadelphia, Mosby, 2004.

Chapter 25
Figure 25-7: From Frazier MS, Drzymkowski JW. Essentials of Human Diseases and Conditions, 4th ed. St. Louis, Saunders, 2009. 25-9: From Canale ST. Campbell's Operative Orthopaedics, 11th ed. Philadelphia, Mosby, 2008. 25-10: From Green NE, Swiontkowski MF. Skeletal Trauma in Children, 3rd ed. Philadelphia, Saunders, 2003.

Chapter 26
Figure 26-1: From Diagnosis Related Groups Definitions Manual, version 14.0. Wallingford, Conn., 3M Health Information Systems, 1996. 26-2: Courtesy U.S. Department of Health and Human Services, Public Health Service, Centers for Medicare and Medicaid Services.

Chapter 27
Figure 27-1: CPT only copyright © 2009. Current Procedural Terminology, 2010, American Medical Association. All Rights Reserved.

Index

Note: Entries followed by "f" indicate figures, "t" tables.